KU-154-528

THE

GUIDING SYMPTOMS

OF OUR

MATERIA MEDICA

BY

C. HERING, M. D.

VOLUME IX.

B. Jain Publishers Pvt. Ltd.

NEW DELHI-110055

Reprinted 1989

Price : **Rs** 600.00 (10 Vols.)

Published by

B. Jain Publishers Pvt. Ltd.
1921, Street No. 10, Chuna Mandi
Paharganj, New Delhi-110 055 (India)

Printed by

J.J. Offset Printers
Multani Dhanda, Paharganj
New Delhi-110 055 (India)

ISBN 81—7021—090—9
ISBN 81—7021—099—2

BOOK CODE B-2277

GUIDING SYMPTOMS

OF OUR

MATERIA MEDICA.

RANUNCULUS BULBOSUS.

The Common Field Buttercup. *Ranunculaceæ.*

Provings by Franz, Archiv für Homœopathische Heilkunst, vol. 7.

CLINICAL AUTHORITIES.—*Hemeralopia* (2 cases), Billig, Rück. Kl. Erf., vol. 5, p. 149; *Neuralgia of stomach*, Custis, Hom. Phys., vol. 2, p. 403; *Jaundice*, Custis, Hom. Phys., vol. 2, p. 403; *Diarrhœa*, Berridge, Hom. Phys., vol. 6, p. 43; *Pains in chest*, Pope, A. H. Z., vol. 107, p. 38; Smith, N. E. M. G., vol. 12, p. 247; *Sore spots after pneumonia*, Ockford, Raue's Rec., 1875, p. 19, from H.W., vol. 9, p. 198; *Pneumonia*, Buchner, Rück. Kl. Erf., vol. 3, p. 328; Smith, N. E. M. G., vol. 12, p. 250; *Pleuritis*, Smith, N. E. M. G., vol. 12, p. 249; *Hydrothorax and pleurisy, pneumonia*, Smith, Times Ret., 1877, p. 40; *Sensation of coldness on chest*, Burnett, B. J. H., vol. 33, p. 730; *Pleurodynia*, Dudgeon, B. J. H., vol. 24, p. 160; Strong, Hom. Rev., vol. 10, p. 753; *Intercostal neuralgia*, Black, B. J. H., vol. 2, p. 274; Gerstel, Times Ret., 1877, p. 119; *Pain at scapula*, Jeanes, Hah. Mo., vol. 6, p. 334; Raue's Rec., 1872, p. 33; *Herpes on hands and fingers*, Schweikert, Haubold, A. H. Z., vol. 107, p. 45; *Wart on thumb*, Chancere, A. H. Z., vol. 102, p. 64, from Bib. Hom., Jan., 1881; *Sciatica*, Smith, N. E. M. G., vol. 12, p. 248; Times Ret., 1877, p. 39, from Mass. Trans., vol. 4, p. 760; *Pain in knee and abdomen*, Heath, Hom. Phys., vol. 6, p. 233; *Cerebro-spinal affection*, Colton, A. H. O., vol. 10, p. 471; *Rheumatism*, Hartmann, Rück. Kl. Erf., vol. 3, p. 536; Black, B. J. H., vol. 2, p. 274; *Herpes zoster*, Marwick, B. J. H., vol. 30, p. 133; *Pemphigus*, Rummel, Rück, Kl. Erf., vol. 4, p. 165; *Eczema*, Pope, A. H. Z., vol. 107, p. 45; *Chilblains, shingles*, Marwick, Hom. Rev., vol. 15, p. 64.

1 **Mind.** Vanishing of thought on reflection; stares at one point.

Obtuseness of senses.

Quarrelsome, angry mood, easily provoked.

Afraid of ghosts; does not like to remain alone.

‖At the beginning of delirium tremens, with talkative mania; unusual exertions and powerful efforts to escape from bed; convulsions of facial and cervical muscles; risus sardonicus; stitches in liver; long-lasting gastralgia, burning changing to a dull pressure, with nausea; vertigo; confusion of head, as if intoxicated.

2 **Sensorium.** ❙Vertigo, with danger of falling, when going from room into open air.

‖Dizziness of head; sensation as if head would be enlarged and distended, making it difficult to think.

3 **Inner Head.** ❙❙Headache over r. eye; < lying down; > walking and standing.

❙Pressing headache in forehead and on vertex, as if pressed asunder, with pressure on eyeballs and sleepiness; > in evening and when entering a room, from cold air, or vice versa.

‖Pain in temples; drawing and pressure in evening while walking, with feverish restlessness and difficulty of breathing.

❙Congestion of blood to head, sensation of fulness and enlargement of head.

‖Headache, with nausea and sleepiness.

❙Headache is caused or aggravated by a change of temperature.

4 **Outer Head.** Head feels too large.

Crawling, creeping, or burning pricking in scalp.

5 **Sight and Eyes.** ❙Mist before eyes.

‖Hemeralopia during pregnancy; heat, biting and pressure in eyes; redness of conjunctiva and lids, especially inner surface of lower lids; lachrymation; pus in canthi; pustules on eyes; eyes look weak; pupils dilated; candlelight appears to her as a bright circle; can see well during day.

‖Sudden hemeralopia in a boy æt. 3¾ years; pupils but slightly dilated; mother similarly affected.

❙❙Pressure and smarting in eyeballs.

❙Painfulness of r. eyeball.

❙Sensation of burning soreness in r. lower eyelid.

❙Smarting and soreness in outer canthus of r. eye.

‖Herpes zoster supraorbitalis, with bluish-black vesicles, high fever and usual pains.

6 **Hearing and Ears.** Sticking in r. ear in region of tympanum.

Stitches in ears, principally in evening.

7 **Smell and Nose.** Redness and inflammatory swelling of nose, with tension.

Scabs in nostrils; sore nose.

▮Hay fever; smarting in eyes; eyelids burn and feel sore; nose stuffed up, especially toward evening, with pressure at root of nose and tingling and crawling sensation within its cavity; sometimes this sensation attacks posterior nares, causing patient to hawk and swallow and endeavor in every way to scratch affected part; hoarseness; sharp, stitching pains in and about chest; general muscular soreness; neck of bladder may be affected, producing some burning in passing water.

8 **Upper Face.** Dry heat in face, with redness of cheeks, evenings.

Tingling in face, especially on nose and chin.

‖ Vesicular eruption on face, as from a burn; smarts as if scalded; eruption in clusters. θEczema.

9 **Lower Face.** Spasms of lips.

12 **Inner Mouth.** White saliva in mouth, tasting like copper.

13 **Throat.** Much viscid phlegm in throat.

‖ Scraping, burning in throat and roof of mouth, inflammatory.

14 **Appetite, Thirst. Desires, Aversions.** ‖ Increased thirst in afternoon.

15 **Eating and Drinking.** ▮▮One of our most effective agents for the removal of bad effects of alcoholic beverages: hiccough; epileptiform attacks; delirium tremens.

16 **Hiccough, Belching, Nausea and Vomiting.** ‖ Frequent eructations.

▮Spasmodic hiccough. θAlcoholism.

‖ Nausea in afternoon, sometimes with headache.

17 **Scrobiculum and Stomach.** ‖ Pressure in pit of stomach.

‖ Violent burning in region of cardiac orifice of stomach.

‖ Sensation of soreness and burning in pit of stomach; < from touch.

‖ Neuralgia of stomach; attacks irregular, coming on without special cause; pain in pit of stomach, with distressing burning and soreness; wanted the clothing all loose and to bend back, with great restlessness and some jaundice; attacks preceded by itching of palms of hands inducing scratching.

18 **Hypochondria.** ▮Sensation of soreness in hypochondria, especially to touch.

▮Stitches in region of liver, extending into chest.

Pulsations in l. hypochondrium.

▮In evening, hypochondria and lowest ribs feel painful as if bruised.

‖ Jaundice; itching of body, especially of palms of hands.

19 **Abdomen.** ‖ Rumbling and movements in abdomen.

▮Stitches in l. side of abdomen, in forenoon when walking.

▮Stitching with pressure, in r. side of abdomen, in region of last true rib, arresting breathing, with stitches and pressure on top of r. shoulder, when walking after having been seated.

▮Sore pain and stitches in l. side of abdomen, immediately after supper.

▮Violent stitches from l. lumbar region transversely through abdomen, especially below umbilicus and toward r. groin, immediately after dinner.

▮Colic and cutting pains in abdomen when pressing on it, sensation as if everything were sore and bruised.

▮Burning soreness in abdomen.

▮Great tenderness of abdomen to touch.

20 **Stool and Rectum.** ‖Diarrhœa for a week; colorless, watery, painless, a little frothy, generally coming in one gush, about six times daily.

‖Acute abdominal and thoracic pains following dysentery; chronic serous discharges of dysentery, with stabbing pains in abdomen and chest.

21 **Urinary Organs.** Ulcers in bladder.

23 **Female Sexual Organs.** ▮Ovarian neuralgia, chronic cases, always excited by atmospheric change.

‖Leucorrhœa, at first mild, then acrid, corroding.

26 **Respiration.** ‖Heavy, short breathing, in evening; must take a deep breath frequently, with burning and fine stitches in l. side of chest.

28 **Inner Chest and Lungs.** ▮Oppression of chest, with much weeping in evening with sore pain in eyes, especially right; as after deep chagrin, had to take a deep breath frequently.

▮Pressure and tightness across lower part of chest, with fine stitches which seem to be felt in outer parts of chest first, but then extend deep into chest, now in r. now in l. side; < moving, stooping, or taking an inspiration; in evening when walking or standing, in open air or in room.

▮Pressing pain in outer parts of chest.

▮Violent pains in chest whole forenoon.

‖Pains in chest, stitches in r. side and pressure in middle chest, continuing uninterruptedly almost all day, with painful inspiration.

‖Pain in morning as if bruised, or as if one had been lying in a wrong position, in region of lowest true rib. l. side.

|Pain in l. side of chest, in morning, in region of pectoralis major, near axilla, < during motion.

||Early in morning, while walking, feels a sticking in region of fifth and sixth l. ribs, with great sensitiveness to touch and debility.

||Sticking pain in l. chest and as if there were subcutaneous ulceration, < from motion.

||Stitches in interior of l. side of chest, when walking in open air, in region of nipple; the stitches disappear when he continues to walk, after which a pain is felt below last true rib in r. side of abdomen.

||Violent sticking pain above l. nipple, near axilla, in morning, when rising; dare not move his arm or raise it; dare not even raise trunk lest he should scream with pain; has to sit or stand stooping, with head and chest forward to l. side.

|Sticking pain in r. side of chest, in region of fifth and sixth ribs, in forenoon.

||Painful soreness under short ribs of l. side, especially when moving trunk, for several days.

||Violent pressure and sensation as if bruised over whole l. side of chest, immediately after rising, in morning; every movement of shoulder causes pain; pain spreads over whole chest, with shortness of breath, is unable to speak long sentences on account of want of breath.

|Pain as if bruised in region of short ribs, with pain in back, lassitude and ill-humor.

|Pressing and pushing in lowest part of r. side of chest, toward liver, in forenoon.

|Pain in chest and restless nights, continuing for weeks.

||Stitches, neuralgic, myalgic, or rheumatic pains in chest.

|Chronic soreness on pressure within thorax or abdomen, as from subcutaneous ulceration.

|Chronic pains in chest, frequently extending toward liver or from liver into chest.

|Chronic cases of internal pains, especially over region of diaphragm; inframammary pains of women.

|Diaphragmitis; sharp, shooting pains, pains from hypochondria and epigastrium through to back.

|Pleurisy and hydrothorax.

|Pneumonia resulting from sudden exposure to cold while overheated, or vice versa; cheeks bright red; tongue clean; respiration difficult, short, oppressed, accompanied by loud râles; dry heat; turgescence of skin without sweat; early prostration, so great at onset that he can hardly walk; small, rapid pulse, with great excitement of heart and circulation; nausea, even fainting when sitting up and on motion.

||Left-sided pneumonia with pleurisy; great soreness just

below l. nipple on drawing a breath, with a sensation as of something tearing, and occasional pleuritic stitches radiating from that point over whole l. side of chest, which was quite sensitive to touch; appetite and strength failing from effects of incessant pain; there was but slight cough; while drawing an unusually full breath a sudden sense of tearing in affected part of chest, followed by expectoration of about two ounces of blood.

▮Small sore spot, as from subcutaneous ulceration; after pneumonia.

▮Acute thoracic pains after pneumonia or pleuritis, suggestive of adhesions.

▮Pain about lungs from adhesions after pleurisy.

29 **Heart, Pulse and Circulation.** Pulse full, hard, rapid in evening, slower in morning.

30 **Outer Chest.** ııWhenever she goes out of doors a sensation as if she had cold wet cloths applied to three different parts of anterior wall of thorax, viz., in both infraclavicular fossæ and just under l. breast; sensation comes on at once on going out of doors, is constant as long as she is out, and disappears immediately on going into house; it prevents her from conversing with any one while out; after a fall two and a half years ago.

▮▮Stitches about chest in every change of weather.

▮External painfulness of whole trunk.

▮External soreness of chest and abdomen, < from touch, motion and coughing, accompanied by tightness of chest as if a full breath could not be drawn on account of acute pain and mental anxiety.

▮▮Chest feels sore, bruised; < from touch, motion, or turning body. θPleurodynia.

▮Sharp, shooting pains about chest. θIntercostal neuralgia.

ııAcute pain principally in shoulder, axilla and mamma, so severe in breast that she dreaded cancer. θIntercostal neuralgia.

ııAfter overstraining himself threw up some blood; it rose into mouth at night or after exertion, and seemed to draw from r. side about hip; bloodspitting ceased, but more or less pain continued in that part ever since, and down into arm toward insertion of pectoral muscle; the breast swells the size of hand and is tender to touch and when arm is moved; < from cold, singing, hard work; feels much depressed, wishes to lie down and give up. θPleurodynia.

ııSlight rigor; pain in l. side about sixth or seventh ribs, increasing during night and following day; sat bent forward in bed and leaning toward l. side; slightest motion caused intense pain like a knife thrust into side and through back; intense dread of any movement; is afraid to take a full breath; unable to lie down for a moment; could not bear least touch on affected side; screamed if compelled to make least movement; pulse 120, small, weak; much exhausted by want of sleep and the awkward position. θPleurodynia.

▮▮Pleurodynia, rheumatic, myalgic or neuralgic.

ǀǀRheumatism of several months standing caused by catching cold during a sea voyage; pains confined almost entirely to trunk; chest and abdomen feel bruised; on least motion pains become cutting and sharp.

31 **Neck and Back.** ▮Pain along inner edge of l. scapula, often extending below its inferior angle or through lower half of l. side of thorax.

▮Stitches in and between shoulder-blades.

▮Muscular pains about lower margin of shoulder-blades in women who follow sedentary employments; pain burning, often over only a small space, greatly < by long-continued needlework or writing.

▮Pain in back, lassitude, and pain as if bruised in region of short ribs, with ill-humor.

▮Stitches in r. lumbar region when walking, with a slight burning sensation.

▮Pain depending upon spinal irritation.

32 **Upper Limbs.** ▮Spasmodic, rheumatic pains in arms.

▮Stitches in arms and hands.

ǀǀJerking pain in r. upper arm.

ǀǀSudden tearings in r. forearm and between thumb and index finger; while writing.

▮Herpes or blisterlike eruption in palms of hands; blue blisters on fingers.

Cold hands.

ǀǀFrequent tingling in single parts of fingers.

ǀǀCauliflower-like wart on outer side of terminal phalanx of r. thumb.

33 **Lower Limbs.** ǀǀGreat weakness in lower limbs, in forenoon, when walking.

▮Sciatica especially in women; pains < moving about, yet not better lying down; < in rainy, stormy weather; stitching-burning pains, radiating from dorsal region of spine.

▮Drawing pain in thighs, extending downward.

ǀǀSevere pain on inner aspect of l. knee, very sore to touch, point of pain easily covered with finger end; sometimes > from motion < from pressure; knee joint cracked on stretching limb; also sore spot on abdomen about two inches above navel and same distance l. of median line; it was sore as a boil, but no external evidence; < from pressure.

|| Stinging and soreness in feet and toes.

|| Pulsative stitches in l. heel, when standing, in forenoon.

| Corns sensitive to touch, smart and burn.

| Chilblains.

|| Stump of amputated leg a mass of chilblains, many places being much ulcerated; intense pain and itching, preventing rest at night.

35 **Rest. Position. Motion.** Lying down: headache over r. eye <.

Could not lie down: pain in side.

Could not lie on side: dyspnœa.

Sitting up: fainting.

Sat bent forward in bed and leaning toward l. side: pain in side.

Has to sit or stand stooping, with head and chest forward to l. side.

Standing: headache over r. eye >; stitches and tightness in chest; stitches in heel.

Indisposition to standing or walking: irritability of cerebro-spinal system.

Change of position: bruised pains <.

Motion: pain in l. side of chest <; of arm or trunk < sticking above l. nipple; causes fainting; soreness of chest <; abdomen <; of arm, tenderness of breast; slightest, causes intense pain in side; sciatica <; sometimes > pain in knee; bruised pains <.

Walking: headache >; pressure in head <; stitches in abdomen; after having been seated stitches in shoulder; stitches and tightness in chest; sticking in l. chest continuous; stitches disappear; weakness in lower limbs.

36 **Nerves.** Tired and broken down all day.

Lassitude, ill-humor; pain in back and as if bruised in region of short ribs.

Twitching of muscles.

|| Epileptiform attacks. θAlcoholism.

Sudden weakness, with fainting.

Trembling of limbs, with oppression of breathing, after fright or anger; < in evening, and sometimes after eating, from change of temperature, especially from heat to cold.

|| Intercostal or spinal neuralgiæ; rheumatic or neuralgic pleurodynia.

|| Great depression of spirits, almost amounting to suicidal mania; constant twitching and jerking of muscles of neck and of face and chest contiguous to this region;

muscles of back, between shoulders, also contributed to increase this jerking movement; the principal direction of the movement was to bring chin directly, or from side to side, toward chest; sterno-mastoid and sterno-hyoid muscles frequently drawn into ridges by tonic contractions of their fibres; < from talking and presence of individuals; while talking, if shoulders were constantly moved up and down, the spasm was considerably > and the articulation easier; marked indisposition to stand up for any length of time, also to walking, even about house. θIrritability of cerebro-spinal system.

37 **Sleep.** ‖ Falls asleep late in evening and wakes several times at night, not from any pain, but because he is not sleepy.

| Disturbed sleep at night.

‖ Sleeplessness, often with dyspnœa, heat and ebullitions; cannot lie on side.

38 **Time.** Morning: pain as if bruised in region of lowest true rib l. side; sticking pain above nipple; pressure and bruised sensation in l. side of chest; pulse slower; sweat scanty.

Forenoon: stitches in abdomen; violent pain in chest; weakness in lower limbs.

Day: tired and broken down.

Immediately after dinner: stitches through abdomen.

Afternoon: increased thirst; nausea; stitches in heel; chilly, with heat in face <.

Evening: pressing headache <; pressure in temples; stitches in ears; nose stuffed up; dry heat in face; hypochondria feel painful; heavy short breathing; oppression of chest; stitches and tightness in chest; pulse full, hard, rapid; trembling of limbs; falls asleep late; chilly, with heat in face <.

Night: sleep disturbed by itching of chilblains; wakes several times.

After midnight: intermittent fever.

39 **Temperature and Weather.** Room: stitches or tightness in chest.

Open air: stitches and tightness in chest, as if she had cold cloths applied to thorax; well-covered chest is chilly.

Change of temperature: causes or aggravates headache; excites ovarian neuralgia; stitches about chest: trembling of limbs.

From room into open air: vertigo; pain in forehead and vertex <.

From cold air into room: headache <.

Sudden exposure to cold while overheated, or vice versa; pneumonia.

Cold: tenderness of breast <; ulcers <

Draft of cold air: bruised pains in different parts of body <.

Rainy stormy weather: sciatica <; rheumatic pains <.

40 **Fever.** ▮Chilly, with heat in face, < afternoon and evening; the well-covered chest is chilly out-doors.

Pulse full, hard and rapid in evening; slower in morning; chill predominates, with heat in face; < in afternoon and evening.

Chilliness and heat in face after dinner.

The fever consists only of a chill.

Heat, with internal chill at same time.

Heat in evening, < on r. side of face, with cold hands and general discomfort.

Sweat scanty, only in morning on waking.

ǁIntermittent fever after midnight; heat and violent thirst, with full, soft, quick pulse, followed by general sweat, mostly on forehead.

Rainy, stormy weather: sciatica, <; rheumatic pains <.

41 **Attacks, Perodicity.** Daily: diarrhœa six times.

For weeks: restless nights and pain in chest.

42 **Locality and Direction.** Right: headache over eye; painfulness of eyeball; soreness of lower eyelid; soreness of outer canthus of eye; sticking in ear; stitching with pressure in side of abdomen; stitches and pressure on top of shoulder; stitches in side of chest; pressing and pushing in lowest part of r. side of chest; blood seemed to draw from side about hip; jerking pain in upper arm; tearing in forearm and between thumb and index finger; wart on terminal phalanx of thumb; heat < side of face.

Left: pulsations in hypochondrium; stitches in side of abdomen; stitches from lumbar region through abdomen toward r. groin; burning and stitches in chest; sticking in region of fifth and sixth ribs; stitches in interior of side of chest; violent sticking above nipple; violent pressure and bruised sensation over whole side of chest; pneumonia; soreness below nipple, along inner edge of scapula, or through lower half of side of thorax; severe pain on inner aspect of knee; pulsative stitches in heel.

43 **Sensations.** Confusion of head, as if intoxicated; as if head would be enlarged; as if head were pressed asunder; hypochondria in lowest ribs painful as if bruised; as if everything in abdomen were sore and bruised; as if there were subcutaneous ulceration; as if bruised in l. side of chest; in region of short ribs, as if bruised; as of something tearing in chest; as if she had cold wet

cloths applied to three different parts of wall of thorax; as if a full breath could not be drawn; as of a knife thrust into side and through back; muscles as if they had been pounded.

Pain: over r. eye; in temples; in pit of stomach; in chest; in region of lowest true rib l. side; in region of pectoralis major; in back; about lungs; along inner edge of l. scapula.

Intense pain: in stump of amputated leg.

Violent pains: in chest.

Acute pain: in chest; in shoulder, axilla and mammæ.

Severe pain: on inner aspect of l. knee.

Cutting pains: in abdomen.

Stabbing pains: in abdomen and chest.

Shooting pains: from hypochondria and epigastrium to back; about chest.

Tearings: in r. forearm and between thumb and index finger.

Stitches: in liver; in ears; from liver into chest; in l. side of abdomen; on top of shoulder; from lumbar region through abdomen; in l. side of chest; in r. side; in interior of l. side of chest; in and between shoulder-blades; in r. lumbar region; in arms and hands.

Pulsative stitches: in l. heel.

Stitching pains: in and about chest; in r. side of abdomen.

Stitching burning pain: radiating from dorsal region of spine.

Jerking pain: in r. upper arm.

Pressing pain: in outer part of chest; in lowest part of r. side of chest.

Drawing pain: in thigh.

Rheumatic pains: in chest; in arms; in muscles about trunk.

Sticking: in r. ear; in region of fifth and sixth l. ribs; in l. chest; above l. nipple; in r. side of chest.

Stinging: in feet and toes.

Smarting: in eyballs; in outer canthus of r. eye; in eyes; of eruption on face; of corns.

Burning soreness: in lower eyeball; in abdomen.

Burning: in region of cardiac orifice of stomach; in pit of stomach; in neck of bladder; of corns; of eczema; of ulcers.

Soreness: of nose; in pit of stomach; in hypochondria; under short ribs in l. side; just below l. nipple; in feet and toes.

Burning pricking: in scalp.

Painfulness: of r. eyeball.

Pressure: in forehead; on vertex; on eyeballs; in

temples; in eyes; at root of nose; in pit of stomach; on top of r. shoulder; across lower part of chest; in middle of chest, over whole l. side.

Pulsations: in l. hypochondrium.

Heat: in face.

Tightness: across lower part of chest.

Oppression: of chest.

Tingling: in face; in single parts of fingers.

Crawling: in scalp; in nose; in skin of fingers.

Creeping: in scalp.

Itching: of palms; of body; of stump of amputated leg; of vesicles on fingers.

Chilliness: in face; in chest.

44 **Tissues.** ‖Inflammation of serous membranes, particularly of pleura or peritoneum; acute stabbing pains in chest in case of pleuritis; effusion of serum, with great anxiety, dyspnœa and distress.

‖‖Rheumatism of muscles, particularly in muscles about trunk; intercostal rheumatism; muscles sore to touch, feel bruised as if they had been pounded.

‖Tearing-stitching bruised pains, now in one then in another part of body; pain < from touch, motion, change of position, draft of cold air; fever; heat of one side of body with coldness of hands and feet.

‖Rheumatic pain < in damp weather, and particularly from change of weather or change of temperature; rheumatic headache.

‖Rheumatic and arthritic soreness, with stitches over whole body.

45 **Touch. Passive Motion. Injuries.** Touch: burning in pit of stomach <; soreness of hypochondria; tenderness of abdomen; sensitiveness of l. side of chest; breast swells and is tender; l. knee very sore to touch; corns sensitive; muscles about trunk sore; ulcers <.

Pressure: on abdomen, bruised feeling; < pain in knee.

After a fall two years ago: as if she had cold wet cloths applied to thorax in open air.

46 **Skin.** ‖‖Coarse itching in hollow of hand.

‖‖Crawling in skin of fingers.

‖Vesicles on fingers, transparent, dark-blue, elevated as large as pin's head; intolerable burning itching; herpetic horny scurf forms after vesicles open; scratching brought on a shining red, loose swelling of fingers, with inflammation; after applying hart's grease the horny scurf no longer formed, but in places, the size of a shilling, crowded groups of small holes of size of pin's head (as if they were the pores) were formed, emitting a yellow lymph in shape of drops of sweat and changing to small, flat, spreading ulcers, healing with difficulty, with corroded sharp borders and intolerable burning-stinging itching, depriving him of rest for weeks.

▮Vesicular eruptions as from burns.

▮Herpes zoster; zona; vesicles filled with serum which burn, may have a bluish-black appearance; especially when following course of supraorbital or intercostal nerves and followed by sharp stitching pains.

▮Herpes: preceding neuralgia costalis; on fingers and in palm of hand; over whole body.

||Pemphigus: large blisters form, burst, and leave raw surfaces; in children, blisters of two, three or four inches in diameter; restlessness; prostration.

||Constantly repeating eruption of blisters, secreting a foul-smelling, gluey matter, forming crusts and healing from centre. θPemphigus.

▮Eczema: vesicles followed by scurfs, then a fresh eruption of vesicles, with burning and itching; attended by thickening of skin and formation of hard, horny scabs.

▮Pain like that of shingles, without eruption.

▮▮Shingles and intercostal neuralgia.

▮Flat, burning, stinging ulcers, with ichorous discharge; pus sanious or acrid; < from touch or cold.

▮Hornlike excrescences.

▮Chilblains.

47 **Stages of Life, Constitution.** Boy, æt. $3\frac{3}{4}$ years, mother affected with same trouble during her pregnancies; hemeralopia.

Lady, æt. 27, three weeks after confinement went out driving; on a cold day and met with an accident which frightened her considerably; affected evening of same day; pleurodynia.

Mary J., æt. 30, teacher, two and a half years ago had a fall, since then suffering; cold sensation on chest.

Man, æt. 30, black hair, irritable temper, blacksmith, four years ago overstrained himself and threw up some blood, since then suffering; pleurodynia.

Woman, æt. 30, pregnant, suffering since seventh month, similarly affected during former pregnancy; hemeralopia.

Mrs. E., æt. 38, widow, mother of three children, nervo-bilious temperament, engaged in nursing, and subjected to care and anxiety; cerebro-spinal affection.

Man, æt. 42, pain in knee and abdomen.

Man, æt. 50, suffering two months; neuralgia of stomach.

48 **Relations.** Antidoted by: *Bryon.*, *Camphor.*, *Pulsat.*, *Rhus tox.*

Incompatible: *Sulphur*, *Staphis.*, *Spir. nitr. dulc.*, alcohol, wine and vinegar.

Compare: *Acon.*, *Arnica*, *Bryon.*, *Cactus*, *Clemat.*, *Crot. tigl.*, *Euphorb.*, *Mezer.*, *Sabad.*

RANUNCULUS SCELERATUS.

Celery-Leaved Crowfoot. *Ranunculaceæ.*

Proved by Y., Archiv für Hom., and Schreter, Neues Archiv für Homöopathie.

CLINICAL AUTHORITIES.—*Inflammation of mouth and tongue, diphtheria,* Rittenhouse, A. O., vol. 7, p. 528; B. J. H., vol. 29, p. 428; *Use in aneurism of aorta,* Searle, A. O., vol. 7, p. 409; *Neuralgia,* Price, Org., vol. 2, p. 118; *Pemphigus,* Elwert, Hom. Cl., vol. 4, p. 147, from A. H. Z., vol. 30, p. 345; *Corns,* Berridge, Hah. Mo., 1874, p. 111.

1 **Mind.** Dulness of head.
Indolence and aversion to mental occupation in morning; low-spirited, depressed in evening.

2 **Sensorium.** Vertigo with loss of consciousness.

3 **Inner Head.** ❙❙Gnawing pain in a small spot on vertex or either temple.

4 **Outer Head.** Sensation as if head were too large and full.
Biting itching on scalp.
Scalp feels tense.

5 **Sight and Eyes.** ❙❙Eyes very weak and watery.
❙❙Pain in eyeballs, when moving them quickly.
❙❙Pressing in eyeballs, periodically.
❙❙Painful pressure in eyeballs.
❙Smarting in eyes and canthi.

6 **Hearing and Ears.** ❙❙Otalgia with pressing or gnawing pain in head, and drawing pain in teeth.

7 **Smell and Nose.** Lachrymation, with watery nasal discharge.
❙❙Ordinary catarrh, with sneezing, fluent coryza, pains in joints, and burning on urination.

8 **Upper Face.** ❙Sensation as if face were covered with spider web.
❙❙Slight drawing with feeling of coldness above r. eyebrow, down cheek, as far as corner of mouth.
Face cold, livid.

9 **Lower Face.** ❙❙Tremulous sensation around corners of mouth and lower lip, preceding vomiting without inclination to vomit.

10 **Teeth and Gums.** ❙❙Drawing, stinging, jerking in teeth.

11 **Taste and Tongue.** ❙Tongue exfoliated in spots, which are raw; mouth inflamed.
❙❙Both sides of tongue denuded, like islands, the remaining parts thickly coated. θDiphtheria.

Tongue coated white, inflamed, red and burning.

‖Tongue cracks and peels off.

Shooting in tip of tongue.

13 **Throat.** Scraping and burning in throat.

‖Swelling of tonsils, with shooting stitches in them.

16 **Hiccough, Belching, Nausea and Vomiting.** ‖Eructations: empty; after meals, with taste of what has been eaten.

17 **Scrobiculum and Stomach.** ‖Pain in stomach, with fainting fits.

‖Pressure and sensation of fulness in pit of stomach, < from external pressure, most violent in morning.

Sensation of soreness and burning in pit of stomach.

Inflammation of stomach.

18 **Hypochondria.** ‖Dull pressure about liver, < from a long breath.

‖Stitches in liver, spleen or kidneys.

‖Long stitches in region of spleen; < during deep inspiration.

▮Spleen swollen after intermittent fever and abuse of quinine.

19 **Abdomen.** ‖Screwing pressure behind umbilicus; sensation as if a plug were lodged there, in morning.

Twitching in abdominal integuments.

20 **Stool and Rectum.** ▮Frequent sensation as if diarrhœa would set in.

‖Frequent soft, or watery, fetid stools.

Hard stool, preceded by colic.

21 **Urinary Organs.** ‖Urine burns; strangury.

22 **Male Sexual Organs.** Stitches in glans penis.

26 **Respiration.** Dyspnœa from gnawing behind sternum.

28 **Inner Chest and Lungs.** ‖Burning soreness behind xiphoid cartilage.

‖Long, frequent stitches behind xiphoid cartilage, in a space as large as palm of hand.

▮Stitches in chest and intercostal muscles.

‖Gnawing in chest; behind sternum (with dyspnœa).

‖Continual pressure, as from dull instrument, below r. false ribs, < from deep inspiration.

‖Painful sticking in r. chest, not < by inspiration.

‖Violent contracting-pinching pain in chest, behind r. nipple.

‖Whole chest feels weak and bruised.

‖Aneurism of descending aorta and varicosities; cold and livid face and ears, with sensation of a cobweb upon face; lachrymation and discharge of watery mucus from nose (much relieved).

29 **Heart, Pulse and Circulation.** ||Stitches in region of heart.

Pulse quick, full, but soft, with heat at night.

30 **Outer Chest.** ||Chest feels bruised, with sensation of weakness therein.

|Stitches in chest and intercostal muscles.

||External chest and sternum painfully sensitive to touch.

31 **Neck and Back.** |Pain in small of back.

||Stitch in r. lumbar region when walking.

||Stitches in region of kidneys.

||Sudden violent jerks in lumbar region during a walk in open air, arresting breathing.

32 **Upper Limbs.** ||Long-continuing boring sticking along whole l. forearm to tip of index finger, where it is most violent.

||Continual gnawing in palm of l. hand.

Itching between fingers, evenings.

Swelling of fingers, mornings.

33 **Lower Limbs.** Stinging, boring and gnawing in legs, especially violent in big toe.

||Boring and gnawing in r. big toe.

|Sudden stitches in forepart of r. big toe, as if a needle were thrust in deep, made him cry out.

|Sudden stitches in r. big toe, passing into a burning.

||For four months two corns on ball of first and second l. toes, sensitive to touch or pressure, smart and burn, and occasionally shock very painful, when letting leg hang down, when they also throb, and especially painful by flexing toes; > by extending them; > by wearing a thick-soled boot; at times numbness in corns; knocking toe against anything so as to cause boot to grate against corns causes great pain and burning.

34 **Limbs in General.** Gout in fingers and toes.

35 **Rest. Position. Motion.** Letting leg hang down: corns painful.

Flexing toes: corns painful.

Extending toes: corns >.

Motion: of eyeballs causes pain.

Walking: stitch in r. lumbar region; jerks in lumbar region.

36 **Nerves.** ||Neuralgia of head, back and cardiac region, with extreme tenderness of whole spinal column; patchy appearance of tongue.

Convulsive twitches of limbs.

Fainting with the pains in stomach.

37 **Sleep.** ||Wakes after midnight, is wide awake and remains so for a long time.

||Half slumber after midnight, frightful, anxious dreams

about corpses, dead bodies, serpents, battles, etc.; constant tossing about in bed.

38 **Time.** Morning: aversion to mental labor; fulness and pressure in pit of stomach; sensation of plug behind umbilicus.

Evening: low-spirited and depressed; heat; itching, biting, tingling <.

Night: heat.

After midnight: wakeful; heat and thirst <.

39 **Temperature and Weather.** Open air: violent jerks in lumbar region while walking; after walking, heat.

40 **Fever.** || Chill or chilliness during meals.

Heat, in-doors evening, after walking in open air.

Dry heat at night, with violent thirst, mostly after midnight.

|| Fever; wakes after midnight, many nights in succession, with heat over whole body and violent thirst; pulse full, soft, accelerated, 80; afterward sweat over whole body, especially on forehead.

41 **Attacks, Periodicity.** Periodical: pressing in eyeballs.

During meals: chilly.

Many nights in succession: wakes after midnight.

42 **Locality and Direction.** Right: coldness and drawing above eyebrows; pressure below false ribs; painful sticking in chest; pinching behind nipple; stitch in lumbar region; gnawing in big toe; stitches in big toe.

Left: continual gnawing in palm of hand.

43 **Sensations.** As if head were too full and too large; as if face were covered with spider webs; as if a plug were lodged in umbilicus; as if diarrhœa would set in; pressure as from a dull instrument; as if a needle were thrust deep into big toe.

Pain: in eyeballs; in joints; in stomach; in small of back; in corns.

Violent contractive pinching pain behind r. nipple.

Shooting: in tip of tongue.

Shooting stitches: in tonsils.

Stitches: in liver, spleen and kidneys; in glans penis; behind xiphoid cartilage; in chest; in region of heart; in r. lumbar region; in region of kidneys; in big toe.

Gnawing pain: in a small spot on vertex or either temple; behind sternum; in palm of l. hand; in legs; in big toe.

Long-continued boring, sticking: along whole l. forearm to tip of index finger.

Boring: in legs; in big toe.

Neuralgia: in head, back and cardiac region.

Drawing pain: in teeth.

Violent jerks: in lumbar region.

Jerking: in teeth.
Stinging: in teeth; in legs.
Smarting: in eyes and canthi; of corns.
Burning: of tongue; in throat; in pit of stomach; of corns.
Burning soreness: behind xiphoid cartilage.
Soreness: in pit of stomach.
Scraping: in throat.
Bruised feeling: in chest.
Biting, itching: on scalp.
Drawing: above r. eyebrow down cheek to corner of mouth; in teeth.
Pressure: in pit of stomach; about liver; behind umbilicus; below false ribs.
Pressing: in eyeballs; in head.
Fulness: in pit of stomach.
Tense feeling: on scalp.
Tremulous sensation: around corners of mouth and lower lip.
Weakness: in chest.
Numbness: of corns.
Itching: between fingers.
Coldness: above r. eyebrow.

45 **Touch. Passive Motion. Injuries.** Touch: external chest and sternum sensitive; first and second toe sensitive.
Pressure: fulness in pit of stomach <.
Knock against boot: corns very painful.

46 **Skin.** ||Itching, boring, biting, tingling, gnawing in various parts of body, now here, now there, especially toward evening.
||Vesciular eruptions, with acrid, thin, yellowish discharges.
||Blisters which leave a raw surface with acrid discharges.
||The body of an infant about three months old was covered all over with pemphigus; continual thirst; very frequent, weak and intermitting pulse; trembling with anxious features; *Arsen.*[4] caused improvement for six days, blisters decreased; here and there ulcers formed on parts covered with blisters, discharging a yellowish fluid; *Ran. scel.*[3] healed them up.

47 **Stages of Life, Constitution.** Infant, æt. 3 months; pemphigus.

48 **Relations.** Compatible: After *Arsen.* in pemphigus; *Laches* follows in diphtheria with denuded tongue.

RAPHANUS SATIVUS.

Radish. *Cruciferæ.*

The tincture is prepared from the fresh root.

Symptoms obtained from the effects of eating the root, also by proving the tincture 2d, 15th and 30th dilutions, by Nusser, Rev. de la Mat. Med. Hom., vol. 1, p 545, 1840; Curie's Journ. de la Soc. Gall., vol. 5, p. 281; Martin, Am. J. of Hom. Mat. Med., 1870, p. 154; Berridge, Am. Observer, 1875, p. 307.

CLINICAL AUTHORITIES.—*Flatulence and diarrhœa after ovariotomy*, Bell, Raue's Rec., 1873, p. 264, from Trans. Am. Inst., 1871, p. 269; *Flatulence*, Hom. Rec., vol. 3, p. 151.

1 **Mind.** Anguish with dread of death, which is supposed to be near.

2 **Sensorium.** Vertigo with dimness of sight.

3 **Inner Head.** Pressure above root of nose.

Stitches on vertex.

Brain feels tender and sore from least jar when walking.

5 **Sight and Eyes.** Pressure above eyes, with difficulty of sight, going off after vomiting.

Œdema of lower lids.

6 **Hearing and Ears.** Heat in l. ear and over whole l. side of face.

7 **Smell and Nose.** Nose somewhat stopped.

8 **Upper Face.** Face pale.

Expression of pain and exhaustion.

Cheeks burn, are red; whole head and face red.

11 **Taste and Tongue.** ▮Taste: bitter; pasty.

Tongue coated thick white.

Tongue pale and purplish, with a deep furrow and pale-red points in middle.

13 **Throat.** Back of throat dry, > holding cold water in mouth.

White tenacious mucus in throat after heavy sleep.

14 **Appetite, Thirst. Desires, Aversions.** Loss of appetite.

▮Thirst: excessive; violent; constant.

15 **Eating and Drinking.** Worse after eating.

16 **Hiccough, Belching, Nausea and Vomiting.** ▮Nausea: with efforts to vomit; when lying down; constant; in paroxysms with faintness and inability to lie down.

Vomiting: of food and white mucus, with oppression of chest, heaving of stomach and coldness; of bile and water.

Shuddering over back and arms before vomiting.

17 **Scrobiculum and Stomach.** ▮Violent pressure in epigastric region.

▮Pain in stomach, obliging one to eat all the time.

19 **Abdomen.** ▮Pain in abdomen.

▮Griping about umbilicus.

Colic: after drinking milk or water; after eating.

Pains in belly constant, but < after motion.

Bowels sore from least jar; can hardly tolerate clothing.

▮Gurgling in abdomen (at night).

▮▮Accumulation and retention of flatus, no relief upward or downward.

▮Distension of abdomen, followed by griping, as if stool would occur.

▮Abdomen much swollen, hard and painful to pressure, especially hypogastrium.

▮Great swelling of abdomen, commencing at stomach; abdomen hard as if filled with air, without pain; cannot bear any pressure on stomach.

▮▮Pains from incarcerated flatus, coming in paroxysms; colon and other intestines project in little tympanitic tumors all over abdomen, which is flaccid in the interval; diarrhœa of yellow brown fluid, with no passage of flatus by mouth or anus for a long time; twenty-two days after performance of ovariotomy.

20 **Stool and Rectum.** ▮Stool: brown or yellow-brown fluid, coming with much force; green, liquid, mixed with mucus and blood; frothy, copious, undigested.

▮Constipation, bloating of abdomen, absence of gases, no emission of gas upward or downward, prompt satiety when eating, sedentary life.

21 **Urinary Organs.** ▮Urine: more copious than the liquid drunk; copious, yellow; yellow, turbid, with a sediment resembling yeast.

▮Phos.-ammon.-magnes. in excess in urine; gravel.

During micturition, burning in urethra.

23 **Female Sexual Organs.** Sexual excitement; nymphomania.

Great aversion to opposite sex.

Constant titillations in genitals.

Sensation of a foreign body rising from uterus to chest.

Mucous leucorrhœa, at times slightly tinged with blood.

25 **Voice and Larynx. Trachea and Bronchia.** Feeling as of something sticking in larynx; after quietly walking or much talking it becomes a dryness and excites a cough.

29 **Heart, Pulse and Circulation.** Pulse: quick, full but soft, with heat at night; small.

35 **Rest. Position. Motion.** Lying down: nausea.

Inability to lie down: nausea and faintness.

Motion: pain in belly <.

Walking: jar from, brain feels tender and sore.

36 **Nerves.** || Great weakness and languor; weakness with tenderness of abdomen.

|| Hysterical attack.

37 **Sleep.** | Sleep restless with distressing dreams.

Awoke in morning with cramping sore pain.

38 **Time.** Morning: awoke with cramping pain; toward, perspiration after heat.

Night: gurgling in abdomen; pulse quick, full, soft, with heat.

After midnight: dry heat, thirst, ebullitions.

39 **Temperature and Weather.** Cold water: held in mouth > dryness of throat.

40 **Fever.** | Chilliness: in back; along back and posterior surface of arms; during meals.

Heat in evening, in room, after walking in open air.

Dry heat at night, with violent thirst and ebullition, mostly after midnight.

|| Disposition to perspire.

Perspiration after heat, toward morning, mostly on forehead.

Intermittent fever after midnight; heat and violent thirst, with full soft, quick pulse, followed by general perspiration, mostly on forehead.

41 **Attacks, Periodicity.** Paroxysms: pain from incarcerated flatus; nausea.

During meals: chilliness.

42 **Locality and Direction.** Left: heat in ear and side of face.

43 **Sensations.** As if stool would occur; abdomen as if filled with air; as of a foreign body rising from uterus to chest; as of something sticking in larynx.

Pain: in stomach; in abdomen.

Stitches: on vertex.

Griping: about umbilicus.

Burning: of cheeks; in urethra.

Heat: in l. ear and over l. side.

Pressure: above root of nose; above eye; in epigastric region.

Tenderness: of abdomen.

Dryness: in larynx; in throat.

Titillation: in genitals.

Shuddering: over back and arms.

Chilliness: in back; along arms.

45 **Touch. Passive Motion. Injuries.** Cannot bear clothing: bowels sore.

46 **Skin.** Vesicular eruption, with acrid, thin, yellowish discharge.

Pressure: abdomen painful; cannot bear it on stomach.
Least jar: bowels sore.

48 **Relations.** Compare: *Anacard.* in stomach symptoms; *Carbo veg.* in flatulence.

RATANHIA.

Rhatany, Mapato, Pumacuchu. *Polygalaceæ.*

A native of Peru, growing in dry, argillaceous and sandy soil.

The tincture is prepared from the dry root.

Hartlaub and Trinks, Arz. M. L., vol. 3, p. 57; Teste, Mat. Med.; Trousseau and Pidoux, Mat. Med.; Gaz. des Hosp.,1843; Berridge, U. S. Med. Times, 1876.

Clinical Authorities.—*Pterygium,* Newton, Hom. Rev., vol. 15, p. 210; *Constipation and fissure of anus,* Allen, N. A. J. H., vol. 26, p. 523; *Fissured anus,* Hibbard, A. H. O., vol. 10, p. 255; *Ascaris vermicularis,* Cushing, N. E. M. G.; *Fissures of nipple,* Allen, N. A. J. H., vol. 26, p. 527.

3 **Inner Head.** Painful sticking in head, here and there.
Headache as if head were in a vise.
Dull, deep stitches in vertex.
Pain in middle of forehead, as if brain would fall out, while straining at stool.

5 **Sight and Eyes.** Sensation of white speck before eyes, impeding sight in evening by candlelight, with constant urging to wipe eyes, > after wiping.
Sensation as of a skin before eyes.
‖ Inflammation of white of eye; a membrane seemed to extend to central point of eye, which burned.
| Pterygium.
‖ Twitching in l. upper eyelid.
Twitching in r. eye and r. upper lid.

6 **Hearing and Ears.** Violent stitch in r. ear.
Chirping in r. ear.

7 **Smell and Nose.** Dryness of nose.
Dry coryza, with complete stoppage of nostrils.
Bleeding of nose.
Scabs on nose.

10 **Teeth and Gums.** The molars feel elongated, with sensation as if coldness rushed out of them.
| Terrible toothache during early months of pregnancy; must get up at night and walk about.
Shooting pulsating pain, with sensation of elongation in

one l. upper incisor (which is painful to touch) in evening; < after lying down, compelling one to rise and to walk about.

Gums exude sour blood on sucking them.

11 **Taste and Tongue.** Burning on tip of tongue.

12 **Inner Mouth.** ‖ Tasteless water collects in mouth.

13 **Throat.** Painful spasmodic contraction in throat, during which he is unable to speak a loud word.

14 **Appetite, Thirst. Desires, Aversions.** Constant desire to eat.

16 **Hiccough, Belching, Nausea and Vomiting.** | Very violent hiccough, so that stomach is painful.

17 **Scrobiculum and Stomach.** Contractive pain in stomach.

Ulcerative pain in region of stomach.

‖ Atonic dyspepsia; accumulation of tasteless water in mouth; flat taste; no appetite, but constant desire to eat; eructations after dinner, empty or tasting of ingesta; vomiting of water, preceded by loathing; bloatedness of stomach > by emission of flatus; cutting in abdomen, going off by eructations; ineffectual urging to stool; hard stool with straining; yellow diarrhœic stools, with burning before and during stool; languor and prostration, with weariness of whole body.

18 **Hypochondria.** ‖ Exudation in pleura with sweat and diarrhœa. θInduration of liver.

20 **Stool and Rectum.** Thin, fetid stools, burning like fire in anus.

‖ Bloody diarrhœa.

| Discharge of blood from rectum with or without stool.

| Urging sensation in small of back, as if there would be stool; hard stool with straining; sudden stitches in anus; fissures of anus.

‖ Stool is accompanied by sweat. θDiarrhœa.

| Hard stool, with straining; ineffectual urging to stool.

| Straining; stool so hard that she cried out; great protrusion of hemorrhoids, followed for a long time by burning in anus.

‖ Inactivity of bowels for a long time, but without large accumulation of hardened feces; constantly increasing distress in rectum and anus, protrusion of rectum after stool; great heat with frequent but ineffectual efforts to evacuate bowels and bladder; three or four deep and angry-looking fissures of anus, also several superficial, but very sore and raw abrasions of mucous membrane, extending as far as sphincter, and a little beyond into rectum; sensation as if rectum and anus were all twisted up, followed by most violent cutting, not only after an evacuation, but at other times; pain after stool as if splinters of glass were sticking in every direction into anus and rectum, with great heat: these pains so intense that she could not keep quiet; sensation after stool as if rectum protruded and then suddenly went back with a jerk and most horrible pain; frequent ineffectual desire to urinate; fluttering of heart; desire to die during pains; relief, after a stool, by hot water, so that he always sat for a quarter of an hour in a sitz-bath as hot as he could endure; relief only while in bath.

|| Fissure of anus; great constriction; stools are forced with great effort, and anus aches and burns for hours.

▮▮ Excruciating pains immediately after stool, especially if bowels are costive. θFissured anus.

▮▮ Fissures of anus, with great sensitiveness of rectum.

▮ Violent itching of rectum.

▮ Dry heat at anus, with sudden stitches, like stabs with a penknife.

Burning in anus before and several hours after stool, with protrusion of varices.

▮ Burning in anus before and during a diarrhœa-like stool.

▮ Burning in anus before and after soft diarrhœic stools.

Protrusion of varices after hard stool, with straining and violent pressing in rectum.

▮ Oozing from anus.

▮ Ascaris vermicularis; severe itching about anus.

▮ Pin-worms in children.

21 **Urinary Organs.** || Diabetes; considerable emaciation and weakness; limbs sore and aching; great appetite; insatiable thirst and constant dryness of mouth; gums livid and swollen; soreness in kidneys; severe pain in small of back, $>$ from motion; hard stool with straining; frequent urging to urinate, with scanty discharge, or passes large quantities of light-colored urine.

Burning in urethra while urinating.

Incontinence of urine.

Frequent urging to urinate, with scanty discharge which soon becomes turbid and cloudy.

23 **Female Sexual Organs.** || Uterine pains following retrocession of eruption on lumbar region.

Menstruation too early, profuse and of too long duration, with pains in abdomen and small of back.

Metrorrhagia.

Leucorrhœa, with itching in rectum and discharge of bloody mucus.

24 **Pregnancy, Parturition, Lactation.** || Threatened miscarriage.

‖Fissures of nipples in nursing women.

27 **Cough.** Dry cough with tickling in larynx and great soreness in chest.

28 **Inner Chest and Lungs.** Congestion of blood to chest, with heat and dyspnœa.

Stitches in chest, especially when ascending steps.

‖Hydrothorax.

‖Exudation in pleural cavities with sweat and diarrhœa.

31 **Neck and Back.** Bruised sensation in back and hips, early on rising, > on motion.

Twitching in small of back.

Pain in small of back during menses.

35 **Rest. Position. Motion.** Lying down: toothache <.

Motion: pain in back >.

Ascending steps: stitches in chest.

39 **Temperature and Weather.** Hot water: relieved pain in rectum and anus.

41 **Attacks, Periodicity.** Several hours: burning of anus.

42 **Locality and Direction.** Right: twitching in eye and upper lid; stitch in ear; chirping in ear.

Left; twitching in upper eyelid; sensation of elongation in upper incisor.

43 **Sensations.** As if head were in a vise; as if brain would fall out; as of a white speck before eyes; as of skin before eyes; as if coldness rushed out of molars; as if there would be stool; as if rectum and anus were all twisted up; as of splinters of glass in anus and rectum; as if rectum protruded and then suddenly went back with a jerk.

Pain: in middle of forehead; in abdomen and small of back.

Excruciating pains: in bowels.

Horrible pain: in rectum.

Severe pain: in small of back.

Cutting: of abdomen.

Shooting, pulsating pain: in l. incisors.

Stitches: dull, deep on vertex; in r. ear; in anus; in chest.

Contractive pain: in stomach.

Ulcerative pain: in region of stomach.

Sticking painful in head.

Aching in limbs.

Burning on tip of tongue; in anus; in urethra.

Soreness of limbs; of kidneys; in chest.

Bruised sensation: in back and hips.

Heat: at anus.

Tickling: in larynx.

Twitching: in l. upper eyelid; in r. eye and upper lid; in small of back.

Chirping: in r. ear.
Dryness: of mouth; of nose.
Itching: of rectum.

41 **Tissues.** ▮Asthenic hemorrhages with exhaustion.
▮Chronic diarrhœa and leucorrhœa.
▮▮Fissures of anus and nipples.

45 **Touch. Passive Motion. Injuries.** Touch: tooth painful.

47 **Stages of Life, Constitution.** Man, æt. 30, suffering over a year; fissured anus.
Man, æt. 47, nervous temperament, spare, overworked; constipation and fissure of anus.

48 **Relations.** Compare: *Iris vers.*, *Canthar.*, *Sulphur*, in rectal symptoms; *Thuja* in sensation of splinters of glass in rectum and anus.

RHEUM.

Rhubarb. *Polygonaceæ.*

Provings by Hahnemann, Gross, Hornburg, Rückert, Teuthorn, etc. See Allen's Encyclopedia, vol. 8, p. 303.

Clinical Authorities.—*Headache*, Fuller, Hah. Mo., vol. 20, p. 539; *Difficult dentition*, Tuller, Hah. Mo., vol. 20, p. 538; *Renal affections*, Tuller, Hah. Mo., vol. 20, p. 542; *Diarrhœa*, Hartmann, Tietze, Weigel, Rück. Kl. Erf., vol. 1, p. 846; Kirsch, Müller, Hartmann, Kafka, Weber, Rück. Kl. Erf., vol. 5, p. 430; Smalls, Raue's Rec., 1873, p. 122, from U. S. Med. and Surg. Jour., vol. 7, p. 428; *Dysentery*, Gauwerky, Rück. Kl. Erf., vol. 5, p. 447.

1 **Mind.** ▮▮Child impatiently and vehemently desires many things and cries; dislikes even its favorite playthings.
▮▮Screaming of children, with urging and sour stools.
Not inclined to talk much; indolent; taciturn; morose.
Restless, with weeping.

2 **Sensorium.** Vertigo and heaviness, with beating in head; $<$ while standing.
Sensation as if brain moved, when standing.

3 **Inner Head.** Beating headache.
Dull, light, dizzy sort of headache, extending over whole brain.
Dull, stupefying headache, with bloated eyes.
Heaviness of head; heat rising up to it.

Pulsation in head, ascending from abdomen.
Pulsative, crampy headache.
Sensation as if brain moved when stooping.
‖ Headache due to gastric derangement; pain on top of head; sour, flat, slimy taste in mouth; bitter taste of food; hunger, but great repugnance to food after eating a little.

[4] **Outer Head.** ▮Sweat on hairy scalp, constant and very profuse; whether asleep or awake, in motion or quiet, the hair is always sopping wet; sweat may or may not be sour.

[5] **Sight and Eyes.** Weak and dull, especially when looking intently at any object.
Swimming eyes full of water, especially in open air.
Pupils dilated, with pressing headache; later contracted, with inward restlessness.
Contracted pupils.
Pulsation in eyes.
Convulsive twitching of eyelids.
Granulated upper lids.

[7] **Smell and Nose.** Stupefying drawing in root of nose, extending to tip, where it tingles.

[8] **Upper Face.** Pale; one cheek red, the other pale.
Muscles of forehead are drawn together and wrinkled.
Tension of skin of face.
Cool sweat on face, most around nose and mouth.

[10] **Teeth and Gums.** Painful sensation of coldness in teeth, with accumulation of much saliva.
▮▮Difficult dentition; restlessness and irritability; child is nervous, with temporary satisfaction after its whims are gratified; pallor of face; occasional twitching of eyelids, corners of mouth, lips and fingers; the child smells sour.

[11] **Taste and Tongue.** ▮Taste: sour; flat, slimy; insipid or nauseous; bitter only of food, even of sweet things.
Tongue numb, insensible.

[12] **Inner Mouth.** ‖ Salivation with colic or diarrhœa.

[14] **Appetite, Thirst. Desires, Aversions.** ▮Desire for various kinds of food, which become repugnant as soon as a little is eaten.

[15] **Eating and Drinking.** After eating prunes, colic.
After a meal, loose stool; colic, which is worse standing.

[16] **Hiccough, Belching, Nausea and Vomiting.** Nausea, as from stomach or abdomen, with colic.

[17] **Scrobiculum and Stomach.** ▮Fulness in stomach, as after eating too much.
Throbbing in pit of stomach.
▮Disordered stomach in children; nervous, irritable, de-

siring many things, with repugnance to food, pale face, sour-smelling breath, nightly restlessness and crying during sleep.

18 **Hypochondria.** ▮Jaundice, in consequence of eating unripe fruit, accompanied by white diarrhœa.

‖Duodenal catarrh and catarrh of biliary ducts, with jaundice; stools whitish, pasty, or clay-colored; skin, earthy, jaundiced.

19 **Abdomen.** ‖Sensation of nausea in abdomen.

▮Abdomen bloated, tense; wind seems to rise into chest.

‖Like a lump around navel.

▮Cutting and rumbling as from flatulence.

▮Griping with great urging to stool.

▮Cutting in umbilical region.

‖Colic: violent pain with cutting; must lie doubled up; < when standing; immediately before stool, not > by stool; before and during stool, > after; a quarter of an hour after dinner; ‖with very sour stools, acid children; in children made < at once by uncovering an arm or a leg, child smells sour; < by eating plums.

20 **Stool and Rectum.** ▮Frequent urging and ineffectual straining; < on motion and walking.

▮Colicky; ineffectual urging; altered fecal stools.

▮Desire for stool after a meal.

▮Stool: brown, slimy; loose, thin, curdled, sour-smelling, fermented; corroding anus; mucous and fecal; pasty; thin, brownish, fecal; whitish, curdy, turning green on diaper on exposure to air; of a pea-green; feces mixed with green slime; fetid; frothy.

▮Before stool: urging; ineffectual urging to urinate; cutting colic.

▮During stool: colic; chilliness, cutting and constricting pains in abdomen; pale face; salivation; screaming (teething infants), with drawing up of limbs or stiffening body.

▮After stool: tenesmus; renewed urging (when moving); constrictive cutting colic, < from motion.

▮Aggravation: when moving about; in infants and children; after eating; during dentition; in childbed; during inflammatory rheumatism; in hot weather; when uncovering (pains).

▮Amelioration: by bending double (colic).

▮Diarrhœa, with sour, slimy stool and tenesmus after abuse of Magnesia.

▮Almost immediately after nursing child has a loose stool, which is sour-smelling, accompanied by colic.

▮Liquid slimy stools, as if fermented, with pale face, ptyalism, colic, crying and restlessness; child draws up legs, smells sour despite all washing.

|| Very severe diarrhœa, with colic and tenesmus; alternate chilliness and heat; great thirst; general sweat; great prostration, restlessness, fear of death.

▮ Diarrhœa of teething children during Summer; extreme emaciation.

▮ Diarrhœa of children who have not cut any teeth; evacuations fluid, greenish, sour-smelling, as if fermented, accompanied by colic, with flexing of thighs upon abdomen; tossing about; paleness of face; ptyalism.

▮ Sour, fetid discharge during dentition; always some congestion about head; fever and dark-colored, smarting urine and dysuria.

| Dysentery; after bloody stools have ceased, tenesmus, with brown, mushlike, slimy, sour stools.

|| During phthisis, greenish diarrhœa, of sour smell, containing much mucus, accompanied by colic and tenesmus.

|| Diarrhœa during inflammatory rheumatism.

▮ Chronic diarrhœa, sour, frothy; with moist tongue, thirst, loss of appetite.

21 **Urinary Organs.** Burning in kidneys and bladder, before and during urination.

Bladder weak, must press hard to urinate.

Urine: increased; red or greenish-yellow.

|| Abdomen distended; urine scanty, burning, reddish, with a pink sediment; face pale and bloated; disposition irritable; very nervous; constant disposition to sweat upon slightest motion; hair wet all the time; severe cutting drawing in l. loin below short ribs, with a drawing, aching, burning sensation in l. ovarian region, sometimes agonizing. *θ*Ascites.

|| Child lay in a stupor, from which he frequently roused and screamed; face pale and covered with cool sweat, forehead and hair sopping wet; lips, eyelids and fingers twitching; urine scanty, hot, with slimy shreds and strings of blood on diaper; renal region tender on pressure, causing child to wince and cry.

|| Eight months pregnant; face and eyes bloated; great pallor of countenance, irritable, nervous, easily startled by noises and apprehensive, twitching of facial muscles; great disposition to sweat on slightest motion; cool sweat on forehead; hair constantly wet; urine scanty and fragrant, high-colored.

23 **Female Sexual Organs.** Bearing down in uterine region, while standing.

24 **Pregnancy. Parturition. Lactation.** || After abortus, urinary complaints.

▮ Milk of nursing women yellow and bitter; infant refused breast.

▮Diarrhœa in first days after confinement, with colic, tenesmus, prostration, restlessness; fear of death; stools watery, offensive.

▮Stitches in nipples.

26 **Respiration.** Dyspnœa, as from a load on upper part of chest.

‖Snoring inspiration during sleep.

29 **Heart, Pulse and Circulation.** Pulse generally unchanged; only a little accelerated, especially in evening.

31 **Neck and Back.** Stiffness in sacrum and hips; cannot walk straight.

Violent cutting, as if in lumbar vertebræ, < by stool.

‖Cutting, drawing in l. lumbar region, beneath short ribs and in forepart of l. side of lower abdomen, just above pubes; digging in intestines.

32 **Upper Limbs.** Darting pains in arms.

Twitching in arms, hands and fingers.

Bubbling sensation in elbow joints.

Veins of hand distended.

Cold sweat on palms of hands.

33 **Lower Limbs.** Twitching of muscles of thighs.

‖Sensation of fatigue in thighs, as after great exertion.

‖Tensive, pressing pain in hollow of l. knee, extending to heel.

Stiffness in bend of knee, with pain on motion.

Bubbling sensation from bend of knee to heel.

34 **Limbs in General.** Limbs fall asleep from lying on them, particularly the lower, in putting one over the other.

‖Simple pain in all the joints during motion.

35 **Rest. Position. Motion.** Takes the queerest positions, in order to rest awhile; restless nights; cannot walk erect; flexes limbs; puts hands over head; must lie doubled up.

Lying on limbs: makes them fall asleep.

Must lie doubled up: colic.

Stooping: as if brain moved.

Standing: vertigo, as if brain moved; colic <; bearing down in uterine region.

Motion: urging and straining <; colic <; slightest disposition to sweat; stiffness in bend of knee painful, pain in all joints.

Walking: urging and straining.

Cannot walk straight: stiffness of limbs, hips and sacrum.

36 **Nerves.** Weakness, exhaustion also of children, with diarrhœa.

Weakness and heaviness of whole body as if one were waking from a heavy sleep.

Restlessness.

Child is pale, quarrels, frets in sleep; with convulsive startings in fingers.

37 **Sleep.** Puts hands over head when falling asleep and in sleep.

During sleep: heat; jerking motion of muscles in face or eyelids; trembling; moving limbs; bending head backward.

▮Children cry and toss about all night; delirious talking; full of fear.

▮▮Vivid, sad, anxious dreams.

Walking in sleep.

On awakening from sleep, headache; bad odor from mouth.

Requires very little sleep and not much food.

38 **Time.** Evening: pulse accelerated.

Night: restlessness; children cry and toss about.

39 **Temperature and Weather.** General aggravation from uncovering, from cold.

Amelioration from wrapping up, from warmth.

Open air: eyes full of water.

Uncovering arm or leg: colic <.

Hot weather: colic <.

40 **Fever.** Chilliness, alternating with heat; internal, with external heat.

Heat all over, mostly on hands and feet, with cold face; no thirst.

Perspiration from slight exertions.

▮Sweats easily without fever.

▮Perspiration on forehead and scalp after slight exertion.

▮Cold perspiration on face, especially about mouth and nose.

▮▮Sweat on scalp and forehead.

Cold sweat about nose and mouth.

Sweat stains yellow.

41 **Attacks, Periodicity.** Alternate: chilliness and heat.

42 **Locality and Direction.** Symptoms mostly left-sided; going (in the sick) downward, or from r. to left.

Left: cutting drawing in loin; drawing, burning in ovarian region; cutting drawing in lumbar region and in forepart of side of lower abdomen; pressing pain in hollow of knee.

43 **Sensations.** As if brain moved; as of a lump around navel; as of a load on upper part of chest; cutting as if in lumbar vertebræ; heaviness, as if one were waking from a heavy sleep.

Pain: on top of head; in all joints.

Violent pain: in abdomen.

Cutting: in umbilical region.

Cutting drawing: in l. loin; in l. lumbar region.
Darting pains: in arms.
Digging: in intestines.
Stitches.: in nipples.
Constricting pains: in abdomen.
Drawing, aching, burning: in l. ovarian region.
Tensive, pressing pain: in hollow of knee.
Beating: in head.
Throbbing: in pit of stomach.
Pulsation: in head; in eyes.
Twitching: eyelids, corners of mouth, lips and fingers; in arms and hands; of muscles of thighs.
Burning: in kidneys and bladder.
Bearing down: in uterine region.
Stupefying drawing: in root of nose.
Dull, stupefying headache.
Dull, light, dizzy sort of headache.
Bubbling sensation: in elbow joints; from bend of knee to heel.
Fulness: in stomach.
Heaviness: in head.
Numbness: of tongue.
Painful coldness: in teeth.

45 **Tissues.** Diarrhœa during dentition.
Acute rheumatism, going from joint to joint, r. shoulder to hip, l. hip to right.
Lameness of wrists and knees after sprains and dislocations.
Anasarca.

46 **Skin.** ▮Sour smell of whole body.
▮Child smells sourish, even if washed or bathed.

47 **Stages of Life, Constitution.** Often suitable for children, sucklings, or during dentition.
Sour-smelling children who cry a great deal.
Child, æt. 5 months, suffering four days; diarrhœa.
Boy, æt. 6 months, after diphtheria; acute nephritis.
Boy, æt. 9 months, ill three days; diarrhœa.
Girl, æt. 2; frothy diarrhœa.
Woman, æt. 35, blonde, lively disposition, delivered several days ago, suffering three days; diarrhœa.
Mrs. W., æt. 47, eight months pregnant; renal disorder.
Mrs. A., æt. 60; renal affection.

48 **Relations.** Antidoted by: *Camphor., Chamom., Coloc., Mercur., Nux vom., Pulsat.*
It antidotes: *Canthar.* and *Magn. carb.*
Compatible: *Ipecac.*
Complementary: after *Magn. carb.*
Compare: *Arsen., Bellad., Chamom., Coloc., Dulcam., Nux vom., Podoph., Pulsat., Rhus tox., Sulphur.*

RHODODENDRON.

Yellow Snowrose. *Ericaceæ.*

A native of Siberia, grows in the mountains and flowers in July.

The tincture is prepared from the fresh leaves.

Provings by Seidel and others, Archiv für Hom., vol. 10, p. 139.

CLINICAL AUTHORITIES.—*Dysecoia, Tinnitus aurium,* Schulz, Kallenbach, Rück. Kl. Erf, vol. 1, p. 379; *Prosopalgia,* Hirschel, Raue's Rec., 1870, p. 292; B. J. H., vol. 27, p. 149; Ussher, A. H. Z., vol. 106, p. 191, from Hom. World; *Toothache,* Gutmann, Altschul, Elb, Rück. Kl. Erf., vol. 1, p. 473; Villers, Oehme, Rück. Kl. Erf., vol. 5, p. 209; Eidherr, B. J. H., vol. 19, p. 133; *Pains in stomach,* Goullon, Meyer, Hom. Clin., vol. 3, p. 117; Raue's Rec., 1871, p. 22; *Dysuria,* Wilson, Med. Adv., vol. 5, p. 375; *Ovarian cyst is caused to discharge into abdomen,* Ozanam, Bulletin de la Soc. de France; *Balanitis,* Gilchrist, Surg. Therap., p. 532; *Induration of testicles,* Hartman, Schreter, Rück. Kl. Erf., vol. 2, p. 210; Berridge, Hom. Phys., vol. 8, p. 553; *Hydrocele,* Seidel, Kallenbach, Rück. Kl. Erf., vol. 2, p. 214; Gross, Rück. Kl. Erf., vol. 5, p. 585; Lilienthal, N. A. J. H., vol. 14, p. 138; Hastings, B. J. H., vol. 18, p. 351; Raue's Rec., 1870, p. 242; *Orchitis, hydrocele,* Ussher, A. H. Z., vol. 106, p. 191; *Cough,* Kafka, Rück. Kl. Erf., vol. 5, p. 694; *Pain in arm,* Allen, A. H. Z., vol. 112, p. 77; *White swelling of knee* (2 cases), Henke, Seidel; *Pain in periosteum,* Waddell, Hom. Phys., vol. 7, p. 427; *Rheumatic pain in l. side,* Goullon, Raue's Rec., 1871, p. 172, from A. H. Z., vol. 80, p. 75; *Rheumatism,* Gross, Hartmann, Rück. Kl. Erf., vol. 3, p. 537; Smith, N. E. M. G., vol. 8, p. 220; Raue's Rec., 1874, p. 254.

1 **Mind.** Leaves out whole words in writing.

Great indifference, with aversion to all occupation.

While talking easily forgets what he is talking about; does not recollect what he had been talking about till he has thought awhile.

| Nervous persons who dread a storm and are particularly afraid of thunder.

2 **Sensorium.** Sensation of stupefaction and drowsiness in head on rising in morning.

Intoxicated from a little wine.

|| Dulness of head.

3 **Inner Head.** Pain in forehead and temples when lying in bed in morning; < from drinking wine and from wet, cold weather; > after rising and moving about.

Early in morning in bed, headache which almost deprives him of his senses, > after rising.

|| Tearing, boring pain in l. temporal region.

4 **Outer Head.** The scalp feels sore and as if bruised.

Violent drawing and tearing in bones and periosteum of cranial bones; < when at rest, in morning; during a thunderstorm and during wet, cold, stormy weather; > from wrapping head up warmly; from dry heat and from exercise.

Biting itching on scalp, especially in evening.

5 **Sight and Eyes.** Dimness of vision when reading and writing.

ǁA man about 40 complained of a gradual failure of sight, accompanied by periodically recurring violent pains, involving eyeball, extending to orbit and head, < at approach of storm, > when storm broke out; rheumatic diathesis; pupils somewhat dilated and sluggish, $T+^{1}$ in both eyes; pulsation of retinal veins, but no excavation of optic nerve; field of vision not circumscribed; Hm. $\frac{1}{30}$; vision improved by glasses, but could not be brought above $\frac{20}{30}$; pain recurred until relieved by the medicine.

Periodical, dry burning in eyes, < in bright daylight and from looking intently.

ǁBurning pain in eyes; when reading or writing he has a feeling of heat in them.

ǁCiliary neuralgia, < before a storm.

ǁInsufficiency of internal recti muscles; darting pains like arrows through eye from head, < before a storm. θAsthenopia muscularis.

ǁOn staring or writing, very hot lachrymation from r. eye, and at same time shooting in r. eye from within outward.

Spasmodic contraction of eyelids.

6 **Hearing and Ears.** Otalgia (r. ear); violent twitching pain.

Sensation in ear as from a worm.

Buzzing in ear, < when swallowing.

Violent pain in r. external ear, commencing in morning and continuing nearly all day.

Tearing sensation in and about r. ear.

Constant buzzing in ears and a sensation as if water were rushing into them; loud sounds re-echo for a long time; humming and ringing before ears.

ǁConstant tearing pain in ears; roaring; stitching, tearing headache; shortness of breath, < from least motion; for several years hardness of hearing.

ǁTinnitus aurium, < r. side; feels pulsation of heart in ear; sounds in ears as of a gentle downpour of rain, < toward evening; hears with difficulty the talking around him; tick of watch not heard 14 inches from r. ear and 11 from l.; flushes of heat at night, pressure in forehead and vertex.

||After an arthritic affection of head, twenty years ago, constant ringing and roaring in ears, followed by hardness of hearing, which gradually grew worse, so that for the last ten years could hear nothing unless one called loudly into her ear. θDysecoia.

||After catching cold, roaring and ringing in ears; can hear in morning on rising, but as day advances the noises in ears gradually grow more intense, so that in evening can scarcely hear those about him; buzzing in ears like that of a bee, or noise like that following the tolling of a bell, at times interrupted by cracking sounds; noises cease for a time, then begin again; tick of watch heard on both sides at distance of two feet and two inches.

7 **Smell and Nose.** Diminished sense of smell.

Bleeding of nose, l. side.

Soreness of inner nose, with yellow or black scurf.

Violent sneezing, when rising in morning, with heat in face.

Thin, fluid and profuse discharge from nose, with rheumatic or gouty symptoms.

||Stoppage of l. half of nose, near root, < in morning before rising; during day stoppage of l. nostril alternates with that of r., but nose is never stopped entirely; > in open air.

8 **Upper Face.** Chilliness over face.

Violent tearing, jerking faceache; < in wind and changes of weather; > while eating and from warmth.

||Prosopalgia; pain begins in temple and extends to lower jaw and chin; acute pain extending from temple to temple, < from motion, talking and cold applications.

||Violent faceache, spreading over r. side of face from teeth and gums, radiating over mouth, eyes and ears, equally violent day and night, during motion and rest; pains drawing, tearing, jerking; < by wind and changes of weather; > from warmth, entirely relieved while eating and for some time after; commonly troublesome in Spring and Autumn, the present very severe attack in Winter.

9 **Lower Face.** Lips dry, burning.

Vesicles on inner side of lower lip, sore when eating.

10 **Teeth and Gums.** ||Toothache: with earache; teeth loose; snags; gums swollen; < from change of weather; > from warmth and after eating; great weakness after pain.

|Toothache; the approach of a thunderstorm or cloudy, windy weather is always preceded by a drawing, aching or cutting pain.

Occasional grumbling and tearing in four first anterior

molars for a short time; now in upper, now in lower jaw; now on r., now on l. side.

|Transient pain in single teeth, recurring especially in damp weather and before a storm.

||Toothache appearing every Spring and Fall during prevalence of a sharp east wind, lasting several weeks; constant boring in a single tooth; stitches extending into ear; pain < on touching tooth; pain at times intermits, < at night from cold drinks, especially inhalation of cold air; > from external heat.

||Toothache especially after a chill, begins with a disagreeable pricking in teeth of one side, gradually increases to a drawing, tearing pain over face and temples on same side; < from warmth, especially warmth of bed; teeth perfectly sound.

||Toothache; pain began in a carious tooth, but finally affected also neighboring teeth; pain > while chewing and for a short time afterward.

||Rheumatic or gouty pains in teeth; drawing tearing in molars, < in cloudy, stormy, rainy weather, also in rest; pain often intermits, generally appears in morning.

|Arthritic toothache, < at night, from cold or warm drinks; > from external application of heat.

||Neuralgia in inferior and superior dental nerves for seven weeks; woman in agony, sleepless; gums had been swollen; had three sound teeth taken out, without relief.

||Rheumatic toothache radiating from r. lower jaw to teeth.

11 **Taste and Tongue.** Taste lost; food has no taste.

Smarting vesicles under tongue.

12 **Inner Mouth.** Increase of saliva in mouth, with dryness of throat.

13 **Throat.** Sore throat.

Constriction and burning in throat.

Scraping and scratching sensation in fauces; sensation as if those parts were lined with mucus.

14 **Appetite, Thirst. Desires, Aversions.** Easily satisfied with a small quantity of food; feels uncomfortable afterward.

16 **Hiccough, Belching, Nausea and Vomiting.** Gulping of a rancid or bitter fluid.

||Empty eructations.

Nausea, waterbrash, pressure at stomach, > by belching.

Vomits after fluids, especially cold water; green, bitter vomit.

17 **Scrobiculum and Stomach.** Sinking at stomach.

Pressure in stomach at night, after cold drinks.

Constriction and pressure at pit of stomach, with dyspnœa.

Pressing in pit of stomach during and after eating.

||After a thorough wetting, pressing pain in l. side under short ribs; > by eating.

||Periodical crampy pain under short ribs; pressing and drawing, with fulness in pit of stomach, with oppression in breathing; pain as from flatulency in different parts, but especially in l. hypochondrium.

||Bellyache after eating; in umbilical region after supper, obliquely over hypochondria; pressing in pit of stomach after dinner, during and after eating.

18 **Hypochondria.** ||Pain as from tension under short ribs; periodical crampy pains.

|Painful incarceration of flatus in hypochondria and in small of back.

Pressing and drawing, with feeling of repletion in stomach, and oppression of breathing.

Stitches in spleen from walking fast; tension from stooping.

19 **Abdomen.** Distension in upper part of abdomen, with dyspnœa; evening and morning.

Much rumbling in abdomen, with eructations and discharge of fetid flatus.

Colic at navel, or feeling of repletion after eating.

20 **Stool and Rectum.** |Stool: papescent, yet tardy, requiring much urging; painless, undigested; thin, brownish, fecal; spurting out with force.

|Diarrhœa: after meals; after fruit; from wet, cold weather; before a thunderstorm; in morning, with much flatus; with pains in limbs.

||Dysentery in summer, renewed before a thunderstorm.

Drawing extending from rectum to genitals.

Pulsation in anus.

21 **Urinary Organs.** Frequent urging to urinate, with drawing in region of bladder.

Greenish urine.

||Somewhat increased pale urine has an offensive, acrid odor.

|Frequent desire to urinate; pain in urethra as from subcutaneous ulceration.

22 **Male Sexual Organs.** Desire weak; aversion to an embrace.

Emissions at night, with amorous dreams, later long-continued erections.

|Testicles: especially epididymis, intensely painful to touch; soreness extending into abdomen and thighs; drawn up, swollen, painful; drawn up when walking, contusive pain.

Violent sticking in r. testicle, as if violently contused, in evening, while sitting; pain disappears when walking, but returns immediately upon sitting down.

▮Violent, painful drawing in hard, somewhat swollen testes, extending as far as abdomen and thigh, especially on r. side.

Drawing, sticking pain in r. testicle and spermatic cord, > from motion; sometimes pain is pricking, commencing in r. testicle and spreading in a zig-zag manner along perineum toward anus, lasting some seconds, and so violent that it arrests breathing.

▮Balanitis; prepuce distended like a bladder, with integument thin, no pain or fever, little discharge, and no annoyance apart from the increased size.

ǀǀScanty, painless, thin discharge from urethra; swelling of l. testicle, with tearing pains therein, extending up spermatic cord; severe, periodic, tearing, throbbing, digging pain in l. hip bone, extending to middle of thigh, becoming almost intolerable when at rest, so that he could not sit or lie in bed at night; after cohabiting with wife who had fluor albus.

ǀǀOrchitis, l. side, smooth, hard swelling; preceded by hydrocele.

▮▮Chronic orchitis; testicle indurated, with tendency to atrophy; feeling in gland as if it were being crushed.

ǀǀSeventeen years ago had orchitis, r. side, after which testicle remained somewhat enlarged, after severe exertion severe pain in small of back, followed in evening by drawing, pressing pain in r. testicle which became swollen; pain > lying with knees drawn up, < standing; pain sometimes extends into abdomen and causes tension at r. inguinal ring.

ǀǀOrchitis with fever, from catching cold while dancing, while recovering from an attack of gonorrhœa; l. testicle swollen to size of hen's egg.

▮▮Induration and swelling of testicles after gonorrhœa, or with blennorrhœa.

ǀǀSwelling and hardness of l. testicle, following gonorrhœa; formerly had headache before a thunderstorm.

ǀǀFarmer, aged 40, without known cause, had orchitis, treated six months without benefit, swelling increased in size and hardness, so that he could not walk, and penis lay hidden in the tumor; l. testicle size of three fists, very tense, hard, painful to least touch. θHydrocele.

▮▮Hydrocele: from birth, r. side, in a child aged 4 weeks; as large as a hen's egg, since birth, in a boy aged 1½ years; left-sided, in a scrofulous child æt. 3 years; r. side, in an infant æt. 1 year; l. side, in a boy æt. 4 years; from birth, increasing from year to year, in a boy æt. 7 years; l. side, in a hemorrhoidal subject æt. 60.

▮Itching and sweating of scrotum.

Soreness or sore sensation between genitals and thighs.

23 **Female Sexual Organs.** Menstruation too profuse and too early; fever and headache at each menstrual period.

Suppressed menstruation.

Pain in ovaries; < in changes of weather.

Serous cysts in vagina.

A country-woman, æt. 35, suffered since five years from a voluminous cyst in r. ovary; *Rhodod.*^{6} was employed internally and externally; about sixth day patient was taken with acute pains in stomach, with a feeling of fluid pouring into abdomen; vomited bile; for three days high fever; the cyst filled up again; repeated *Rhodod.* next month, again a rupture took place in about eight to ten days, with symptoms of subacute peritonitis, after cure of which patient refused to continue treatment.

24 **Pregnancy. Parturition. Lactation.** After parturition, burning in uterine region, alternating with pains in limbs, fingers spasmodically flexed.

26 **Respiration.** Dyspnœa from constriction of chest.

27 **Cough.** Cough: dry, exhausting, morning and evening, with oppression of chest and rough throat; with escape of urine; dry, excited by tickling in trachea.

‖ Attacks of dry cough; after an attack has lasted four to five hours, during which time she coughs constantly, there follows either vomiting of a serous, bitter, somewhat slimy fluid, containing no particles of food, or she is so prostrated that she has to lie down and sleep; for the next four or six hours feels well and has no cough; suddenly and without apparent cause sensation of severe pressure and constriction in region of stomach, as if some one was pressing forcibly with fist against stomach, accompanied by a constant and uncontrollable irritation to cough, arising from epigastrium; with the pressure in stomach there is a similar, but less severe, sensation in lumbar region of spine, from which place extend drawing, tearing pains at one time into upper, then into lower limbs; appetite impaired.

28 **Inner Chest and Lungs.** Shooting through l. chest to back, when bending back and to right.

‖ A very transient dull pain extending from chest to l. hypochondrium, almost like splenetic stitches, when walking fast.

‖ Breath and speech fail from the violence of pleuritic stitches running downward in anterior l. chest, after standing on cold ground and getting chilled.

‖ Rheumatic pain in l. side below short ribs, continuous and of a pressing nature, after taking cold by getting wet; > from eating.

29 **Heart, Pulse and Circulation.** Boring pain in region of heart.
Heart's beat stronger.
Pulse slow and weak, or unchanged.

30 **Outer Chest.** Chest sensitive to touch.

31 **Neck and Back.** Stiffness of nape of neck, in morning.
▮Stiffness of nape of neck; tearing pains in nape of neck, extending thence gradually half-way down back; < at night and in bed, so that she must rise.
▮Rheumatic pains in back and shoulders.
▮Stiff neck, gums and teeth sore, pains fly about everywhere.
Shooting from back to pit of stomach.
Pain from small of back into arms.
▮Small of back pains, < when sitting and in wet weather.

32 **Upper Limbs.** Paralytic, rheumatic pain in r. shoulder upon which he rests, sometimes extending below elbow and going off by turning to other side.
▮Violent tearing, boring pain in l. shoulder joint.
‖Severe pain in deltoid muscle, < from motion and from vexation before a thunderstorm.
Drawing pain in arms, < in wet weather.
Sensation as if blood ceased to circulate in arms, hands feel warm.
▮Sensation of weakness and formication in arms, as if they were asleep, < from heat of bed, exposure to cold and stormy weather.
▮Tearing: in l. forearm, at night; in r. forearm.
‖About 6 P.M., tearing, cramplike drawing in forearm, as if in periosteum, during wet, cold weather; violent tearing, boring pain in l. shoulder joint, with prickling in fingers. θChronic rheumatism.
▮Sensation as if wrists were sprained.
▮Pain as if sprained in r. wrist joint, impeding motion, < when at rest, in rough weather.
Intensely painful drawing and digging in l. wrist joint, in evening, when at rest.
‖Sudden swelling with tearing pains in r. wrist, extending to dorsum of hand; in a man suffering from condylomata.
Increased warmth in hands.
Itching, obliging to scratch, of middle and ring fingers of l. hand, with erysipelatous redness.

33 **Lower Limbs.** Sensation of soreness in thighs near genitals.
‖Severe tearing pains beginning in upper and posterior portion of r. thigh and extending down into foot, with sensation of formication in whole limb; pain < during rest, drives her out of bed early in morning; foot im-

mediately "goes to sleep" when sitting down after walking; must move foot constantly; pain and stiffness of leg, < mornings.

‖ Periodical tearing pains in lower limbs, particularly about hip joint, < in stormy weather, in rest and at night; at times swelling and painfulness of finger joints.

‖ Stitching pains in knee and ankle joints; tension in legs when walking; constant sensation as if feet and legs were asleep; < after sitting still, and early in morning on rising; after an attack of influenza.

‖ White swelling of knee, with intolerable tearing pains, < during rest and at night.

| Rheumatic pains in lower extremities and feet, as if in periosteum, < when at rest and during wet, cold weather.

Sensation of coldness, skin wrinkles on legs.

Dropsical swelling of lower legs and feet.

| Sensation in lower legs and feet "as if asleep."

Unusual coldness of feet.

| Gout, when there is a fibrous deposit in great toe joint, not the usual deposits of urate of soda.

| Affection of great toe joint, often mistaken for bunion, but of rheumatic character.

34 **Limbs in General.** Heavy, weak feeling and formication in back and limbs; < at rest and in rough weather.

Sensation in joints as if sprained, with swelling and redness; with arthritic nodosities.

| Drawing, tearing pain in periosteum, < at night, in wet, stormy weather and in rest; > in motion; mostly in forearms and lower legs.

Erratic tearing pains in limbs.

Pains in limbs felt especially in forearm and legs down to fingers and toes; they soon pass off, and resemble a cramplike drawing.

| Pains in limbs seem to be seated in bones or periosteum; they are mostly confined to small spots and reappear on change of weather.

‖ Tearing pain beginning at outer side of r. arm, extending to nape of neck and into back, then down into thigh, where it becomes stitching in character; heels are particularly painful; walking difficult, feels as if heavy weights were hanging to feet; < in rest and change of weather. θRheumatism.

‖ For twelve years, periodical, severe, tearing pains in limbs; for six days r. forearm and foot affected; no swelling or redness; < at night, she cannot remain in bed.

‖ Severe tearing pains in limbs, with swelling and redness of several joints; r. knee, elbows, l. finger joints affected; pains < at night, particularly toward morning, with tension and stiffness in joints; after syphilis treated with large doses of Mercury.

|| After catching cold, paralytic condition of limbs; severe drawing, pinching, stitching pains in limbs; fever; could not walk or stand, neither could he move his arms or hands; sleep disturbed at night by pain.

| Chronic rheumatism affected the smaller joints and their ligaments.

35 **Rest. Position. Motion.** Rest: gouty pains in teeth <; pain in hip bone intolerable; pain in wrist <; pain in thigh; pains in lower limbs <; paralytic weakness; heavy, weak feeling and formication.

Lying with knees drawn up: pain in r. testicle.

Shoulder on which he rests, rheumatic pain; goes off when turning.

Cannot get to sleep or remain asleep unless her legs are crossed.

Rising: headache >.

Sitting: severe pain in testicles; after walking, feet go to sleep.

Stooping: tension.

Standing: pain in testicle <.

Motion: pain in ears <; prosopalgia <; pain in deltoid muscle; pains in limbs >; in open air causes profuse debilitating sweat.

Must move foot constantly.

Walking: stitches in spleen; testicles drawn up; pain in testicles >; tension in legs.

Chewing: pain >.

Exertion: pain in back; slight, causes great weakness.

Exercise: headache >.

Could not walk or stand, neither move his arms nor hands on account of severe pain.

36 **Nerves.** Paralytic weakness during rest.

Great weakness after slight exertion.

Heavy, weak feeling and formication in back and limbs, < in rest and in rough weather.

Painful sensitiveness in windy and cold weather.

|| Paroxysmal chorea in l. arm, leg and face, on approach of a storm.

37 **Sleep.** Awakes as if called.

Great sleepiness during day, with burning in eyes.

Deep, heavy sleep before midnight, with sleepiness early in evening, but sleepless after midnight; morning sleep disturbed by pain and restlessness in body.

|| Cannot get to sleep or remain asleep unless her legs are crossed.

38 **Time.** Morning: on rising, stupefaction and drowsiness in head; when lying in bed, pain in temples and forehead; pain in external ear; violent sneezing when rising; toothache generally; distension in abdomen; diarrhœa; dry cough; stiffness of nape of neck; tearing in thigh; stiffness of leg <; in bed, chilliness.
During day: alternate stoppage of l. and r. nostril; great sleepiness; if cold air blows on him, chilliness.
All day: severe pain in external ear.
About 6 P.M.: tearing, cramplike drawing in forearm.
Toward evening: sounds in ears <.
Evening: itching of scalp <; distension in abdomen: pain in testicle; dry cough; pain in wrist joint; early, sleepiness; persistent ice-cold feet; heat.
Night: flushes of heat; toothache <; pressure in stomach; emissions; pain in hip bone; pains down back <; pain in lower limbs <.
Before midnight: deep, heavy sleep.
After midnight: sleepless.

39 **Temperature and Weather.** Almost all symptoms reappear with rough weather.
Open air: stoppage of nostril >; moving in, profuse sweat.
Dry heat: headache >.
Heat of bed: formication in arms <.
Warmth: faceache >; toothache >; toothache < from warmth of bed.
Wrapping up warmly: head >.
Wind and changes of weather: violent faceache <; toothache <; pains in ovaries <; painful sensitiveness.
After thorough wetting: pressing pain in l. side; rheumatic pain in l. side.
Wet, cold weather: pain in head <; transient pain in single teeth; gouty pains in teeth <; diarrhœa; small of back pains <; drawing pain in arms <; exposure to, weakness and formication in arms; tearing in forearm.
Cold: prosopalgia <; toothache < from cold drinks and inhalation of air; water, vomits after; standing on ground, stitches in chest; increased warmth of hands.
External heat: toothache >.
Stormy weather: rheumatic pains <.
Before a storm: ciliary neuralgia <; pains through eye from head <; toothache; diarrhœa; dysentery; pain in deltoid muscles <; paroxysmal chorea in l. arm, leg and face.
After catching cold while dancing: orchitis.

40 **Fever.** Chilliness in morning in bed and during day if cold air blows on him.

Chilliness alternating with heat.

Persistent ice-cold feet in evening, continuing long after lying down in bed.

Heat in evening with cold feet.

Sensation of heat, especially in hands, although they feel cold to touch.

||Frequent increase of warmth of hands, even in cold weather.

Feverish heat in evening, with burning in face.

Profuse debilitating sweat, especially when moving about in open air.

Offensive smelling sweat in axillæ.

Formication and itching of skin, with sweat.

Perspiration has an odor of spice.

41 **Attacks, Periodicity.** Alternate: l. and r. nostril stopped; burning in uterine region and pains in limbs; chilliness and heat.

Periodical: pains in eyeballs; crampy pain under short ribs in l. hip bone; tearing pains in lower limbs; in limbs.

Spring and Autumn: faceache; toothache during sharp east wind.

For several years: hardness of hearing.

42 **Locality and Direction.** Right: hot lachrymation; shooting in eye; otalgia; pain in external ear; tearing sensation in and about ear; tinnitus aurium <; violent faceache; toothache from lower jaw to teeth; sticking in testicle; tension at inguinal ring; voluminous cyst in ovary; rheumatic pain in shoulder upon which he rests; tearing in forearm; pain in wrist joint; tearing in thigh; knee and elbow, tearing pain.

Left: pain in temporal region; bleeding of nose, side; stoppage of side of nose; pain in hypochondrium; swelling of testicles; pain in hip bone; orchitis; testicle swollen to size of hen's egg; testicle size of three fists; shooting through chest to back; stitches in anterior chest; rheumatic pain in side below short ribs; boring pain in shoulder joint; tearing in forearm; digging in wrist joint; itching of fingers; finger joints, tearing pains; chorea in arm, leg and face.

Within outward: pain in r. eye.

43 **Sensations.** Scalp as if bruised; as of a worm in ear; as if water were rushing into ear; as if throat were lined with mucus; as from tension under short ribs; testicle as if violently contused; or as if it were crushed; as of fluid pouring into abdomen; as if some one were forcibly pressing with fist against stomach; as if blood ceased to circulate in arms; as if arms were asleep; as if wrists

were sprained; as if feet and legs were asleep; rheumatism as if in periosteum of lower extremities; as if heavy weights were hanging to feet.

Pain: in forehead and temples; in limbs; in urethra; in ovaries; from small of back into arms; in r. wrist joint; of leg.

Violent pain: in eyeball, orbit and head; in external ear.

Severe pain: in small of back; in deltoid muscle.

Acute pain: from temple to temple; in stomach.

Cutting: in teeth.

Darting pains: like arrows through eye from head.

Shooting: in r. eye from within outward; in upper and lower limbs; through l. chest to back; from back to pit of stomach.

Stitching: in head; from teeth into ears; in knee and ankle joints.

Tearing: in l. temporal region; in bones and periosteum of cranial bones; in and about r. ear; in head; in molars; in testicle and spermatic cord; in l. hip bone; in nape of neck; in l. shoulder joint; in forearms; in upper posterior portion of r. thigh into foot; in lower limbs.

Jerking, tearing pain: in face.

Violent, twitching pain: in r. ear.

Boring: in l. temporal region; in a single tooth; in region of heart; in l. shoulder joint.

Digging: in l. hip bone.

Throbbing: in l. hip bone.

Pulsation: in anus.

Crampy pains: under short ribs.

Cramplike drawing: in forearm.

Drawing, sticking pain: in r. testicle and spermatic cord.

Sticking: in r. testicle.

Burning pain: in eyes.

Rheumatic pain: in l. side below short ribs; in back and shoulder.

Rheumatic or gouty pains: in teeth.

Transient dull pain: from chest to l. hypochondrium.

Drawing: in bones and periosteum of cranial bones; in teeth; from rectum to genitals; in stomach; in region of bladder; in arms.

Pressing pain: in l. side under short ribs.

Pressing: in pit of stomach; in stomach.

Pressure: in forehead and vertex; in stomach.

Soreness: of inner nose; of throat; extending into abdomen and thighs; between genitals and thighs; of teeth.

Burning: in uterine region; in face.

Dry burning: in eyes; in lips; in throat.
Heat: in eyes.
Warmth: in hands.
Stiffness: of nape of neck; of leg; in joints.
Tension: in legs.
Constriction: in throat; at pit of stomach.
Fulness: in pit of stomach.
Dulness: in head.
Stupefaction: in head.
Pricking: in teeth.
Scraping: in fauces.
Dryness: of throat.
Formication: in whole limb; in back and limbs.
Biting, itching: on scalp.
Itching: of scrotum; of middle and ring fingers of l. hand.
Coldness: in legs.

44 **Tissues.** ▮Acute inflammatory swelling of joints, wandering from one joint to another, and at times reappearing in joint first affected; pains particularly severe at night; < in rest and during rough, stormy weather.

▮General rheumatic pains, brought on by damp, cold weather and < during wet.

▮Rheumatism of cervical and thoracic muscles; rheumatic neuralgia of extremities; pains < at rest and in cloudy and stormy weather.

▮Rheumatic pains especially in all the aponeuroses, < in rest; < at night; pains do not admit of the limbs being at rest; desire to move, and moving relieves; < before change of weather, particularly before a thunderstorm; especially r. side; pains < in night, but more toward morning; in hot season.

▮Arthritic nodes.

▮Orchitis and hydrocele.

Dropsical swellings.

45 **Touch. Passive Motion. Injuries.** Touching: toothache <; testicles very sensitive; chest sensitive.

46 **Skin.** Burning and tearing, with erysipelas.

47 **Stages of Life, Constitution.** Boy, æt. 7, suffering since birth; hydrocele.

Boy, æt. 14, good constitution; swelling of knee.

Woman, æt. 22, delivered a short time ago, after an attack of influenza; rheumatism.

Girl, æt. 26, servant; toothache.

Man, æt. 28, strong, after catching cold while dancing, while recovering from an attack of gonorrhœa; orchitis.

Man, æt. 30, thin, tall, good constitution; weakness and formication in arms.

Man, æt. 31, strong, under treatment for condylomata; pain and swelling of wrist.

Man, æt. 33, printer, for last six months suffered from syphilis, after being apparently cured by large doses of mercury present attack came on; swelling and pain in joints.

Woman, æt. 34, working out by the day, suffering six days; rheumatism.

Woman, æt. 35; ovarian cyst discharged.

Woman, æt. 35, weak, mother of several children; cough.

Woman, æt. 36, good constitution, violent temper, married fifteen years, suffering three weeks; tearing in leg.

Man, æt. 37, good-humored, well built, seven days ago caught cold, since then suffering; rheumatism.

Man, æt. 38, strong and healthy, after cohabiting with wife who was suffering with fluor albus; orchitis and pain in leg.

Farmer, æt. 40; hydrocele.

Man, æt. 41, two years ago caught cold, since then suffering; dysecoia.

Man, æt. 48, laborer, had orchitis seventeen years ago; orchitis.

Woman, æt. 50, suffering twenty years; dysecoia.

Woman, æt. 51, suffering twelve years; rheumatism.

Woman, æt. 54, suffering fourteen days; earache.

Man, æt. 55, laborer, strong constitution, suffering fourteen days; rheumatism.

Man, æt. 64, after catching cold; tinnitus aurium

Man, æt. 64 suffering ten months; enlargement of testicle.

Old lady, irritable, suffering six years; rheumatism.

48 **Relations.** Antidoted by: *Bryon.*, *Camphor*, *Clematis*, *Rhus tox.*

Compare: *Aurum*, *Bryon.*, *Calc. ost.*, *Clematis*, *Conium*, *Kalmia*, *Ledum*, *Lycop.*, *Mercur.*, *Nux vom.*, *Phosphor.*, *Pulsat.*, *Ranunc.*, *Rhus tox.*

RHUS TOXICODENDRON.

Poison Oak or Ivy. *Anacardiaceæ.*

Provings by Hahnemann and his provers, R. A. M. L., vol. 2, p. 357; Helbig, Heraclides, vol. 1, p. 53; Robinson, Br. J. of Hom., vol. 25, p. 330; Joslin, Am. Hom. Rev., vol. 1, p. 553; Berridge, N. A. J. of Hom., N. S., vol. 3, p. 501; and numerous involuntary provings from coming in contact with the plant, or being exposed to its exhalations, see Allen's Encyclopedia, vol. 8, p. 330.

Clinical Authorities.—*Melancholia*, Sorge, A. H. Z., vol. 93, p. 109; *Mental disorder*, Hartlaub, Rück. Kl. Erf., vol. 1, p. 44; *Fear of being poisoned*, Dulac, Hom. Cl., vol. 3, p. 75; *Vertigo*, Goullon, A. H. Z., vol. 88, p. 132; *Headache*, Stens, A. H. Z., vol. 91, p. 188; *Migraine*, Hs., A. H. Z., vol. 109, p. 207; *Meningitis*, Sturm, Rück. Kl. Erf., vol. 1, p. 128; *Eruption on head and Ozœna*, Pulte, Rück. Kl. Erf., vol 1, p. 398; *Irido-choroiditis*, Norton, Raue's Rec., 1874, p. 80, from N. Y. J. H., March, 1873, p. 30; *Opacity of cornea*, Stens, Raue's Rec., 1875, p. 58, from A. H. Z., vol. 89, p. 156; *Ophthalmia: rheumatic, catarrhal, scrofulous, exanthematous-scrofulous, erysipelatous*, Kammerer, Schelling, Gross, Nehrer, Thorer, Lichtenfels, Lobethal, Mschk., B. J. H., vol. 6, pp. 517–23, Rück. Kl. Erf., vol. 1, p. 239; *Conjunctivitis*, B., Med. Inv., vol. 6, p. 204; *Ptosis*, Le Beau, N. A. J. H., vol. 19, p. 572; *Swelling under eyes*, Munroe, Mass. Trans., vol. 4, p. 374; *Affection of eye*, Martin, Hom. Cl., vol. 4, p. 149; Buchner, B. J. H., vol. 2, p. 209; *Epistaxis*, Gross, Ng., Rück. Kl. Erf., vol. 1, p. 414; *Facial neuralgia*, Schrön, Rück. Kl. Erf., vol. 5, p. 189; B. J. H., vol. 11, p. 299-301; *Diphtheria of lips*, Nichol, T. H. M. S. Pa., 1887, p. 279; *Parotitis*, Fielitz, Hirsch, Rück. Kl. Erf., vol. 4, p. 374; *Rheumatism of lower jaw*, Von Tagen, Hom. Cl., vol. 3, p. 142; *Toothache*, Hartman, Schelling, Rück. Kl. Erf., vol. 1, p. 474; *Sore throat*, Baylies, Hom. Cl., vol. 1, p. 219; *Œsophagitis*, Griesselich, Rück. Kl. Erf., vol. 1, p. 540; *Pain in r. hypochondrium*, Kirkpatrick, Hah. Mo., vol. 10, p. 167; *Pain in abdomen*, Berridge, Hom. Phys., vol. 8, p. 554; *Colic*, Hegewald, A. H. Z., vol. 113, p. 31; *Physconia peritonealis* (3 cases), Gauwerky, Rück. Kl. Erf., vol. 1, p. 728; *Enteritis*, Kirsch, Schelling, Rück. Kl. Erf., vol. 5, p. 356; *Intestinal catarrh*, Molin, B. J. H., vol. 32, p. 696; *Hernia*, Schelling, Rück. Kl. Erf., vol. 5, p. 384; *Diarrhœa*, Martin, Hom. Cl., vol. 1, p. 137; Mann, Hom. Rev., vol. 16, p. 482; *Chronic diarrhœa*, Madden, B. J. H., vol. 28, p. 717; *Dysentery*, Bowie, T. H. M. S. Pa., 1886, p. 154; Smith, U. S. M. and S. Jour., Oct., 1870, Raue's Rec., 1872, p. 145; Pröll, A. H. Z., vol. 113, p. 186; *Fissure of anus*, Macfarlan, Hom. Cl., vol. 4, p. 73; *Bright's disease* (2 cases), Bürkner, Rück. Kl. Erf., vol. 5, p. 524; *Weakness of bladder*, Jacobi, B. J. H., vol. 33, p. 548; *Incontinence of urine*, Sonnenberg, Rück. Kl. Erf., vol. 2, p. 45; *Urinary difficulty*, Diez, Rück. Kl. Erf., vol. 2, p. 386; *Metastasis of mumps to testicle*, Fisher, Bib. Hom., vol. 8, p. 140; *Œdema of scrotum and penis*, Gross, Rück. Kl. Erf., vol. 4, p. 62; *Ovarian tumor*, Chauvet, A. J. H. M. M., vol. 3, p. 65; *Prolapsus uteri*, Southwick, T. A. I. H., 1888, p. 411; *Polypus of uterus*, Cuntz, Raue's Rec., 1873, p. 169, from I. H. Pr., 2, p. 60; *Metrorrhagia*, Kershaw, Org., vol. 3, p. 368; *Amenorrhœa*, Thorer, Rück. Kl. Erf., vol. 2, p. 252; *Use in dysmenorrhœa*, Gorton, Hah. Mo., vol. 7, p. 513; *Influenza*, Hooper, A. J. H. M. M., vol. 9, p. 128; Payne, N. E. M. G., vol. 4, p. 232; Rück. Kl. Erf., vol. 3, p. 48; *Cough*, Miller, Hah. Mo., vol. 7, p. 403; *Pain in chest*, Gregg, Griggs Ill. Rep. (R. radicans), p. 96; *Hæmoptysis*, Diez, Rück. Kl. Erf., vol. 3, p. 224; *Pneumonia*, Gross, Diez, Rück. Kl. Erf., vol. 3, p. 330; Sherbino, Hom. Phys., vol. 7, p. 120; *Use in phthisis*, Payne, N. E. M. G., vol. 6, p. 167; *Cardiac neurosis*, Pellicer, Raue's Rec., 1875, p. 130, from El. Crit. Med., June, 1874; *Affection of heart*, Cochran, Hah. Mo., vol. 6, p. 397; *Swelling of glands of neck*, Guernsey, M. I., vol. 3, p. 281; *Spinal irritation*, Miller, T. H. M. S., Pa., 1885, p. 181; Dittrich, Raue's Rec., 1873, p. 189, from A. H. Z., 85, 78; *Lumbago*, Drysdale, B. J. H., vol. 1, p, 36; Brewster, Hah. Mo., vol. 10, p. 14; Greenleaf, A. H. O., vol. 10, p. 258; Glover, Hom. Phys., vol. 8, p. 618; *Affection of back*, Wesselhoeft, Hom. Cl., vol. 3, p. 61; Martin, Hom. Cl., vol. 4, p. 149; *Strain of shoulder*, Stens, A. H. Z., p. 85, vol. 189; *Burning in hand and arm*, Hesse, A. H. Z., vol. 112, p. 68; *Pain in wrist*, Smith, Hom. Cl., vol. 1, p. 125; *Strain of wrist, strain of thumb*, Gallupe, M. I., vol. 6, p. 442; B. J. H., vol. 24, p. 309; *Warts on hands*, Gross, Rück. Kl. Erf., vol. 4, p. 311; *Injury of hip*, Gallupe, B. J. H., vol, 24, p. 308; M. I., vol. 6, p. 442; *Inflammation of hip joint*, Hiller, N. A. J. H., vol. 26, p. 375; *Coxalgia*, Weber, A. H. Z., vol. 89, p. 123; *Sciatica*, Villers, B. J. H., vol. 11, p. 146; from Hom. Vierteljahrsch., vol. 2, p. 425; Bürkner, A.H.Z., vol. 111, p. 109; Gordon, Hom. Cl., vol. 4, p. 29; Pratt, M. I., vol. 4, p. 132; Seip, T.H.M.S. Pa., vol. 2, p. 269; Martin, Hom. Rec., vol. 3, p. 69; Carter, Hom Rec., vol. 3, p. 165; Peck, Org., vol. 3, p. 376; *Ischias*, Hendrichs, A. H. Z., vol. 109, p. 126; Roberts, A. O., vol. 4, p. 237; *Rheumatic sciatica*, Hughes, B. J. H., vol. 22, p. 238; *Hydrarthros genu*, Sulzer, Raue's Rec., 1874, p. 256, from A. H. Z., vol. 87, p. 84; *Gonagra*, Hartmann, B. J. H., vol. 12, p. 294; *Swelling of knee joints*, Klauber, A. H. Z., vol. 112, p. 140; *Swelling in popliteal space*, Miller, Hah. Mo., vol. 10, p. 163; *White swelling of knee*, Thomas, A. H. Z., vol. 106, p. 46; *Suppuration of knee*, Müller, Rück. Kl. Erf., vol. 4, p. 289; *Pains in legs*, Goodno, Hom. Cl., vol 3, p. 140; *Ulcer on leg*, Brewster, Hom. Phys., vol. 8, p. 267; *Sprain of ankle*, Helmuth, N. Y. J. H., vol. 2, p. 272; *Swelling of foot*, E. B. S., Hom. Cl., vol. 1, p. 198; *Fetid foot sweat*, Gorton, U. S. M. and S. J., vol. 9, p. 13; *Chronic inflammation of joints*, Sircar, Calcutta Jour., vol. 2, p. 220; *Eruption on limbs*, Norton, Hah. Mo., 1875, Times Ret., 1875, p. 135; *Hysteria*, Schrön, Rück. Kl. Erf., vol. 2, p. 288; *Chorea*, Wesselhoeft, Mass. Trans., vol. 4, p. 363; *Epilepsy*, Sircar, Calcutta Jour., vol. 1, p. 458; *Restlessness of legs*, Rushmore, Org., vol. 3, p. 356; *Loss of co-ordination in legs*, Searle, Hom. Cl., vol. 1, p. 101; *Paraplegia*, Smith, N. Y. St. Tr., 1869, p. 519, Raue's Rec., 1871, p. 192; *Paralysis*, Rau, Payr, Aegidi, Valenti, Schelling, Rück. Kl. Erf., vol. 4, p. 476; *Paresis*, Sorge, Fischer, Schoff, B. J. H., vol. 33, p. 548; Peters, N. A. J. H., vol. 4, p. 349; *Rheumatic lameness*, Bolle, B. J. H., vol. 25, p. 661; *Rheumatic paralysis*, Hughes, B. J. H., vol. 28, p. 793; *Paralysis agitans*, Payr, Rück. Kl. Erf., vol. 4, p. 479; *Ague*, Müller, Gross, Battmann, Mschk, B. in D. Rück. Kl. Erf., vol. 4, p. 979; A. H. Z., vol. 107, p. 148, Elb., A. H. Z., vol. 110, p. 11; Skeels, Hah. Mo., vol. 2, p. 493; Mann, Hom. Rev., vol. 16, p. 483; Pearson, M. I., vol. 5, p. 433; Hills, Med. Inv., vol. 7, p. 583; Miller, Org., vol. 1, p. 324; Martin, Org., vol. 2, p. 108; Ayres, Org., vol. 2, p. 117; Sarchet, Org., vol. 2, p. 135; *Catarrhal fever*, Mann, Hom. Rev., vol. 16, p. 482; *Rheumatic fevers*, Kunkel, Raue's Rec., 1874, p. 251, from J. Pr., 1873, p. 237; *Typhoid fever*, Dunham, Hom. Rev., vol. 15, p. 148; (5 cases), Wurmb & Caspar, B. J. H., vol. 12, pp. 13–23; *Rheumatism*, Dixon, B. J. H., vol. 28, p. 383; Sorge, B. J. H., vol. 33,

p. 549; H. H., Hom. Cl., vol. 1, p. 13; Hall, Hom. Rev., vol. 16, p. 485; Hupfield, T. A. I. H., 1880, p. 224; Smith, Med. Inv., vol. 4, p. 277; *Inflammatory rheumatism*, Baxter, Proc. H. M. S., Ohio, 1874, p. 110; *Anasarca*, Weber, Rück. Kl. Erf., vol. 4, p. 354; Newton, Hom. Rev., vol. 14, p. 340; Searle, A. H. O., vol. 6, p. 225; *Dropsy*, Hesse, Hom. Phys., vol. 7, p. 25; *Boils*, Mooers, Am. Hom., vol. 1, p. 215; *Boils and abscesses*, Chamberlain, N. E. M. G., vol. 12, p. 107; *Carbuncle*, Gross, Rück. Kl. Erf., vol. 4, p. 194; *Induration of glands*, Hartmann, Rück. Kl., Erf., vol. 4, p. 410; *Syphilitic nodes*, Peters, N. A. J. H., vol. 4, p. 535; *Secondary syphilis*, Berridge, Hah. Mo., vol. 10, p. 78; *Erysipelas*, Holeczek, Gross, Bethmann, Goullon, Kapper, Schwarze, Rück. Kl. Erf., vol. 4, p. 147; Berridge, Hah. Mo., vol. 9, p. 344; Brewster, Hah. Mo., vol. 10, p. 14; W. J. B., A. J. H. M. M., vols. 2, p. 265; Payne, N. E. M. G., vol. 4, p. 235; *Erysipelatous inflammation*, Walker, Med. Inv., vol. 5, p. 323; *Erysipelas bullosum*, Goullon, N. A. J. H., vol. 4, p. 547; *Herpes zoster* (2 cases), Burnett, Raue's Rec., 1874, p. 291, from H. W., vol. 8, p. 37; Blake, B. J. H., vol. 30, p. 119; *Zona*, Russell, B. J. H., vol. 30, p. 119; Hawley, Hom. Phys., vol. 5, p. 168; *Erythema nodosum*, Newton, Hom. Rev., vol. 15, p. 212; *Urticaria*, Kent, Hom. Phys., vol. 4, p. 262; Rück. Kl. Erf., vol. 4, p. 200; *Eczema*, Blake, B. J. H., vol. 30, p. 118; Elb, A. H. Z., vol. 111, p. 164; Hedges, U. S. M. and S. J., vol. 8, p. 441; *Eczema rubrum, Eczema impetiginoides, Arcularius*, N. A. J. H., vol. 20, p. 145–6; *Crusta lactea*, Hooper, A. J. H. M. M., vol. 9, p. 128; *Psoriasis*, Preston, Org., vol. 3, p. 373; *Purpura*, Müller, H. in F., Rückert, Rück. Kl. Erf., vol. 4, p. 206; *Chronic eruptions*, Stapf, Jahr, Trinks, Lindner, Rück. Kl. Erf., vol. 4, p. 256; *Itching eruption*, Stowe, Org., vol. 2, p. 220; *Scarlet fever*, Müller, Rück. Kl. Erf., vol. 4, p. 63; Farrington, Hah. Mo., vol. 7, p. 378; *Measles*, Goullon, B. J. H., vol. 30, p. 587, from A. H. Z., Jan., 1872; *Smallpox*, Mayrhofer, Rück. Kl. Erf., vol. 4, p. 114; *Rhus poisoning*, Miller, T. H. M. S. Pa., 1886, p. 152.

1 **Mind.** ▮Absence of mind; forgetfulness; difficult comprehension, cannot remember recent events; recalls with difficulty things and names.

▮Languor of the mind, is unable to hold an idea.

▮Stupefaction, with tingling in head and pains in limbs, $>$ in motion.

Illusions of the fancy; visions.

▮Low, mild delirium, thinks he is roaming over fields, or hard at work.

▮▮Incoherent talking; answers hastily or reluctantly, thought seems difficult; answers correctly but slowly.

▮Anxiety, timidity; $<$ at twilight; restless change of place; wants to go from bed to bed.

▮Apprehensive, anxious and tremulous.

Inexpressible anxiety, with pressure at heart and tearing at small of back.

▮▮Great apprehension at night; cannot remain in bed.

▮Anxiety: while sitting was obliged to take hold of something because she did not think she could keep up on account of the beating and drawing pains in limbs; and apprehension as if he wished to take his own life; with loss of strength as if he would die.

Fear and despair on account of sad thoughts, which she could not get rid of.

▮Fear: that he will die; with anxiousness and sighing; of being poisoned.

▮Fretful; general unhappiness of temper.

Ill-humored, depressed; easily moved to tears.

Impatient and vexed at every trifle; she does not endure being talked to.

▮Great despondency, with prostration; inclination to weep, especially in evening, with desire for solitude.

▮Disgust for life: thoughts of suicide; wants to drown himself; with fear of death; with desire to die, without sadness.

Depression and discouragement and dissatisfaction with the world, in the evening.

▮Sad, begins to weep without knowing why.

▮Melancholy, ill-humor and anxiety, as if a misfortune would happen, or as if she were alone and all about her were dead and still, or as if she had been forsaken by a near friend; < in house, > walking in open air.

‖Melancholia after suppression of menses by fright and sorrow; great restlessness and anguish as if she had committed a crime, or as if she thought some terrible calamity impended; these feelings drove her from one place to another; could not rest quietly at night in bed; was robbed of sleep and all desire to live; slight pain in temples; a little vertigo; head cool; much depressed in mind; spoke but little.

‖Restlessness and anxiety about heart as if she had committed a crime or as if some great misfortune was in store for her, is driven from one place to another; deprived of sleep and all desire to live; always depressed, speaks little, no appetite, sometimes belching which relieves; slight vertigo and pain in temples. θAmenorrhœa from fright.

‖After fright heavy feeling in forehead; a week later she told her mother not to look at her; seemed to be distrustful and did not wish to see any one; she came running in from the street and said people were looking at her; sat quietly alone; her eyes dim, shunned the light; since this time the symptoms have returned three times, lasting six weeks each time; this time eight weeks, symptoms as before but without the complaint of the eyes; cries without cause, imagines people are finding fault with her because she is earning nothing, acts in a childish manner; heaviness of head when head is in a low position; beating in temple on which she is lying; after taking cold, diarrhœa; for past week coughed when lying down, with stitches in pit of stomach; chilly hands and feet; frequent motion in bowels.

[2] **Sensorium.** ▮Vertigo: and dulness of head; as if intoxicated when rising from bed; with chilliness, and pressure behind eyes; in the aged, < when rising from lying, turning or stooping; when standing or walking; while lying down.

Weakness of head; whenever she turned the head she quite lost consciousness; on stooping it seemed as if she could never rise again.

▮Head confused and dull.

Dulness of head: pressure in r. temple, and just above and behind r. orbit a pressing downward as from a weight; disinclination for literary work; and an intoxicated feeling, in morning; as if intoxicated while sitting, on rising such dizziness that it seemed as if she were going to fall forward and backward.

Heaviness and dulness of head on turning eyes; even the eyeball hurts.

Head so heavy that she was obliged to hold it upright in order to relieve the weight pressing forward into forehead.

[3] **Inner Head** Burning in forehead when walking.

▮Feeling as of a board strapped across forehead.

❙❙Pain in l. temple and orbital region, appearing daily for three months, and lasting until evening; caused by getting wet; > from rapid motion.

▮▮Brain feels loose when stepping or shaking head.

▮A sensation of swashing and jarring in brain; each step concusses brain.

▮Pain as if brain were torn, < when moving eyes.

▮Headache: stupefying, with buzzing; < when sitting or lying, in cold, in morning, from beer; > from warmth and motion; must lie down; returns from least chagrin; immediately after a meal.

▮Stitches in head extending to ears, root of nose and malar bones, with toothache.

▮Feeling as if parts were screwed together in muscles of back part of head.

❙❙Dull pain beginning in occiput extending to vertex and thence to forehead, there attaining an intolerable degree of severity; at times vomiting of bile which relieves the pain but exhausts the patient; pain begins in morning, lasts until 5 P.M., and is particularly severe after 3 o'clock, > by walking rapidly in open air; paroxsyms every week. θMigraine.

❙❙Periodical attacks of headache; pain particularly in

back part of head, so severe that she cannot speak and must go to bed for 24 hours, during which time she neither speaks, eats nor drinks; the slightest vexation or least exercise in open air, particularly if she amused herself at same time, brought on an attack next day. θHysteria.

▮Occipital headache; muscles sore, > from moving and warmth; caused by draught, dampness, or by internal causes, as in typhoid.

▮Headache in occiput, > by bending head backward.

▮Painful tingling in head, especially of occiput.

▮Aching in occipital protuberances.

▮Rush of blood to head, with humming, formication and throbbing; face glistening and red; restless moving about.

▮▮Meningitis in exanthematous fevers, or after getting wet; tingling limbs; high fever; restlessness.

▮▮For two days complete loss of consciousness; r. upper and lower extremities paralyzed; pulse rapid, trembling, scarcely perceptible; involuntary escape of urine; respiration very gentle, with frequent moaning; appearance cadaverous; œdematous swelling of lids; body cold to touch. θMeningitis.

▮Cerebro-spinal meningitis; anxiety, restlessness, stupefaction, vertigo; fulness and bruised pain in head, extending to ears; bleeding of ears and nose; dry cough, with perhaps bloody sputa; pain in back as if sprained; tearing tensive pains, with stiffness of muscles and joints; vivid dreams; various eruptions.

[4] **Outer Head.** ▮Head painful to touch, sore as a boil.

▮Scalp sensitive, < on side not lain on, when growing warm in bed, from touch and combing hair.

▮Violent tearing and drawing pains in periosteum of cranial bones; < at rest and in damp, stormy cold weather; > wrapping head up warmly and by dry heat and exercise.

▮Headache as if occipital tissues were screwed together.

▮Liability to take cold from having the head wetted.

▮Vesicular erysipelas of scalp, going from l. to right.

Biting itching on scalp, forehead, face and about mouth, with eruption of pimples like nettlerash.

▮▮Thick scurf over hairy whole scalp, from under which a greenish pus discharges; severe itching at night under the scurfs; hair eaten away.

▮▮Eruption on head, eating into surrounding parts, with violent itching at night; discharge of greenish pus from r. nostril; l. nostril excoriated, with discharge of bloody mucus on blowing nose.

▮Eruption suppurating, moist, forming thick offensive-smelling crusts; itching < at night; hair is eaten off; extends to shoulders. θScald-head.

‖Dry herpes on hairy scalp.

5 **Sight and Eyes.** ▮Aversion to light; scrofulous affections.

▮Extreme confusion of sight.

▮Obscurity of vision; sensation as of a veil before eyes.

▮Lids red, swollen, œdematous, especially the upper, and spasmodically closed, with profuse gushes of hot tears on opening them; saclike swelling of conjunctiva; yellow, purulent, mucous discharge; swelling around eyes; burning pain in eye, with much photophobia; stitches in eyes and temples, with vertigo; lids cannot be opened; < in evening; pressive burning pain in r. eye, so intense he could not bear slightest touch; child lies constantly on its face with its hands to its head; head hot and face red. θIrido-choroiditis.

‖Mr. S., æt. 66, rheumatic diathesis; had a cataract removed by Graefe's modified linear extraction; on second night after operation, sharp pains in eye, restless, fever and thirst; upper lid œdematous, lids tightly closed, on opening a profuse gush of hot tears followed; chemosis, haziness of aqueous, suppuration commencing. θIrido-choroiditis suppurativa traumatica.

‖Miss D., æt. 18; had discission made of capsule remaining after extraction of cataract; nausea, vomiting; 1 A.M., sharp shooting pain in eye, lids spasmodically closed, œdematous, profuse hot lachrymation on opening, photophobia, chemosis.

▮▮Iritis: either of rheumatic or traumatic origin or from exposure to wet; inflammation may extend to and involve choroid: pains shoot through eyes to back of head, < worse at night; profuse flow of hot tears on opening eyes; in some cases inflammation may go on to suppuration; in rheumatic or gouty subjects; suppurative, or where the ciliary body and choroid are involved, especially if of traumatic origin.

▮Mydriasis from exposure to cold and dampness.

▮Pustules and superficial ulcers on cornea, with great photophobia; conjunctiva quite red, even to chemosis.

▮Suppuration of cornea, especially when consequent upon cataract extraction.

‖Totally blind; cornea filled between its lamellæ with a thick whitish exudation; iris distorted; iridectomy of no avail; has been subject to facial erysipelas; cold water had suppressed eruption; since then weak sight, gradually total blindness, until relieved. θOpacity of cornea.

▮Kerato-iritis, especially if rheumatic in character, from cold, damp atmosphere.

Glaucoma.

▮Orbital cellulitis.

‖Pain in r. eyeball, of such intensity that she could not bear even a slight touch; redness of sclerotic, and development of numerous bloodvessels; dulness of cornea, great sensibility to light; iris of affected eye, which in its natural state was blue, is now green, pupillary margin not well defined, pupil itself does not move when exposed to light, lens appeared of a smoky dimness; an eruption of red pimples and pustules on nose and cheek increased as action of eye declined, and vice versa; a burning tearing pain in neighborhood of diseased eye, < morning and night, depriving patient of rest and sleep.

Itching in eyes on exerting vision.

▮Aching or pressive pain in eyes.

Left eye felt enormously swollen and enlarged, though this was not the case.

Sharp pains run from eyes into head.

Biting as from something sharp and acrid in r. eye.

Biting in eyes; lids agglutinated in morning.

Drawing and tearing in region of brows and in malar bones.

▮▮Eyes are closed and greatly swollen and inflamed.

▮Acute conjunctivitis from getting wet.

▮Great photophobia, profuse acrid lachrymation in morning and in open air; cheek under eye dotted with red pimples; lids spasmodically closed.

‖Violent inflammation of r. eye. θConjunctivitis.

▮Saclike swelling of conjunctiva, with yellow purulent discharge.

▮Eyes red and agglutinated in morning.

‖Catarrhal ophthalmia; lids swollen and completely closed, from under which escaped, from time to time, purulent mucus; on attempting to open lids there flowed out a quantity of water, and the conjunctiva covering the lids was loose, swollen, projecting betwixt the lids and prevented the eyeball from being seen.

Arthritic ophthalmia, from working in water or getting wet, with tearing pain in eyes, especially at night.

▮Scrofulous ophthalmia; phlyctenules on and about cornea; intense photophobia; eyelids involved and spasmodically closed; yellow pus gushes out when they are forced apart; pains < at night.

‖Scrofulous ophthalmia; r. eye affected; not much photophobia; lids slightly swollen; on cornea a small scrofulous ulcer surrounded by fasciculi of vessels.

‖Scrofulous ophthalmia, with phlyctenulæ on edge of cornea of l. eye; pain and photophobia not very great; scrofulous eruption on internal nose, which was much swollen.

‖Conjunctiva of l. eye very red and studded with small ulcers; great photophobia; frequent lachrymation; eruption behind ears and beneath scalp, exuding plentifully. θScrofulous ophthalmia.

‖Violent inflammation of eyeball; two dirty-looking ulcers on cornea of l. eye, size of hemp seeds; great photophobia; thick scabs around alæ nasi and angles of mouth. θScrofulous ophthalmia.

‖Scrofulous ophthalmia; excessive photophobia, child lies all day with face resting on floor; constant restlessness, loss of appetite; emaciation.

‖Right eye surrounded by an œdematous swelling, from border of orbit to alæ nasi; eyes slightly red, lachrymose by day, closed up by night; child constantly rubbing its eyes, restless and sleepless. θOphthalmia erysipelatous.

‖Conjunctivitis granulosa; < in right eye; heaviness of lids; < in stormy weather, with pannus.

▮Ophthalmia neonatorum; lids red, œdematously swollen and spasmodically closed; restlessness at night.

▮▮Pains in eyes when moving or turning eyeballs.

▮Paralysis of any of muscles of eyeball, resulting from rheumatism, exposure to cold or getting feet wet.

Burning in inner canthus of r. eye.

▮Weeping eyes; bleareyedness.

▮Epiphora of long standing, with an apparent stricture of lachrymal duct.

▮▮Inflammation of lids; lids much swollen.

‖Right upper lid much swollen, hard; pains < from 5 to 7 P.M.; walking around does not relieve; when she moves her eye it feels as if there was a hard ball moving around; burning, itching, shooting pains around lid; < in cold air.

▮Erysipelas of lids, sometimes of traumatic origin; profuse lachrymation, spasmodic closure of lids.

▮Eyelids œdematous, or erysipelatous, with scattered watery vesicles; meibomian glands enlarged, cilia fall out.

▮Œdematous erysipelatous swelling of lids and face, with small watery vesicles scattered over the surface, and drawing pains in cheek and head.

▮Lids look red and fiery, like erysipelas, and itch greatly.

▮Violent burning, itching and prickling in swollen lids.

▮Uncomplicated blepharitis, especially of acute form, with

a tendency to formation of abscess; lids highly œdematous, profuse lachrymation with pain; < at night, > from warm applications.

▮Simple œdema of lids.

▮Eyelids present a bladder-like appearance, and the lids are closed from the great swelling.

▮Lids œdematously swollen, copious, acrid, serous discharge, corrodes adjacent parts. θBlepharitis.

▮Chronic inflammation of lids; puffiness of lids and face; meibomian glands enlarged; falling out of ciliæ; itching and biting in lids; sensation of dryness of eyes; burning in internal canthus; acrid lachrymation in morning and in open air, or constant and profuse lachrymation which may be acrid or not.

Relaxation of eyelids, with puffiness of lids and hot, flushed face.

▮Heaviness and stiffness of lids, like a paralysis, as if it were difficult to move lids.

||Ptosis of r. eyelid in a girl, æt. 5, first noticed when five days old; whenever she wished to open her eye to look at anything, she involuntarily opened widely her mouth, which made her look ludicrous.

▮▮Ptosis, also paralysis of muscles of eyeball, from exposure to cold or wet; in rheumatic patient.

▮▮Lids agglutinated with purulent mucus, in morning.

||Eruption on l. lower lid; inflammation of conjunctiva; burning and painful twitching in affected part.

A red, hard swelling, like a stye, on lower lid, toward inner canthus, with pressive pain, lasting six days.

▮Styes on lower lids.

▮Symptoms of lids dependent upon inflammation of deeper structures.

6 **Hearing and Ears.** Hardness of hearing, especially of human voice.

▮Otalgia, with pulsation in ear at night.

▮Excoriating discharge of bloody pus from ear in acute inflammation.

▮Erysipelatous inflammation of external and internal ear, vesicular, with excessive otalgia.

▮Inflammatory swelling of glands beneath ears. θAfter scarlatina.

▮Lobule of l. ear swollen.

▮▮Parotitis, l. side; especially suppuration. θScarlatina.

7 **Smell and Nose.** ||Loss of smell.

▮Nosebleed: frequent; on stooping; in morning; at night; coagulated blood; at stool, or from exertion; in typhus, with some relief.

▮Spasmodic sneezing.

‖ Sudden cessation of cough followed by most outrageous sneezing, all night; in morning face red, swollen, cannot talk for sneezing; points to head and abdomen. θInfluenza.

▮ Dryness and stoppage of nose.

▮ Sensation of soreness in nostrils.

▮ Discharge from nose: of thick, yellow mucus; of nasal mucus without coryza; of green, offensive pus; of yellow ichor, with swollen cervical glands; hot, acrid from nares.

Hot burning beneath l. nostril so that the breath seemed to come out of it hot.

▮ Swelling of nose.

▮ Tip of nose red and sensitive; nose sore internally.

▮ Puffiness of nose.

▮ Fever blisters and crusts under nose.

‖ Eczema on both sides below nose; nose swollen, now and then bleeding.

▮ Eruption in corners of nose.

Upper Face. Face: fiery red; pale, sunken, nose pointed, blue around eyes; red, with heat.

▮ Burning, drawing, tearing in face; teeth feel too long; restlessness.

‖ For several successive nights, awoke after having been asleep about an hour, with pain in temporal region of l. side, extending toward head, cheeks and teeth of same side; pain increased from minute to minute, was of a glowing, tearing character and forced him to quit his bed and walk about the room for three hours during the night; went to bed exhausted, fell asleep, but awoke again in half an hour and was obliged once more to walk about until 7 or 8 A.M.; during day teeth of affected side felt too long and were loose so that he could masticate but little; felt very weak and cold. θFacial neuralgia.

‖ Facial neuralgia; feeling of great coldness; < in open air; violent evening exacerbation; dysenteric diarrhœa.

‖ From having been in a cellar, where he perspired much, especially on head, old neuralgic pains reappeared; patient pressed hand on l. cheek, pressed teeth together and had a distorted painful face.

▮ Tension and swelling of face.

▮ Great swelling of face, especially of eyelids and ears.

Violent burning in swollen face, lids and ears.

▮▮ Erysipelas from l. to r.; face dark-red, covered with yellow vesicles; burning, itching and tingling with stinging; delirium and high fever.

‖ Whole face swollen, eyes nearly closed; ears swollen;

swelling of face red, hot, with tension and burning, r. side being covered with vesicles, some of which had burst; hairy part of scalp very sensitive to touch, particularly in region of occiput, which was the seat of pressing pains; ringing in ears with hardness of hearing; frequent short naps; delirium at night; slow, complaining speech; great despondency; constantly lies on back, at rare intervals sluggish movements of limbs; no appetite; great thirst; frequent, deep inspirations with sighing; diarrhœa; cough with expectoration of blood; urine bluish-red. θErysipelas.

|| Whole face, except forehead, greatly swollen, hot, harsh to touch, bright-red, shiny and covered with vesicles; lids greatly swollen, cannot open eyes; auditory meatus on both sides swollen; stitching pains in throat on swallowing; sides of back painful to touch, without swelling or hardness; tongue red, dry; great thirst; frequent yawning; painful pressure on chest and about heart; at rare intervals cough with expectoration of blood; tearing pains in all the limbs; skin dry, hot; urine scanty, dark; pulse rapid, weak. θErysipelas.

|| Erysipelas bullosum; the spots had spread over forepart of scalp, entire face covered with large blisters; heat, swelling and intense pain; tongue smooth, very red; much thirst; anxiety; restlessness; sleeplessness; very quick pulse.

|| Inflammation commenced in outer ear and gradually spread to cheek and forehead of same side, then to opposite ear, cheek and side of head, with blistering, burning and itching. θErysipelas.

▮▮ Acne rosacea.

▮ Milk crust; thick crusts and a secretion of fetid, bloody matter.

▮ Impetigo on face and forehead.

|| Forepart of head and r. side of face covered with a thick, moist crust, from under which an ichorous, frequently sanious, offensive discharge oozes; underlying skin rough, excoriated; lids of r. eye red, swollen; conjunctiva red; skin of whole body, but particularly of arms and feet, rough and scaly, often covered with thick moist crusts; intolerable biting-itching in affected parts, < toward evening, at night and from warmth; on scratching a sanious pus is discharged with momentary relief; an intolerable odor arises from the patient.

▮ Crusta lactea; crusts on cheeks, extending up to temples over hairy part of scalp, even eyelids being covered; on several fingers painful ulcerations about nails.

▮ Chronic suppurating eruptions on face.

9 **Lower Face.** Cramplike pain in articulation of lower jaw, close to ear, during rest and motion of part, > from pressure and warmth.

Pressive and digging pain in glands beneath angle of lower jaw.

▮Pain in maxillary joints as if the jaw would break.

▮▮Stiffness of jaws, cracking in articulation of jaw when moving it; jaw easily dislocated.

▮Dull, aching cramplike pain in articulation of r. lower jaw when at rest, and when in motion, accompanied by a crackling sound and severe pain as if jaw would break, > by pressure and warm food and drinks.

▮Rheumatism of maxillary joint.

▮▮Parotitis after catching cold; suppuration was feared and an incision made; swelling then somewhat subsided but became more indurated, particularly around scar; if exposed to north and east winds inflammation and swelling occurred, at which time she could hardly open mouth.

▮▮Corners of mouth ulcerated, fever blisters around mouth.

▮Exanthema on cheeks, chin and around mouth.

▮Herpetic, crusty eruptions around mouth and nose with itching and burning.

▮Pimples about mouth and chin.

▮Lips dry and parched, covered with reddish-brown crusts. θTyphus.

10 **Teeth and Gums.** ▮Teeth painful with stinging at root of nose, extending to malar bones.

Toothache, in evening, first in a hollow tooth, which became elongated and loose, then also in other teeth in which the pain was partly sticking and partly crawling.

Jerking toothache at night (about 10 P.M.); the jerking extending into head; > from application of cold hand.

Tearing pain in teeth, > by hot applications.

▮Jumping, shooting, as if teeth were being torn out; or slow, pricking, throbbing or tearing, extending into jaws and temples; face sore; < at night, from cold, from vexation, > from external heat; crusty caries.

▮Gnawing sensation in hollow teeth < from cold.

▮Teeth feel too long and too loose, feel as if asleep.

Looseness of lower incisors; she cannot bite upon them.

11 **Taste and Tongue.** ▮Taste: putrid, mornings after eating; ▮▮metallic; food, especially bread, tastes bitter; disgusting, bitter, with a sensation of dryness in mouth, frequently awoke her at night.

▮▮Tongue: dry; sore, redness at tip; not coated but very dry, which provoked drinking; dry, red, cracked; has a triangular red tip; white, often on one side; yellowish;

covered with brown mucus; takes imprint of teeth; blistered; coated at root, yellowish-white; thickly coated; brown mucus, excepting on edges, in morning on rising.

12 **Inner Mouth.** Sleeps with open mouth.

▮Breath: putrid, excessively so in typhoid fever and diphtheria.

▮Mouth dry, with much thirst.

Water accumulates in mouth, is frequently obliged to spit.

▮Saliva bloody; runs out of mouth during sleep.

▮Much tough mucus in mouth and throat.

‖Both lips large, prominent, tender and of an ashy-gray color from infiltration beneath mucous membrane of an albuminous-looking matter behind which was a layer of dark-colored fluid, probably blood; face, especially forehead, bluish and cool; features drawn and pinched; submaxillary glands greatly swollen; pulse 96, small and thready; temperature 97.3°; tongue swollen, pale and covered with an offensive mucus similar in odor and hue to lips; extreme prostration. θDiphtheria of lips.

13 **Throat.** ▮Sensation of dryness in throat.

▮▮Great thirst and dryness in throat, in typhoid conditions.

Unable to drink; at every swallow the drink chokes her as if pharynx were inactive or paralyzed; associated with a sensation of dryness in throat posteriorly.

▮Difficult swallowing of solids, as from contraction.

▮Painful swallowing, particularly when swallowing empty or saliva.

Sore throat; deglutition difficult, with stitching pains, throat much swollen externally, maxillary and parotid glands greatly enlarged.

▮Sore throat as from an internal swelling, with bruised pain, also when talking, with pressure and stinging when swallowing.

▮▮Throat sore, feels stiff; after straining throat.

▮Sticking or stinging pains in tonsils, < on beginning to swallow.

▮Erysipelatous inflammation; parotids swollen; cellulitis of neck; drowsiness.

Tonsil (right) covered with yellow membrane.

‖Fever < toward night; pains in back of neck with stiffness, < on turning, > on change of position; restlessness; inflammation of r. tonsil, with a patch like chamois leather, yellowish-white, thick; tongue white, heavily coated, top and edge red, almost sore, raw-looking; fetid breath; sticking pain on swallowing, < when first beginning to swallow; loathing of food. θDiphtheria.

▮Diphtheria; child restless, wants to be carried about

wakes up every now and then complaining of pain in throat; bloody saliva runs out of mouth during sleep; parotid glands swollen; transparent, jelly-like discharges from bowels at stool or afterward.

▮▮Pain in back, in a spot corresponding with about centre of œsophagus, < eating and drinking; when food reaches this spot it refuses to go further, so that she can take only fluids; seeks to force food past affected spot by twisting body about or assuming some favorable position, after which she is relieved. θŒsophagitis.

▮Œsophagitis, especially after corrosive substances.

▮▮Parotid and submaxillary glands highly inflamed and enlarged; swallowing nearly impossible. θDiphtheria. θScarlatina. θVariola.

▮Mumps on left side.

14 **Appetite, Thirst. Desires, Aversions.** ▮Hunger without appetite.

Loss of appetite in palate and throat, with emptiness in stomach, and at same time ravenous hunger, that disappeared after sitting awhile.

▮Complete loss of appetite for all food; nothing tastes well, neither food, drink nor tobacco.

▮No appetite, or wants only dainties.

▮▮Thirst with dryness of throat.

▮Unquenchable thirst, wants only cold drinks; < at night, from dryness of mouth.

▮Desire for: oysters; sweets; beer; cold milk.

▮Aversion to: spirituous liquors; to meat; to beer.

15 **Eating and Drinking.** ▮After eating: great sleepiness; fulness in stomach; giddiness; heaviness in stomach as from a stone.

From drinking ice-water: pain in stomach and nausea.

16 **Hiccough, Belching, Nausea and Vomiting.** ▮Eructations: seem to become incarcerated and remain in r. side of chest; with nausea; with tingling in stomach, < when rising from lying.

▮Nausea: after ice-water; after eating, with sudden vomiting; with inordinate appetite and inclination to vomit; < at night and after eating.

17 **Scrobiculum and Stomach.** Violent throbbing in epigastric region.

▮Stinging or pulsation in pit of stomach.

▮Ulcerative pain in pit of stomach.

Fulness in stomach, as if overloaded.

▮Fulness or heaviness, as from a stone in stomach; after eating.

▮Pressure in pit of stomach, as if swollen or as if drawn together.

Oppression in stomach toward evening.

▮▮Pain in stomach and nausea, after ice-water.

18 **Hypochondria.** ▮▮Soreness as if beaten in hypochondriac region and abdomen, < on side on which he lies, < when turning and worst when beginning to move.

Pressing drawing, from below upward, in l. hypochondrium, with anxiety and nausea in chest.

| |Severe pain in r. hypochondriac region with high fever, was hardly able to breathe; kept moving about; > after eating.

| |Shooting pains of two weeks standing. θAbscess of liver.

19 **Abdomen.** ▮Abdomen bloated: especially after eating; all day a sensation of fermentation in it.

Griping and jerking pain in abdomen.

Pain in region of ascending colon.

Pain and contraction in abdomen, she was obliged to walk bent over.

| |Pains like a knife in r. abdomen on walking.

▮Soreness of navel.

▮▮Soreness in walls of abdomen, especially in morning when stretching; after physical strain.

▮Sensation as if something were torn loose in abdomen.

▮Visible contractions of abdomen above navel.

| |Pains in stomach and abdomen after drinking ice-water; since then whenever she eats anything has colic, which is followed by a normal stool, with relief.

▮Colic, he must walk bent; < at night; after getting wet.

| |Violent colic, > only by lying on back with legs elevated vertically.

▮▮Typhlitis.

| |Constant pressing, burning pains in whole r. side of abdomen, < rising from a seat, but particularly severe when sitting down, with sensation as if a lump lay like a pressing heavy weight in abdomen; on this account and because of a tension and disturbance in whole r. side of abdomen which extended to groin, she could not stand erect, or easily lift r. foot or propel it forward, whole r. side of abdomen very tense and painful to pressure; a broad flat tumor could be detected extending from crest of ilium to linea alba, upward to liver, downward to region of groin, feeling as if it rounded itself inward and backward; face sunken, pale, distorted, with suffering expression; anorexia; aversion to food; moderate thirst; chilliness mixed with heat; rapid hard pulse; emaciation; despondency; feeling of extreme prostration. θPhysconia peritonealis.

| |Vomiting of mucus, bile and food; sleeplessness; fever;

belching of wind; loss of appetite; mouth dry, pappy; dirty white coating on tongue; abdomen distended, painful, very sensitive to pressure; stitches below r. ribs on inspiration; pain < on eating; on fourth night recurrence of chill; unquenchable thirst; skin burning hot and dry; pulse rapid, small and hard; pain in limbs as if constricted; feet and ankles numb, as if asleep; eyes dull; face pale, pointed, expressive of suffering.

‖ Enteritis; tearing, stitching, burning pains; grass-green vomiting; cannot tolerate least touch; whitish stools containing pus; burning fever, < 1 P.M.; burning in and beneath eyes; dryness of gums; throbbing in temples; tickling in throat; gurgling in abdomen followed by stools which are not fecal; difficult urination; extremely sensitive spot, r. side, one inch below navel, which when touched causes nausea.

‖ Enteritis or peritonitis, with typhoid symptoms; involuntary stools.

▮ Incarcerated hernia.

▮ Inflammatory swelling of inguinal glands.

20 **Stool and Rectum.** ▮ Stools: watery, mucous and bloody, with nausea, tearing down thighs, and much tenesmus; frothy; white; painless and undigested; bloody water like washings of beef; yellowish brown, bloody, cadaverous smelling and involuntary at night [typhoid]; dark, yellow, watery; thin, mucous, red or yellow; jelly-like, streaked white and yellow; greenish, mucous, with jelly-like globules or flakes; lumps of transparent mucus; yellowish white, fecal; yellow, fluid; dark red [brick-colored] fluid; otter-colored fluid [typhoid]; profuse, yellow, watery; scanty, frequent bloody water; alternating with constipation; involuntary (at night while sleeping); fetid; frothy and painless [yellow fluid]; very offensive [dark yellow, watery]; odorless [bloody, watery or yellow fluid].

▮ Before stool: constant urging, with nausea and tearing colic; cutting colic.

▮ During stool: cutting colic; nausea; urging; tenesmus; tearing pains down thighs; shortness of breath.

▮ After stool: remission of pains and urging; tenesmus.

▮ Nightly diarrhœa, with violent pain in abdomen, > after stool or while lying prone.

‖ Diarrhœa after marching through moist ground with bare feet.

‖ Dark brown, thin, and very fetid stools eight or ten imes daily, especially in early morning and between 4 and 6 P.M.; stools often contained mucus, occasionally pus and frequently lentil-shaped clots of blood; very weak, could not sit up, except in bed, because hanging down feet always brought on urging to stool, with involuntary evacuation if not at once responded to. θChronic diarrhœa.

॥Intestinal catarrh during subsidence of cholera epidemica; twenty to thirty motions in twelve hours; vomiting frequent; cyanosis of hands and face; corpselike coldness of forearms, forehead and cheeks; bowels emitted a splashing sound when pressed, showing an admixture of fluid and wind; asphyxia; prostration of strength; apathy of mind; liquid stools mixed with some firmer lumps, strong smelling; vomiting of whitish fluid, with a shade of green, with a sickly smell and mixed with mucus; headache; incessant thirst; frequent sighing; tenesmus; bowels distended with wind; sickly taste in mouth.

▮▮Involuntary stools, with great exhaustion. θTyphoid fever. θGastro-enteritis.

▮Cholera infantum, typhoid type; very restless at night, has to be moved often to get relief.

▮Dysentery; tenesmus, with nausea, tearing and pinching in abdomen; tenesmic stools, followed by involuntary discharges from bowels.

▮Dysenteric discharges since early in morning; extremely severe and constant tenesmus; great chilliness; constant restlessness.

▮Hemorrhage of black blood from bowels. θTyphoid.

▮Sense of constriction in rectum as if one side had grown up.

▮Shooting pain up rectum.

॥Fissure of anus, with periodical profuse bleeding.

▮Hemorrhoids: sore, blind; protruding after stool, with pressing in rectum, as if everything would come out.

21 **Urinary Organs.** ▮Tearing pain in region of kidneys; œdema; after exposure to wet.

॥In a miner exposed to much dampness, œdema of face and feet developing into a general anasarca; urine full of albumen. θBright's disease.

॥Severe tearing pains in small of back; urine contains blood and albumen; anasarca; in a man exposed to heat. θBright's disease.

▮Urine: hot; white; muddy; pale, with white sediment; dark, becoming turbid; high-colored, scanty and irritating; turbid when passed; red and scanty; snow-white sediment [urate of ammonia]; bloody, discharged drop by drop, with straining; **diminished, though he drinks much; passes in a divided stream.**

▮Tenesmus vesicæ; discharges a few drops of blood-red urine.

▮Retention of urine; backache; restless, cannot keep quiet.

▮Urine voided slowly; spine affected; from getting wet.

||Urine escapes in drops, flow interrupted; burning in small of back; constipation; paralytic weakness with coldness and numbness of l. arm and foot; during sixth month of pregnancy.

▮Frequent urging day and night, with increased secretion.

▮Urine involuntary, at night, and while at rest.

▮Weakness of bladder in girls and women, with frequent desire to urinate; also constant dribbling in boys.

22 **Male Sexual Organs.** ▮Erections at night with desire to urinate.

▮Pains in glans penis on account of swelling of prepuce, causing paraphimosis.

▮▮Swelling of glans and prepuce, dark red, erysipelatous.

Stinging itching on inner surface of prepuce.

▮Humid vesicles on glans.

▮Red blotches on inner surface of prepuce.

▮▮Humid eruption on genitals and between scrotum and thigh.

▮Eruption on genitals, closing urethra by swelling.

▮▮Scrotum becomes thick and hard, with intolerable itching.

▮▮Œdema of scrotum and penis.

||Enormous œdema of scrotum and penis after scarlet fever, with recurrence of fever; penis assumed a spiral form.

▮Humid eruptions or erysipelas of scrotum.

||Metastasis of mumps to r. testicle.

||Gonorrhœa; repeated urging to urinate; burning in urethra; scanty, very thick discharge.

||Sweat in second sleep for a month; aching in glans penis; after urination a few drops escape. *θ*Secondary syphilis.

23 **Female Sexual Organs.** ||Ovarian cyst, had existed eighteen months in a laboring woman æt. 20, brunette; fresh, rosy complexion; strained herself lifting shortly after first appearance of tumor.

||Consciousness of uterus feeling sore and low down in pelvis, so as to seriously interfere with walking; micturition frequent and painful; much burning and itching of skin all over body; soreness in back and hypogastrium; subject to rheumatism. *θ*Prolapsus.

||Bearing down in pelvis when walking; itching in rectum; desire for acids; pains are most in r. ovarian

region; feels as if her back would break; > by lying on a hard floor or with pillow under back; stiffness in joints when at rest, goes off during motion.

▮Prolapsus: after parturition; from straining or lifting; in rheumatic women whose pains compel them to shift about in order to get relief; < in damp weather or before a storm.

▮Laborlike pains and pressure in abdomen while standing.

▮Metrorrhagia, blood clotted with laborlike pains.

‖The flow following last confinement never ceased, at times amounting to a severe hemorrhage; when lying or sitting quietly extreme vertigo came on, which only passed away on rising and walking.

‖Polypus of uterus after getting chilled from a sea-bath, felt benumbed after the bath and had a pain in shoulders as if sprained, < at night toward 3 A.M.; lost her memory and was almost paralyzed in her limbs; headache and vertigo; soon afterward uterine hemorrhage; twice there had been removed from her womb masses of polypous growth, but the bleeding returned soon after; uterus low down in pelvis and retroverted, its posterior wall softened and swollen, filling almost entire cavity of pelvis; os dilated, cicatriced, discharging thin blood; leucorrhœa; turbid urine.

▮▮Menses: too early, profuse and protracted; flow light-colored, acrid, causing biting pain in vulva.

▮Menorrhagia: from a strain; in rheumatic women; < at night, demanding constant change of position to find relief.

▮Membranous dysmenorrhœa in rheumatic women.

‖Obstructive dysmenorrhœa; pains cramping, bearing down; backache, < in horizontal position and by lying on back.

▮Amenorrhœa: from getting wet; with milk in breasts after catching cold, with frequent affections of chest and epistaxis.

‖Amenia, after getting wet in a rainstorm, followed by hydrometra.

▮Discharge of offensive, blackish water from vagina, with bursting feeling in head as if head was swelling out.

▮Shooting pains by spells through head; < when lying and > when head is raised.

▮Soreness in vagina shortly after an embrace, or hindering an embrace.

Sticking pain in vagina, not increased by contact.

▮▮External genitals inflamed, erysipelatous, œdematous.

▮Uterine complaints resulting from exposure to cold, damp weather, from getting wet, particularly while perspiring.

24 **Pregnancy. Parturition. Lactation.** ▮During pregnancy: discharges of blood; pelvic articulations stiff when beginning to move.

▮Abortion impending from straining or overexertion.

▮Lochia vitiated and offensive, lasting too long, or oft returning, she is well-nigh exhausted.

▮A vitiated discharge from vagina with shooting upward in parts, with a bursting sensation in head.

▮After-pains of too long duration, after severe labor, with much and excessive straining.

▮▮Milk leg, also metritis after delivery; with typhoid symptoms.

▮Mammæ: swell from catching cold, streaks of inflammation; galactorrhœa; milk vanishes with general heat.

‖For weeks after delivery has much pain in r. limb, with numbness from hips to feet.

‖For weeks after delivery has a terrible cough, it seems as if something would be torn out of chest.

25 **Voice and Larynx. Trachea and Bronchia.** ▮▮Hoarseness: with roughness, scraping, or raw sensation in larynx; roughness and soreness in chest; from overstraining voice.

▮Muscular exhaustion of larynx from prolonged and loud exercise of voice; hoarseness, after being silent awhile, > talking; < in evening, and from change of weather.

Frequent tickling, irritability in air-passages, as if it would provoke cough.

▮Cold sensation in larynx, when breathing.

‖Burning rawness in larynx.

▮Hot air arises from trachea.

▮Influenza; air-passages seem stuffed up; aching in bones; sneezing and coughing, < from uncovering body; arising from exposure to dampness; dry, hard, tickling cough, < evening until midnight; stiffness in back and limbs.

26 **Respiration.** ▮Respiration hurried; very short at night.

▮Oppression: as if breath were stopped at pit of stomach; < after a meal; anxious, as if not able to draw a long breath.

▮Dyspnœa from pressure and painfulness in pit of stomach.

▮Hot breath.

27 **Cough.** ▮Cough: dry, teasing; caused by tickling in bronchia; from uncovering, even a hand; with tearing pain in chest, stitches, profuse sweat and pain in stomach; < evening until midnight, or in morning soon after waking, from talking, lying down or sitting still; from tickling under sternum; preventing sleep at night; frequent hacking in evening after lying down,

with bitter taste in throat till he falls asleep, and in morning a similar hacking cough and a similar taste, lasting till he rises; short, from severe tickling and irritation behind upper half of sternum, followed by feeling of discouragement and apprehension; whenever he puts his hands out of bed; spasmodic, shatters the head; short, anxious, painful, frequently awakens her from sleep before midnight with very short breath; dry, during day, wrenching epigastrium, excited by talking or singing, shoulders and cervical muscles stiff and lame on first moving; > during exercise.

▮▮During convalescence from pneumonia, when coughing, terrific pain in l. shoulder, as if shoulder would fly to pieces, and his wife would have to hold his shoulder with her hand and pinch as hard as she could; pain was brought on by a fit of coughing, and he had to get out of bed and swing his arm back and forth as fast as he could to relieve it.

▮Acute cases of cough with much prostration of whole system.

▮Dry, hard, racking, rheumatic coughs; the case is apt to take on a low typhoid form, and is greatly aggravated at night.

▮▮A dry teasing cough coming on before the chill and continuing during it.

▮Nocturnal dry cough with insufficiency of mitral valve.

▮▮Cough with taste of blood, although no blood is to be seen.

▮Cough with expectoration of bright-red blood and qualmish feeling in chest.

▮Sputa: acrid pus; grayish-green cold mucus of putrid smell; pale, clotted or brown blood.

28 **Inner Chest and Lungs.** Oppression of chest: at night with sticking pains, especially on breathing; anxiety with weight on lower portion of chest.

Tension across chest, in evening very short breath and weakness in all the limbs.

In morning on rising, drawing and stitching pains in l. nipple through to scapula, gradually increasing until it caused severe suffering; face pale.

▮Stitches in chest and sides of chest, especially when sitting bent, talking, sneezing or taking long breath; < when at rest.

▮Tingling in chest, with tension in intercostal muscles.

▮Acute pleurisy with typhoid symptoms.

▮Acute catarrh; the nasal, laryngeal, tracheal and bronchial passages seem stuffed up, commencing at about sunset, with sneezing and dry, hard, tickling cough, continuing very severe until midnight, when all the sufferings are >; renewed next morning.

|| After exposure, chilliness, headache, oppressed breathing, catching pains in r. side of chest, cutting off breath on deep inspiration; anxiety and apprehension that unless relieved he would only be able to breathe but a short time; restless at night; plentiful crop of vesicles around mouth, which had appeared over night. θInfluenza.

|| Pneumonia after exposure to rain while overheated; short, oppressed respiration; cough with stitches in sides; skin hot, dry; tongue red, dry; pulse rapid, hard; urine dark, becoming turbid on standing, and depositing a sediment; diarrhœa; impaired appetite; considerable thirst; sleep restless, full of dreams; languid and weak.

|| Stitches in r. side of chest, < coughing and breathing; short, anxious respiration; deep respiration impossible; severe cough with expectoration of mucus and brownish blood; partly crepitant and partly bronchial râles; bronchophony r. side and dulness on percussion; lies upon back or on r. side; burning, dry heat; pulse tense, frequent; anxious sleep; transient delirium; circumscribed redness of cheeks with yellowness of alæ nasi, corners of mouth and sclerotica; unquenchable thirst; loss of appetite; yellowish-brown coating on tongue; bitter taste; nausea, inclination to vomit, diarrhœa; dark brown urine. θPleuro-pneumonia biliosa.

|| Pneumonia, relapse; restless tossing about at night; acute pain in r. side of chest in locality previously affected, very sensitive to touch; pulse again rapid, strong and full; cough severe, with scanty expectoration of bloody mucus; on breathing, sensation as if air became imprisoned in epigastrium, causing great anxiety.

| Pneumonia: adynamic type; free expectoration of thin, puslike secretion stained deeply with blood.

Brickdust expectoration of bloody sputa, raised with great difficulty, and accompanied by high fever, involuntary diarrhœa, in the worst cases; with typhoid symptoms, often from resorption of pus; with tearing cough and restlessness, because quiet makes pain and dyspnœa worse; pneumonia nervosa.

|| Frequently recurring short cough, with blood-streaked expectoration; stitches in l. side and oppression of chest; menses scanty but regular; for last 8 days, after catching cold, erysipelatous on dorsum of r. hand, with burning and stitching, and formation of a flat ulcer which began as a vesicle. θHæmoptysis.

▮Hæmoptysis: expectoration of blood becomes nearly a habit, so that patient gradually becomes anæmic, weak, and the blood itself poor; from overexertion, blowing wind instruments; blood bright; pain in lower part of chest; renewed from least mental excitement.

29 **Heart, Pulse and Circulation.** ▮Weak and tremulous feeling about heart; chest and heart feel weak after a walk.

▮Dragging and stiffness of cardiac region, especially on beginning to move.

▮Stitches in heart with painful lameness and numbness of l. arm.

▮Palpitation: violent, when sitting still, pulsations moving body; anxious in morning on awaking; following overexertion.

▮▮Uncomplicated hypertrophy, from violent exercise.

||Enlargement of heart with dilatation; pain in l. shoulder and down l. arm, which felt cold and numb; pain < at 4 A.M. faint, fluttering sensation in stomach and l. chest; sensation of gurgling in heart region, with soreness in l. side; lying on it causes severe palpitation and pain in heart.

||Difficult breathing on ascending stairs; a deep inspiration, or raising l. arm suddenly, caused a momentary, acute, stabbing pain in middle anterior portion of fourth intercostal space on same side; heart beats slightly accelerated; some time previous was wet for several hours.

▮▮Organic diseases of heart, with sticking pain and soreness; numbness and lameness of l. arm.

▮▮Aching in l. arm, with disease of heart.

▮▮Myalgia cordis.

▮Pulse: accelerated, weak, faint and soft; trembling or imperceptible; sometimes quicker than heart's beat; irregular; affected by beer, coffee or alcohol.

30 **Outer Chest.** Numb sensation in chest.

Pain in chest as if sternum were pressed inward.

▮Myalgia or muscular rheumatism of chest.

31 **Neck and Back.** ▮▮Stiff neck with painful tension when moving; of rheumatic origin; from a draft.

Pain in cervical muscles as if parts were asleep, and as if one had been lying for a long time in an uncomfortable position, toward evening.

Hard swelling on l. side of neck under ramus of lower jaw increased to size of a man's fist, so large that it turned face directly to one side, causing chin to rest on r. shoulder.

▮Swollen or inflamed glands of neck, with red streaks, as in scarlet fever.

‖Carbuncle on nape of neck near spinous process of upper cervical vertebra; swelling brownish-red, with several small openings, discharging offensive-smelling pus; great pain: fever; sleep disturbed.

▮▮Pains in shoulders and back, with stiffness as from a sprain.

▮Pain between shoulders on swallowing food.

Sticking in back while stooping, in evening.

Pressive stitches in back, < while walking or stooping but more on rising up again.

Constrictive pain in dorsal muscles, while sitting, > bending back, < bending forward.

Violent rheumatic pain between scapulæ, neither > nor < by motion or rest, only > by warmth, < by cold.

▮Painful tension between shoulder-blades.

▮▮Stiffness in small of back, painful on motion.

Sensation as if bruised, in r. side of lumbar vertebræ and in small of back.

▮▮While sitting small of back aches, as after long stooping or bending.

▮▮Pain as if bruised, in small of back, whenever he lies quietly upon it or sits still; > on moving about.

▮Pain in small of back, on grasping it, as if the flesh had been beaten.

▮▮Heaviness and pressure in small of back, as if one had received a blow, < while sitting.

Pressure as with a cutting edge, across small of back, while standing or bending backward.

▮▮Pain in small of back, < when sitting still or when lying; > when lying on something hard, or from exercise.

‖Sudden acute pain in small of back while lifting a light board so that he could raise himself only with difficulty; next day paralysis of arms, with burning on urination, scanty discharge, and vesical tenesmus.

▮Violent pain "as if back were broken" in lumbar region, on least movement or coughing, from straining back by lifting.

▮Lumbago; pain < after, not during motion.

‖Lumbar pain of three weeks duration after a strain; great pain and soreness, < after getting warm in bed and on beginning to move.

‖Sensitive spot in spine between shoulder-blades; when spot is touched, he has waterbrash, afterward nausea and vomiting; easily tired and then can swallow nothing without vomiting it up directly; before vomiting, burning sensation in stomach and between shoulder-blades; must make great effort to vomit; cannot eat meat, it distresses him; numbness of middle finger of r. hand; has not done a day's work for six years, on account of weakness, a kind of paralytic feeling in arms, and increased pain in back and consequent nausea; < in damp, rainy, cold weather, particularly east wind; can only drink coffee, tea makes him worse; vomits cold water immediately; bowels move only every five or seven days, very costive; strained himself lifting an invalid wife eight or nine years ago, but felt no immediate symptoms after it, except pain in back; Spring of 1862, during a northeast rainstorm, he endeavored to assist in moving a heavily laden team of lumber, after which felt something giving way between his shoulders.

|| Violent pain in head, from back to front and down spine; lies on her back, head and back drawn backward; slightest move or touch causes excruciating pain; pulse slow; action of bowels almost paralyzed; urine voided daily but slowly; complete sleeplessness; pain in paroxysms; caused by getting wet. θSpinal irritation.

|| Great pain in small of back; < in bed, > on pressure. θSpinal irritation.

|| Severe pain over crest of l. ileum, between crest and posterior superior spine, > by pressure and heat. θSpinal irritation.

▮▮ Spinal membranes inflamed, even myelitis; from getting wet or sleeping on damp ground.

Burning feeling in loins.

▮ Stiffness and lameness in sacrum, < on resting after exercise.

▮ Curvature of dorsal vertebræ.

32 **Upper Limbs.** Pressure on shoulders like a heavy weight.

Left shoulder seems paralyzed.

Sensation as if some one were pressing upon l. shoulder, by the clavicle.

Rheumatic pain in l. shoulder and arm in region of deltoid muscle.

Severe pain at top of l. shoulder.

Tearing in shoulder joint and on top of scapula.

Shooting inward and throbbing in left shoulder.

Stitches in shoulders while lying, > on moving about.

▮ Tearing and burning in shoulder, arm lame, < in cold, wet weather, in bed, and at rest.

|| Pain in muscles of l. shoulder and arm, also in bones of arm while joints remain unaffected; numb sensation about hands and fingers, after a wetting.

|| Strain of l. shoulder joint very painful for a long time; became at last immovable; sleepless at night.

▮ Painful swelling of axillary glands; suppurating.

▮Trembling of arms after moderate exertion.

▮Violent tearing pain in arm, most violent while lying still.

The arm upon which he rests the head in sleep becomes numb.

Shooting pains through arms.

▮Drawing, paralyzed sensation in l. arm, at night.

▮Sticking and drawing in l. arm extending downward to tips of fingers.

Drawing stitches in arms, from shoulders downward.

▮Tensive aching pains as if arms were luxated.

Pain in l. upper arm as if muscles or tendons were unduly strained, when limb is raised.

▮▮Numbness or aching in l. arm, with heart disease.

Cramplike drawing or tension in elbow joint.

▮Chronic inflammation of articular structures, especially when resulting from blows, sprains, etc.

Drawing and tearing extending from elbow joint into wrist.

▮Jerking tearing in elbow and wrist joints, during rest, > during motion.

||Loss of power and stiffness of forearms and fingers on moving them.

▮Paralysis of arm, with coldness and insensibility.

||Sudden paralysis of l. arm while in open air on a rainy day; arm cold without sensation or motion; pulse on affected side small, almost trembling; dull headaches roaring in ears; lachrymation and pressure in eyes a from sand; dryness of gums; offensive taste in mouth clean, dark red tongue; diarrhœa with tenesmus and frequent urging to urinate; restless sleep; constant chilliness; melancholy.

▮▮Erysipelatous swelling of arms.

▮Pain in r. wrist.

▮Sensation on upper surface of l. wrist on bending it as if it had been sprained.

||For six months stiff wrist joint, swollen and painful; pain < after rest when first beginning to move the joint, after washing in cold water, by cold generally, change of weather, in a feather bed, by exertion in morning after night's rest, and in evening.

||Rheumatic pains darting through wrist joint from side to side after a sprain.

||Tenderness of carpal articulation; could not bear any shaking of wrist from forearm, or any pressure over articulation of wrist or any sideway motions of hand; inflamed state of articular surfaces of wrist, probably of synovial membrane; after sprain.

Drawing pain in palm of r. hand.

▮Rheumatic pains in hands.

||Pains, aching, drawing with numbness; began in r. hand, extended to all parts; stiff in morning on beginning to move; must change position frequently at cost of pain; < after midnight. θRheumatism.

▮Rheumatism with great swelling of hands, brought on by wet weather.

▮Hot swelling of hands in evening.

||Burning in palm of r. hand and sensation as if hand were being held in hot water, < in rest, in cold, holding anything cold, but particularly from cold water, and from midnight toward morning; > from motion, letting hand hang, warmth and warm water; at 3 A.M. whole hand and forearm burn, driving her nearly to distraction, must get out of bed and walk about till morning; hand as if lame and during day often "goes to sleep" for hours; hand dry as if withered, unless it is rubbed with fat; must constantly carry something in hand.

▮Rhagades on backs of hands.

Swollen veins on hands.

▮Warts particularly on hands and fingers.

▮Cold, sweaty hands.

▮Fingers can be moved only with pain, on account of great swelling.

Tearing in joints of all fingers.

A fine sticking pain in fingers.

Index and middle fingers of one hand feel numb and asleep in morning.

Severe pain at phalanges of several fingers, about midway between joints, in evening.

▮When grasping anything, feeling as if pins were pricking tips and palmar surfaces of first phalanges of fingers.

▮Crawling as if asleep, in tips of fingers.

||Strained middle joint of thumb severely eight days before; had been quite sore and painful, < nights; could not use it without increasing painful state.

▮Inflammatory swelling of finger tips with formication.

||Acute pain in middle finger of r. hand while working, which disappeared as he continued his occupation; thereupon a sensation of numbness and formication appeared in finger, which gradually extended along median nerve to elbow; this sensation grew more pronounced from day to day, and hand began to lose its strength, middle finger particularly seeming lamed.

▮▮Swelling of fingers.

▮Hangnails.

||Eczema impetiginoides; angry eruption on r. forearm,

extending from elbow to phalangeal joints; surface raw and excoriated and covered with yellow scabs and eliminates a sero-purulent discharge; infiltration of areolar tissue, with much swelling; general health affected; fever at night, with chilliness, etc.

▮Chronic psoriasis covering arms, especially left, exterior surface of arms and dorsa of hands; violent itching, but not the cloud of branlike scales.

38 **Lower Limbs.** Drawing pain in r. natis, just below small of back, > on pressure.

▮Pressive pain in hip joints at every step, and a paralyzed sensation in anterior muscles of thigh.

Tension and drawing in r. hip.

▮Tension in l. hip joint while sitting.

▮When lying upon side hip hurts, and when lying upon back small of back hurts.

▮Tearing and drawing from hip to knee while walking or standing.

▮▮Sciatica: r. side, dull aching pain, < at night, in cold or damp weather; > by rubbing, from heat and when warmed by exercise; numbness and formication.

‖Severe attack every few weeks, crippling him for days at a time; r. thigh and hip affected; pains < when keeping still and on attempting to move, in wet, damp weather; > after moving around and from warm applications; attacks brought on by overwork and exposure. θSciatica.

‖Violent tearing, burning pain proceeded from tuberosity of r. ischium, followed course of sciatic nerve and spread over thigh, knee and leg; generally came at night, increased in intensity every minute, until obliged to get up and walk about, when pain went off. θSciatica.

‖Acute pain in l. hip, particularly when rising from a seat, pain then extending toward spine, into abdomen, and at times to knee; shortness of breath; pains about heart, at times very severe, as if something would burst in chest, hard pressure over painful spot, and entire quietness relieves. θSciatica.

‖Sciatic neuralgia for twelve years; pain occupied whole l. lower limb, particularly posterior part of thigh; drawing, burning, lancinating pains, < at night, so as to prevent sleep; also < in cold wet weather.

‖Sciatica, l. side; intense pains gradually increasing in severity; lightning-like pains shoot through limb; sensation of coldness in limbs; < in rest, > from continued motion; sleeplessness at night.

‖Sciatica with tenderness about knee joint; pain constant when walking; could rise from bed or chair only with great effort and care.

‖ Sciatica, r. side; pain extremely violent, makes him scream, < when at rest; > by walking when able to walk.

‖ Stinging pain, < during rest in bed; has to turn over, or change position of leg every few minutes, which relieves pain for a short time; heaviness, when he undertakes to run, leg lacks power; cramps in calves obliging him to get out of bed and walk the floor.

‖ Excessive nervousness; sleeplessness; inability to rest in any position; muscular twitching in all parts of body, especially in affected leg, at night. θSciatica.

‖ Rheumatic sciatica; pain < after rising from his box (he is a coachman); urine thick.

‖ Coxalgia in r. hip-joint along ischiatic nerve to ankle; > from warmth, < from cold; first motion very painful, gradually getting > from continued motion.

| Coxalgia: involuntary limping; pains felt mostly in knee; < from overexercise; < at night; with lengthening of limb.

| After exposure, pain in hips, thence to lower part of thigh, only on external side; leg lame and stiff; pain < in change of weather, from cold and exercise.

| Pain as if sprained in hip, knee or ankle joint.

| A sense of stiffness in pelvic articulations on first attempting to walk; > after getting warm in walking.

| Much pain continues in r. limb, with numbness from hips to feet. θAfter parturition.

‖ Drawing pain with crepitation in hip joints; pain < by leaving chair after long sitting, by sitting down in the cold, by exerting leg during walking, in the Autumn and by change of weather; > from warmth of stove, in sun, and by continued gentle motion; leg is so lame that he is obliged to take hold of the pantaloons near knee, in order to lift it and move it on; when limping in this manner the leg was always bent in the knee-joint, and every attempt to extend it caused pain, complete extension was impossible; the limb being stiff in hip joint every motion was painful and imperfect; after exposure to snow-storm while overheated. θRheumatism.

| Traumatic cases of inflammation of hip joint; frequently after *Arnica*, in bad effects from contusion and from straining of capsular ligaments and of tendons and muscles of thigh, with swelling and great pain in affected parts; or when caused by exposing perspiring skin to sudden cold, or by getting wet, or from lying on wet ground after body has been in perspiration; aching, drawing, tearing, tensive pains with a sensation as if

skin around diseased parts were too tight; pain < in recumbent posture.

‖ Four years ago was thrown from a wagon and much injured about hips and small of back; was very lame and unable to move much or sit up any length of time; has been in feeble health ever since; it has affected her very much to stand or walk since the injury; thinks she has not been able to bear her weight on her limb since, without more or less suffering through the hips; cannot endure walking, even for a short distance, without suffering for a week or more, and at times is confined to bed in consequence; riding or any jarring affects her in much the same way; much tenderness to pressure about heads of both femora and edges of acetabulum, joint of coccyx and sacrum; pressing head of femur against acetabulum produces much pain and aching, and she feels it so constantly while bearing any weight upon limbs; sleep restless and unquiet, especially first part of night.

‖ Man of sanguine temperament, had been injured by the caving in of a gravel bank, injuring his r. hip; no sleep for three nights; unable to move or have the leg stirred; groaning under severe pain and suffering; whole hip and thigh quite hot and inflamed.

| Aching pain in both hip joints at every step, and a paralytic feeling in anterior muscles of thighs.

Right rectus cruris muscle very sensitive on pressure, as if bruised.

Tension on posterior surface of thigh while riding one leg over the other.

Tension in l. thigh, extending downward from hip-joint.

Jerking and tearing in r. thigh, somewhat above knee.

Tearing pain in middle of outer portion of thigh, while sitting, > on motion.

Tearing, dragging pains in muscles of l. thigh.

| The pain runs in streaks down limbs with every evacuation.

‖ From a severe wetting all over, was seized with terrible pains in lower extremities, paroxysmal in character, driving him to desperation; could remain in no position, but resembled a dancing monkey.

☞ Lameness and stiffness and pain on first moving after rest, or on getting up in the morning, > by continued motion.

‖ After becoming thoroughly chilled a year and a half ago during a long railroad journey, legs had gradually become stiff and weak; numbness of feet with tingling; every now and then attacks of painful stiffness in back, which would lay her up for two or three weeks; urine thick. θRheumatic paralysis.

▮▮Restlessness of lower limbs in bed at night, > by motion.

▮Spasmodic twitching in limbs when stepping out.

Jerking in thigh, with tremor of knees.

▮▮Paralysis of lower extremities.

▮Lower extremities feel bruised, they are so weary.

▮Heaviness of lower limbs.

▮Powerlessness of lower limbs, she can hardly draw them up; nurse has to move them. θAfter parturition.

‖On rising from seat after sitting about four hours, loss of power of co-ordination in lower extremities, staggers, takes longer strides than he intends, steps higher than usual; feels strangely; symptoms return after sitting or lying down.

▮Scrofulosis and rachitis; tensive feeling in diseased limb, as if tendons were too short; bruising pains, causing patient to scream; < when touched.

‖For some years swelling of feet in warm weather; finally limbs began to enlarge; no evidence of any organic disease; both legs much swollen and pit upon pressure; prickling heat in limbs and after walking, surface of them becomes red and hot; on first attempting motion limbs are stiff, but become more supple after continued exercise; tongue yellowish, with red points at tip. θAnasarca.

▮After scarlet fever anasarcous condition of lower limbs, with diminished secretion of urine.

▮Painful swelling above knee.

A pulling with tension in tendons on inner side of r. knee, causing uneasiness in foot.

Pains under patella.

Burning pain in knee joints and lower extremities.

▮Tearing in knee and in ankle, < during rest.

A stitch across knee on standing up after sitting.

A sticking from within outward in side of knee, while walking.

▮▮Stiffness, especially of knees and feet.

▮Tension in knee, as if it were too short.

Heaviness like a hundredweight, in hollows of knees and in calves, so that he could not move feet along.

A crawling with tension in tendons on inner side of r. knee.

‖After catching cold, swelling of knee, followed by suppuration; after eight weeks surgical treatment, there were around the patella three openings with elevated edges, from which an unhealthy thin pus was discharged;

fever; continuous pain; sleeplessness; looks as if he had consumption.

|| Swelling of knee, with violent gnawing pains. θRheumatic gout.

|| Groaning with pain in l. knee joint, which extends down leg; begged to have the limb cut off. θAcute rheumatism.

▮ Shooting and deep cutting pains in leg. θAcute rheumatism.

|| Pain in r. knee; < when straining knee; often a cracking in joint when stretching limb; exudation in joint; change of weather, especially rain or storm < pain, when at rest there is no pain. θHydrarthrus genu.

|| Painful swelling in popliteal space of one limb, occasioned by a cold, preventing extension of leg; pain in tumor, particularly after walking and exercising leg.

|| After exposure to dampness, swelling of finger joints, followed by a pale, rather painless, somewhat fluctuating swelling of r. knee; leg flexed, cannot be extended; emaciation; paleness of face; no fever. θWhite swelling of knee.

|| Erysipelatous inflammation and swelling of both knee joints; second sound of heart impaired.

▮▮ Great heaviness, weakness and weariness of legs.

Great inclination to stretch out leg and foot, in morning.

▮▮ Aching pains in legs, inability to rest in any position but for a moment.

Tension in calves while walking and a sensation as if the hamstrings were too short.

Cramps in calves after midnight, while lying in bed and while sitting after walking.

Pain in inner, lower and posterior part of calf of leg, felt during earlier portion of a walk, whenever the heel was raised by the action of the calf; > after walking a few minutes.

On rising from a chair, sudden and severe pain as from a sprain, at insertion of ligamentum patellæ into tibia.

A stitch in hamstrings just above calves, on violent motion, on rising from a seat and on touch.

Stitches just below r. knee.

▮ Pain like a tingling, in tibiæ at night, while feet are crossed; she is constantly obliged to move legs back and forth, and on this account is unable to sleep.

▮ When walking legs feel as if made of wood.

▮▮ Paroxysmal pains in legs from getting wet, especially when warm and sweaty.

▮ Cramps in legs and feet, must walk about.

| Ulcers: on legs, discharging profusely; on dropsical legs, discharging serum.

|| Intolerable itching of legs and feet at night; old rash.

|| Erysipelas, red, itching, phlegmonous swelling, with vesicular eruption extending like a band around r. ankle; large open ulcer on ankle; pain < after, not during motion (*Rhus rad.* cured after failure of *Rhus tox.*).

|| Four weeks ago, while running fast, was suddenly taken with a very acute pain in ankle-joint; pain > when at rest, but is felt as soon as he attempts to walk fast, obliging him to stand still.

|| Sprain of ankle, could not touch foot to ground for six weeks, or expose it to dampness, or be out nights.

| Aching pains in ankles and hollow of feet on walking, so that he must lie down after the least walk.

| Swollen about ankles after sitting too long, particularly in traveling; feet swell in evening.

|| Ulcer as large as a silver dollar on internal malleolus, with itching, stinging, darting pains; < after motion.

| Swelling of feet, painless to touch in evening.

Weariness of feet so that she could not easily go up stairs.

Deadness and numbness of lower part of r. foot, which seemed made of wood.

| Heaviness and tension of feet while sitting.

Feet painful as if sprained or wrenched, in morning on rising.

A paralytic drawing in whole of foot, while sitting.

Crawling in feet in morning, while lying in bed and after rising.

Aching pains in hollow of feet.

Pains in both heels as if stepping upon pins, on first standing, in morning.

Sharp pain in heels at times, like running nails under skin.

Stitching in heels when stepping upon them.

Spasmodic contraction in inner side of sole of foot, > by stretching it out and bending sole upward.

Stitches in soles of feet as if he were walking upon needles, in evening.

| Fetid perspiration of feet in men of a rheumatic tendency much exposed to weather and devoted to hard manual labor.

| Corns, with soreness and burning.

| Eczema on inner side of thighs after vaccination, much itching and thirst.

| Eczema rubrum; leg, from knee joint to toes, exhibits a dark, purplish aspect and emits a musty odor, together with copious serous discharge; intense burning and

itching, particularly on exposure to cold; extreme irritation of mind; general debility; sleeplessness; loss of appetite; distress when eating; constipation; headache.

‖ Child, æt. 1½, has had hives, which were very itchy, scratching developed them into large blisters; very uneasy and restless at night; has now erysipelas on l. leg, which is swollen and dark purple.

‖ Erythema nodosum on legs; large painful protuberances over each tibia.

34 **Limbs in General.** | Great weakness in limbs; they tremble.

All the limbs feel stiff and paralyzed during and after walking, with a sensation of a hundredweight on nape of neck.

‖ Sensation of stiffness on first moving limb, after rest.

‖ Limbs upon which he lies, especially arms, fall asleep.

A sensation similar to a trembling in arms and lower extremities, even while at rest.

‖ Drawing or tearing pains in limbs during rest.

‖ Pains as if bruised, or sprained, in joints.

‖ Cracking of joints when stretched.

| Tension, stiffness and stitches in joints; < when rising from a seat.

‖ Rheumatoid pains in limbs: with numbness and tingling; joints weak, stiff, or red; shining swelling of joints, stitches when touched; < on beginning to move, after 12 P.M., and in wet, damp weather or places; > from continued motion.

‖ Pain, swelling and stiffness of joints from sprains, overlifting or overstraining.

‖ Inflammatory rheumatism, from exposure to cold, followed by paralysis of r. side; pains almost constant in r. side; marked periodicity, coming on at 10 P.M. and lasting until 6 A.M.; < in winter and before a storm, during a storm pains over whole body; intense pain on moving after rest, but continued motion relieved.

| Chronic inflammation of articular structures, especially when resulting from blows, strains, etc.

| Synovitis; spurious anchylosis.

| Swelling of hands and feet.

| Phlegmonous erysipelas of limbs.

| Eruption on limbs, with intense itching, < at night, and when putting hands in hot or cold water.

35 **Rest. Position. Motion.** Rest: tearing pains in cranial bones <; pain in jaw; involuntary urination; stiffness of joints; stitches in chest <; tearing and burning in shoulders <; tearing in elbow and wrist joints <; sciatica <; stiffness and lameness in sacrum <; tear-

ing in knee and ankle joint <; no pain in knee tearing and drawing in limbs; weakness of limbs.

Lying: cough; vertigo; headache <; diarrhœa >; extreme vertigo; shooting through head <; cough <; pain in small of back <; stitches in shoulders; tearing in arms <; symptoms return.

Lying on back: colic > with legs elevated; obstructive dysmenorrhœa <; pain in small of back <; pain in head and down spine; small of back hurts; rheumatic fever <; trembling of paralysis >.

Lying in bed: cramps in calves.

Lies on back constantly: erysipelas.

Lies on its face with hands to head: sore eyes.

Lying on hard floor with pillow under back: backache >.

Lying on side: hip hurts.

Lying on l. side: causes palpitation and pain in heart.

Side on which she lies: beating in temple; scalp sensitive; soreness of abdomen <.

Lying upon limbs: they fall asleep; no sweat on parts.

Head low: heaviness <.

Head raised: shooting pains through head >.

Must hold head to relieve weight in it.

Bending head backward: pain in occiput >; pain in head and down spine.

Bending back: pain in dorsal muscles >; pressure in small of back.

Bending forward: pain in dorsal muscles <.

Sitting: headache <; hunger >; pains in abdomen <; extreme vertigo; cough <; palpitation; pain in dorsal muscles; small of back aches; heaviness and pressure in small of back <; tension of l. hip-joint; symptoms return; after walking, cramps in calves; too long, ankles swollen; heaviness and tension of feet; paralytic drawing in whole foot.

Sitting bent: stitches in chest.

Could not sit still: on account of general uneasiness, must turn in every direction on chair and move limb.

Rising from seat: pain in hip <; loss of power of co-ordination in lower extremities; severe pain at insertion of ligamentum patellæ into tibia; stitch in hamstrings; tension, stiffness and stitches in joints.

Rising from bed: vertigo; eructations <.

Rising from stooping: stitches in back <.

Stooping: vertigo <; nosebleed; pain in back; stitches in back <.

Standing: vertigo <; laborlike pains and pressure in abdomen; pressure in small of back; tearing from hip to knee; after sitting, a stitch across knee; pain in both heels; could not stand erect, or easily lift r. foot or propel it forward.

Raising l. arm suddenly: causes stabbing pain in fourth intercostal space; pain in arm.

Bending wrist: as if sprained.

Riding one leg over other: tension of thigh.

Bending sole of foot upward: contraction >.

Hanging down feet: caused urging to stool.

Change of position: > pain in back of neck; frequent, in cholera infantum; constant, to > menorrhagia; > pain in leg; rheumatic fever; during typhoid; zona, necessitates.

Beginning to move: soreness in abdomen worst; pelvic articulations stiff; shoulders and cervical muscles stiff, lame; stiffness of cardiac region; lumbar pain <; pain in wrist joint <; sciatica <; limbs stiff; rheumatism in limbs <.

Motion: stupefaction in head, with tingling and pains in limbs >; rapid, > pain in temple; of eyes, painful; of eyes, < pain in head; headache >; pain in jaw; cracking of jaw; stiffness of joints >; painful tension of neck; stiffness of back painful; pain in small of back >; lumbago < after, not during; slightest, causes excruciating pain in back; stitches in shoulders >; tearing in elbow and wrist joints >; loss of power and stiffness of forearms and fingers; sciatica >; continued, > coxalgia; gentle continued, > pain in hip joints; restlessness of legs >; violent stitch in hamstrings; pain in ankle, < after, not during; pain in ulcers on feet <; continued, > rheumatism; produces cold feeling; causes shuddering; slight chills.

Swallowing food: pain between shoulders.

Stretching: limb, cracking sound in knee joint; inclination for, leg and foot; sole of foot, contraction >; cracking of joints.

Stretching: soreness of abdomen.

Turning: vertigo <; pain in back of neck <; soreness in abdomen <.

Swinging arm back and forth: > pain in shoulder.

Stepping out: spasmodic twitching in limbs.

Stepping: brain feels loose.

At every step: pain in hip joints; stitches in heels.

Walking: vertigo <; burning in forehead; pains in abdomen; bearing down in pelvis; vertigo >; heart feels weak after; stitches in back <; tearing from hip to knee; > sciatica; surface of feet becomes red and hot; sticking in side of knee; tumor of knee, pains; tension in calves; a few moments, pain in heel >;

pain in ankle returns; pain in ankles and hollows of feet; all limbs feel stiff and paralyzed.

Must walk bent over: pain in abdomen.

Must shift about to get relief: prolapsus.

Could remain in no position: terrible pain in legs; tingling in tibiæ.

Cannot remain quiet a moment.

Inclination to move affected parts, continued motion: > soreness of nipples.

Ascending stairs: difficult breathing.

While running fast sudden acute pain in ankle joint.

Exercise: pain in cranial bones >; stiffness of cervical muscles >; violent, uncomplicated hypertrophy; pain in small of back >; trembling of arms; stiffness and soreness of muscles pass off.

Unwonted exertion: paralysis.

Overexertion: palpitation; coxalgia <.

36 **Nerves.** ▮▮Great restlessness: inclination to move affected parts; at night; has to change position frequently; it seemed as if something forced him out of bed; could not sit still on account of internal uneasiness, but was obliged to turn in every direction on chair and move limbs.

▮Weakness: with desire to lie down; over whole body; weary as if deprived of sleep; of limbs, mostly during rest; in morning does not wish to rise and dress; feels as if sinking through bed; as if bones ached; constantly desires to sit or lie down; especially on walking in open air.

▮▮Great debility with soreness and stiffness, < on beginning to move; > from continued motion, but soon fatigued, requiring rest again.

▮▮Numbness: in extremities, with previous twitching and tingling in them; in the parts on which he lies.

▮Paresis of limbs with numb sensation and difficulty of moving the back, in consequence of a wetting.

ǀǀParesis of lower extremities, with commencing amaurosis so that patient could not distinguish large objects.

ǀǀPainless paresis in legs in a girl æt. 14.

▮▮Paralysis: after unwonted exertion; after parturition; rheumatic, from getting wet or lying on damp ground; from sexual excesses; after ague or typhoid; parts painless, or painfully stiff and lame, with tearing, tingling and numbness.

ǀǀSudden paralysis of lower half of body, in a girl who was being treated by an extension apparatus for curvature of spine; obstinate constipation; legs numb, cold, emaciated.

|| On third day after a natural labor, the mother being only thirteen years and six months old, r. side became entirely paralyzed; there was an apparent total abolition of functions, of voluntary motion and special sensation; could not articulate so as to be understood.

| Hemiplegia, right-sided; sensation as if "gone to sleep."

|| Paraplegia in a woman following an attack of apoplexy five years previously; she was unable to stand or rise up.

| Acute spinal paralysis of infants.

|| Sits upon a stool and keeps it in constant motion; cannot remain quiet a moment; head and body hang forward, the former oscillating continually; violent trembling of extremities; cannot raise himself into erect sitting posture, or hold anything, so that he must be fed; on attempting to walk legs are extremely unsteady, although he can stand a short time, the knees meanwhile shaking constantly; if he takes a few steps falls over his feet and is not able to rise again without assistance; trembling > in horizontal position; during sleep, frequent spasmodic starting unnoticed by himself; muscles flabby; emaciation; constipation; urine clear as water; pulse small, soft, 70. θParalysis agitans.

|| After falling down steps the following condition gradually developed: lies upon abdomen, with head retracted so that it almost touches spine; face pale, distorted, covered with cold sweat; goitre-like swelling of neck due to tonic spasm of cervical muscles; spine drawn from normal position; crackling sound on bending lumbar vertebræ; great swelling of bone in region of sacrum; complete paralysis of lower extremities; retention of urine, or discharge of bloody urine in drops with vesical tenesmus; retention of stool; no appetite; great thirst; fever with evening exacerbation; but little sleep, and if he falls asleep is restless and disturbed by frightful dreams; violent jerks through body awake him frequently.

|| Twitchings of limbs and muscles.

|| Chorea-like twitching; skin red, hard, itching, < from scratching; great anguish.

|| Chorea with pruritus vulvæ with intense itching, redness and hardness.

| Chorea caused by a cold bath, getting drenched or after repression of measles.

|| Epilepsy after childbirth, brought on by a fall immediately before delivery.

87 **Sleep.** || Spasmodic yawning, yet not sleepy, with stitching and pain as from dislocation of jaw.

| Great sleepiness and lassitude after eating.

▮Heavy sleep, as from stupor.

▮Somnolence with snoring, muttering and grasping at flocks.

When intoxicated with beer, sleeps with mouth open and head thrown back.

▮▮Restless at night, has to change position frequently.

At night it seemed as if something forced him out of bed.

After midnight, restless slumber filled with fretful, disagreeable thoughts and events.

▮Restless sleep, with tossing about, raising and throwing off covers.

Was unable to sleep after 3 A.M., rose very anxious, restless and weak, constantly trembled, especially in knees.

Unable to fall asleep after 3 A.M., but after awhile fell asleep and then dreamed very vividly and on awaking it seemed as if he had not slept.

No sound sleep after midnight; she tossed about uneasily on account of a distressing sensation as if whole body were burning, without thirst; with dreams full of anxious agitations.

She did not sleep for half the night, was despondent, apprehensive and full of anguish about the heart.

▮Sleepless for four nights; she could not remain in bed.

▮Sleeplessness: from pain, more before 12 P.M., must turn often to find any ease.

As soon as he wished to fall asleep his business came to him in anxious dreams.

Fearful dreams, for example, that the world was on fire, with palpitation on awaking.

▮▮Dreams of great exertion; rowing, swimming, walking, climbing or working hard.

38 **Time.** 3 A.M.: sleepless after.

4 A.M.: pain in shoulder and arm <.

Morning: as if intoxicated; headache <; tearing pain near eye <; lids agglutinated, photophobia and lachrymation; nosebleed; tongue coated; soreness in walls of abdomen; cough <; on rising, drawing and stitching pains in l. nipple through to scapula; anxious; after night's rest stiffness of wrist joints <; inclination to stretch leg and foot; feet painful as if sprained; crawling in feet while lying in bed and after rising; pain in heels; sweat.

9 A.M.: chill came on.

10 A.M.: drowsy, weary, with yawning.

All day: child lies with face resting on floor (ophthalmia).

During day: dry cough; anxious palpitation; tenacious expectoration.

1 P.M.: burning fever <.

2 P.M.: red flush all over body.

5 P.M.: paroxysms appear.

Twilight: anxiety, timidity <.

Evening: inclination to weep <; depression; eyes <; facial neuralgia <; biting itching of face <; toothache; oppression in stomach; hoarseness <; till midnight cough <; hacking cough; tension and short breath; pain in cervical muscles; pain in back; stiffness of wrist joints <; feet swell; stitches in soles of feet; fever < toward, creeping coldness all over; heat; chill <; fever commencing with a short chill; quartan fever in paroxysms.

7 P.M.: as if blood were running cold through veins; severe chill.

10 P.M.: jerking toothache.

Night: great apprehension; severe itching of scalp; crusta lactea <; pain in eyes <; iritis <; tearing pain near eye <; otalgia; sneezing;. nosebleed; delirium; biting itching of face; shooting toothache <; awoke with dryness in mouth; fever <; nausea <; colic <; involuntary stool; involuntary urination; pain in shoulders < toward 3 A.M.; menorrhagia <; oppression of chest; restless; sleepless from pain in shoulder; paralyzed sensation in arm; sciatica <; coxalgia <; restlessness of legs; tingling in tibiæ; itching of legs and feet; pain between shoulders and stretching of limbs during fever; rheumatic fevers <; general perspiration; itching of rash in joints <; itching <.

12 P.M.: rheumatism <.

About midnight: quotidian fever.

After midnight: cramps in calves; restless slumber; great restlessness; itching of rash <.

39 **Temperature and Weather.** Sensitiveness to cold open air.

Sufferings during raw, cold weather and the prevalence of northeasterly winds.

Sufferings after drinking cold water.

‖Bad consequences from getting wet, especially after being heated.

From cold bathing, convulsive twitches.

Heat: pain over crest of l. ilium >; sciatica >; gives general relief.

Exposed to heat: tearing pains in small of back.

Hot application: pain in eyes >; pain in teeth >; shooting toothache >; sciatica >.

Warm weather: swelling of feet.

Warmth: headache >; of bed, < sensitiveness of scalp; biting-itching of face; pain in jaw >; rheumatic pains between scapulæ >; coxalgia >; of stove > pains in hip joints; burning and itching of erysipelas; crusta lactea <.

Getting warm in bed: lumbar pain <.

Getting warm from exercise: sciatica >.

Feather bed: stiffness and pain in wrist joints <.

Whenever he puts his hands out of bed he is seized with a convulsive cough.

Uncovering body: influenza <; cough.

In house: melancholy, ill-humor, anxiety <; chilliness.

Open air: melancholy >; lachrymation; facial neuralgia <; during rain sudden paralysis of l. arm; walking, weakness; acrid lachrymation.

Change of weather: stiffness of wrist joints <.

Damp, stormy weather: pain in cranial bones <; conjunctivitis <; paralysis of muscles of eyeball from exposure to cold or wet; prolapsus <; uterine complaints; paralytic feeling in arms <; rheumatism <.

Before a storm: inflammatory rheumatism <.

Putting hands in hot or cold water: eruptions on limbs <.

Exposure to wet: tearing pain in region of kidney; œdema of face and feet; burning and sticking in skin.

From getting wet: causes pain in l. temple; liability of taking cold; iritis; conjunctivitis; arthritic ophthalmia; colic <; urine voided slowly; amenorrhœa; amenia; difficult breathing and pain; pneumonia; spinal irritation; spinal membranes inflamed; pain in shoulder and arm; terrible pains in lower extremities; paroxysmal pains in legs; paresis of limbs; paralysis; erysipelatous inflammation.

Washing in cold water: pain in wrist joint.

Getting chilled: from sea bath, polypus of uterus; on a long journey, legs become weak and stiff.

Lying on damp ground: paralysis.

Marching through moist ground with bare feet: diarrhœa.

Cold or dampness: mydriasis; ptosis; influenza; rheumatic pain between scapulæ; tearing in shoulder; pain in wrist; sciatica; coxalgia; swelling of finger joints; erysipelatous inflammation <; urticaria <.

Exposure to cold: eczema rubrum itches and burns; inflammatory rheumatism; erysipelatous inflammation <.

Cold air: pains in eyelid <.

Cold drinks: desire for; vomits water immediately.

Cold application: of hand, toothache >; shooting toothache <.

Ice-water: causes pain in stomach and nausea.

After exposure to snowstorm when overheated: rheumatism.

East wind: < paralytic feeling in arms and weakness.
In Autumn: dragging pains in hip joints.
In Winter: inflammatory rheumatism <.

40 **Fever.** ▮Chilliness: in house, toward evening, creeping coldness all over; and heat in evening, face seemed very hot, though cheeks were cold to touch, and pale, breath hot; in back and head, heat on anterior part of body; as if cold water were poured over him, or as if blood were running cold through veins, 7 P.M., feels cold when he moves.

▮Chill: over back, < evenings; with pains in limbs, restlessness; face pale, or alternating red and pale; begins in the legs, usually in thighs, or between scapulæ.

▮Shuddering on moving or uncovering.

▮Sensation of internal coldness in limbs.

Coldness on l. tibia.

▮Stretching and pain in limbs, shivering over whole body, with much thirst, cold hands, heat and redness of face.

▮Shivering, heat and perspiration over body at same time.

‖Severe chill at 7 P.M., as if dashed with ice-cold water, or as if blood were running cold through vessels; cold when he moves; < eating and drinking; became hot by lying down and covering up; pain between shoulders and stretching of limbs during fever at night, sweat in morning.

▮▮Cough during chill; dry, teasing, fatiguing.

‖Great restlessness during chill.

During chill, pains in limbs, and during fever twitchings.

▮Chill increased by drinking.

▮Heat: with great thirst; after the chill, with sweat which relieves; general, as from hot water, or hot blood running through veins; general, with slight chills during motion, face livid; urticaria breaks out over whole body, with violent itching, < by rubbing.

▮During fever, nettlerash; thirst, drinking little and often.

▮Drowsy, weary, with yawning; 10 A.M. excessive heat, without thirst.

▮Evening fever, with diarrhœa.

Sweat: with pains, often with violent trembling; even during heat, except on face; with violent itching of eruption; sour; musty, putrid; with or without thirst; from warm drinks; profuse in morning; profuse, odorless, not exhausting; general, except on head.

▮▮During sweat: sleep; urticaria passes off with violent itching.

▮Night sweat, with miliary itching eruption.

▮Suppressed foot sweat.

Checked perspiration by rain or dampness, when patient

has become warm from exercise and has been in a free perspiration.

▮Dry, teasing, fatiguing cough, coming on sometimes hours before, and continuing during chill. θAgue.

‖Chill comes on about 9 A.M.; during chill seemed almost frantic, frequently changing his position in bed, groaning and complaining of intense drawing, tearing, crampy pains in muscles of both hips running down posterior thighs to calves of legs; fever intensely high, pulse accelerated but weak, face and whole body red; slight thirst during both chill and fever, most during chill; fever followed by sweat and headache. θAgue.

‖Fever commencing with a short chill in evening; every day the chill and heat being mixed up at the commencement, the fever continuing during the night with restlessness and tossing about in bed and a profuse sour sweat toward morning; prostration, great weakness, loss of appetite, vomiting and inability to take food during day. θIntermittent fever.

‖Chill every morning, 3 A.M., beginning in r. thigh, and thence spreading over whole body; during chill, dry, hacking cough; immediately after chill, vomiting followed by fever; during fever, thirst; no sweat; great exhaustion. θAgue.

‖Paroxysms appear about 5 P.M., preceded by great yawning and pain in the maxillary joint, as if dislocated; chill long and severe, with shivering and chattering of teeth; during chill pain in small of back, as if bruised, compelling him to change position constantly, also peculiar drawing in arms, with formication and numbness of fingers; heat great, with great dryness of lips and mouth, but lies quietly, without drinking, in a half stupid condition; answers questions slowly and despondingly; there also occur regularly two or three diarrhœic stools with some colic; passes night in sleep, disturbed only by thirst and sweat; spleen enlarged. θQuotidian ague.

‖Ague: double tertian; diarrhœa during day of paroxysm; high fever with lassitude and somnolence; spleen enlarged; loss of appetite; constipation; had taken much Quinine.

‖First chill at 5 A.M., second at 6 A.M.; with chill pain in limbs, great restlessness and stretching; fever with thirst, drinks little but often; colic, diarrhœa; great nausea and vomiting of bile; during fever, nettlerash. θAgue.

‖Chills coming on every afternoon, followed by heat and then sweat; dry, racking cough during chill. θAgue.

‖Quartan fever: paroxysm came on in evening, with predominating chill; much thirst during chill and heat: throbbing pain in forehead before and after heat; chronic miliary eruption on back of l. hand.

|| Chill 7 P.M., very cold even to shaking, fever and sweat in regular succession; no thirst. θAgue.

|| Quotidian fever about midnight, with pressure and swelling at pit of stomach and anxious palpitation during day.

|| First headache (throbbing in temples), afterward chilliness with thirst and tearing pains in limbs as from fatigue; afterward general warmth, with slight chills during motion and livid face; finally profuse, sour-smelling perspiration.

|| Tertian fever with nettlerash, which disappears after attack; during apyrexia burning and redness of sclerotica.

|| Ague commencing in r. side (first arm, then leg gets cold).

▮ Hydroa on upper lip. θAgue.

▮ Rheumatic fevers prevalent and characterized by drawing, tearing pains in limbs; < at night, with constant change of position, < lying on back; lame feeling in lower extremities; frequent desire to urinate; fever < at night; vertigo, occipital pain; tension in nape of neck and between shoulders; diarrhœa; erysipelas bullosum.

▮▮ Slow fevers; tongue dry and brown, or red as if it had been skinned; sordes on teeth; bowels loose; great weakness; powerlessness of lower limbs, can hardly draw them up; great restlessness after midnight; must move often to get relief.

▮▮ Acute diseases take on a typhoid form. θDysentery. θPeritonitis. θPneumonia. θScarlatina. θDiphtheria.

|| For nine days great weakness and mental dejection; loss of appetite; vertigo; confusion of head; sleeplessness; attacks of fever returning every afternoon, consisting of coldness, followed by heat lasting for a long time and abundant sweat; delirium at night of eighth day; on ninth day fever; face red; tongue dry, red; breathing quickened, sharp; pulse 88; abdomen slightly tympanitic; spleen enlarged, reaching to anterior border of ribs; no stool for three days; urine scanty, turbid; skin moist; several small red spots on chest, disappearing on pressure of finger; vertigo; roaring in ears; confusion and heat of head; pressive pain in region of forehead; dryness of mouth and throat; pappy, bitter taste; loss of appetite; great thirst; abdomen painful to touch; feeling of great

weakness; general feeling of illness; sleeplessness on account of many and perplexing dreams, occurring at moment he falls asleep. θTyphoid fever.

‖ Shivering followed by heat; feels himself very ill; pressive pain in occiput; weariness and aching in all the limbs; want of sleep; on third day temperature, especially of head, elevated; skin bedewed with perspiration; face very red; tunica albuginea of a yellowish color; lips dry; tongue dry and coated; voice rough and hoarse; some small red spots on chest, disappearing under pressure of finger, and some small pustules; respiration quicker, sharper; an occasional dry cough; heart normal, pulse 108; abdomen tympanitic; spleen reaching nearly to anterior border of ribs; stools liquid; is uneasy; reflects with difficulty; answers very slowly but correctly; complains of a feeling of great prostration and debility; sleeplessness and dreamy doziness; aching of whole body; oppression of chest and slight burning behind sternum; inclination to cough; abdomen sensitive to touch. θTyphoid fever.

‖ Typhoid fever: patient is of a mild temperament; delirium mild and not violent; at times may exhibit a disposition to jump out of bed or try to escape, but when more or less conscious, manifests little petulance or irritability; mental or physical restlessness, constantly tosses about bed, first lying on one side then on other, one moment sitting up, the next lying down; or, at beginning of disease, wants to lie perfectly quiet on account of the great weakness, feels completely prostrated, is indifferent to everything, this sense of debility is out of proportion to all other symptoms; hallucinations; fears he will be poisoned, refuses medicine and food; as the stupor progresses, he answers very slowly, reluctantly, or petulantly, but is not violent; violent headache, as of a board strapped to forehead, often associated with rush of blood to head and sudden flushing of face; epistaxis, which relieves headache, blood dark; pneumonic cough, dyspnœa, rust-colored sputum; tongue dark-brown, dry, cracked, cracks gape considerably and even bleed at times; sometimes tongue and mouth are covered with a brownish tenacious mucus; at other times tongue takes imprint of teeth; tongue shows a triangular red tip; disturbance of stomach and bowels; diarrhœa with yellowish-brown stools of cadaverous odor; involuntary stool during sleep; urine escapes involuntarily, and sometimes leaves a reddish stain; tearing pains in limbs with almost intolerable backache; if he falls asleep he is restless and dreams of roaming over fields and undertaking arduous labors; sometimes dreams of business of day, surface of body dry and hot and often redder than natural; red spots on skin; if he has sweat, it is copious and sour-smelling and is accompanied by a miliary rash; abdomen tympanitic; r. iliac region and region of spleen especially sensitive; spleen swollen; stools scanty and greenish, unattended by tenesmus; in women uterine hemorrhages may appear, but give no relief to symptoms; symptoms of pulmonary congestion appear; râles all through chest; lower lobes especially affected; cough at first dry, then more frequent and loose, with expectoration of blood-streaked sputa.

41 **Attacks, Periodicity.** Periodical attacks: of headache; profuse bleeding from anus.

Alternating: stool and constipation; red and pale face.

Every few minutes: changes position of leg on account of pain.

Daily: for three months pain in temple and orbital region; thin stools eight or ten times; chill and heat mixed at commencement.

Every morning 3 A.M.: chill.

From morning till 5 P.M.: headache.

Every afternoon: attacks of fever.

Nightly: diarrhœa.

For four whole nights: sleepless.

For several successive nights: awoke after one hour's sleep with pain in l. temporal region.

For twenty-four hours: neither speaks, eats, nor drinks.

Between 4 and 6 P.M.: thin stools.

5 to 7 P.M.: pain in eye <.

From 10 P.M. to 6 A.M.: inflammatory rheumatism lasts.

For six days: swelling on l. lower lid.

Every 3, 5 or 7 days: bowels moved.

For nine days: great weakness and mental dejection.

Every week: paroxysm of headache.

For three weeks: lumbar pain.

Every few weeks: sciatica.

For a month: sweat in second sleep.

For six weeks: could not touch foot to ground on account of sprain.

For six months: stiff wrist joints.

Every year on 13th of May: seized with burning itching of skin, lasting twenty-four hours.

For six years: has not worked on account of weakness in arms.

For twelve years: sciatica.

42 **Locality and Direction.** Right: pressure in temple above and behind orbit; burning pain in eye; ophthalmia; œdematous swelling around eye; conjunctivitis granulosa; burning in canthus; upper lid swollen; pain in eyeball; biting in eye; inflammation of eye; ptosis of eyelid; side of face covered with vesicles; side of face covered with thick crust; lid of eye red, swollen; inflammation of tonsil; tonsil covered with yellow membrane; pain in hypochondriac region; like a knife in abdomen; side of abdomen very tense; stitches below ribs; side, an inch below navel, sensitive spot; metastasis of mumps to testicle; pains in ovarian region; pain in limb; catching pains in chest; bronchophony; acute pain in chest; erysipelas on dorsum of hand; side of lumbar vertebræ as if bruised; pain in wrist; pain in nates; tension in hip; sciatica; tearing from tuberosity of ischium spreading over thigh, knee and leg; coxalgia in hip joint; rectus cruris muscle very sensitive; jerking and tearing in thigh; pulling and tension in tendons on inner side of knee; crawling with tension in tendons on inner side of knee; fluctuating swelling of knee; stitches just below knee; eruption like a band around ankle; deadness and numbness of lower part of foot; paralysis of side; constant pain in side; chill begins in thigh, ague commencing in arm and leg; zona, pain going down leg.

Left: pain in temple and orbital region; nostril excoriated; eye felt enormously swollen; phlyctenules on edge of cornea; conjunctiva red and studded with small ulcers; ulcers on cornea; eruption on lower lid; swelling on lower lid; lobule of ear swollen; parotitis; hot, burning beneath nostril; mumps; pressive drawing in hypochondrium; coldness and numbness of foot and arm; terrific pain in shoulder; pain in nipple through to shoulder; stitches in side; numbness of arm; fluttering sensation in chest; lameness and aching in arm; hard swelling on side of neck; shoulder seems paralyzed; pain over crest of ileum; as if some one were pressing upon shoulder; rheumatic pain in shoulder and arm; severe pain in top of shoulder; shooting and throbbing in shoulder; pain in muscle of shoulder: strain of shoulder joint; paralyzed sensation in arm; sticking and drawing in arm down to finger tips; as if muscles of upper arm were strained; numbness and aching in arm; sudden paralysis of arm, wrist as if it had been sprained; tension in hip; acute pain in hip; in whole lower limb; tension in thigh; tearing in muscles of thigh; acute rheumatism in knee joint;

erysipelas on leg; tibia cold; chronic miliary eruption on back of hand; felt a shock in external orbital integuments; excoriation at inner side of nates: skin peeled from hand entirely; wheals more numerous on index finger; on thigh there is a round elevated red blotch; enlargement of parotid.

Right to l.: erysipelas travels.

Left to r.: vesicular erysipelas of scalp; erysipelas in face.

From front to back: pain in head.

From within outward: stitching in knee.

43 **Sensations.** As if intoxicated; as of a weight behind r. orbit; as if she were going to fall forward or backward; as of a board strapped across forehead; brain as if loaded; as if brain were torn; as if muscles in back of head were screwed together; back as if sprained; as if occipital tissues were screwed together; as of a veil before eyes; as if it were difficult to move lids; as if jaw would break; as if teeth were being torn out; teeth feel too long and too loose; as if asleep; as if pharynx were inactive or paralyzed; stomach as if overloaded; as of a stone in stomach; as if pit of stomach were swollen or drawn together; hypochondriac region and abdomen as if beaten; as of a knife in r. abdomen; as if something were torn loose in abdomen; as if a lump lay like a pressing heavy weight in abdomen; limb as if constricted; feet and ankles as if asleep; as if one side of rectum had grown up; as if everything would come out of rectum; shoulders as if sprained; as if head were swelling out; as if something would be torn out of chest; as if breath were stopped at pit of stomach; as if not able to draw a long breath; as if shoulder would fly to pieces; as if air became imprisoned in epigastrium; as if sternum were pressed inward; as if cervical muscles were asleep; as if one had been lying in an uncomfortable position; as if bruised in r. side of lumbar vertebræ and in small of back; as if flesh of small of back had been beaten; as if back were broken; as if some one were pressing upon l. shoulder; as if arms were luxated; as if muscles and tendons of l. upper arm were unduly strained; as of sand in eyes; as if wrist had been sprained; as if hand were held in hot water; hand as if lame; hand dry, as if withered; as if pins were pricking point and palmar surfaces of first phalanges of fingers; finger tips as if asleep; as if something would burst in chest; hip, knee, or ankle joint as if sprained; as if skin around diseased parts were too tight; r. rectus cruris muscle as if bruised; as if tendons of limb were too

short; as if knee were too short; as if hamstrings were too short; legs as if made of wood; lower part of r. foot as if made of wood; feet as if sprained or wrenched; heels as stepping upon pins; as if running nails under skin in heels; as if walking upon needles; as of a hundredweight on nape of neck; as of a trembling in arms and legs; joints as if bruised; as if sinking through bed; as if bones ached; as if jaw were dislocated; as if something forced him out of bed; as if whole body were burning; as if cold water were poured over him; as if blood were running cold through veins; as if maxillary joints were dislocated; as if back were bruised; as if tongue had been skinned; as of a board strapped to forehead; as if flesh were torn loose from bones, or as if bones were being scraped; pains as if sprained in outer parts; as if inner parts were grown together; as if something in inner parts were torn loose; face and hands as if covered with suggillations.

Pain: in l. temple and orbital region; in back part of head; in eyes; in r. eyeball; in temporal region of l. side, thence to head, cheeks and teeth; in maxillary joints; in back of neck; in back; in stomach; in region of ascending colon; in abdomen; in glans penis; in r. limb; in lower part of chest; in l. shoulder and arm; in heart; in cervical muscles; in shoulder and back; between shoulders on swallowing; in muscles of l. shoulder and arm, also in bones of arm; in r. wrist; in hips; down thighs; in streaks down limbs with every evacuation; under knee-pan; in l. knee joint; in inner, lower and posterior part of calf of leg; in heels; in jaw; about umbilicus.

Terrific pain: in l. shoulder.

Terrible pains: in lower extremities.

Violent pain: in abdomen; in lumbar region; in head; in l. leg.

Intense pain: in l. leg.

Acute pain: in r. side of chest; in middle anterior portion of fourth intercostal space, l. side; in small of back; in middle finger of r. hand; in r. hip; in ankle joints.

Great pain: in small of back.

Severe pain: in jaw; in r. hypochondriac region; over crest of ileum; at top of l. shoulder; at phalanges of several fingers; sudden, at insertion of ligamentum patellæ into tibia.

Sharp pain: in eye; from eyes into head; in heels.

Tearing: at small of back; in periosteum of cranial

bones; in neighborhood of diseased eye; in region of brows and malar bones; in face; in teeth; down thighs, in region of kidneys; in chest; in shoulder joint and on top of scapula; in shoulder; violent, in arm; from elbow joint into wrist; in joints of all fingers; from hip to knee; from r. ischium following sciatic nerve in r. thigh; in middle of outer portion of thigh; in muscles of l. thigh; in knee and in ankle.

Bursting pain: in head.

Deep cutting pains: in leg.

Lancinating pain: in l. leg.

Beating pain: in limbs; in temple.

Darting pains: in ulcers.

Jerking pain: in teeth; in abdomen; in elbow and wrist joints; in r. thigh.

Catching pains: in r. side of chest.

Throbbing: in temples; from teeth into temples and jaws; violent, in epigastric region; in l. shoulder; centrifugally in inflamed integuments of face and forehead.

Digging pain: in glands beneath angle of lower jaw.

Gnawing pain: in swelling of knee.

Ulcerative pain: in pit of stomach.

Laborlike pains: in abdomen.

Shooting pain: in teeth; in eyelid; up rectum; through head; in l. shoulder; through arms; in leg.

Stupefying pain: in head.

Stitches: in head to ears, root of nose and malar bones; in eyes and temples; below r. ribs; in stomach; in chest and sides of chest; in l. side; in heart; in shoulders; just below r. knee; in soles of feet; in joints.

Stitching pains: in throat; in l. nipple through to scapula; on dorsum of r. hand; in heels.

Drawing stitches: in arm.

Pressive stitches: in back.

A stitch: across knee; in hamstrings just above calves.

Stinging pain: in leg.

Sticking pain: in throat; in vagina; in chest; in l. side; in back; in l. arm; in fingers; in side of knee.

Constrictive pain: in dorsal muscles.

Bruised pain: in head; in throat; in limb.

Burning pain: in knee joints and lower extremities; in corns; of sclerotica; in eruption around mouth and nose.

Drawing pains: in cheek and head; in limbs; in region of brows and malar bones; in face; in l. nipple through to scapula; in l. arm; cramplike, in elbow joint; from elbow joint into wrist; in palm of r. hand; in r. natis; in hips; from hip to knee in l. leg; in hip joints; paralytic, in whole foot; in arms.

Rheumatic pain: violent, between scapulæ; in l. shoulder and arm and in region of deltoid muscles; through wrist joints; in hands.

Pressing pain: in eyes; in stye; in glands beneath angle of jaw; in hip joints; in region of forehead; in occiput.

Dull pain: in occiput, vertex and forehead.

Tensive aching pains: in arms.

Aching: in occipital protuberances; in eyes; in articulation of r. lower jaw; in teeth; in glans penis; in bones; of l. arm; in elbow joint; in r. limb; in legs; in ankles and hollows of feet; of whole body.

Paroxysmal pains: in legs.

Cramplike pain: in articulation of jaw.

Cramp: in calves; in legs and feet.

Jerking: in thigh.

Stinging: in throat when swallowing; in tonsils; in stomach; on inner surface of prepuce; in ulcers; in skin.

Burning: in forehead; in eye; in and beneath eyes; in inner canthus, r. eye; in eyelid; in swollen lids; beneath nostril; in face; of eruption around mouth and nose; in whole r. side of abdomen; behind sternum; in small of back; in urethra; in stomach and between shoulder blades; in loins; in shoulder; in dorsum of r. hand; in palm of r. hand, forearm and hand; in l. leg; of skin; in pustules on chin; in ulcers.

Burning rawness: in larynx.

Burning itching: here and there; of skin.

Biting: in r. eye; in vulva; on lower lids.

Excoriation: feeling of, on inner side of l. natis.

Soreness: of head; of nostrils; of tongue; in abdomen; of navel; in walls of abdomen; in back and hypogastrium; of vagina; in chest; in l. side; of lumbar region; in corns.

Pricking: from teeth into jaws and temples; in swollen lids.

Prickling heat: in limbs.

Tenderness: of carpal articulation about knee joint.

Gnawing sensation: in teeth.

Dragging: of cardiac region; in muscles of l. thigh.

Pressive drawing: in l. hypochondrium.

Tingling: in head; in limbs; in stomach; in chest; of feet; in tibia; in limbs; in skin.

Tickling: in throat; in air passages; in bronchia; under sternum.

Pressure: at heart; behind eyes; in r. temple; on chest and about heart; in throat when swallowing; in rectum; in abdomen; in small of back; on shoulders; in eyes.

Tension: of face; across chest; in intercostal muscles; of neck; painful, between shoulder blades; in elbow joint; in r. hip; in l. hip joints; on posterior surface of thigh; of diseased limb; in tendons on inner side of r. knee; of knee; of calves; of feet; in joints; of nape of neck and between shoulders.

Constriction: in rectum.

Heaviness: of head; of lids; in small of back; of lower limbs; in hollows of knees and calves; of legs; of feet.

Fulness: of stomach.

Anxiety: in chest.

Oppression: in stomach; of chest.

Dryness: of mouth; of tongue; of throat; of gums; of eyes.

Restlessness: of lower limbs.

Pulsation: in pit of stomach.

Trembling: of arms; of knees.

Tremulous feeling: about heart.

Fluttering sensation: in stomach and l. chest.

Gurgling sensation: in heart region.

Swashing, jarring sensation: in brain.

Lameness: of l. arm; of sacrum; of leg.

Paralytic feeling: in arms; in l. shoulder; in anterior muscles of thighs.

Weakness: of lower limbs.

Weariness: of legs; of feet.

Stiffness: of lids; of jaws; in back of neck; of joints; in back and limbs; of cardiac region; of shoulder and back; in small of back; of sacrum; of forearms and fingers; in pelvic articulation; painful, of back; of knees and feet; in joints.

Numbness: of l. arm and foot; from hips to feet; in l. chest; of finger; of hands and fingers; from finger to elbow; of r. leg; of feet; of lower part of r. foot; in limbs; of fingers.

Deadness: of lower part of r. foot.

Crawling: in finger tips; from finger to elbow; of r. leg; in tendons of knees; in feet.

Biting, itching: on scalp, forehead, face and about mouth; of eruption on hand and face.

Itching: under scurfs on head; in eyes; of eruption around mouth and nose; inner surface of prepuce; of scrotum; in rectum; of eruption of arms and hands; intolerable, of legs and feet; of ulcers; of eruption on limbs; of urticaria; intolerable, of rash all over skin; of hairy parts; of small pimples; of eczema; of eruption about nipples, breast, back, chest, forehead, scalp and hair.

Chilliness: in back and head.

Coldness: of forearms, forehead and cheeks; of l. arm and foot; of larynx; of arm; of l. leg; of legs; all over internal of limbs.

44 **Tissues.** ||Acts on fibrous and muscular tissues.

▮▮Soreness and stiffness in muscles, pass off during any exercise.

▮▮Flesh of affected parts sore to touch.

▮▮Pain as if flesh were torn loose from bones; or as if the bones were being scraped.

▮▮Pains as if sprained in outer parts; disposition to sprain a part by lifting heavy weights, or stretching arms high up to reach things.

▮▮Inflammation of tendons of muscles, from overexertion or sudden wrenching as in case of a sprain.

▮Affections of ligaments, tendons and membranes, connected with joints.

▮▮Bad effects of getting wet, especially after being heated.

▮In inner parts sensation of fulness; or as if they were grown together (adhesion) or as if something in them were torn loose.

▮Dropsy, with turbid urine.

||Abdomen and legs greatly enlarged; from some points of legs water trickles down; appetite good, no thirst, passes little urine; after eating, pains in stomach; sensitive to cold, damp weather; preferred to lie propped up in bed.

||General dropsy; scrotum swollen, from prepuce there hung a long-shaped blister.

▮Dropsy resulting from amenorrhœa, caused by being drenched in rain.

▮▮Smooth, red and shining swellings, the inflamed skin being covered with small painful white vesicles.

▮Inflammatory swellings.

▮Cellulitis; accompanying diphtheria; orbital cellulitis with formation of pus.

▮Boils and abscesses.

||Child emaciated; covered with abscesses, most of them of a bloody character; child appeared as if it would shortly die.

▮Carbuncle, in beginning, when pains are intense, and the affected parts are dark red; if given early may abort whole trouble.

▮▮Glands swollen, hot, painful; indurated; suppurating.

▮Abscesses of axillary and parotid glands, swelling painful to touch, and discharging a bloody serous pus, with stinging and gnawing pains.

▮Scrofulous induration of glands of neck, nape of neck and lower jaw.

▮Prominent projections of bones, are sore to touch; as, for example, the cheek bones.

▮Inflammation and swelling of long bones.

▮Crusty caries, always combined with tetter, in rheumatic or gouty subjects.

▮Scrofulous and rickety affections.

45 **Touch. Passive Motion. Injuries.** Touch: head painful; cannot bear slightest, on eye; on sore spot below navel causes nausea; chest very sensitive; sensitive spot in spine; causes waterbrash; causes excruciating pain in back; scrofulosis and rachitis < ; stitch in hamstrings; stitches in limbs; abdomen sensitive; flesh of affected parts sore; abscesses of axillary and parotid glands painful; prominent projections of bones sore; eruption near corners of mouth on margin of lower lip sore; pustules on chin pain.

Pressure: pain in jaw > ; abdomen painful; pain in back > ; pain over crest of l. ileum > ; drawing pain in r. natis > ; hard, on hip and leg > pain; rectus cruris muscle sensitive; pain in eruption <.

Resting head upon arm: causes numbness of arm.

Rubbing: > sciatica; itching of urticaria < ; affected parts increases eruption.

Scratching: developed blisters from hives; itching < ; causes burning; causes an agonizing pleasure; causes smarting and itching of pimples.

Grasping and pinching: > pain in l. shoulder; pain in small of back as if flesh had been beaten.

Riding or jarring: affects injured hip.

Blows or sprains, etc.: cause chronic inflammation of articular structures.

After a sprain: pains in wrist from side to side.

A fall immediately before delivery: epilepsy.

Thrown from carriage: injured about hips and small of back.

Traumatic: erysipelas of lids.

46 **Skin.** ▮Intolerable itching; red, measly rash all over skin.

▮Itching all over, < on hairy parts; burning after scratching.

Violent burning in skin, twitching, general perspiration at night; whenever he puts his hands out of bed he is seized with a convulsive cough.

Burning itching here and there.

▮Stinging and tingling in skin, burning after scratching.

▮▮Burning itching eruptions.

▮Humidity of skin.

▮Rubbing affected parts increases eruption.

Red flush over whole body, at 2 P.M.

Covered from head to foot with a fine red vesicular rash, itching and burning terribly, especially in joints; < at night, causing constant scratching, with little or no relief, felt very hard upon pressure with finger; skin burning hot.

Some small pimples, coalescing into blisters the size of a split pea, filled with yellow watery fluid, with intense itching; < at night after 12 P.M.; the only relief he can get is to rub it with something rough until the blisters are open.

Numerous vesicles appear on different parts of body, varying from two or three lines to one-fourth inch in diameter; vesicles dry and disappear by desquamation.

A burning eruption of small blisters, filled with water, with redness of skin of whole body, except on scalp, palms of hands and soles of feet.

Vesicles, most of which contain a milky, but some of which also contain a clear liquid, become confluent; this condition lasts three days, after which the skin desquamates.

Clusters of vesicles, filled at first with a watery substance, near both corners of mouth on margin of lower lip, with a salty biting sensation, and soreness to touch.

Large blisters containing yellowish liquid, with swelling of arm; blisters were ruptured carelessly and the liquid flowed over whole arm, after which a very large number of vesicles appeared, so that after eight days whole forearm seemed to be one mass of blisters; anointing with olive oil seemed to have no effect upon the complaint; soon the upper arm and then r. arm and other parts of body became affected; whole trouble lasted four weeks.

An eruption of an erysipelatous nature upon face; the inflammation had extended over forehead and into scalp, both eyes were closed, both ears, cheeks and lips were very much tumefied and pitted on pressure, and the patient's features were so much disfigured that he was not at all recognizable.

Erysipelatoid eruption affecting hands and arms, feet and legs, face and sometimes the whole person; it varied in extent and in severity from a small patch, with trivial itching, to an extended surface with enormous swelling and excruciating suffering; pruritus, tingling, smarting, stinging burning were the sensations described; on a red and swollen base of inflamed skin, vesicles and blebs, from the size of a pin's head to a pea, were crowded together, and when these broke and dried, eczematous crusts remained; sufficient irritation carried the inflammation on to ulceration.

Bright redness of scrotum and penis; scrotum extremely flaccid and relaxed, falling half-way to knee.

After the lapse of about twenty-four hours, itching and burning commenced, lasting from half an hour to two hours; after about thirty-six hours, swelling of the parts, with violent itching and burning, increased on touching or moving parts affected, as if pierced by hot needles; white transparent vesicles appeared on the highly red and inflamed skin.

▮Erythema, rapidly progressing to vesication, often accompanied with œdema and with the final formation of pus and scabs; surface about eruption is red and angry-looking.

▮Eruption herpetic; with incessant itching, burning and tingling; alternates with pains in chest and dysenteric stools.

‖Scalp, abdomen, lower portion of chest and part of legs and back covered with a moist, burning, itching eruption, which eats into surrounding parts; large vesicles form which are filled with clear serum, later becoming turbid, which burst and become confluent.

‖After being poisoned while gathering blackberries; face presented a perfect picture of facial erysipelas of vesicular type; hands and forearms were covered with patches of vesicles.

▮Herpes zoster (shingles); burning and neuralgic pains after it.

▮Herpes preputialis and axillaris.

▮Pemphigus, each bulla with a red areola.

‖Erysipelatous swelling under eyes and red blotches over body.

▮Erysipelatous inflammation: hardness of skin, with thickening; urticaria; from getting wet; during rheumatism; with chills and fever; < in cold air; burning, drawing; tearing in face; teeth feel too long; restlessness; face dark red, covered with yellow vesicles; burning, itching and tingling with stinging; < in cold, open air, wet weather, getting wet, or damp, in cold places.

▮Vesicular erysipelas; scalp, face and genital organs particularly affected; affected parts dark red; inflammation travels from r. to left.

‖Capt. S., six years ago, kissed a child who had scarlatina, and felt it burn his lips; in a few weeks had boils on his back; after this was costive; once fainted, bruising his forehead; during faint had an involuntary stool; soon erysipelas appeared on bruised forehead, spreading over face, appearing on scrotum and penis, which suppurated; has had several attacks since, impairing his sight for near objects; felt a shock in l. external orbital integuments; about noon, red erysipelatous swelling began there, extending over whole face, neck and scrotum; vesicles form exuding a fluid which stains linen yellow; affected parts burn and itch; when lying at each beat of heart there is a throbbing centrifugally in inflamed integuments of face and forehead; any moisture to skin brings out erysipelas there, as it always did in those attacks; must scratch parts, which causes an "agonizing pleasure;" scratching of scrotum causes sexual pleasure and an escape of semen, which weakens him; photophobia; very restless all last night, no sleep; walking about stamping, shaking arms, and striking about; large yellow crusts from discharge on chin; eyelids closed from swelling; hands and feet cold; pulse 50, intermitting in volume and rhythm; burning and itching < from warmth.

|| Zona, r. side, pain going down to r. leg, < at night, necessitating constant change of position.

Cutaneous inflammation and feeling of excoriation at inner side of l. natis.

Scurfy eruption over body; fine scurf on face.

Back of hand is covered with cracks and is hot; skin hard, rough and stiff.

Epidermis peeled from cheeks, leaving parts hot and rough.

Skin peeled from l. hand entirely; intolerable itching; skin peeled from all parts affected.

▮▮ Eczema: surface raw, excoriated; thick crusts, oozing and offensive; if face is attacked there is œdema of loose cellular tissue about eyelids; burning, itching, tingling pains; incessant itching and scratching; the more they scratch the greater the urgency to scratch.

▮ Crusta lactea characterized by thick, heavy scabs, on an inflamed base, with much itching and restlessness, < at night and from becoming too warm; green slimy diarrhœa.

|| Very sore nipples after confinement and an itching, burning papular eruption about nipples on breast, neck, chest, forehead, scalp and hair; the itching kept just ahead of the scratching, disappearing and burning after, < during sweat; profuse sweat on exterior parts of body, but not on parts on which she lay; restless, continually sought new positions; > after moving about.

|| Forehead, face and particularly sides of neck, covered with red nodules, apices being filled with pus; severe burning.

Pimples like the itch, with burning itching and smarting after scratching, on inner surface of wrist, and on lower portion of cheek.

Hard pimples on hands, with burning-biting itching.

Pimples large, deep-seated and irritable to touch, on nates, especially on median line near os coccygis.

Tetter-like eruption around mouth and nose, at times with jerking and itching burning pain in it.

Pustules, with pus at tips on side of chin, with pain only when touched, as from pressure of a sharp edge and a persistent burning.

▮Pustulous eruption.

Black pustules, with inflammation and itching, rapidly spreading over whole body.

▮▮Urticaria from getting wet; during rheumatism; with chills and fever; < in cold air.

‖On the 13th of May, every year, for several years, had been seized with a burning itching of skin that drove her nearly to distraction; eruption so confluent not a healthy spot could be seen; eyes closed with œdema of lids; seemed suffocating and threw off bed coverings; whole paroxysm lasted twenty four hours. θUrticaria.

‖Upper and lower limbs and l. side of throat covered with hard, dark-red, circular elevated blotches, in groups and isolated; skin of affected parts tense and shining, while surrounding skin is swollen and shows an erysipelatous redness; the wheals are particularly numerous on l. index finger, dorsum of hand and forearm; on neck and l. thigh there is a round, elevated red blotch, around which larger and smaller patches were closely crowded; intolerable itching in affected parts, particularly on index finger; fine stitching pain in the eruption itself, produced or aggravated by pressure; patient appears depressed; eyes closed as in sleep; fever; skin moist; respirations increased, at times râles; cough not frequent, with tenacious expectoration during day; pulse 104; feeling of weakness; great heat of head; vertigo; nausea; vomiting; constant pain about umbilicus. θUrticaria.

‖Bluish red, lentil-sized spots over body, with lassitude and repeated hemorrhages from nose and mouth. θPurpura.

‖Face and hands appear as if covered with suggillations. θPurpura.

‖After catching cold, by exposure to rain, burning and sticking in skin, which began to swell up here and there, particularly on hands, arms and legs; bright red spots appear, of various shapes and sizes; rheumatic tearing pains in hip, particularly when at rest. θPurpura.

‖ Full of bluish dark blood, spots all over body except face and hands; bleeding from gums; ice-cold temperature; pale face and skin; small pulse.

| Carbuncles, bluish, gangrenous.

| Hardness of skin with thickening.

| Warts: especially on hands and fingers; large, jagged, often pedunculated, exuding moisture and bleeding readily.

‖ Rhagades, chaps; chilblains.

| Ulcers: as if gangrenous, arising from small vesicles, attended with violent fever; burning in them or sensation of coldness.

| Scarlatina: miliary, rash dark, fever high, drowsiness and restlessness; especially adynamic forms, child grows drowsy and restless; tongue red, sometimes smooth; fauces dark red and have a peculiar œdematous appearance, cervical glands enlarged, and there may be enlargement of l. parotid, there may even be impending suppuration of these parts; cellular tissue of neck inflamed, cutaneous surface having a dark-red or bluish erysipelatous hue; delirium, mild in character; secretions altered, acrid; glands in all parts of body may become enlarged, especially those of axillæ; emaciation; prostration; the rash itches violently and there is much restlessness at night; there is an ichorous or yellow, thick discharge from nose, with swelling of glands of throat; a bright edge of inflammation surrounds every portion of eruption, and there is much itching, particularly at night; cases complicated with erysipelatous inflammation.

‖ Skin dark red from head to foot and covered with small vesicles, containing a yellow pus-like fluid; burning heat; great thirst; sopor; starting and fright; restlessness; painful ineffectual urging to urinate; bowels constipated. θScarlatina.

‖ A child, æt. 13, threw a shawl, belonging to a child who had died of scarlet fever, over her shoulders; next day she had high fever; pulse 140; sore throat; vomiting; backache; next day rash appeared on neck and chest, extending gradually over body and becoming red, after pressure, from periphery to centre. θScarlet fever.

| Delirium, dry tongue, almost complete loss of sleep, repeated bilious vomiting, frequent diarrhœa, temperature of skin 40° C. θMeasles.

| Variola: eruption sinks and turns livid; typhoid symptoms.

| Smallpox: typhoid condition; eruption illy developed; livid; burning fever; extreme prostration; burning

thirst; roaring in ears; dry, cracked tongue; lips and teeth covered with tenacious brown mucus; meteoric distension of abdomen.

▮Variola: pustules turn black from effusion of blood within; diarrhœa, with dark, bloody stools.

[47] **Stages of Life, Constitution.** ▮▮Rheumatic diathesis.

Child, æt. 6 months, scrofulous; catarrhal ophthalmia.

Infant, æt. 8 months, badly nourished, afflicted with ascarides which had been relieved by *Podoph.;* abscesses.

Child, æt. 1½, has had hives; erysipelas.

Child, æt. 2, scrofulous, suffering since birth; eruption on head and ozæna.

Boy, æt. 2, suffering nine months; ague.

Boy, æt. 2; scarlet fever.

Boy, æt. 2½; ophthalmia erysipelatosa.

Boy, æt. 3, delicate, pale, head and face covered with an eruption, scrofulous; ophthalmia.

Girl, æt. 3, suffering one year; scrofulous ophthalmia.

Boy, æt. 3, stout, otherwise healthy; strumous ophthalmia.

Boy, æt. 4; scrofulous ophthalmia.

Girl, æt. 5, scrofulous; ophthalmia.

Lizzie B., æt. 5, healthy child from birth, trouble first noticed five days after birth; ptosis.

Child, æt. 5; scrofulous induration of glands.

Boy, æt. 6, several weeks ago fell down a high flight of steps; paralysis.

Boy, æt. 7; inflammation of knee joints.

Girl, æt. 8, ill ten days; meningitis.

Boy, æt. 8, strong, suffering since four weeks old; eruption.

Girl, æt. 9, scrofulous; ophthalmia.

Girl, æt. 10; diphtheria of lips.

Boy, æt. 10; five months ago fell while carrying a bundle of straw, since then suffering; lameness of leg.

Girl, æt. 12, slender, lymphatic, nervous, had rheumatic pains the year before; diphtheria.

Boy, æt. 12, suffering six months; ague.

Girl, æt. 13; affection of eye.

Girl, æt. 13, has curvature of spine; paralysis of lower portion of body.

Girl, æt. 13; scarlet fever.

Young woman, æt. 13½, on third day after a natural labor; paraplegia.

Boy, æt. 14; crusta lactea.

Boy, æt. 14, blonde, suffering four years; eruption on head and body.

Boy, æt. 14; dysentery.

Boy, æt. 15, from a violent sprain two months ago; swelling in elbow joint.

C. P., æt. 16, badly-nourished and overworked needle-girl; erythema nodosum.
Youth, æt. 17; ulceration of cornea.
Boy, æt. 17, after exposure to snowstorm while overheated two and a half years ago; rheumatic lameness.
Girl, æt. 18, small, lateral curvature of spine; mental disorder.
Girl, æt. 18, menstruation not yet established; influenza.
Girl, æt. 18, after nursing a person with typhoid fever; smallpox.
Girl, æt. 19, quiet, calm, strongly-built, blonde, rosy-cheeked; intestinal catarrh.
Man, æt. 19; measles.
Girl, æt. 19½; enteritis.
Laboring woman, æt. 20, brunette, fresh, rosy complexion, strained herself lifting shortly after first appearance of tumor, father had scirrhous tumor of groin; ovarian cyst.
Girl, æt. 20, blonde, caught cold year and a half ago, since then suffering; amenorrhœa.
Young woman, æt. 21; parotitis.
Man, æt. 23, weak, delicate, after typhoid fever; epistaxis.
Baker, æt. 23, of phthisical family, after severe labor in a damp cellar; swelling of knee.
Man, æt. 23, suffering twelve days; quotidian ague.
Mrs. E. D., æt. 24, colored, hysterical, hypochondriacal, suffering since puberty; dysmenorrhœa.
Miss M., æt. 24, slender form, lymphatic temperament, never in good health, suffering four years; injury to hip.
Miss E. H., æt. 24, blonde, clerk in a store, suffering three weeks; swelling of foot.
Artilleryman, æt. 24, small stature, full habit, brown hair; quartan ague.
Miss C., æt. 25; dysmenorrhœa.
Man, æt. 25, strong, caught cold by exposure to rain; purpura.
Mrs. H., æt. 26; boils.
Woman, æt. 28; rheumatic ophthalmia.
Tailor, æt. 28, suffering twelve years; sciatica.
Man, æt. 28; several years ago had ague, then smallpox; typhoid fever.
Woman, æt. 30, sanguineous temperament; inflammation of eye.
Man, æt. 30; œsophagitis.
Woman, æt. 30, thin, healthy, menses absent five years; pleuro-pneumonia.
Woman, æt. 30, married, two years ago sprained wrist, since then suffering; pain in wrist.

Woman, æt. 30, single; warts on hands.
Woman, æt. 30, colored, suffering five years; rheumatism.
Man, æt. 31, slender, muscular, dark complexion, after exposure; rheumatic lameness.
Man æt. 32, robust; erysipelas.
Man, æt. 32, fifteen years after an attack of syphilis; syphilitic rheumatism and formation of soft nodes.
Woman, æt. 33, negro, suffering five years; rheumatism.
Woman, æt. 35, rheumatic, after lifting heavy furniture; affection of back.
Man, æt. 35, sanguine, nervous temperament, suffering six months; sciatica.
Woman, æt. 35; erysipelas.
Man, æt. 36, lively, intellectual, active, brown complexion, black hair, sparkling black eyes; facial neuralgia.
Woman, æt. 36; œsophagitis.
Woman, æt. 36, single, blonde, delicate, irritable disposition, lives by needlework; abdominal inflammation.
Woman, æt. 36, poorly nourished, cachectic, six months pregnant; urinary difficulty.
Josefa Fluchà, æt. 36, married, born in Spain; cardiac neurosis.
Woman, æt, 37, medium height, corpulent, ill half year; hæmoptysis.
Man, æt. 37, professor, nervous temperament; loss of coordination in legs.
Lady, æt. 38, mother of six children; ague.
Woman, æt. 38, well built; urticaria.
Woman, æt. 40, hysterical; headache.
Woman, æt. 40; eruption on eyelid.
Man, æt. 40, suffering several months, had rheumatism previous to attack; diarrhœa.
Woman, æt. 40, brunette, slender figure, mother of many children, suffered six months; rheumatic pain and stiffness in wrist.
Man, æt. 40, sandy complexion, strong, athletic and vigorous constitution; strain of thumb.
Man, æt. 40, large, muscular, had former attacks, after walking fourteen miles; sciatica.
Man, æt. 40, suffering eight weeks; suppuration at knee joint.
Man, æt. 40, after severe wetting; pains in legs.
Woman, æt. 40, wife of clergyman, has had an attack annually for last seven years; urticaria.
Woman, æt. 40, Irish; eczema impetiginodes.
Man, æt. 41, strong and healthy, works in sugar factory and is exposed to great heat; Bright's disease.

Mrs. B., æt. 42, six years previously took a sea-bath and became chilled through and through, since then suffering; polypus of uterus.

Man, æt. 42; typhoid fever.

Man, æt. 43, small, dark complexion, weight 90 pounds, cabinet-maker, suffering eight or nine years; lameness of back.

Woman, æt. 43, suffering eighteen years; rheumatism.

Woman, æt. 44; paralysis of arm.

Woman, æt. 44, Irish, married, suffering four months; eczema rubrum.

Man, æt. 45; opacity of cornea.

Man, æt. 45, small, choleric temperament, nurse, after recovering from an attack of typhoid; paralysis agitans.

Man, æt. 45, strong, confined to bed last three months after exposure; pneumonia.

Man, æt. 46–49, tall, slender, muscular, dark complexion, leather manufacturer, suffering several years with rheumatism of l. arm, after exposure to rainstorm; rheumatism.

Lady, æt. 50; fear of being poisoned.

Woman, æt. 50, pale, emaciated, for years has had a slight hacking cough in Winter, strained back by lifting a heavy weight fortnight ago, since then suffering; lumbago.

Jewess, æt. 51; melancholia.

Woman, æt. 52, year and a half ago became chilled during a railway journey, since then suffering; rheumatic paralysis.

Woman, æt. 53, mild disposition, small stature; suffering two weeks; epistaxis.

Woman, æt. 55, strong, stout, subject to erysipelatous swellings of face, suffering ten days; erysipelas bullosum.

Man, æt. 55, farmer, strong, large, muscular, sufferer from sciatic rheumatism, which was contracted in the army 1862–63, would have severe attacks every few weeks, induced by overwork and exposure; sciatica.

Coachman, æt. 55, some years ago had a similar attack; rheumatic sciatica.

Man, æt. 56, cabinet-maker, athletic figure, otherwise always well, suffering eight months; sciatica.

Man, æt. 62, five years ago similarly affected; dropsy.

Woman, æt. 63; pneumonia.

Woman, æt. 64; sciatica.

Man, æt. 64; ague.

Man, æt. 66, tall, thin, delicate frame; facial neuralgia.

M. K., æt. 66, German, from exposure to cold; rheumatism.

Mrs. C. K., æt. 67, suffering several years; anasarca.

Lady, æt. 80, suffering five months; diarrhœa.

Young man, retired habits, affected with acne punctata, after exposure; influenza.

Mrs. C., sick for twenty years; affection of heart.

Bridge-builder, nervous temperament, suffering three weeks, caused by a strain; lumbago.

Woman, large, strong, suffering six months; burning in hand.

Stout phlegmatic man, frequently subject to attacks of rheumatic gout; gonagra.

48 **Relations.** Antidoted by *Bellad.*, *Bryon.*, *Camphor.*, *Coffea*, *Crot. tig.*, *Mercur.*, *Tenacet.*, *Sassaf.*, *Sulphur*, *Verbena hastata*, *Virginiana serpentaria.*

It antidotes: *Bryon.*, *Ranunculus*, *Rhodo.*, *Tart. em.*

Compatible: *Arnic.*, *Arsen.*, *Bryon.*, *Calc. ost.*, *Calc. phos.*, *Chamom.*, *Conium*, *Lach.*, *Phos. ac.*, *Pulsat.*, *Sulphur.*

Incompatible: *Apis.*

RHUS VENENATA. (Rhus Vernix.)

Poison Sumach. *Anacardiaceæ.*

Grows in swampy localities in Canada and the United States.

The tincture is prepared from the fresh leaves and bark.

Provings by Bute, Archiv für Hom., vol. 15, p. 179; Kunze, N. Zeit. für Klinik, vol. 12, p. 155; Burt, Am. Hom. Rev., vol. 5, p. 23; Oehme, N. E. Med. Gaz., vol. 1, p. 121; Butman, N. E. Med. Gaz., vol. 4, p. 200; McGeorge, H. M., vol. 7, p. 315.

Clinical Authorities.—*Sore mouth*, Burt, A. H. O., vol. 2, p. 66; *Ulceration of cervical glands*, Thomas, B. J. H., vol. 14, p. 350; *Swelling on wrist*, Thomas, B. J. H., vol. 14, p. 349; *Chronic rheumatism*, Thomas, B. J. H., vol. 16, p. 329; *Use in suppuration, etc.*, Thomas, B. J. H., vol. 14, p. 350; *Erythema nodosum*, Œhme, N. E. M. G., vol. 1, p. 152; Pfander, A. H. Z., vol. 108, p. 36; *Impetigo*, Œhme, N. E. M. G., vol. 1, p. 151; *Erysipelas*, Small, Raue's Rec., 1873, p. 240, from U. S. M. and S. Jour., vol. 7, p. 156; *Rhus poisoning* (2 cases), McGeorge, Hah. Mo., vol. 7, p. 322.

1 **Mind.** Great sadness, no desire to live, everything seems gloomy.

Inability, at times, to connect ideas; forgetfulness; dull and stupid feeling.

2 **Sensorium.** Vertigo; < in evening; intolerable heaviness of head.

3 **Inner Head.** Dull heavy, frontal headache, < walking and stooping.

4 **Outer Head.** ‖ Great swelling of head, face and hands, with sharp, irritating fever.

‖ Vesicular erysipelas of face and scalp.

5 **Sight and Eyes.** ‖ Eyes closed from great swelling of cellular tissue about them.

‖ Profuse lachrymation; constant dull, aching pains in eyeballs.

‖ Chronic inflammation of eyes.

6 **Hearing and Ears.** ▮ Vesicular inflammation of ears, exuding a yellow watery serum.

7 **Smell and Nose.** ▮ Erysipelatous redness of nose.

8 **Upper Face.** ▮ Nose and r. side of face much swollen, especially under r. eye.

▮ Face hot, itching and burning in different parts of face, especially l. cheek.

‖ Vesicular eruption about face and hands accompanied

by much swelling and an intolerable itching and burning. θErysipelas.

[9] **Lower Face.** Drawing pains in upper and lower jaw.

[10] **Teeth and Gums.** ||Red vesicular eruption on gums of upper incisors.

[11] **Taste and Tongue.** ||Scalded feeling of tongue, salty, flat, rough taste.

||Centre and base of tongue coated white, sides very red.

||Vesicles on under side of tongue, with a scalded feeling.

|Tongue red on tip, or red and cracked in middle.

Distress in root of tongue and fauces.

[12] **Inner Mouth.** ||Mucous membrane of mouth very red.

||Sore mouth; intense redness of mucous membrane of tongue, cheeks and fauces, with appearance of small vesicular points, accompanied by intense burning, as if mouth and throat had been scalded; this condition, if allowed to go on, seemed to extend wherever there was mucous membrane, even to rectum and vagina; several such attacks every year.

[13] **Throat.** Difficult deglutition.

[17] **Scrobiculum and Stomach.** ||Dyspepsia, with red tongue and tendency to erysipelas.

[19] **Abdomen.** Abdomen bloated and exceedingly painful to least pressure.

Constant rumbling and griping in bowels.

Constant dull pains in umbilicus, with rumbling in bowels, followed by a soft diarrhœic stool.

Pains < before stool, but an evacuation does not stop the pain.

Pains in umbilicus with dry, lumpy, dark-colored stools.

Intolerable itching and burning of anus; neuralgic pains in anus.

Pains in bowels < in morning.

[20] **Stool and Rectum.** Stool almost white, thin, papescent.

Large watery stool, passed with great force and attended with violent colicky pains, at 4 A.M.; during next two hours had three more profuse stools of this character.

[21] **Urinary Organs.** Burning in urethra.

[22] **Male Sexual Organs.** ||Scrotum much swollen, deep red, covered with vesicles.

[25] **Voice and Larynx. Trachea and Bronchia.** Dryness and pain in larynx; hoarseness.

[27] **Cough.** Harsh, dry cough, continuing for more than two weeks.

[28] **Inner Chest and Lungs.** Violent stitches through chest with great suddenness.

[30] **Outer Chest.** |Stiff neck or "crick in neck" and rheumatic pains between shoulders.

▮Lumbago from a strain or a cold.

31 **Neck and Back.** ||Ulceration of cervical glands, which discharged a very offensive, dark-colored pus; dark red areola around ulcers.

32 **Upper Limbs.** Paralytic drawing in r. arm, especially in wrist, extending to tips of fingers.

||Synovial swelling on wrist joint, of nine months' growth, large as a walnut, dark-colored, so as to look like a suppurating tumor; on holding to light it appeared translucent; not much pain.

33 **Lower Limbs.** Paralyzed and bruised sensation in legs.

Paralytic drawing, with pains in bones of l. leg.

Great weakness of knees and ankles; they ache constantly.

||Chronic rheumatism; pain centred in heel; is lame, walks with two sticks; great pain on first putting foot down to stand upon it; shooting pain in bone and sore pain in ball of foot; foot œdematous.

34 **Limbs in General.** Trembling of limbs with twitching of muscles.

35 **Rest. Position. Motion.** Stooping: frontal headache <.

When first putting down foot to stand upon it: great pain.

Walking: frontal headache <.

36 **Nerves.** ▮Great restlessness.

▮Lassitude; very weak and languid; stretching.

37 **Sleep.** Many dreams during sleep.

38 **Time.** Aggravation of all symptoms in morning after waking.

4 A.M.: large watery stools with pain <.

Morning: pain in bowels <.

Evening: vertigo <.

39 **Temperature and Weather.** Warm room: chills.

40 **Fever.** Chills: over whole body; run up back even when warm and in a warm room.

Intermittent without sweat.

▮Typhus and typhoid fevers.

41 **Attacks, Periodicity.** Intense itching periodically; returning every hour or two.

For more than two weeks: harsh, dry cough.

For nine months: a synovial swelling on wrist joint.

Every year: several attacks of sore mouth, burning of mucous membrane.

42 **Locality and Direction.** Right: side of face much swollen, especially under eye; paralytic drawing in arm; erythema nodosum below knee.

Left: itching and burning of cheek; pains in bones of leg; erythema nodosum on leg.

43 **Sensations.** As if mouth and throat had been scalded.

Pain: in bowels; in larynx; in bones of l. leg; in ankles, wrists and elbows.

Violent stitches: through chest.
Shooting pains: in bone of foot.
Neuralgic pains: of anus.
Rheumatic pains: between shoulders; in heel.
Drawing pains: in upper and lower jaw.
Griping: of bowels.
Colicky pains: in bowels.
Dull, aching pains: in eyeballs.
Dull, heavy pain: in forehead.
Dull pains: in umbilicus.
Aching: in knees and ankles.
Paralytic drawing: in r. arm; in l. leg.
Distress: in root of tongue and fauces.
Sore pain: in ball of foot.
Burning: in face; of mouth and throat; of anus; in urethra.
Bruised sensation: in legs.
Scalded feeling: of tongue.
Heaviness: of head.
Great weakness: of knees and ankles.
Trembling: of limbs.
Dryness: of larynx.
Itching: in face; of anus; under and about vesicles on forearms and hands of Rhus poisoning.

44 **Tissues.** Affects all parts of the body where bones are directly covered with the cutis and nothing more; back of fingers, forehead, etc.

Phagedenic ulcers of legs and arms, syphilitic or scrofulous, having a dark red blush.

▮Ulcerations of lymphatic glands; lymphatic abscesses.

45 **Touch. Passive Motion. Injuries.** Touch: erythema nodosum painful.

Pressure: abdomen exceedingly painful to least.

46 **Skin.** A fine white rash keeps under the skin.

▮▮Erythema nodosum: on r. leg below knee, seven such spots; on l. three, all in different stages, the largest one over two inches in diameter.

▮▮Erythema nodosum during an invasion of an attack of typhoid fever; pain in ankles, wrists and elbows, followed by an eruption of red patches, these also soon appear on anterior surface of thighs and forearms; these spots are painful to touch, new ones are constantly forming, some of which are bluish.

▮▮On forearms and hands, especially on r. side, little vesicles formed, the contents of which soon changed to pus, but as itching was very violent, they were almost always destroyed by scratching, before the transformation into pus was complete; these efflorescences were soon covered with thin, brownish, cracked, firmly adhering scabs, and increased in circumference; the largest was about six lines in diameter; under the scab is a sore, even with the skin and covered with a thin layer of pus; violent itching under and about the vesicles. θImpetigo.

‖Phlegmonous erysipelas.

▮Rhus tox. poisoning: eruption on face, hands, genitals and thighs; red and rough; scabs at corners of mouth; intolerable itching.

▮Ulcers, cuts and other lesions of skin surrounded by a miliary, whitish rash.

[47] **Stages of Life, Constitution.** Girl, æt. 5, during invasion of typhoid fever; erythema nodosum.

Boy, æt. 13; Rhus tox. poisoning.

Boy, æt. 16, suffering two years; ulceration of cervical glands.

Lady, æt. 22, suffering several weeks; impetigo.

Man, æt. 30, fifteen months ago had rheumatism in shoulders and arms, pain disappeared from these parts and became fixed in heel; chronic rheumatism.

Lady, æt. 38, lymphatic temperament; erysipelas.

Man, æt. 40; Rhus rad. poisoning.

[48] **Relations.** Antidoted by: *Phosphor.*, *Bryon.* Blue clay applied externally relieves itching and burning entirely.

Compare: *Anac.*, *Clematis*, *Comoclad.*, *Crot. tig.*, *Ranunculus*, *Rhus tox.*, *radicans* and *vernix*.

ROBINIA.

Locust. *Leguminosæ.*

The common locust tree, indigenous to the southern part of the United States.

The tincture is prepared from the fresh bark of the young twigs.

Provings by Burt, Am. Hom. Obs., 1864, p. 61; Spranger, Am. Hom. Obs., vol. 1, p. 271; Ball (poisoning), Am. Hom. Obs., 1865, vol. 2, p. 327; Houatt, Nouvelles Données, Paris, 1866.

Clinical Authorities.—*Headache*, Burt, A. H. O., vol. 1, p. 62; *Pain in stomach*, Burt, A. H. O., vol. 1. p. 62; *Pyrosis*, Peck, T. A. J. H., 1883, p. 676; *Sour stomach*, Burt, A. H. O., vol. 1, p. 62; Kippax, Org., vol. 3, p. 96; Smedley, A. H. O., vol. 5, p. 24; *Dyspepsia*, Blake, Hom. Rev., vol. 16, p 405; *Chronic affection of stomach*, Shafer, A. H. O., vol. 4, p. 277; *Ague*, Funk, A. H. O., vol. 3, p. 555.

1 **Mind.** ▮Very low-spirited; excessive irritability. θIndigestion.

2 **Sensorium.** Vertigo and dulness of head, in whatever posture it is placed.

Sensation as if brain revolved, especially when lying down.

Vertigo with unsteadiness and nausea.

3 **Inner Head.** Dull frontal headache; much < by motion, with neuralgic pains in temples; migraine.

Steady headache, with sensation as if head were full of boiling water, and when moving head sensation as if brain struck against skull.

▮Gastric headache from a sour stomach, caused by fat meat, gravies, flatulent food, cabbage, turnips, warm bread, pastry, ice cream, raw fruit, etc.

▮Sick-headache, with eructations and vomiting of excessively acid secretions; irritable and desponding.

▮▮Chronic sick-headache.

8 **Upper Face.** Neuralgic faceache, spreading to eyes, forehead, ears and teeth, changing the whole features; sensation of disarticulation and fracture of jawbone; l. side.

9 **Lower Face.** ▮Jawbone feels as if disarticulated; intensely sour taste and vomiting. θNeuralgia.

10 **Teeth and Gums.** Burning, lancinating pains, especially in carious teeth, spreading to cheeks, eyes and temples, < at night, or when coming in contact with food, especially cold or spiced food; teeth become loosened from the spongy and easily bleeding gums.

16 **Hiccough, Belching, Nausea and Vomiting.** ▮Heartburn and acidity of stomach, at night on lying down.

▮Regurgitation of acid and bitter substances, everything turning to acid.

‖Sour vomiting of infants; the whole child smells sour.

▮Nausea, with vomiting of intensely acid fluid. θMigraine

Water taken before eating, at night, returned in morning green and sour.

Vomiting of intensely sour fluid, setting the teeth on edge.

17 **Scrobiculum and Stomach.** ▮Heartburn and acidity of stomach at night on lying down.

▮Dull, heavy, aching distress in stomach.

‖Acidity of stomach; food turns sour soon after eating; constant feeling of weight, fulness and tension in stomach; eructations accompanied by a sour liquid, and at times portions of ingesta; burning pain in stomach and between scapulæ; thirst; constant frontal headache; water taken before retiring at night, returns in morning green and sour.

‖Constant dull headache, < by motion and reading; at times dull, heavy aching distress in stomach, with sensation as if scalded; sour stomach every night.

‖Intensely acid condition of stomach often occurring suddenly after taking food, however carefully selected; period between eating and onset of attack not constant; frequent acid, fluid and flatulent eructations, with slight temporary relief; feeling of distension and weight, like a stone, in epigastrium; nausea; palpitation; constipation; severe lancinating pains in epigastric, l. inframammary and l. infrascapular regions; pains of same character, though less severe, in l. side of head and l. extremities; integument of l. temple and side painfully sensitive to contact; pallor of face; shivering, with coldness of l. side, particularly of l. extremities, which were bluish around nails; temperature of r. side normal; then considerable heat of surface and flushed face; with establishment of reaction symptoms subsided; during attack great mental depression; an anxious longing for and expectation of speedy dissolution; at times sudden vanishing of ideas; occasionally very violent and often repeated acid vomiting so sour as to set teeth on edge; matter ejected frequently streaked with blood; after violent attack of vomiting there was entire cessation of pain for half an hour or longer; tongue slightly furred; appetite good; continued eating sometimes seemed to postpone attack; attack usually lasts several hours; suffering almost continuous for last fifteen years.

▮Constant, dull, heavy, squeezing pain in stomach after every meal, causing great distress and making her cry every day; stomach sour; constipation; much pain in lumbar region; obliged to keep her bed most of day; hands and feet very cold; cannot eat more than one meal a day, it puts her in such agony.

▮Fulness and oppression in pit of stomach; bitter, flat or foul taste, excessively acid eructations; long-continued nausea, finally > by vomiting, which is so fatiguing that it may cause fainting; constant inclination to stool, finally black, fetid stools, with great relief. θGastric derangement.

▮Dyspepsia manifesting itself at night and preventing sleep.

19 **Abdomen.** ▮Great distension of stomach and bowels, with flatus; intestines distended almost to point of rupturing, with severe colic and acid diarrhœa.

▮Flatulent colic and pinching in abdomen, corresponding to pains in head; severe colic, with ineffectual desire for stool; tympanitic colic, accompanied by great weakness and < from least motion.

20 **Stool and Rectum.** ▮Desire for stool, but only flatus passes; finally constipated stools; from indigestion.

▮Sour stools of infants, with sour smell from body, and vomiting of sour milk.

▮Diarrhœic stools, yellow, green, burning, with nervous agitation, weakness, cold sweat and dyspnœa.

▮Stools, loose, black, fetid, with great tenesmus.

▮Diarrhœic stools, black, fetid or watery, whitish, excessively frequent and generally involuntary, with sensation as if whole body would pass away with stool; heat and pressure in epigastrium; cramps in extremities; weakness and extreme prostration; acid dyspepsia; putrid emanations from body; suppression of urine; fear of death.

▮Cholera infantum; child smells intensely sour; stools green and watery; with much tympanitis; colic; accompanied by excessive irritability.

21 **Urinary Organs.** Urine scanty and painful; or profuse and turbid.

23 **Female Sexual Organs.** Nymphomania; whitish, greenish, yellowish, thick, acrid, purulent leucorrhœa, with tumefaction and bruised feeling in neck of womb and general prostration; ulcerative pains in vagina, with acrid yellowish leucorrhœa, of most fetid smell.

Hard swelling of womb.

Cramps in womb.

Menses too late; black.

Discharge of blood, like a hemorrhage, between menstrual periods accompanied by purulent leucorrhœa.

Eruption and ulcers like herpes on vagina and vulva.

35 **Rest. Position. Motion.** Lying down: as if brain revolved; heartburn and acidity of stomach.

In whatever position: vertigo and dulness of head.

Motion: dull frontal headache <; of head, as if brain struck against skull; colic <.

38 **Time.** Night: neuralgic pains in teeth and face <; heartburn and acidity of stomach; water taken before eating returned in morning green and sour; dyspepsia at night.

40 **Fever.** || Paroxysms every day, late in afternoon, lasting until 3 or 4 o'clock next morning; during attack entire loss of consciousness; flatulence, eructations; at last with emission of flatus the paroxysms gradually faded away; on third day of treatment, very severe paroxysm followed by collapse, eyes sunken, face hippocratic, rattling of mucus in throat and chest, threatened suffocation; *Carbo veg.* removed the most imminent danger; during next three days had three more attacks, also very severe; high fever with delirium, flatulence with unconsciousness, followed by great prostration, dulness and heaviness of head, distressing dreams when shutting eyes; flatulence seems to be chief cause of fever. θAgue.

|| Hectic fever, with night sweats.

41 **Attacks, Periodicity.** For several hours: attack of vomiting.

Every day: paroxysms of fever late in afternoon, lasting until 3 or 4 o'clock next morning.

Every night: sour stomach.

Last fifteen years: attacks of sour stomach and vomiting.

42 **Locality and Direction.** Right: temperature of side normal.

Left: sensation of disarticulation of jawbone; pain in inframammary, infrascapular regions and in side of head and extremities; integument of temple and side painfully sensitive to contact; coldness of side and extremities.

43 **Sensations.** As if brain revolved; as if head were full of boiling water; as if brain struck against skull; jawbone as if disarticulated; stomach as if scalded; as if whole body would pass away with stool.

Pain: in lumbar region.

Lancinating pains: severe in epigastric, l. inframammary and l. infrascapular regions; in l. side of head and l. extremities.

Burning-lancinating pain: in teeth and face.

Burning pain: in stomach and between scapulæ.
Ulcerative pains: in vagina.
Neuralgic pain: in temples; in face.
Pinching: in abdomen.
Dull, heavy, squeezing pain: in stomach.
Cramps: in extremities; in womb.
Dull, heavy, aching distress: in stomach.
Heat: in epigastrium.
Bruised feeling: in neck of womb.
Pressure: in epigastrium.
Weight: in stomach; in epigastrium.
Heaviness: of head.
Oppression: in pit of stomach.
Dulness: of head.
Tension: in stomach.
Fulness: in stomach; in pit of stomach.
Distension: in epigastrium.
Coldness: of l. side, l. extremities.

45 **Touch. Passive Motion. Injuries.** Contact: neuralgia in face < from food; integument of temple and side painfully sensitive.

47 **Stages of Life, Constitution.** Young man, suffering four months; acidity of stomach.

Miss L., æt. 26, temperament nervo-bilious, with a little of the lymphatic; menstruates every three weeks profusely; pains in stomach.

Mrs.——, æt. 45, dark eyes and hair, nervo-bilious temperament, mother of eight children; suffering since fourteen years old, attacks at first every Spring and Fall, continuing for about three months, for last fifteen years suffering almost continuous; pain in stomach, etc.

Man, æt. 45, suffering three years from enlargement of liver and sympathetic cough; ague.

48 **Relations.** Compare: *Bryon.*, *Cinchon.*, *Carbo veg.*, *Lycop.*, *Nux vom.*

RUMEX CRISPUS.

Yellow Dock. *Polygonaceæ.*

A native of Europe introduced into this country, where it grows wild in fields and waste places.

The tincture is prepared from the fresh root.

Provings by Houghton, Thesis, Hahn. Med. College of Penna., 1852; Joslin, Trans. Am. Inst., 1858.

The provers were E. M. K., H. M. Paine, Wm. E. Payne, Edw. Bayard, Wallace, Bowers and Rhees; Preston, U. S. J. of Hom., vol. 1, 1860; Wright, Am. Inst. of Hom., 1860.

Clinical Authorities.—*Pain in epigastrium*, Morgan, Hom. Cl., vol. 4, p. 137; *Gastralgia, Dyspepsia*, Joslin, Hom. Rev., vol. 2, p. 529; *Morning diarrhœa*, Preston, H. M., vol. 7, p. 139; *Diarrhœa*, Morrison, Hom. Rev., vol. 18, p. 687; Joslin, Hom. Rev., vol. 2, p. 529; Dunham, Hom. Rev., vol. 2, p. 533; Hale, Therap., p. 641; *Aphonia*, Shelton, Hom. Cl., vol. 3, p. 92; *Asthma*, Morgan, Hom. Cl., vol. 4, p. 137; *Catarrhal affections of larynx, trachea and bronchi*, Dunham, Hom. Rev., vol. 2, p. 530; *Cough*, Williamson, Raue's Rec., 1874, p. 133; Shelton, Hom. Cl., vol. 3, p. 91; Smith, A. H. Z., vol. 108, p. 190, from Hom. World, Dec., 1883; Hughes, B. J. H., vol. 23, p. 260; Joslin, Hom. Rev., vol. 2, p. 529; Dunham, Wells, Hom. Rev., vol. 2, pp. 534–5; *Cough* (during pregnancy), Wells, Hom. Rev., vol. 2, p. 535; Blake, Hom. Rev., vol. 16, p. 406; Berridge, Org., vol. 1, p. 437; Dunham, N. Y. S. Trans., 1876–7, p. 41; Farley, M. I., vol. 6, p. 404; Moore, M. I., vol. 6, p. 344; Tinker, Hale, Therap., p. 646; *Incipient phthisis*, Schmucker, N. Y. J. H., vol. 1, p. 372; *Pain in cardiac region*, Rhees, Hom. Rev., vol. 2, p. 535; *Prurigo*, Bernard, Hom. Rec., vol. 3, p. 152, from Pop. Zeit. Hom., No. 15, vol. 13; *Gastralgia*, Knowles (3 cases), N. E. M. G., vol. 14, p. 107.

1 **Mind.** Low-spirited: with serious expression of face; with suicidal mood.

Irritable; disinclined to mental exertion.

2 **Sensorium.** Dull feeling in head (with the cough).

3 **Inner Head.** Headache after waking in morning, preceded by a disagreeable dream.

Dull pains: on r. side; in occiput; in forehead, with bruised feeling, < on motion.

Darting pain, or sharp piercing, in l. side of head.

‖ Catarrhal headache, with great irritation of larynx and trachea, clavicular pain and soreness behind sternum.

5 **Sight and Eyes.** Pain in eyes as from dryness; lids inflamed, < in evening.

Sore feeling in eyes, without inflammation.

6 **Hearing and Ears.** Ringing in ears.

Itching deep in ears.

7 **Smell and Nose.** Great desire to pick nose.

▮Nose obstructed; dry sensation, even in posterior nares.

Sudden, sharp tingling sensation in Schneiderian membrane, followed by violent and rapid sneezing, five or six times in succession, with a watery discharge from nostrils.

▮Violent sneezing; with fluent coryza < in evening and at night.

▮Coryza: fluent, with sneezing; with headache; < evening and night.

Accumulation of mucus about posterior nares.

▮Yellow mucus discharged through posterior nares.

▮Epistaxis, violent sneezing and painful irritation of nostrils.

▮Influenza with violent catarrh, followed by bronchitis.

8 **Upper Face.** Heat of face: redness < evenings; dull headache; with pulsation over whole body.

11 **Taste and Tongue.** Bitter taste (morning).

Dry tongue and mouth; tongue feels as if burned.

Tongue coated: white; yellow; yellowish-brown or reddish-brown.

12 **Inner Mouth.** ǀǀUlceration of mouth and throat.

13 **Throat.** ▮Scraping in throat; excoriated feeling with secretion of mucus in upper part.

▮Sensation of a lump in throat, not > by hawking or swallowing, it descends on deglutition, but immediately returns.

▮Aching in pharynx, with collection of tough mucus in fauces.

▮Catarrhal affections of throat and fauces.

15 **Eating and Drinking.** After meals: flatulency; heaviness in stomach or epigastrium; aching in l. breast; pressure and distension in stomach.

16 **Hiccough, Belching, Nausea and Vomiting.** Nausea in night, before diarrhœa.

17 **Scrobiculum and Stomach.** Sensation of heaviness in epigastrium, immediately after eating.

Sensation as of a hard substance in pit of stomach.

Weight, pressure and distension in stomach after meals.

ǀǀFulness and pressure in pit of stomach extending toward throat pit; descends with every empty deglutition, but immediately returns.

▮Tight, suffocative, heavy ache in epigastrium, through to back; clothes seem too tight; weak feeling in epigastrium, all < when talking; frequently takes a long breath.

▮Shooting from pit of stomach to chest; sharp in l. chest; slight nausea; dull aching in forehead.

▮Aching and shooting in pit of stomach and above it on each side of sternum.

॥Distress in stomach pit, < after eating, especially apples; once after an apple such distress that she became cold and unconscious and seemed to be dying; at times sharp pains in chest and abdomen; at times very distressing sensation as of a bunch either in throat or behind sternum; emaciated; could scarcely find anything she could eat without distress.

॥Pain in pit of stomach; aching in l. chest; flatulence; eructations; pressure and distension in stomach after meals.

॥Aching in pit of stomach, and aching and shootings above it in chest, at, and especially on each side of lower end of sternum; after a cup of tea, in a man unaccustomed to its use.

॥Aching pain in pit of stomach, gradually becoming very severe; sharp stitching pains in stomach extending into chest, and below a sensation of pressure like a lump in pit of stomach, sometimes rising up under sternum, greatly < from motion and somewhat from taking a long breath; generally < after eating; > lying perfectly quiet.

॥Distress in stomach becoming so severe that she could not sit up; severe aching pains in stomach pit and above it; occasional spells of sharp shooting pains in chest, sides and abdomen; some headache and nausea after eating; all symptoms < from motion and eating; sensation as of a lump or pressure sometimes in throat, sometimes behind sternum.

॥Tight, suffocative, dull, heavy ache in epigastrium, through to back; clothes seem too tight; weak feeling in epigastrium; all < by talking; frequently obliged to get a long breath and to yawn, with watering of eyes; stitching pains in back of r. hip; limping walk.

18 **Hypochondria.** ▮Pain in hypochondrium from walking or deep inspiration.

19 **Abdomen.** Griping near navel, partially > by discharge of offensive flatus; flatulent colic soon after a meal.

Pain occurring, or < during deep inspiration.

Sensation of hardness and fulness in abdomen, with rumbling.

॥Pain in abdomen in morning, followed by a stool.

॥Colic from a cold, with cough.

20 **Stool and Rectum.** ▮Stools: painless, offensive, profuse; brown or black, thin or watery; preceded by pain in abdomen; before stool, sudden urging, driving him out of bed in morning.

▮Morning diarrhœa, with cough from tickling in throat pit.

‖Brown, watery diarrhœa, chiefly in morning, having five stools from 5 to 9 A.M., attended by moderate griping pain in lower part of abdomen; cough.

‖Diarrhœa every morning for four days; evacuations profuse, offensive and thin, even watery; cough excited by tickling in throat pit, usually dry; when expectoration occurs it is tasteless; cough shocks the stomach and is attended by a sensation of excoriation in chest; it keeps her awake at night.

‖Diarrhœa in morning; four evacuations between 6 and 10 A.M.; very thin, painless; nausea on movement in night preceding evacuation; mouth dry; tongue coated slightly yellow; day previous had dull pain on r. side of sternum, sharp pain on l.; during climaxis.

‖Serious attack of diarrhœa in an old man of 70, after failure of *Sulphur;* early morning aggravation; nausea; colic; tickling cough, < by cool air and talking.

Feces hard, tough, brown; costive.

Itching at anus with discharge of offensive flatus.

Sensation as from pressure of a stick in rectum.

21 **Urinary Organs.** Sudden urging.

Frequent inclination to urinate, with sensation as if urine could not long be retained.

Involuntary micturition, with cough.

Copious, colorless urine, in afternoon.

25 **Voice and Larynx. Trachea and Bronchia.** ▮Hoarseness, < evenings; voice uncertain.

Sudden change of voice at different times, or at same time on each day, or with cough.

▮Voice: higher, as with catarrh; nasal; hoarse, especially in evening.

▮Aphonia after exposure to cold.

‖Reflex aphonia due to infiltration of tubercle in apex of l. lung.

▮Catarrhal aphonia, with irritation in suprasternal fossa, exciting a distressing cough.

▮Tenacious mucus in throat or larynx, constant desire to hawk.

▮Hawking of mucus from larynx.

▮Desire to hawk phlegm, which is felt in larynx like moving to and fro, without succeeding; < in cold air; < at night.

‖Much tough mucus in larynx, with a constant cough and desire to raise it, but without relief; morning diarrhœa.

‖Tenacious mucus in throat or larynx; a constant desire to hawk; coughing and hawking < at night; scraping in throat; cough excited by tickling or irritation behind sternum; cough attended with pain in head; sudden change of voice at same hour on consecutive days; change of voice at different times.

Hawking of mucus from upper part of larynx and throat; with burning soreness; extending later to l. bronchus; renewed by a stronger exhalation or scraping.

|| Hawking of mucus from larynx, with burning soreness; voice hoarse, especially in evening; tickling in throat; coughing < by pressure on larynx; forced, barking cough, with soreness of larynx and chest.

|| Tickling in throat pit causing cough.

Violent irritation to cough in larynx while eating.

Pain in larynx: while eating; in top of larynx; mostly on l. side; with excoriating cough.

| Raw sensation in larynx, when coughing.

|| Acute catarrhal affections of larynx, trachea and bronchi; dry, frequent, continuous cough, in long paroxysms, or, under certain circumstances, almost uninterrupted, and out of proportion to degree of organic affection of mucous membrane; induced, or greatly < by any irregularity of respiration, such as a little deeper or more rapid inspiration than usual, by inspiration of air a little colder than that previously inhaled, by irregularity of respiration and irregular motions of larynx and trachea, such as are involved in the act of speech, and by external pressure upon trachea in region of suprasternal fossa; great irritability of mucous membrane of larynx and trachea; rawness and soreness in trachea, extending a short distance below suprasternal fossa and laterally into bronchi, chiefly l.; tickling in suprasternal fossa and behind sternum provokes cough; this tickling is very annoying and persistent and is often, but momentarily, and sometimes only partially, > by coughing; cough occurs chiefly, or is much < in evening after retiring, and at that time the membrane of trachea is particularly sensitive to cold air and to any irregularity in the flow of air over its surface, so that patient often covers head with bedclothes to avoid the cold air and refuses to speak or even listen to conversation, lest his attention should be withdrawn from the supervision of his respiratory acts, which he performs with the most careful uniformity and deliberation.

|| Has not been able to speak above a whisper for nearly three months; soreness in throat < during empty deglutition, but is not < by swallowing food; posterior surface of pharynx irritated and in places excoriated,

edges of soft palate and uvula red and swollen, and covered with an eruption of minute red pimples; slight hacking cough, produced by tickling in larynx and upper part of trachea; after taking cold.

26 **Respiration.** Frequent feeling as if she could not get another breath.

Sensation of breathlessness, as if air did not penetrate chest, or like what is felt when falling or passing very rapidly through air.

Breathing causes soreness behind sternum.

❚❚ Rattling in windpipe; frequent feeling as if she could not get another breath (compare *Apis*), coughing spells several times a day, lasting one and a half hours at a time and originating in a sense of great accumulation of tough mucus in chest, with increased dyspnœa and desire to cough it up, causing a general hot sweat half an hour before spell (increasing during it); cough very hard, with feeling of suffocation, reaching to epigastrium, as if tough phlegm must work up; severe soreness behind whole sternum, spreading to each side; constant but < during cough; much tough mucus is brought up during spell; during its continuance feels like killing herself in despair; afterward prostrate and tearful. θAsthma.

❚ Asthma of consumptives; aggravation 2 A.M.

27 **Cough.** ❚ Hoarse, barking cough; in attacks, every night at 11 P.M., and at 2 and 5 A.M. (children).

❚ Cough, with pain behind mid-sternum.

❚❚ Dry, incessant, fatiguing cough, caused by tickling in throat pit, extending to behind sternum and to stomach; soreness in larynx and behind sternum; rawness under clavicles; pain in stomach; stitches in l. lung; cough < from changing rooms, evening after lying down, touching or pressing throat pit, from slightest inhalation of cool air, covers head with bedclothes to make air warmer.

❚ Hawking with burning soreness in larynx; later in l. bronchus, renewed by strong exhalation and scraping.

Dry spasmodic cough, simulating early stage of whooping cough, at first dry, coming on in paroxysms preceded by tickling in throat pit, attended by congestion and slight pain in head and wrenching pains in r. side of chest; the most violent paroxysm began a few moments after lying down at night, usually at about 11 o'clock; this paroxysm lasted ten or fifteen minutes, after which he slept all night; a less severe paroxysm occurred in bed, in morning after waking, and at various times through day; after two weeks, expectoration of adhesive mucus in small quantities, detached with difficulty.

▮Hacking cough.

Pressure on throat causes cough.

Cough as soon as he turns on l. side.

▮The most violent cough occurs a few moments after lying down and at night; in some cases complete aphonia.

‖Severe cough, provoked by pressure on trachea, deep inspirations, inhalation of cold air and talking; cough severe, explosive and continuous, hurts the head, accompanied by involuntary micturition; < latter part of night.

‖Dry, tickling, spasmodic, cough, with tenderness in larynx and trachea, rendering cough quite painful.

▮▮Teasing, persistent cough, < in cool air, or by anything which increases the volume or rapidity of inspired air.

▮Dry, hacking, incessant, very fatiguing cough, excited by tickling in suprasternal fossa, extending downward to middle of sternum, with a sensation as if a feather were swaying to and fro in bronchi with respiration, causing a tickling which provokes cough.

‖Cough begins with tickling behind top of sternum and sometimes in paroxysms of five to ten minutes duration; trachea sore to outward pressure, feels excoriated through its whole extent, as do also the whole fauces; cough excited by pressure on throat pit; cough is violent with scanty, difficult expectoration, shocks head and chest, head as if it would fly into pieces and he feels as if he might raise blood any minute; greatly exhausted after the paroxysms of coughing; head aches during cough.

‖Dry cough; tickling in throat pit; continued desire to cough on breathing cold air, < after retiring to bed; obliged to cover mouth with bedclothes and use every effort to prevent coughing; occasional pains through both lungs extending up into trachea; feels weak and exhausted in morning; very frequently a rawness in throat in morning.

‖Is very nervous; confusion of head; hoarseness in evenings; cough; excoriation behind whole of sternum on coughing and on inspiration; coldness of fingers.

‖Cough originally produced by inhalation of extremely cold air during Winter; cough < lying down, and especially at 11 o'clock at night; excited by tickling behind sternum and attended by a sprainlike aching near sternum and with accumulation of mucus in fauces near posterior nares.

‖Cough about 11 P.M. when lying on l. side; awoke between 1 and 2 A.M. with cough in any position; it made the chest feel bruised and seemed as if it did not reach low enough down to raise the phlegm, and when it did loosen it, it caused soreness of chest; after catching cold from exposure to cold early morning air.

|| Severe cold for several days; pulse quick, not hard, 110, skin moderately hot and dry, face somewhat flushed; respiration embarrassed not so much by any constriction of chest as by violent and long-continued cough, which follows any attempt to make a full inspiration; physical examination of chest reveals nothing abnormal; roughness and soreness in lower part of trachea and behind upper third of sternum much more perceptible when she coughs; cough dry, slightly hoarse, very violent and fatiguing; it is provoked by a tickling in suprasternal fossa, is induced by pressure upon trachea in that region and especially by talking and by deep inspiration or by inspiration of cool air; this irritability of trachea increases very markedly after 7 P.M., so that she suffers exceedingly from the constant tickling and violent cough; she can prevent it only by respiring with great caution and deliberation, by avoiding all distractions of speech and conversation, and finally she draws bedclothes over head in order to avoid inhaling cool air of chamber.

|| Severe dry cough at times for several years; cough < in evening; unable to breathe the cold air of his bedroom and has a severe coughing spell in morning on rising and at times during day, especially on taking a deep inspiration; is thin and rather emaciated; has frequent night sweats; tickling in throat and at top of sternum; after coughing some time, rawness in throat of a very disagreeable character, extending from pharynx down beneath upper portion of sternum, accompanied by a burning sensation through upper lobes of both lungs (clavicular region), with loss of appetite and considerable prostration, on examination no indication of presence of tubercles.

|| Contracted cold in head, throat and lungs; cough hard, dry and explosive, provoked by tickling in throat, talking, deep inspiration, inhaling cold air, < in lying; hurts the head and is accompanied by involuntary micturition.

|| Contracted cold; cough dry, hoarse, barking, sounding like croup, accompanied by fever.

|| Constant dry, barking, spasmodic cough. θChronic pneumonia.

|| Cough originating in larynx, where loud mucous rat-

tling could be heard; returns every ten seconds during day, less frequent at night.

||Subject to eight miscarriages, all in early stage of pregnancy, which in each case was early attended by dry, shaking, spasmodic cough, in paroxysms of great violence, instrumental in producing the abortions; at beginning of ninth pregnancy had her cough, which was very dry, harsh, loud, shaking, < at night, preventing sleep, excited instantly and violently by pressure on trachea.

▮▮Cough provoked by change from warm to cold, or cool to warm air, also by change in rhythm of respiration.

||Constant dry cough lasting many months in a woman disposed to consumption.

Aching from shoulder blades down back or kidneys.

▮In women every fit of coughing produces the passage of a few drops of urine.

▮Dry cough commencing at 2 A.M.

▮Cough on changing rooms.

▮Night cough of phthisis, with or without clavicular pain.

28 **Inner Chest and Lungs.** ▮Pain in chest: in both sides.

Dull aching in anterior portion of both lungs day and night, for five days, accompanied by headache and pain in stomach, also belching of wind.

Fine stitches in l. lung, at 3.30 P.M., while writing.

▮Sharp stitching or stinging pains through l. lung; when patient turns l. side feels sore; early stages of phthisis. θPleurodynia.

Very acute stitch along l. margin of sternum on inspiration, in afternoon while riding.

Burning-stinging pain in l. side, near heart, soon after lying down in bed; gradually moved up into great pectoral muscles about two inches above and to l. of nipple and continued for a long time; < from deep inspiration and by lying on back or r. side; > lying on l. side.

Burning-stinging pain in whole l. side of chest, suddenly when taking a deep inspiration, while in the act of lying down in bed at night.

Stinging, almost itching pain in l. side of chest, just below nipple, followed and accompanied stinging, burning pain in back.

Burning pain in l. side of chest, just below nipple, < on taking a deep inspiration.

Severe pain in both sides and felt as if in lungs.

▮Clavicular pain; raw pain just under each clavicle while hawking mucus from throat.

Burning-sticking or burning-stinging pain in l. chest

near heart; < from deep breathing and lying down in bed at night; rheumatism.

Burning, shooting pain in r. chest.

Sharp pain near l. axilla.

Pain in centre of l. lung.

The sternum feels sprained.

|| Great dyspnœa; constant, dry, hacking cough; mucous rale at apex of r. lung, with slight dulness; haggard countenance; commenced coughing two years before; sometimes pain in l. side just below nipple; cannot expectorate; cough excited by tickling in larynx and suprasternal fossa; sensation of a lump in throat not > by hawking or swallowing; tough mucus in larynx with desire to raise it, but without relief; diarrhœa; thighs and back covered with small red pimples; night sweats and restless nights; cough < in morning, on entering warm room from cold air, on stopping after a walk, on first lying down at night, in smoke, or in kitchen where cooking is being done. θIncipient phthisis.

29 **Heart, Pulse and Circulation.** Heart feels as if it suddenly stopped beating, followed by a heavy throbbing through chest.

Burning in region of heart.

Dull pain in region of heart; stinging; < when lying down and breathing deeply.

|| Violent palpitation of heart with throbbing of carotids and throughout body, visible to eye and shaking bed; pulse 120; violent aching pain in region of heart; great dyspnœa, especially while lying so that he had to be propped up in a sitting posture; face red and puffed, especially about eyes, which were red, heavy and lustreless; tongue coated with white fur, red tip and edges; excessive thirst; no appetite; costive.

Pulse accelerated, mostly when going up stairs.

31 **Neck and Back.** Pressing aching in back, at lower border of scapula.

Sore or burning pain near sacro-iliac symphysis.

32 **Upper Limbs.** Pains in shoulder down to elbow, arms feel strained.

Hands cold when coughing.

33 **Lower Limbs.** Stitching in back of r. hip; limping walk.

Legs ache.

Stitchlike pain in knee joint, when standing.

Legs covered with small red pimples.

Feet cold.

Feet sensitive; stinging in corns.

35 **Rest. Position. Motion.** Lying down: cough <; soon

after burning pain near heart; while in the act, burning pain in chest; stinging in region of heart <.

Lying quiet: distress or pain in pit of stomach >.

Lying on l. side: pain near heart >.

Standing: stitchlike pain in knee joint.

Motion: pains in head; pressure in pit of stomach <; causes nausea.

Talking: tight, suffocative, heavy ache in epigastrium <.

Turning on l. side: cough <.

Walking: pain in hypochondrium.

Going up stairs: pulse accelerated.

36 **Nerves.** Great debility; averse to work; indifferent to his surroundings.

Restlessness in evening.

‖Sensitive to open air.

37 **Sleep.** Sleep disturbed; wakeful, restless; short naps and unpleasant fancies, even when awake.

Unpleasant dreams.

Unquiet sleep, dreams of danger and trouble.

Wakes early, with headache.

38 **Time.** Morning: headache after waking; bitter taste; sudden urging to stool drives him out of bed; diarrhœa; rawness in throat; weak and exhausted.

2 A.M.: dry cough commences.

Afternoon: copious, colorless urine; stitch on margin of sternum; fever.

3.30 P.M.: stitches in l. lung.

Evening: lids inflamed <; fluent coryza <; heat of face <; hoarseness <; cough <; hoarseness.

Day and night: aching in lungs.

Night: fluent coryza <; nausea; desire to hawk phlegm; latter part, cough <; burning, stinging pain in chest <.

39 **Temperature and Weather.** Warmth: prurigo >.

Covering mouth with bedclothes: prevents cough.

While undressing: itching on various parts, < in lower limbs.

Changing rooms: cough <.

Change from cold or cool to warm air: provokes cough.

Open air: sensitive to; urticaria <.

Cool air: cough <; vesicular eruption itching when exposed.

Exposure to cold: aphonia.

Cold: prurigo <.

Cold air: desire to hawk phlegm <; cough <; inhalations cause cough.

40 **Fever.** Chilly, < on back; colic, nausea, stitches near middle of chest.

Increased frequency of pulse, and afternoon fever.

Sensation of heat, followed by that of cold, without shivering.
Flushes of heat < on cheeks.
Sweat on waking from a sound sleep.

41 **Attacks, Periodicity.** From 5 to 9 A.M.: five stools.
From 6 to 10 A.M.: four stools.
Every ten seconds: cough.
Every morning for four days: diarrhœa.
After 7 P.M.: irritability of trachea <.
At same time each day: sudden change of voice.
Several times a day: coughing spells lasting one and a half hours at a time.
Every night at 11 P.M., between 1 and 2 A.M. and at 2 and 5 A.M.: attacks of cough.
For several years: at times dry cough.

42 **Locality and Direction.** Right: pain in side of occiput; pain in hip; dull pain on side of sternum; pains in side of chest; shooting pain in chest; mucous râle at apex of lung; stitches in back of hip.

Left: sharp pain in side of head; aching in breast; sharp pain in chest; tubercles in apex of lung; burning soreness of bronchus; pain in side of larynx; stitches in lung; soreness in bronchus; when turning on side, cough; fine stitches in lung; stitching or stinging pains through lung; side feels sore when turning; stitch along margin of sternum; burning, stinging pain near heart; burning stinging near nipple; > lying on side; burning stinging pain in whole side of chest; almost itching pain in chest; sharp pain in axillæ; pain in centre of lung.

43 **Sensations.** Eyes pain as if from dryness; tongue as if burned; as of a lump in throat; as of a hard substance in pit of stomach; as of a bunch in throat or behind sternum; as of pressure of a stick in rectum; as if urine could not long be retained; as if she could not get another breath; as if air did not penetrate chest; as if a feather were swaying to and fro in bronchi; as if head would fly into pieces; as if he might raise blood any minute; as if cough did not reach low enough down to raise phlegm; as if heart suddenly stopped beating.

Pain: in pit of stomach; in hypochondrium; in abdomen; in head; in larynx; in stomach; through both lungs; in chest; in centre of l. lung; in l. side just below nipple; in shoulder down to elbow.
Severe pain: in both sides as if in lungs.
Sharp pains: in chest and abdomen; on l. side of sternum; near l. axilla.

Darting pain: in l. side of head.
Piercing: in l. side of head.
Shooting: from pit of stomach to chest; in l. chest; on each side of lower end of sternum; in abdomen.
Burning, shooting pain: in r. chest.
Wrenching pains: in r. side of chest.
Stitches: in l. lung; very acute along l. margin of sternum; in back of r. hip.
Sharp stitching pains: in stomach into chest; in back of r. hip; through l. lung.
Stitchlike pain: in knee joint.
Burning-stinging pain: in l. side, near heart; in back.
Stinging, almost itching pain: in l. side of chest.
Burning pain: in l. side of chest near sacro-iliac symphysis.
Raw pain: just under each clavicle.
Griping: near navel; in lower part of abdomen.
Aching: in pharynx; in l. breast; in epigastrium; in forehead; in pit of stomach and above it on each side of sternum; from shoulder blades down back or kidneys; in anterior portion of both lungs; in region of heart; in legs.
Tight, suffocative, dull, heavy ache: in epigastrium through to back.
Sprainlike aching: near sternum.
Pressing aching: in back at lower border of scapula.
Dull pains: on r. side; in occiput; in forehead; on right side of sternum; in region of heart.
Burning: in region of heart.
Burning sensation: through upper lobes of lungs.
Sharp, tingling sensation: in Schneiderian membrane.
Stinging: in region of heart; in corns.
Soreness: behind sternum; in eyes; burning of larynx and throat; of larynx and chest; of trachea; lower part of trachea.
Raw sensation: in larynx; in trachea; under clavicles.
Excoriated feeling: in upper part of throat; in chest; behind sternum.
Bruised feeling: in forehead.
Scraping: in throat.
Tenderness: in larynx and trachea.
Distress: in stomach pit.
Tickling: in throat pit; in suprasternal fossa and behind sternum.
Heavy throbbing: through chest.
Heaviness: in stomach or epigastrium.
Pressure: in stomach; in pit of stomach, extending toward throat.

Hardness: in abdomen.
Dull feeling: in head.
Distension: in stomach.
Fulness: in abdomen.
Weak feeling: in epigastrium.
Dryness: of tongue and mouth.
Dry sensation: in nose.
Itching: deep in ears; at anus; in various parts on lower limbs.
Coldness: of fingers; of hands; of feet.

45 **Touch. Passive Motion. Injuries.** Touch: on throat pit; cough <.
Pressure: on larynx, cough <; on throat pit, cough <; on trachea causes severe cough.
Riding: stitch along margin of sternum.

46 **Skin.** ▮Itching in various parts, < on lower limbs, while undressing.
‖Eruption covered uniformly several regions of skin with exception of face; itching more of a pricking than a burning character; < by cold, and > by warmth. θPrurigo.
▮Contagious prurigo or "army itch."
▮Stinging-itching, or prickling-itching of skin.
▮Vesicular eruption, itching when uncovered and exposed to cool air.
‖Prairie itch.
Urticaria; < in open air.

47 **Stages of Life, Constitution.** Boy, æt. 4; cough.
Boy, æt. 5; diarrhœa.
Girl, æt. 6, suffering three weeks; cough.
Girl, æt. 6, after catching cold; cough.
Girl, æt. 12, suffering four days; diarrhœa.
Joseph H., æt. 13, subject to violent attacks of inflammatory rheumatism, heart being implicated; pain in cardiac region.
Miss C., æt. 20, robust, healthy, after exposure; aphonia.
Woman, æt. 22, feeble constitution, strumous, subject for several years to subacute rheumatism; cough.
Miss W., young lady of highly nervous temperament; cough.
Man, æt. 23, nervous temperament, suffering several years, thinks himself consumptive; cough.
Miss B., æt. 25, clear, white, very smooth skin, rather pale, dark-auburn hair, full round figure, after catching cold three months ago; sore throat, aphonia.
Man, æt. 26, nervous, sanguine temperament; cough.
Man, æt. 26, dark complexion, married; incipient phthisis.
Mrs. G., æt. 30, suffering five days; cough.

Woman, æt. 35, married, suffering four days; diarrhœa.
Mrs. A., æt. 45; cough.
Lady, æt. about 50, suffering three weeks; pain in stomach.
Lady, æt. about 50, suffering four days; diarrhœa.
Man, æt. 70; diarrhœa.
Farmer, suffering three years; prurigo.

48 **Relations.** Antidoted by: *Camphor.*, *Bellad.*, *Hyosc.*, *Conium*, *Laches.*, *Phosphor.*
Compare: *Apis*, *Bellad.*, *Calc. carb.*, *Caustic.*, *Cistus*, *Dulcam.*, *Eryngium*, *Hepar sulph.*, *Iris*, *Iodium*, *Juglans*, *Laches.*, *Lycopod.*, *Lobelia*, *Mercur.*, *Nuphar*, *Phosphor.*, *Podoph.*, *Rheum*, *Sanguin.*, *Spongia*, *Sulphur.*

RUTA GRAVEOLENS.

Rue. *Rutaceæ.*

A native of the South of Europe, cultivated in Northern gardens. The leaves are acrid, hot and bitter, the flowers yellow. The tincture is prepared from the fresh herb, gathered shortly before blooming.

Proving by Hahnemann, Franz, Gross, Hartman, Herrman, Hornburg, Langhammer, Stapf, Wislicenus, R. A. M. L., vol. 4; Hartlaub and Trinks, R. A. M. L., vol. 1; Hering, Archiv für Hom., vol. 15.

Clinical Authorities.—*Amblyopia*, Bethmann, Lobethal, Rück. Kl. Erf., vol. 1, p. 338; *Pain in eyes*, Cowperthwaite, M. I., vol. 1, p. 96; *Dyspepsia*, Farrington, Raue's Rec., 1874, p. 171; from A. J. H. M. M., vol. 7, p. 25; Hah. Mo., vol. 10, p. 45; *Chronic prolapse of rectum*, Spooner, N. E. M. G., vol. 4, p. 409; *Polypus and prolapsus of rectum*, Gerstel, A. H. Z., vol. 106, p. 83; *Prolapsus ani*, Müller, Rück. Kl. Erf., vol. 1, p. 994; *Urinary difficulty*, Koch, Hom. Cl., vol. 1, p. 220; *Pain in back*, Kirsch, Rück. Kl. Erf., vol. 5, p. 877; Berridge, N. A. J. H., vol. 22, p. 494; *Pain below scapula*, Berridge, Hom. Cl., vol. 4, p. 113; *Soreness in bones of hands*, Libby, M. I., vol. 3, p. 205, 1876; *Ganglia*, Gregory, Hom. Phys., vol. 2, p. 164; *Bursitis*, Smith, M. I., vol. 4, p. 266; *Sciatic rheumatism*, Miller, H. M., vol. 8, p. 199; *Rheumatism*, Nankivell, Raue's Rec., 1873, p. 192, from H. W., vol. 7, p. 278; *Injury to bones*, Hrg., Rück. Kl. Erf., vol. 4, p. 1029.

1 **Mind.** Inclination to contradict and quarrel.
Dissatisfied with himself and others.
Anxious and low-spirited, with mental dejection.
Melancholy disposition toward evening.

2 **Sensorium.** Vertigo: in morning when rising; when sitting; when walking in open air.

3 **Inner Head.** ||Sticking drawing pain extending from frontal to temporal bone.

||Stitches in l. frontal bone, only while reading.
Pulsative pressing pain in forehead.
Heat in head, with much restlessness.
||Rhythmical pressive pain in head.
||Pain as from a fall, in periosteum, extending from temporal bones to occiput.
Headache: as if a nail were driven into head; like a stupefying pressure on whole brain; after excessive use of intoxicating drinks.

[4] **Outer Head.** Large painful swelling on scalp, as if originating in periosteum, sore to touch and preceded by rending pain.
|Head externally painful, as if bruised or beaten.
Erysipelas of scalp, arising from wounds.
Humid scabs on head.
|Periosteum from temples to occiput, pains as if bruised.
Corrosive itching on scalp.
Twitching in muscles of brow.

[5] **Sight and Eyes.** Vision very weak, as if eyes were excessively strained.
Objects seem dim before eyes, as if a shadow were flitting before them.
|Dulness of sight, brought on by taxing or straining eyes.
|As if sight had been strained by too much reading.
Letters seem to run together.
Pain like a pressure in r. eye, with obscuration of vision, as if one had looked too long and intently at an object.
||Aching in and over eyes, with blurring of vision, after using eyes and straining them at fine work.
|Amblyopia: dependent upon overexertion of eyes, or anomalies of refraction; from writing by artificial light; fine needlework, etc.; in a weaver, could with difficulty distinguish one thread from another, and could not read at all; mistiness of sight, with complete obscuration at a distance.
||Asthenopia: irritability of every tissue of eye from overwork or from using eyes on fine work; heat and aching in and over eyes, eyes feel like balls of fire at night, blurring of vision, letters seem to run together, lachrymation, etc.
||Choroiditis in a myopic eye, caused by straining eyes; much pain in eyes on trying to look at objects, heat in eye though it seems cold, and twitching in balls.
|Asthenopia; more often indicated in weakness of ciliary muscles than of internal recti.
|Loss of power over internal rectus.
||Burning in eyes in evening, especially when trying to sew or read; eyes feel strained; read too much by artificial light.

Green halo around light in evening.

Spots on cornea.

Itching on inner canthus and on lower lid, smarting after rubbing, eye becomes full of water.

▮Eyes burn, ache, feel strained, sight blurred; < using them in evening.

Burning beneath l. eye.

Sensation of heat and fire in eyes and aching while reading (in evening by light).

Eyes appear irritable and run water, especially toward evening after working all day.

Pressure deep in orbits.

‖Pain as from a bruise in orbicular cartilages.

Pressure on inner surface of l. eye, with profuse lachrymation.

▮Eyes feel hot like balls of fire.

Eyes water in open air, not indoors.

Spasms of lower eyelids, afterward lachrymation.

6 **Hearing and Ears.** Sensation in ear as if one were digging about with a blunt piece of wood, a kind of scraping pressure.

Pain as if bruised in cartilage of ear, and under mastoid process.

7 **Smell and Nose.** Sweat on dorsum of nose.

Bleeding of nose, with pressure at root of nose.

8 **Upper Face.** Erysipelas and swelling on forehead.

Pain, as if bruised, in periosteum of facial bones.

Facial paralysis after catching cold.

9 **Lower Face.** Lips dry and sticky.

Pimples on lips.

‖Pain as from a blow beneath mastoid process.

10 **Teeth and Gums.** Pain in lower teeth.

Gums painful and bleed readily.

11 **Taste and Tongue.** Spasm of tongue, with difficulty of speech.

13 **Throat.** Sensation as from a lump in throat on empty deglutition.

14 **Appetite, Thirst. Desires, Aversions.** Appetite normal, but aversion to everything as soon as he begins to eat.

Unquenchable desire for cold water, drinks much and often without being incommoded.

Violent thirst for cold water in afternoon.

15 **Eating and Drinking.** After eating: sudden nausea; pinching in stomach after bread and butter; eructations and itching of skin after meat; replete as soon as he eats.

16 **Hiccough, Belching, Nausea and Vomiting.** Hiccough, with depression.

Frequent odorless eructations.

A kind of nausea in pit of stomach.

Nausea, sudden, while eating, with vomiting of food.

17 **Scrobiculum and Stomach.** Epigastric region sensitive.

Tension at stomach in great measure appeased by drinking milk.

Burning gnawing in stomach.

Gnawing sensation in stomach as from emptiness or hunger.

Pruritus of stomach and intestines showing itself by pricking, gnawing pains.

||Dyspepsia of fifteen years, caused by straining stomach when carrying heavy weight; pulse soft, and every attempt to eat meat would be followed by headache; eructations and itching all over, like an undeveloped nettlerash; he could eat fat meat and drink milk.

18 **Hypochondria.** Gnawing pressing pain in region of liver.

Painful swelling of spleen.

19 **Abdomen.** Gnawing pain about navel.

Colic: with burning or gnawing pain; in children, from worms.

20 **Stool and Rectum.** Stool: soft, discharged with difficulty, from inactivity of rectum; |rectum protrudes immediately on attempting a passage; lumpy, slimy or bloody, with much flatus; seemingly only flatus; empty eructations, distended abdomen; feces often escape when bending over.

Frequent urging to stool with small, soft discharges.

|Frequent unsuccessful urging, with prolapsus ani.

Constipation, alternating with mucous, frothy stools.

Scanty, hard stool; stool like sheep's dung.

Constipation from inactivity of bowels or impaction of feces following mechanical injuries.

Difficult expulsion of large-sized feces.

Tearing in rectum and urethra, while urinating.

Tearing stitches in rectum while sitting.

Frequent pressure to stool, with prolapsus of rectum, also with emission of much flatus; the slightest stooping, or still more crouching down, caused rectum to protrude.

||Prolapsus of rectum; frequent, lumpy, slimy stool, bloody at times; much flatus; stool often unsatisfactory, passing nothing but flatus; empty eructations and distended abdomen; feces often pass involuntarily while bending over; weakness in lumbar region; frequent urination; prolapse always with and sometimes without stool; after sitting a long time at stool the prolapsed bowel becomes much swollen and difficult to replace; four or five stools a day; of years standing.

|Protrusion of rectum, after confinement.

||Prolapsus ani, after an attack of dysentery, half a year previously.

||Frequently itching in rectum; at times expulsion of thread worms; slightly constipated; abdomen somewhat bloated; poor appetite; sudden prolapsus recti, with tenesmus, after eating grapes; prolapsus frequently recurred, especially after stool; after four weeks' use of *Ruta*, a mucous polypus was discharged from rectum, since then entirely well.

||Worm complaints of children.

21 **Urinary Organs.** Tearing pains in urethra while urinating.

Pressure on bladder, as if continually full; the pressure to urinate continues after micturition; at every step after urinating, she feels as if bladder were full and moving up and down.

Great pressure to urinate, as if bladder were constantly full, yet but little urine is passed, and micturition is followed by dragging as if much should be passed, which, however, does not occur.

||Constant urging to urinate, could hardly retain urine; when that feeling occurred she had to hurry to water-closet; if she forcibly retained the water she could not pass any afterward and suffered severe pains.

Frequent pressure to urinate, with scanty green urine.

Spasmodic stricture of neck of bladder.

Frequent micturition.

Involuntary micturition at night in bed, and during day when walking.

22 **Male Sexual Organs.** Varicocele following a strain; hæmatocele in which the effusion is small and firmly coagulated.

23 **Female Sexual Organs.** Menses: too early and too profuse; feeble, followed by leucorrhœa.

Corrosive leucorrhœa after irregular or suppressed menses.

24 **Pregnancy. Parturition. Lactation.** Lameness and soreness all over; weak, feeble contractions during labor.

25 **Voice and Larynx. Trachea and Bronchia.** Sensation in larynx as from a bruise.

26 **Respiration.** Short breath with tightness of chest.

27 **Cough.** Awakened about midnight with a choking cough.

Cough with copious expectoration of thick yellow mucus, with weak feeling in chest after it.

Violent cough with expectoration of tough mucus and nausea.

28 **Inner Chest and Lungs.** Pressure on sternum seeming to be internal and external.

A painful spot on sternum, painful to pressure.

Gnawing pain, associated with some biting and burning in r. side of chest.

▮Phthisis after mechanical injuries to chest.

Sensation of coldness or heat in chest.

29 **Heart, Pulse and Circulation.** Anxious palpitation.

Pulse unchanged; or, somewhat accelerated only during heat.

30 **Outer Chest.** On sternum a painful spot; also painful to pressure.

31 **Neck and Back.** || For twelve days pain below r. scapula < in evening, after exertion, by deep inspiration and by moving r. arm; > by pressure and lying down, especially on r. side; the pain extends over a spot as large as the palm; when severe it extends to corresponding part of l. side.

Pain as if sprained or bruised in nape and shoulders.

Bruised pain extending along back.

Drawing, bruised pain in spine, frequently taking away breath.

Pain as if beaten and lame in spine.

Pressive drawing, very acute pain in r. side of spine, opposite liver, especially on inspiration.

Pain as from a fall in dorsal vertebræ.

Severe pressure in small of back, from within outward, as if bruised; pain appears 5 o'clock in morning, and is > by moving about and by passage of flatus.

Stitches in small of back when sitting, stooping or walking; > by pressure and when lying down.

Stitches in spine while sitting; is suddenly overcome by anxiety.

▮Rheumatic pains in back, < in morning before rising.

▮Pain as if bruised in lumbar vertebræ.

▮Weakness in lumbar region; prolapsus recti.

▮Pain in back or coccyx, as from a blow or fall, or as if bruised.

Bruised sensation in hip bones.

Cramplike contraction or pulsation ascending from thighs into small of back.

32 **Upper Limbs.** Pain in l. elbow joint as from a blow; arm weak.

Wrists feel as if sprained, stiff; < in wet, cold weather.

Bones in wrist and back of hand painful, as if bruised, during rest and motion.

πGanglionic swelling on front of l. wrist.

Hands numb and tingle after exercise.

|| Soreness through small bones of hands.

|| Ganglia on sheath of flexor tendons of fourth finger, situated in palm of r. hand, as large as a hickory nut, greatly interfering with use of hand; rheumatism of r. leg.

Flat, smooth warts on inside of hands.

Contraction of fingers.

▮Bursitis.

33 **Lower Limbs.** On rising, after sitting, he cannot walk; he falls back again.

While walking he falls from side to side; the feet will not support him; there is no power or steadiness in thighs.

Ascending or descending a hill is difficult, the legs give out.

▮Hip bones feel bruised; as if from a blow or fall.

The painful parts, especially hips and bones of legs, are sore, as if beaten, whenever touched.

▮Sciatica; pain deep-seated as if in marrow of bone, or as if bone were broken; obliged to walk about constantly during paroxysms; pain < sitting or lying down; constantly complaining about his sufferings; burning, corrosive pains, < in damp or cold weather, or from cold applications.

‖Shooting pains from back down outside of l. thigh, sometimes down sciatic nerve on first moving or on rising after sitting; hamstrings, chiefly outer, feel shortened and sore. θSciatic rheumatism.

▮Ischias arising from injuries and contusions.

Anterior surface of thigh feels bruised and painful to touch.

Whenever he stretches out the limbs, even a little, the thighs are painful, as if beaten.

▮Hamstrings feel shortened and weak, knees give way going up or down stairs.

Posterior portion of thigh above knee seems bruised.

▮Pain and lameness in ankles after a sprain or dislocation.

Throbbing and hacking pain as if there were an ulcer on anterior portion of l. ankle.

He dare not step heavily upon feet, on account of pains in bones of feet, with a sensation of heat.

Burning and biting pains in bones of feet during rest.

Fistulous ulcers on lower legs.

34 **Limbs in General.** Is unable to bend on account of pains in all the joints and hip bones.

Inflammation of larger joints, especially in upper extremities.

‖Since five weeks severe rheumatism of r. wrist and in both feet from heels to toes; has been in bed for a month; puffy swelling of instep; sour sweat.

▮▮Lameness after sprains, especially of wrists and ankles.

35 **Rest. Position. Motion.** Rest: wrist and back of hand painful; pains in bones of feet.

Lying down: pain below r. scapula >; stitches in small of back >; parts on which he lies sore.

Sitting: vertigo; tearing stitches in rectum; stitches in rectum; stitches in small of back in spine; on rising cannot walk, falls back again; sciatica <; pains down sciatic nerve on rising.

Lies in one position, then in another, turns from side to side; uneasiness of legs; rheumatism.

Bending over: feces often escape.

Slightest stooping or crouching down: causes rectum to protrude; stitches in small of back.

Is unable to bend: pains in all joints.

Stretching out limbs even a little: thighs painful.

Motion: of r. arm, pain below r. scapula <; > pain in small of back; wrist and back of hand painful.

Exertion: pain below scapula <.

Exercise: hands numb and tingle.

Walking: vertigo; involuntary micturition; stitches in small of back; falls from side to side; short distance, great weakness; limbs painful.

Ascending or descending a hill is difficult, legs give out.

Going up and down stairs: hamstrings feel shortened and weak.

36 **Nerves.** Great weakness after a short walk; the limbs feel bruised; small of back and loins are painful.

Tottering, as if thighs were weak; limbs pain when walking.

Does not know where to lay his legs on account of uneasiness and heaviness; he lies now in one place, now in another, and turns from side to side.

All parts of the body upon which he lies, even in bed, are painful as if bruised.

||Restless, turns and changes position frequently when lying. θRheumatism.

Facial paralysis after catching cold; suits robust and sanguineous persons.

Rheumatic paralysis of tarsal and carpal joints.

37 **Sleep.** Yawning and stretching, indoors.

Sleepiness during day.

Frequent waking at night, feeling as if it were time to rise.

||Vivid confused dreams.

38 **Time.** Morning: vertigo on rising; rheumatic pains in back < before rising; sweat in bed.

At 5 o'clock A.M.: pressure in small of back.

During day: involuntary micturition; sleepiness.

Afternoon: thirst for cold water; heat with anxiety.

Toward evening: eyes irritable and run water.

Evening: melancholy disposition, burning in eyes; green

halo around light; sight blurred, eyes ache; pain below r. scapula.

Night: eyes feel like balls of fire; involuntary micturition in bed; feeling as if it were time to rise.

About midnight: awakened with a choking cougn.

39 **Temperature and Weather.** Near warm stove: chill; chilliness.

Indoors: yawning and stretching.

Open air: vertigo when walking, eyes water; after walking, general sweat.

Cold applications: sciatica <.

Cold water: thirst for.

Wet, cold weather: wrists feel stiff, sprained; sciatica <.

40 **Fever.** Coldness running over one side of head.

|| Coldness down spine.

Chill mostly left-sided; < up and down back; shakes even near a warm stove.

Chill with heat of face and violent thirst.

External and internal heat of face with red cheeks and cold hands and feet.

Frequent attacks of quick flushes of heat.

Heat, mostly afternoons, with anxiety, restlessness and dyspnœa; no thirst.

Sweat, cold on face; morning in bed.

General sweat after walking in open air.

|| Chilliness through whole body even when near a warm stove, hands and feet cold, confusion and heat in head, great thirst which disappears immediately after drinking, frequent sneezing, pain in eyes as if strained, lachrymation, pain in larynx as if bruised, hoarse cough awakening him at midnight, and causing by its continuation vomiting and pain in sternum, expectoration seldom and scanty. θCatarrhal fever.

41 **Attacks, Periodicity.** Day: four or five stools.

For twelve days: pain below r. scapula.

Since five weeks: severe rheumatism of r. wrist, both feet.

Years standing: prolapsus of rectum.

42 **Locality and Direction.** Right: pain like a pressure in eye; biting and burning on side of chest; pain, below scapula; acute pain in side of chest; ganglion on sheath of flexor tendon of fourth finger in palm; rheumatism of leg; rheumatism of wrist.

Left: stitches in frontal bone; burning beneath eye; pressure on inner surface of eye; ganglionic swelling on front of wrist; pain down outside of thigh; as of an ulcer on ankle; chill mostly side.

From within outward: pressure in small of back.

43 **Sensations.** As if from a fall, pain in periosteum; as if a nail

were driven into head; head as if bruised or beaten; pains as if bruised in periosteum; as if eyes were excessively strained; as if a shadow were flitting before eyes; as if one had looked too long and intently at an object; eyes as if balls of fire; as if one were digging about in ear with a blunt piece of wood; as of a lump in throat; bladder as if continually full; spine as if beaten and lame; wrists as if sprained; as if pain were in marrow of bone or as if bone were broken; thighs as if beaten; as if there were an ulcer in ankle; as if thighs were weak; all parts of body as if bruised at night, feeling as if it were time to rise.

Pain like a pressure: in r. eye; in orbicular cartilages; in lower teeth; below l. scapula; in ankles; in bones of feet; in all joints and hip-bones; in nerves and tissues.

Shooting pains: from back down outside of l. thigh.

Rending pain: on scalp, preceding swelling.

Tearing: in rectum and urethra.

Hacking pain: in anterior portion of l. ankle.

Throbbing pain: in anterior portion of l. ankle.

Tearing stitches: in rectum.

Stitches: in l. frontal bone; in small of back; in spine.

Stitching-drawing pain: from forehead to temples.

Pressive-drawing, very acute pain: in r. side of spine.

Pain as if bruised.

Bruised pain: in orbicular cartilages; in cartilage of ear and under mastoid process; in periosteum of facial bones; in larynx; in nape and shoulders; along back; in spine; in small of back; in lumbar vertebræ; in coccyx; in hip bones, in bones of wrists and back of hand.

Pain as from a blow: below mastoid process; in coccyx; in l. elbow joint.

Pain as from a fall: in dorsal vertebræ; in back or coccyx.

Pinching: in stomach.

Pulsative pressing pain: in forehead.

Rhythmical pressive pain: in head.

Gnawing pain: in stomach, about navel; in r. side of chest.

Pricking, gnawing pains: in stomach and intestines.

Burning gnawing: in stomach.

Gnawing, pressing pain: in region of liver.

Burning: in eyes; beneath l. eye; in r. side of chest; in bones of feet.

Biting: in r. side of chest; in bones of feet.

Cramplike contraction or pulsation: ascending from thighs into small of back.

Soreness: all over; through small bones of hands; in hamstrings; of parts on which he lies.

Rheumatic pain: in back; of r. leg; of r. wrist, both feet from heels to toes.
Aching: in and over eyes.
Pressure: deep in orbits; on inner surface of l. eye; at root of nose; on bladder; on sternum; in small of back.
Painful spot: on sternum.
Twitching: in eyeballs.
Tension: at stomach.
Lameness: all over; in ankles.
Heaviness: of legs.
Uneasiness: of legs.
Heat: in head; in eyes; in chest; in feet; of face.
Weak feeling: in chest, in lumbar region.
Corrosive itching: on scalp.
Itching: on inner canthus and on lower lid; of skin after meat; in rectum.
Coldness: in chest; over one side of head; down spine; of hands and feet.

44 **Tissues.** ▮Bruised feeling all over as from a fall or blow, < in limbs and joints.
Sensation of soreness of parts on which he lies.
Pain in nerves or tissues that have been stretched, as in sprains.
Pain in long bones as if they were broken.
▮▮Bruises and other mechanical injuries of bones and periosteum; sprains; periostitis; erysipelas.
Dropsy.
▮Periostitis and pains in consequence of external injury, with erysipelatous inflammation of parts.
▮In dislocations where the inflammation is fully under control, it hastens the curative process in the joint.
▮▮Bone lesions and fractures; scrofulous exostoses.
▮Swelling of ankles.
▮▮Small epithelial swellings on joints of toes.

45 **Touch. Passive Motion. Injuries.** Touch: swelling on scalp sore, painful parts sore; anterior surface of thigh feels painful.
Pressure: a spot on sternum painful; pain below r. scapula >; stitches in small of back >.
Rubbing: smarting of lower lid and inner canthus.
Scratching: > itching.
Walking or riding: causes chafing of skin.
Straining stomach when carrying a heavy weight: caused dyspepsia.
Mechanical injuries: inactivity of bowels or impaction of feces; to chest, phthisis.

46 **Skin.** ▮Itching over whole body, > scratching.
Itching of skin after eating meat.

Jaundice from liver complaints.
Skin becomes easily chafed, from walking and riding; also in children.
Acne rosacea.
Erysipelas: after mechanical injuries; of hands.
Ulcers and scabs on scalp, with copious discharge.
Ulcerations; gnawing, jerking pains; pus sanious.
Fistulous ulcers on lower legs.
Inflamed ulcers.
Warts; with sore pains; flat, smooth on inside of hands.

47 **Stages of Life, Constitution.** In robust, sanguineous persons.
Child, æt. 1½, suffering half a year after an attack of dysentery; prolapsus ani.
Girl æt. 6, pale, delicate, subject to slight catarrhal attacks, which generally yielded to *Acon.;* polypus and prolapsus of rectum.
Man æt. 27, nervous temperament, dark hair, blue eyes, troubled for years, it is a family complaint; prolapse of rectum.
Weaver, æt. 29; amblyopia.
Woman, æt. 34; pain in back.
Mrs. H., æt. 36, suffering a long time; urinary difficulty.
Man æt. 53, suffering five weeks; rheumatism.

48 **Relations.** Antidoted by: *Camphor.*
It antidotes: *Mercur.*
Compatible: *Calc. ost., Caust., Lycopod., Phos. ac., Pulsat., Sepia, Sulphur, Sulph. ac.* (diseases of bones).
Compare: *Arnic., Argent. nit.* (asthenopia), *Bryon., Calc. ost., Conium* (asthenopia), *Euphras., Lycopod., Mercur., Mezer., Phosphor., Phytol., Pulsat., Rhus tox., Sepia, Silica, Sulphur.*

SABADILLA.

Cebadilla. *Liliaceæ.*

Indigenous to Eastern Mexico, Guatemala and Venezuela. It is a bulbous plant bearing greenish-yellow flowers on a spikelike raceme. The tincture is prepared from the powdered seeds.

Provings by Hahnemann, Gross, Hartlaub, Hromada, Langhammer, Rückert, Schultz, Schönke, Stapf, etc., Archiv für Hom., vol. 4.

Clinical Authorities.—*Vertigo*, Deck, Hom. Phys., vol. 8, p. 463; *Lachrymation*, Boyce, N. Y. S. Tr., 1870, pp. 214, 217, Raue's Rec., 1870, p. 130; *Toothache*, Oehme, H. M., vol 9, p. 319; *Sensation of a body in throat*, Fanning, N. Y. S. Tr., 1870, p. 793, Raue's Rec., 1871, p. 15; *Sore throat*, Hirsch, Rück. Kl. Erf., vol. 5, p. 250; *Tænia*, Fielitz, Rück. Kl. Erf., vol. 1, p. 808; *Worm affections*, Müller, Rück. Kl. Erf., vol. 5, p. 390; *Ovaritis*, Doury, Raue's Rec., 1873, p. 146, from Med. Inv., vol. 9, p. 51; *Influenza*, Rückert, Croserio, Rück. Kl. Erf., vol. 3, p. 49; *Spinal affection*, Lobethal, Rück. Kl. Erf., vol. 3, p. 472; *Ague*, Sonnenberg, Lobethal, Tripi, Escalier, Neumann, Müller, Hartlaub, Seidel, Rück. Kl. Erf., vol. 4, p. 983; Segin, Gueyraid, Allen's Int. Fever, p. 218, from Hom. Clinique; *Rheumatism*, Berridge, Time's Ret., 1875, p. 110, from N. Y. J. H., vol. 2, p. 312; *Measles*, Fornias, Hah. Mo., vol. 15, p. 533.

1 **Mind.** No response to questions, loss of consciousness; afterward jumps up and runs recklessly through room.

▮Erroneous impressions as to the state of his body.

▮▮Imagines: himself sick; parts shrunken; that she is pregnant, when she is merely swollen from flatus; that she has some horrible throat disease which will end fatally.

▮Delirium during intermittents.

Mania; rage, quieted only by washing head in cold water.

Melancholy from deep-seated abdominal irritation.

Anxious sensation with restlessness and qualmishness.

Easily frightened; startled by noises.

Thinking produces headache.

Mental exertion aggravates headache and produces sleep.

After fright hysteric paroxysms.

2 **Sensorium.** Vertigo: things turn black before eyes, sensation of fainting; as if things were turning, especially when rising from a seat; more sitting than walking; felt stupid.

Dulness of head. θInfluenza.

Beclouded, as after intoxication, without vertigo or pains.

▮▮Vertigo with sensation as if all things were turning around each other.

ǁ Attacks of giddiness coming generally in evening; in one attack fainted, then vomited food and bile; during attacks felt suddenly as if she would fall if she did not hold on to something; felt glad to get into open air; gastric disturbance, felt sick after meals.

ǁ Attacks of giddiness; of short duration, affected suddenly; everything seems to be whirling round her; she has to hold on to something, otherwise she would fall down; if in the house the whole house seems to be coming down upon her; if in the street the houses seem to be falling upon her, and unless she can hold on to some support she falls down; sometimes awakes at night with the whirling sensation; attacks come on without warning, last but a few moments, and are followed by a weak, tired feeling; at other times suffers from attacks of longer duration, sometimes lasting greater part of forenoon, accompanied by nausea and visual disturbance; brain seems to go round and round, and eyes move to and fro, as if they went round with the whirling sensation; if she shuts her eyes the whirling seems to go in the opposite direction and she becomes sick; she likes to lie perfectly still and to look fixedly at one object; if she turns her eyes to look at any other object, or if she shuts her eyes she becomes sick; feels < in mornings, very weak in forenoon and > in afternoon; the sudden giddy attacks come on at any time, the attacks with nausea mostly in the mornings; has a depressed, anxious look; appetite very poor; likes milk, feels soon satisfied; some nausea after meals; mouth when she wakes very dry and burning, tongue dry and thickly coated; bad taste; palms of hands dry and horny and inclined to scale; at night they are so burning that she has to keep them outside the bedclothes; the top of her head is hot; she feels best out of doors.

3 **Inner Head.** ▮ Pressure in head < in forehead and temples. θ Hay fever.

Stitches in temples.

Headache after a walk; on returning to room a twisting, screwing pain from r. side of head to both temples, spreading over whole head, after going to bed, returning daily.

▮ Hemicrania with tænia.

▮ Headache from much thinking or too close attention.

Stupefying, oppressive sensation in forehead, producing a reeling sensation.

Corrosive, burning point on top of head.

Head feels dull and heavy.

Painful heaviness, first in forepart of r. side of forehead, whence it extends more and more toward l. side.

‖Headache and vertigo, > while eyes are steadily fixed upon an object and while patient is thinking of one subject.

▮Stupefying headache with coryza, itching and burning of scalp, general heat of whole body; < in forenoon.

4 **Outer Head.** Fine prickling stitches in skin of forehead and scalp, when becoming warm.

Burning, crawling itching on hairy scalp, > from scratching, < from getting into a sweat while walking.

Burning and tingling itching on scalp, as from lice.

Burning itching most on front of head and behind ears; feeling of heat spreading thence over whole body; after scratching violent tickling and stinging; red spots, later with a scurf, < when overheated or sweating during day.

Forehead covered with cold sweat.

5 **Sight and Eyes.** ▮Lachrymation: when walking in open air, on looking at light, sneezing, coughing or yawning; as soon as least pain is felt in some other part of body, for instance in hand.

Pressure on eyeballs when looking upward.

Margins of lids red.

Blue rings under eyes.

6 **Hearing and Ears.** Difficulty of hearing.

Severe stitches in l. ear.

Tickling in ears.

Jerking pains with itching in ear.

Itching of ears, with worms.

7 **Smell and Nose.** ▮Spasmodic sneezing. θHay fever. θInfluenza.

▮Fluent coryza. θInfluenza.

▮Either nostril stuffed up, inspiration through nose labored, snoring.

Itching in nose; agreeable titillation in alæ.

Profuse bleeding from nose.

Bright red blood comes from posterior nares and is expectorated.

Very sensitive to smell of garlic.

Violent sneezing from time to time, shaking abdomen; followed by lachrymation.

▮Coryza with severe frontal pains and redness of eyelids; violent sneezing; copious watery discharge from nose.

8 **Upper Face.** ▮Face feels hot, as after wine, face and eyes are red. θHay fever.

Face deadly pale and sunken, features distorted, great anxiety.

Beating and jerking in muscles of l. upper jaw.

Intermittent neuralgia, beginning with a shaking chill of great severity; twitching, convulsive trembling.

Swelling of face, with spotted eruption.

9 **Lower Face.** Can hardly open mouth from pain in joints and muscles; with sore throat.

Lips hot, dry, burn as if scalded.

Cracking of articulation of jaw on opening mouth wide.

10 **Teeth and Gums.** ‖ Remittent or intermittent toothache, often extending over whole side of face; < from hot or cold food or drink, from walking in cold air, even with closed mouth.

Dull, troublesome pain in carious teeth, with sore throat.

Gums: swollen; bluish.

11 **Taste and Tongue.** Taste: bitter; sweet; lost.

Tongue: sore, coated thick yellow; white in centre; moist, during fever; feels sore as if full of blisters; burning on tip.

Cannot protrude tongue, with sore throat.

Pain in tongue and down throat, deglutition difficult.

12 **Inner Mouth.** Cannot bear anything hot in mouth.

Anything cold in mouth causes pain during sore throat.

| Mouth dry; throat sore.

Saliva: seemingly hot during pyrosis; copious with nausea, vomiting and vomiturition; sweetish, collects in mouth; jellylike; ptyalism.

Frequent spitting of insipid water.

13 **Throat.** | Sensation of a skin hanging loosely in throat, must swallow over it; as if uvula were down.

| Much tough phlegm in throat; must hawk.

‖ Hawks bright red blood from posterior nares.

| Stitches in throat, only when swallowing; tonsils swollen and inflamed, nearly suppurating; l. to right.

| Tonsillitis after coryza; suppuration; r. tonsil remains somewhat swollen and indurated.

‖ Dryness of fauces and throat.

| Constricted feeling deep in throat, as if œsophagus would be closed, as after swallowing an astringent drink.

| Continual desire to swallow, deeply cutting pains, whole body writhes.

| Cannot swallow saliva on account of pain, must spit it out.

| While swallowing, or not, feeling in throat of a body which he must swallow.

Can swallow warm food more easily, in sore throat.

| Sensation of a lump in throat with inclination to swallow.

| Sore throat, continual desire to swallow, pale redness and slight swelling of mucous membrane; in children affected with worms.

| Roughness in throat, as if a morsel of food had lodged there, causing cough.

▮In an epidemic of sore throat, all cases which commenced on l. and extended to r. side.

▮▮Angina; hydrophobia.

14 **Appetite, Thirst. Desires, Aversions.** ▮Morbid hunger or loathing of food. θIntermittent.

▮Disgust: for all food; for meat; for sour things; for coffee; for garlic.

▮No relish for food until she takes the first morsel, when she makes a good meal. θPregnancy.

Canine appetite, especially for sweets, farinaceous food, puddings, alternating with disgust for meat, wine or sour things.

No thirst, with moist tongue.

▮Desire for hot things. θAngina.

▮Great thirst. θAngina.

▮▮Thirstlessness, with exception of desire for milk.

16 **Hiccough, Belching, Nausea and Vomiting.** Eructations: in intermittents; rancid; sour.

Pyrosis, heat comes up into throat; copious salivation, saliva seemingly as hot as the body, but it is not.

Constantly spits insipid water.

Nausea: before eating; with chilliness; regurgitation, vomiturition in intermittents; regurgitation of bitter mucus, leaving fatty taste; constantly spits insipid water.

Vomiting: of bile; with whooping cough; of lumbrici; or frequent nausea and vomiturition, with feeling of foreign body in œsophagus.

Nausea and retching, with feeling of worm in œsophagus.

Much nausea and vomiting, with heat in abdomen.

17 **Scrobiculum and Stomach.** Coldness in stomach.

Empty feeling in stomach.

Spasm of stomach, with short breath and dry cough.

Troublesome bloatedness of stomach, with loss of appetite.

Beating in l. side of gastric region toward back.

Burning in œsophagus and stomach, vomiturition, cutting in abdomen; loose stool; nervous debility, twitchings.

Corroding, burning pain in stomach, when walking.

πHeat in stomach and through whole body.

Burning pain in stomach and along chest, as high as pit of throat.

A peculiar pain as if a sore spot were pressed upon, below pit of stomach on pressure and during inspiration.

Gastric symptoms, < in morning.

18 **Hypochondria.** Stitching pains in hypochondria.

19 **Abdomen.** Turning and twisting through whole abdomen, as from a lump.

Spasmodic contraction of abdominal muscles, l. side, with burning pains; he bends over to l. side.

Sensation as if a ball of thread were moving and turning rapidly through abdomen.

Cutting in bowels as with knives.

Burning, boring, whirling in region of navel. θWorms.

Bloated abdomen.

Sensation as if abdomen were sunken.

Rumbling in abdomen as if empty.

Colic: with sensation as if a ball were moving and turning through abdomen, cries out, "O my bowels, they go like a wheel;" with violent urging to stool and borborygmus; from worms.

20 **Stool and Rectum.** Emission of much flatus.

Violent urging to stool with croaking as of frogs; sits a long time, then passes immense quantities of flatus, which is followed by an enormous evacuation; after that burning in abdomen; stool mixed with blood.

Diarrhœa: ▮stool fermented, brown, floating on water; liquid, mixed with blood and slime.

Very difficult stools, with much burning in abdomen and a sensation as of something alive in abdomen.

Before stool: pinching around umbilicus; loud rumbling; urging; emission of flatus; drawing in spermatic cords; burning in anus; shuddering.

After stool: burning in abdomen and rectum.

▮Crawling, itching in anus; ascarides.

▮Lumbrici; tænia; worm fever.

▮▮Vomiting of lumbrici, or nausea and retching, with sensation of a foreign body in œsophagus.

▮▮Tapeworm with severe burning-boring pains in abdomen, accumulation of saliva in mouth, great chilliness and sensitiveness to cold; sensation as if abdomen were sunken, or stomach gnawed; vomiturition and sensation of foreign body in throat.

▮▮Tænia; flushed face; one-sided headache with drawing extending into shoulders, and one-sided convulsive throwing about and involuntary rotations of arm of same side; *Sabad.* cured, and after a few weeks administration caused discharge of a large mass of tapeworm, with complete relief.

21 **Urinary Organs.** Urging to urinate, especially in evening.

Burning in urethra when urinating. θGonorrhœa.

Urine thick and turbid like muddy water.

22 **Male Sexual Organs.** Pollutions, followed by loss of power in extremities.

Lascivious dreams and emissions, with relaxed penis; afterward painful erections with extraordinary lassitude.

23 **Female Sexual Organs.** ▮Nymphomania from ascarides.

Before menses: painful pressure downward.

▮Cutting pains, as from knives, in ovary. θOvaritis.

▮Menses: too late, with painful bearing down a few days previous; decrease, flow by fits and starts, sometimes stronger, sometimes weaker, blood bright red.

24 **Pregnancy. Parturition. Lactation.** ▮Gastric symptoms during pregnancy.

25 **Voice and Larynx. Trachea and Bronchia.** Hoarseness when pressing on larynx, throat feels sore.

▮Influenza; violent spasmodic sneezing and lachrymation on going into open air; tonsillitis begins on l. side and extends to r.; pain < when swallowing empty; sensation as of a thread or string in throat, or a sense of constriction as if it were tied by a string.

▮Epidemic influenza: great sleepiness during day; chilliness, shivering and horripilations, particularly toward evening; chilliness running upward, from feet to head; lachrymation and redness of eyelids; pressure in eyes, particularly when moving them and when looking upward; pressing headache, particularly in forehead; sore pain in tongue, which is covered with a thick yellow coating; pain in tongue extends into throat; difficult deglutition; frequent sensation as if a skin were hanging loosely in throat; bitter taste in mouth; complete loss of appetite; nausea; dryness of mouth; thirstlessness; constipation with rumbling of flatus or diarrhœa of brown fermented stool, which floats upon the water; urine yellow and turbid; cough with vomiting, headache, sharp stitches in vertex, pain in region of stomach; hoarse cough, often with hæmoptysis; painful paralytic weakness of limbs, particularly of knees; all the symptoms < from cold; aggravation toward afternoon, reaching its height in evening; heat of face with chilliness and coldness of limbs or chilliness running up back, returning every ten minutes; skin dry as parchment; sleep restless; disturbed by anxious dreams; cough immediately on lying down.

26 **Respiration.** Sensation of narrowness in throat.

Shortness of breath, cardialgia, dry cough.

Breathing: heavy; anxious, during heat.

Wheezing in chest.

Sudden oppression of breathing, in pit of stomach, with anxiety.

27 **Cough.** ▮Cough: dry, from scratching or roughness in throat; in children, with lachrymation; during chill, also during apyrexia; hoarse sounding with hæmoptoë; nightly, dry; short, dry, produced by a scraping in throat; as soon as one lies down; dry, with perspiration and lachrymation; with stitch in vertex, vomiting and pain in stomach.

|Cough $<$: from cold, or becoming cold; as soon as he lies down; violent spells recur at same hour or at new and full moon.

Expectoration: of tenacious, yellow mucus, of a repulsive sweet taste; of bright red blood, especially when lying down.

28 **Inner Chest and Lungs.** Pain and oppression in chest during apyrexia. θIntermittent.

Stitches in side of chest, especially when inspiring or coughing.

Pleuritis, great paralytic debility.

Complains of coldness, with hot flashes intervening. θPleuritis.

Burning and stitches in chest.

29 **Heart, Pulse and Circulation.** Pulse small, spasmodic.

Sensation as if circulation were suspended.

30 **Outer Chest.** Red spots on chest.

31 **Neck and Back.** |Spine affected; after pollutions excessive weakness shows itself in legs.

Bruised feeling in back and spine; also in sacral region.

32 **Upper Limbs.** Sweat in axillæ.

Convulsions in arms.

Trembling of arms and hands.

Stitches in muscles of arms.

Red spots and stripes on arms and hands.

When writing trembling of hand; old people.

Thick, crippled nails.

Pain in r. shoulder extending to chest, with sensation as if a tape prevented circulation of blood.

Blisters on hands and fingers from little work.

33 **Lower Limbs.** Rheumatic pains in hips; severe stitching; $<$ during rest, $>$ from motion.

Stinging sensation in both thighs at same time.

‖Smarting in r. hypochondrium; shooting down in front of thigh and up to r. scapula; pain makes her twist around; numbness and tingling down r. leg and foot. θRheumatism.

|Loss of power in legs. θSpermatorrhœa.

Boring, tearing in thighs.

Stitches in muscles of thighs.

Severe burning and inflammation of tibia.

Feet swell, are painful on walking; feels every pebble.

Heaviness of feet.

Thick, inflamed, crippled toe nails.

Horizontal fissures between and under toes.

Swelling of feet with tenderness or profuse sweating of soles.

34 **Limbs in General.** Paralytic drawing through limbs.

Stitches in flesh of arms or thighs.

Weariness in limbs.

Continuous heaviness in limbs, obliging one to lie down all day, but especially in later hours of forenoon and toward evening.

35 **Rest. Position. Motion.** Lying perfectly still: vertigo >.

Lying down: cough immediately; expectoration <.

Sitting: vertigo <.

Rising from a seat: vertigo.

He bends to l. side: contraction of muscles of abdomen.

Opening mouth wide: cracking of articulation of jaw.

Writing: trembling of hands.

Walking: vertigo; afterward headache, getting into sweat < itching of scalp; pain in stomach.

36 **Nerves.** Lassitude.

Great debility of knees with relaxation or heaviness of body.

Great debility in intermittents.

Great paralytic weakness in pleuritis.

Intense but transient bruised pain in various parts of body.

Intense pain in all the bones, especially in joints, as if interior of bones were scraped and cut with sharp knife.

Hysteria after a fright.

▮Twitchings, convulsive tremblings, or catalepsy from worms.

▮Nervous diseases from worms or deeply seated abdominal irritation.

37 **Sleep.** Sleepiness: in forenoon; all day; can hardly overcome the inclination; before chill; during heat.

Sleep disturbed by confused unremembered dreams.

Drowsy during day, restless at night.

Many ideas occupy mind, prevent sleep or make it light; evenings.

Sleep restless, tosses about; interrupted by frightful dreams.

In morning starts up from sleep as from a fright.

38 **Time.** Morning: feels <; vertigo and nausea; gastric symptoms <; heat on rising, mouth dry and sticky; sweat.

Forenoon: attacks of giddiness last greater part; very weak; stupefying headache <; later hours, weariness of limbs; sleepiness.

Day: itching on front of head; great sleepiness; drowsy.

Afternoon: feels >; influenza <; chill.

Evening: attacks of giddiness, urging to urinate <; toward, shivering and horripilations <; influenza <; toward, heaviness of limbs; many ideas occupy mind, prevent sleep; chill.

9 P.M.: paroxysms of tertian ague.

Night: awakes with a whirling sensation; palms burn; restless; heat, only tertian ague paroxysms.

39 **Temperature and Weather.** Hot drinks: toothache < ; cannot bear anything hot in mouth.

When overheated: itching on head <.

Warm stove: chilliness >.

Warmth: stitches in forehead and scalp.

Returning to room: twisting, screwing pain from r. side of head to temple.

Open air: vertigo > ; feels > ; when walking, lachrymation; spasmodic sneezing and lachrymation.

Anything cold in mouth causes pain.

Cold drinks: toothache <.

Cold air: toothache < from walking.

Cold: < all symptoms; cough < ; sensitive to.

40 **Fever.** Chilliness and sensitiveness to cold.

Frequently recurring fits of shuddering, passing off quickly without being immediately followed by heat or thirst; suddenly feels hot, especially in face; feels as if a hot breath came out of mouth and nose and heated neighboring parts; no thirst; very comfortable feeling in whole body, and clearness of head; fits of shuddering recur eight or ten times at intervals; paroxysms of heat less frequent but last longer.

▮Chill without thirst, often without subsequent heat.

Violent chilliness, as if dashed with cold water, > by a warm stove.

▮Dry spasmodic cough with pain in ribs and tearing in all bones, during chill.

▮Thirst begins as chill leaves.

▮Thirst for warm drinks before heat.

▮Chill: afternoon or evening, returning at same hour; often without subsequent heat; predominates particularly on extremities, with heat of face; runs from below upward.

▮Evening fever with cold hands and feet and burning face.

▮Whole body feels hot during coryza. θInfluenza.

▮Heat mostly of head and face, often interrupted by shivering, always returning at same hour.

▮Feverish; he feels sick, anxious, starts easily, trembles, breathes short and hot.

Febrile condition, an unwell, sick feeling, restless anxiety, easy startings, short hot breath, trembling, great orgasm of blood, eyes weak and unsteady, as if everything were in motion, as if air itself were in tremulous motion; irresistible desire to sleep, with yawning, icy-cold, shivering without shaking, constant nausea.

▮Heat: only at night and after rising in morning, more internally or only hands, forehead, lips and cheeks feel hot; hands are constantly dry and rough; mouth completely dried up and sticky, in morning; moderate thirst, desire for juicy food; no perspiration, daily for two weeks; head and face, as if he had taken wine, not perceptible to hand, for three hours.

Heat in head not felt externally; internal chilliness.

▮Sweat of soles of feet.

Apyrexia: constantly chilly; loss of appetite; eructations sour, rancid; vomiting of bile and bitter mucus; oppressive bloatedness of stomach; pain in chest; debility; sour eructations.

▮Sweat often during heat; in morning hours with sleep; on face, rest of body cold.

॥Tertian ague of several months' duration which had been treated with Cinchona; chill predominates; thirstlessness and bulimia alternating with aversion to food.

॥Violent shaking of limbs as in a severe chill, so that she could not stand and hardly speak, without any sensation of coldness, although surface was cold to touch; then heat and thirst followed by sweat; twelve to eighteen attacks during twenty-four hours, < every other day. θAgue.

॥Tertian ague, paroxysms at night, after use of household remedies paroxysms ceased for a short time; finally returned and set in daily, always at same hour; chill moderate, followed by thirst and severe long-continued fever with headache.

॥Stages not well marked, shivering often recurs after onset of heat, or there are heat and coldness at same time in different parts of body, thirst at one time present, at another absent, little alteration in pulse, sweat profuse but of short duration; transient nausea; aversion to food during paroxysm; accumulation of water in mouth; belching; scratching in throat as from something sharp, and sensation as if a soft body in throat must be constantly swallowed; paroxysms appear at 9 P.M. θTertian ague.

॥Intermittent fever during Spring; severe chill without subsequent heat or sweat; during apyrexia great weakness of limbs.

॥Ague with regurgitation of food and nausea; thirst between chill and heat.

॥Paroxysms recur at same hour; chill predominates; thirst only between chill and heat; during apyrexia constant chilliness, cough, oppressed breathing and pain in chest.

||Ague paroxysms consisting only of a cold stage; after abuse of Quinine.

||Paroxysm invariably at 3 P.M., chill lasted two hours, with some thirst; heat violent of three hours' duration, and sweating for four hours; no thirst in heat or sweat. θQuartan ague.

|Fever where gastric symptoms prevail, with dry, convulsive cough in cold stage. θQuartan ague.

41 **Attacks, Periodicity.** Alternating: canine appetite and disgust for meat and sour things; thirstlessness and bulimia with aversion to food.

At intervals: eight or ten times fits of shuddering.

Every ten minutes: chilliness up back.

At same hour: cough; chill.

Invariably at 3 P.M.: paroxysms of chills.

Daily: twisting pain in head; for two weeks heat in head and face; twelve to eighteen attacks; shaking.

Nightly: cough.

Every other day: attacks of shaking <.

At new or full moon: cough <.

Ague: of several months' duration.

Spring: intermittent fever.

42 **Locality and Direction.** Right: screwing pain, in side of head; heaviness in side of forehead; pain in shoulder; smarting in hypochondrium; numbness and tingling down leg and foot.

Left: severe stitches in ear; jerking in muscles of upper jaw; beating in side of gastric region; spasmodic contraction of abdominal muscles; he bends to side.

Left to r.: stitches in throat, sore throat; tonsillitis.

Upward: chilliness running from feet to head.

From below upward: chill.

43 **Sensations.** As if things were turning around each other; as if she would fall if she did not hold on to something; as if eyes went round with the whirling sensation; lips as if scalded; tongue as if full of blisters; as of a skin hanging loosely in throat; as if uvula were down; as if œsophagus would be closed; as of a body in throat which he must swallow down; as of a lump in throat; as if a morsel of food had lodged in throat; as of a worm in œsophagus; as if a sore spot were pressed upon; as of a lump in abdomen; as if a ball of thread were moving and turning rapidly through abdomen; as if knives were cutting abdomen; as if abdomen were sunken; abdomen as if empty; croaking as of frogs in abdomen; as of something alive in abdomen; as if stomach were gnawed; as of a thread or string in throat; as if throat were tied with a string;

as if circulation were suspended; as if tape prevented circulation in chest; as if interior of bones were scraped and cut with a sharp knife; as if hot breath came out of his mouth and nose; as if dashed with cold water; as if everything were in motion; as if air itself were in tremulous motion; as if he had taken wine; shaking as if in a severe chill; as of something sharp in throat; as if a soft body in throat must be constantly swallowed.

Pain: in joints and muscles, in tongue and down throat; in region of stomach; in chest; in r. shoulder into chest; in ribs.

Intense pain: in all bones and joints.

Severe pains: in frontal region.

Boring, tearing: in thighs.

Tearing: in all bones.

Cutting pains: in throat; in abdomen; in ovary.

Shooting: down in front of thigh and up to r. scapula.

Stitches: in temples; fine prickling, in skin of forehead and scalp; in l. ear; in throat; in vertex; in side of chest; in muscles of arms; in hips; in muscles of thighs.

Stitching pains: in hypochondria.

Boring, cutting, or scraped feeling: in bones.

Twisting, screwing pain: from r. side of head to both temples.

Pinching: around umbilicus.

Dull pain: in carious teeth.

Rheumatic pains: in hips.

Burning-boring pains in abdomen.

Burning pain: in stomach; along chest as high as pit of throat.

Burning: of mouth; of hands; in point on top of head; of scalp; of face; on tip of tongue; in œsophagus and stomach; in region of navel; in abdomen; in anus; in rectum; in urethra; in chest; in tibia.

Burning itching: most on front of head and behind ears.

Smarting: in r. hypochondrium.

Sore pain: in tongue.

Stinging: in both thighs.

Soreness: of throat; of tongue.

Bruised feeling: in back and spine and sacral region.

Drawing: in spermatic cords into shoulders; through limbs.

Stupefying oppressive sensations: in forehead.

Heat: spreading from head over whole body; of lips; in abdomen; in stomach; in head.

Tingling: down r. leg and foot.

Tickling: in ears.
Scraping: in throat.
Roughness: in throat.
Jerking: in muscles of l. upper jaw.
Beating: in muscles of l. upper jaw; in l. side of gastric region.
Pressure: in head; on eyeballs; in eyes.
Heaviness: of head; r. side of forehead, then to left; of feet; of limbs.
Oppression: of chest.
Dulness: of head.
Sensation of narrowness: in throat.
Constricted feeling: deep in throat.
Turning and twisting: through whole abdomen.
Boring, whirling: in region of abdomen.
Weariness: of limbs.
Empty feeling: in stomach.
Dryness: of mouth; of tongue; of palms; of lips; of fauces and throat.
Crawling: of scalp; like ants in skin.
Numbness: down r. leg and foot.
Itching: of scalp; in ears; in nose; in anus.
Coldness: in stomach; of limbs.

44 **Tissues.** Boring, cutting or scraped feeling in bones.
Inflammation of internal organs.

45 **Touch. Passive Motion. Injuries.** Pressure: on larynx, throat sore.
Scratching: itching of scalp >; violent tickling and stinging on head and behind ears.

46 **Skin.** Crawling sensation like ants in skin.
Red spots and stripes, more marked in cold.
Gray dingy color of skin.
Red spots on face or on chest.
Parchment-like dryness of skin.
ǀMeasles.

47 **Stages of Life, Constitution.** Suited to persons of light hair, fair complexion, with a weakened, relaxed muscular system.
Children; old people.
Boy, æt. 6; ague.
Young man, æt. 16, plethoric; tænia.
Mrs. R., æt. 28, suffering more or less for about three months; she could only ascribe her condition to some extra strain, mental and physical, to which she had been exposed; there is a tendency to neurotic disease in her family; one brother has lately died in an insane asylum, and another has shown symptoms of mental weakness.

Man, æt. 48, suffering 8 days; ague.
Gardener, æt. 55, large, robust, jaundiced hue, suffering several weeks; quartan ague.

48 **Relations.** Antidoted by: *Conium*, *Pulsat.*
Compatible: After *Bryon.* in pleurisy; *Arsen.*, *Bellad.*, *Mercur.* and *Nux vom.* follow well.
Compare: *Verat. alb.*, *Colocyn.* (ovaritis); *Colchic.*, *Lycopod.*, < 4–8 P.M. *Pulsat.* > open air.

SABINA.

Savine. *Coniferæ.*

An evergreen shrub native of the south of Europe. The tincture is made from the young fresh tops of the branches.

Proved by Hahnemann, Gross, Fr. H., Herman, Hartmann, Stapf, etc.; Archiv für Hom., vol. 5; Hering, Prak. Mittheilungen, 1827; Buchner, A. H. Z., vol. 20.

CLINICAL AUTHORITIES.—*Toothache*, Bönninghausen, Rück. Kl. Erf., vol. 1, p. 476; *Hemorrhoids*, Hartmann, Rück. Kl. Erf., vol. 1, p. 1003; *Gleet*, Gollman, Rück. Kl. Erf., vol. 5, p. 550; *Condylomata*, *Exuberant granulations*, *Uterine displacements*, Kurtz, Rück. Kl. Erf., vol. 5, p. 635; *Uterine affection*, Lietzkau, Rück. Kl. Erf., vol. 2, p. 356; *Menorrhagia*, *Metrorrhagia*, *Abortion*, Hartmann, Weber, Rau, Lobethal, Griessel, Nenning, Knorr, Genzke, Attomyr, Schrön, Emmrich, Sturm, Pleyel, Schüler, Tietze, Rück. Kl. Erf., vol. 2, p. 325; *Metrorrhagia*, Löw, Battman, Huber, Rück. Kl. Erf., vol. 5, p. 628; Hahnemann, B. J. H., vol. 12, p. 270; Huber, B. J. H., vol. 16, p. 303; Eidherr, B. J. H., vol. 27, p. 51; Terry, N. A. J. H., vol. 25, p. 317; Ludlam, M. I., vol. 4, p. 278; *Uterine hemorrhage*, Burchfield, Med. Ad., vol. 20, p. 350; *Menorrhagia*, Patzak, Rück. Kl. Erf., vol. 2, p. 253; Wesselhoeft, Hom. Cl., vol. 4, p. 20; Cowperthwait, A. J. H. M. M., vol. 8, p. 11, Raue's Rec., 1875, p. 177; Frost, H. M., Nov., 1874, p. 145, Raue's Rec., 1875, p. 176; Waddell, Hom. Phys., vol. 8, p. 445; *Dysmenorrhœa*, Johnson, T. H. M. S. Pa., 1887, p. 328; Fanning, Hom. Rev., vol. 3, p. 30; *Amenorrhœa*, Watzke, A. J. H. M. M., vol. 4, p. 55, from Œstr. Zft. f. Hom., vol. 2, p. 1; *Amenorrhœa and anœmia*, Madden, B. J. H., vol. 24, p. 301; *Leucorrhœa*, Wood, Hom. Cl., vol. 3, p. 93; Boynton, Hah. Mo., vol. 10, p. 412; *Threatened abortion*, Gibson, M. I., vol. 6, p. 141; Lindsay, Org., vol. 1, p. 472; Fleming, T. H. M. S. Pa., 1887, p. 282; Barretti, Riv. Om., 1874; (2 cases), Slocomb, Mass. Trans., vol. 4, p. 810; *Premature rupture of the membranes*, Streeter, M. I., vol. 4, p. 371; *Dystocia*, Adams, Med. Adv., Jan., 1890, p. 35; *Retained placenta*, Schrön, Rück. Kl. Erf., vol. 2, p. 404; Eaton, Hom. Phys., vol. 9, p. 140; *Arthritis*, Hartmann, Rück. Kl. Erf., vol. 5, p. 546; *Rheumatism*, Wells, Hom. Rev., vol. 3, p. 259; *Chronic rheumatism*, Ægidi, A. J. H. M. M., vol. 3, p. 90.

1 **Mind.** Music is intolerable to her.
Much irritability of temper, hysteria.

Hypochondriacal mood.

Great tiredness and laziness, with a feeling of deep-seated inward trouble, which makes him melancholy and sad.

Irritability of temper, with sour stomach and great anxiety; hypochondriacal mood; rheumatic subjects.

[2] **Sensorium.** Vertigo: especially in morning, fears she will fall; everything turns black before her eyes; suppressed menses; with congestion to and heat in head; when standing; as if he would fall; with obscuration of vision.

[3] **Inner Head.** Headache, especially in temporal eminences, as if parts were pressed asunder; it comes suddenly, disappears gradually and recurs frequently.

Frontal headache, pressing down on eyes as if they would be pressed out; < in morning on rising; > in open air.

Transitory tensive pain in forehead, as if skin had grown fast, with tension in eyes.

Pressure and dulness in head, especially in forehead.

Sense of painful stricture over temples.

Circumscribed pain in each temporal region.

[5] **Sight and Eyes.** Lustreless eyes.

[6] **Hearing and Ears.** Buzzing in ears.

[7] **Smell and Nose.** Dry coryza.

Epistaxis, preceded by dulness and pressure in forehead.

Redness of skin around alæ nasi, painful to touch.

[8] **Upper Face.** Flushes of heat in face, with chilliness all over and coldness of hands and feet.

Pale face; eyes lustreless with blue rings around them.

Pimples on cheeks and forehead.

Black pores in face and on nose.

[10] **Teeth and Gums.** Drawing toothache caused by masticating.

||Throbbing toothache, appearing toward evening and at night, < after eating and from warmth of bed; sensation as if tooth would burst; throbbing in all the bloodvessels; belching; profuse discharge of bright red blood from genitalia between periods.

||Toothache after a gouty pain in great toe had been driven away by external applications.

Toothache evening and night.

Tearing pain in roots of molars.

Swelling of gums around broken teeth.

[11] **Taste and Tongue.** Bitter taste of food, of milk and coffee.

[12] **Inner Mouth.** Offensive breath.

Dryness of mouth and œsophagus without thirst.

Dryness of mouth and throat; the saliva is quite white, and becomes frothy while talking.

[13] **Throat.** Dryness in throat with drawing pain.

Sensation of swelling in throat, as if he had to swallow over a foreign body.

Sensation of a lump in throat; when trying to swallow, cannot; can swallow food.

14 **Appetite, Thirst. Desires, Aversions.** Constant desire for acids (especially lemonade) and roasted coffee.

Appetite poor.

16 **Hiccough, Belching, Nausea and Vomiting.** Burning in stomach; morning sickness.

Heartburn and sour eructations, especially when sitting bent, which position also aggravates other symptoms.

Paroxysms of nausea and qualmishness when she is in a crowd.

Frequent empty retching.

Vomiting: of bile; of undigested food eaten day previous.

17 **Scrobiculum and Stomach.** Stitches in pit of stomach, extending to back.

Frequent burning in pit of stomach, with drawing, twisting and gurgling in bowels, bearing down toward sexual organs.

19 **Abdomen.** Tympanitis; bloatedness of abdomen; rumbling in evening, in a warm room.

Writhing and pinching in abdomen, in umbilical region; frequently recurring with increasing violence and a sensation as if vomiting would come on, without nausea.

Slight sensation of motion in abdomen, as if something were alive.

Quivering in abdomen, as if there were something alive in it, resembling fœtal movements.

Laborlike pains in abdomen, down groins.

Soreness of abdominal muscles.

Pressing down toward genitals.

20 **Stool and Rectum.** Diarrhœa: with pain extending from back through to pubes; in rheumatic or gouty women; with much flatulence.

Stools: of blood and mucus; frequent urging, finally a liquid portion is discharged, followed by a hard portion.

| Constipation: stools hard, difficult and painful; pain from back to pubes.

| Hemorrhoids with discharge of bright red blood, causing pain in back, from sacrum to pubes, biting sore pain in the varices, especially during morning stool.

|| Hemorrhoids with excessive discharge of bright red blood or blood mixed with mucus; cutting, pressive pain low down in abdomen; pressing, urging pain in sphincter ani; constant urging to stool; itching and burning in anus; paroxysmal stitching pain in small of back.

21 **Urinary Organs.** ▮Nephritis, with retention of urine, or discharge by drops, with burning; ardor urinæ in rheumatic subjects.

▮Vesical irritability, depending on gouty diathesis.

Diminished discharge of red urine, with strangury.

Frequent violent urging to urinate, with profuse discharge.

Urine bloody and albuminous.

22 **Male Sexual Organs.** Sexual desire increased, with violent continuous erections.

▮Inflammatory gonorrhœa, with discharge of pus.

▮Rheumatic gonorrhœa.

| |Glans penis dark red, with burning soreness to touch; painfulness of prepuce, cannot retract it; attacks of pain in frænum præputii. θGleet.

Hard swelling on penis.

▮Sycotic excrescences, with burning soreness.

▮Fig-warts with intolerable itching and burning; exuberant granulations.

23 **Female Sexual Organs.** Increased sexual desire almost amounting to nymphomania; almost insatiable desire for an embrace.

Ovaritis, stitches in vagina, deep from before backward.

▮▮Inflammation of ovaries or uterus after abortion or premature labor.

Contractive pain in region of uterus.

▮Uterine pains running from back to groins.

▮Painful active congestions of uterus.

▮Acute metritis; metritis hæmorrhagica.

▮Lateral and posterior displacements of uterus from general atony.

| |Remittent but fixed pain in uterus, at times stitching in character; $<$ during menstruation; colic with the menses; long-continued leucorrhœal discharge after menses; pain during an embrace; uterus enlarged or swollen (mother died of carcinoma uteri).

▮The os tincæ is open, the blood looks red, the discharge is profuse and paroxysmal, especially during motion. θThreatened abortion.

▮Discharge of blood between periods, with sexual excitement.

▮Copious hemorrhages, accompanied by uterine colic; contractive laborlike pains extending from back to pubes and great urging to urinate.

| |Pain or feeling of malaise, extending between sacrum and pubes and experienced in those points. θMetrorrhagia.

▮▮Metrorrhagia: resulting from plethora; clotted and fluid

blood, pain extending from sacrum or lumbar region, to pubes; with severe bearing down, extending from lower part of back around abdomen and down thighs, blood bright red, thin, liquid; laborlike pains in lumbar and uterine region, discharge of large clots of blood, bright red, coming in gushes, particularly profuse on motion, os uteri being constantly open; < by least motion, often > by walking; produced by great irritability of organism, in patients who have menstruated very early in life and very freely, and have always had more or less tendency to miscarriage

|| Without any apparent cause menses recurred three times during the month, each time very abundant and lasting three days; the following month while carrying a heavy burden a stream of blood suddenly gushed from genitals, attended with violent hypogastric pains, weakness of head almost amounting to vertigo; paleness of face; eyes heavy, lustreless; great thirst; little appetite, loose stool; urine red by admixture of blood; drawing, bearing-down pains from fundus of uterus toward sacrum and along broad ligaments to each side, appearing periodically, accompanied at one time by a discharge of black fluid, at another, of coagulated blood; when the pains are absent she has constant hemorrhage; pains > by pressure; least motion increases discharge; hypogastrium distended, has a doughy feeling, but only tender on firm pressure; temperature of skin not elevated, that of extremities lowered; pulse full, soft, quick; sleep uneasy; frequent shivering and mental anxiety. θMetrorrhagia.

|| After miscarriage (two months ago) placenta remained fourteen days; had a constant hemorrhage which could not be stopped; a tampon relieved, but when removed hemorrhage returned; had occasional laborlike pains which caused some strings and shreds to pass.

▮ Protracted uterine hemorrhage arising from a loss of tone in vessels of uterus, whether from disease or weight and pressure of fœtus in utero; blood dark and clotted; gouty subjects.

▮▮ Menses: too profuse, too early; last too long; partly fluid, partly clotted and offensive; flow in paroxysms; with colic and laborlike pains; pains from sacrum to pubes.

|| Low grade of asthenic fever, violent menorrhagia; set in with great violence, discharge red, clotted, partly fluid, accompanied by a pain running from back through to pubes; the noise of the piano seemed to set her distracted.

‖In poor health for two years, from living in a damp house in an ague neighborhood; had chills several times; menses profuse, with large coagulated, conical clots. θMenorrhagia.

‖Girl, æt. 14, had menstruated for more than a year and always irregularly; there was an almost incessant discharge of bright-red blood for four weeks, so that it was impossible to determine the actual periods of commencement of menstruation; walking very much lessened the hemorrhage, but it returned again very soon. θMenorrhagia.

‖Five months after delivery, very profuse discharge of blood, with pains in back and laborlike pressing toward pubes; for six days constant dribbling interrupted by profuse gushes of blood with discharge of large masses of dark coagula accompanied by laborlike pains; < from motion; rapid prostration: pale face; vertigo; chilliness; uterus prolapsed, os pointing to l. side while fundus lay on opposite side. θMenorrhagia.

▮▮Menorrhagia during climacteric period in women who formerly aborted.

‖Dysmenorrhœa accompanied by violent headache; menses generally delayed, lasting about seven days, scanty, coming for a few minutes at a time, then ceasing for six or eight hours, bright, clotted, without flow; pain in hypogastrium going to back; feeling of obstruction internally; dragging pain in back and pain throughout lower extremities which seems deep seated; easiest position is on flat of back with limbs extended; pain < walking, > from warmth; severe pain in head principally in anterior part and eyes, < stooping, walking, > from pressure; nausea, at times vomiting; feverishness; cold hands and feet; pulse 120; violent rapid pulsation felt throughout body, except in head; no premonitory symptoms, pain coming about two hours after menses and ceasing on second day.

▮Dysmenorrhœa with violent pain extending from back through to pubes, rheumatic in origin.

‖Kate R., 16 years old, has not yet menstruated, suffered three years ago from intermittent fever, and since then complained of frontal headaches pressing down on eyes as if it would push them out; < in morning when rising, > in fresh air; cachectic features with blue rings around eyes, especially in morning, toothache most severe at night in bed, > walking about, < by eating; paroxysms of nausea and qualmishness when in a crowd; frequent burning in pit of stomach, drawing, twisting and gurgling in bowels, lasting for hours;

bearing down toward sexual organs; shortness of breath; palpitation at every motion, especially when ascending; pressing pains in chest; heaviness of lower extremities, with painfulness of thighs when walking; drawing; tearing pains in extremities, especially at night; great lassitude and sleepiness. θChlorosis primaria amenorrhœica.

||Anna L., 17 years old, strong constitution, menstruated in her thirteenth year; menses returned regularly until they became suppressed about 18 months ago from immoderate dancing; complains since of severe vertigo, especially in morning and after exertion, so that she is afraid of falling, and everything turns black before her eyes; pressing pains in forehead; burning in ears, greenish-yellow corroding leucorrhœa; shortness of breath, palpitation, sweats easily, painful lassitude; leuco-phlegmatic expression; cheeks and forehead covered with pimples; constant desire for acids and roasted coffee. θChlorosis secundaria metastatica.

||Yellowish, ichorous, fetid leucorrhœa, and painful discharges of fetid blood every two weeks; at climaxis.

▮▮Leucorrhœa: of pudenda; of consistence of starch; copious, milky, causing itching; ropy, glairy from cervical canal; with drawing pains in broad of back through to pubes.

||Corrosive leucorrhœa since commencement of first pregnancy, causing soreness and itching of thighs.

▮Stitches from below upward deep in vagina.

▮Condylomata which itch and burn.

▮Cysts in vulva, sensitive or with tearing pains during rest.

||Stitches in l. nipple.

Voluptuous itching in nipples.

24 **Pregnancy. Parturition. Lactation.** ▮Promotes the expulsion of moles.

||Tendency to abortion, especially at third month; discharge of bright-red, partly clotted blood, < from any motion; pain from sacrum to pubes.

||Greatest anxiety; constant fear that she will abort; for last two days on slightest motion, discharge of blood, alternately bright red, fluid and dark or in clots; labor-like pains from back to pubes; external genitals hot to touch; os uteri dilated half an inch. θThreatened abortion.

||During fifth month of pregnancy labor pains come on at regular intervals of about fifteen minutes, with a slight but unceasing flow of bright-red blood. θThreatened abortion.

|| Profuse flow of blood from vagina; os considerably dilated; vagina filled with dark coagulated blood; chilly; nausea; great thirst; much prostration; third month of pregnancy.

|| Hemorrhage of dark-red blood, at times fluid, at others clotted; not the slightest pain in back or hypogastrium; great prostration. θThreatened abortion.

| Miss Rose L., about 22 years old, a thin, delicate female of nervous temperament, forsaken and unhappy; seven months pregnant; morning sickness with loss of appetite and diarrhœa; some blood has passed at intervals of two and three weeks; profuse metrorrhagia and diarrhœa; flooding much < by moving or going to chamber, when it flows profusely and is of an arterial color; constant pain from sacral region to pubes; child has not moved since two days; face pale, she begins to feel faint; os dilated and patulous (delivered two months later of a healthy child).

|| After a miscarriage violent hemorrhages, lasting each time eight to ten days; during first five days profuse discharge of bright-red fluid blood, without pain.

|| Uterine hemorrhage of four weeks' duration after abortion.

|| Retained placenta after abortion; free discharge of blood; mouth of uterus closed; patient very nervous.

|| Premature rupture of membranes and free escape of liquor amnii; occurred forty days previous to labor, caused by overwork and followed by labor pains and discharge of blood.

|| On eighth day after labor, reappearance of blood, lochial discharge having already ceased; on ninth day three attacks of hemorrhage, discharge profuse, containing a large number of clots, < on rising, causing loss of consciousness; heat over whole body with sweat, face cold and pale.

| Atony of uterus; painless loss of dark-red blood immediately after delivery; discharge of fluids and clots with each pain.

| Retained placenta; pain, or an uneasy, bad feeling, extending from sacrum to pubes; a slight sensation of motion in abdomen; intense after-pains, notwithstanding the retention, with discharge of fluid blood and clots in about equal proportion with every pain.

| Retained placenta from atony of uterus.

| After-pains with sensitiveness of abdomen.

| Metritis after parturition.

25 **Voice and Larynx. Trachea and Bronchia.** Crawling and tickling in larynx exciting cough and mucous expectoration.

Dry, hacking cough and tickling in trachea; expectoration streaked with blood next day.

26 **Respiration.** Shortness of breath.

28 **Inner Chest and Lungs.** Intermittent stitches in clavicle.

Tensive pain with pressure in middle of sternum, neither increased by expectoration nor inspiration.

Pressing pains in chest.

▮Hæmoptysis.

29 **Heart, Pulse and Circulation.** Palpitation at every motion, especially when ascending.

Pulse unequal; generally quick, strong and hard.

Violent beating of bloodvessels in whole body.

31 **Neck and Back.** Constant pain in small of back, obliging him to bend the back inward.

Paralytic pain in small of back; would like to stretch; > bending backward.

▮▮Drawing pains in small of back, extending to pubic region.

▮Indescribable uneasiness in lumbar vertebræ; dragging sensation from behind forward resembling weak labor pains.

Weariness in lumbar region.

Laborlike pains drawing down into groins.

32 **Upper Limbs.** Pain as if sprained, in r. shoulder joint, even during rest.

▮▮Pressive pain in both upper arms, near elbow joint, from without inward, < on touch and motion.

Paralytic tearing along r. upper arm as far as hand.

Stinging in both upper arms, from within outward, near elbow joints.

Aching pain in right radius, < from motion or touch.

▮Arthritic stiffness and swelling of wrist joint, with tearing and stinging, made almost insupportable when hand hangs down.

33 **Lower Limbs.** Rheumatism of metatarso-phalangeal joint of big toe, characterized by great swelling, bright shining red; intense sensibility to touch and motion; < at night; high fever.

Heaviness of legs, with painfulness of thighs when walking.

Stinging pains in hip joints, in morning and when breathing.

Sensation of coldness in whole (r.) leg.

Ulcers on tibia, with a lardaceous base.

Swelling, redness and stitches in big toe. *θ*Gout.

The middle of anterior surface of his thighs feels bruised and painful.

Tearing pain with pressure in metacarpal bones of both feet.

Sharp stitches from within outward in heels.

Painful drawing in joints of r. toes, < during a walk.

34 **Limbs in General.** Drawing, tearing pains in extremities, especially at night.

‖ A man æt. 42; haggard, emaciated, stooping gait, thin, grey hair, hollow eyes, skin of an ashy hue; from time to time dry cough, with dyspnœa; complains of weakness and decrepitude, no strength to work, little appetite, slow digestion, sleep restless and full of dreams, sticky sweat toward morning; here and there through joints a gouty lamelike pain, now in shoulder and elbow joint, now in hip and knee; pains < in a warm room and > in open air; pains usually in one side of body, mostly r.; troublesome pulsation in different bloodvessels, especially when taking a deep breath, < in evening in bed, which he has to leave again, not being able to return until morning; transitory, tensive pain in forehead, with sensation as if skin had grown fast, with tension in eyes; redness of skin around alæ nasi, painful to touch; dryness of mouth and œsophagus without thirst; collection of white frothy mucus, filling corners of mouth when talking; sensation of a body in throat, which he tries to swallow but cannot, it offers no impediment to swallowing of food; heartburn and sour eructations, especially when sitting bent, which likewise aggravates the other symptoms; > from sitting erect, from moving and stretching limbs, for which he has an involuntary desire; rumbling and gurgling in abdomen, especially in evening, in warm room; great tiredness and laziness, with a feeling of deep-seated inward trouble, which makes him melancholy and sad. θChronic rheumatism.

Great weakness and weariness of limbs, with tearing pains at night; when very warm; > in cold air.

‖ Red and shining swelling of great toe, with excessive pains, < by least touch or motion; heaviness of affected limbs; fever < in evening; wandering pains, burning, affecting one joint after another, especially big toe and hand; > by cool applications; changes her position often to get relief. θArthritis.

35 **Rest. Position. Motion.** Rest: tearing pains in cysts; pain in shoulder joint.

Lying on flat of back with limbs extended, easiest position during dysmenorrhœa.

Must lie down: heaviness of body.

Sitting bent: heartburn and sour eructations <.

Standing: vertigo.

Stooping: pain in head <.

When hand hangs down: tearing and stinging in wrist joint <.
Must bend the back inward: pain in small of back.
Elevating limbs: > pain in ulcers.
Rising: discharge of clots <.
Changes position often to get relief: arthritis.
Motion: profuse discharge from uterus: palpitation; always increases discharge; palpitation; pain in upper arms <; pain in r. radius <; pain in big toe <.
Moving and stretching limbs: eructations and heartburn >.
Walking: metrorrhagia >; lessened hemorrhage; dysmenorrhœa <; pain in head <; painfulness of thighs; drawing in toes <.
Ascending: palpitation <.
Lies on l. side: during sleep.

36 **Nerves.** Feels weary and weak in all her limbs with great despondency.
‖Heaviness and indolence of body, obliging him to lie down.
Great lassitude and heaviness.
Very tired and lazy.
Is very nervous and hysterical, and if she becomes pregnant is almost sure to abort about third month.
▮Nervousness so great that music becomes unbearable, it goes through bone and marrow.

37 **Sleep.** Sleeplessness and restlessness after midnight, with heat and profuse perspiration.
Lies on l. side during sleep.

38 **Time.** Morning: vertigo <; frontal headache <; pain in varices during stool: pain in hip joints; toward, sticky sweat; tenseness in ulcer <.
During day: great chilliness.
Toward evening: toothache.
Evening: rumbling in abdomen; pulsation in different bloodvessels < in bed; fever <; chill with shivering; tenseness in ulcer <.
Night: toothache; pains in extremities <; pain in great toe <; drawing and tearing in extremities <.
After midnight: sleepless and restless.

39 **Temperature and Weather.** Warmth of bed, toothache <; pain (dysmenorrhœa) >; pain in ulcer <.
Warm room: rumbling in abdomen; rheumatic pains <; gout <.
Open air: frontal headache >; rheumatic pains >; tenseness in ulcer >.
Cool applications: wandering pains in joints >.
Cool air: weariness and weakness of limbs >; gout >.

40 **Fever.** Chill in evening with attacks of shivering.
Great chilliness during day.
Shivering with obscuration of sight, followed by sleepiness.
Burning heat of whole body, with great restlessness.
Flushes of heat in face, rest of body chilly, hands and feet cold.
Sweats easily; sweat every night.

41 **Attacks, Periodicity.** Paroxysms: discharge from uterus; of nausea and qualmishness.
At intervals of fifteen minutes: labor pains.
Periodically: pains in uterus.
Every night: sweat.
Three times during month: menses.
Every two weeks: painful discharge of fetid blood.

42 **Locality and Direction.** Right: pain in shoulder joint; tearing in upper arm; aching in radius; coldness in leg; painful drawing in joints of toes.
Left: stitches in nipple; lies on side during sleep.
From before backward: stitches in vagina.
From behind forward: dragging in lumbar vertebræ.
From below upward: stitches in vagina.
From within outward: stinging in upper arms; stitches in heels.
From without inward: pressive pain in arms.

43 **Sensations.** As if she would fall; as if parts of temporal eminence were pressed asunder; as if eyes would be pressed out; as if skin had grown fast on forehead; as if tooth would burst; as if he had to swallow over a foreign body; as of a lump in throat; as if vomiting would come on; as if something were alive in abdomen; r. shoulder joint as if sprained.
Pain: in temporal eminences; from back through to pubes; in frænum; in uterus from back to groins; throughout lower extremities; from sacral region to pubes; in small of back.
Violent pains: in hypogastric region; from back to pubes.
Severe pain: in head and eyes.
Tearing pain: in roots of molars; in cysts, in vulva; in wrist joints; in metacarpal bones of both feet; in extremities.
Paralytic tearing: along upper arm as far as hand.
Throbbing pain: in teeth.
Stitches: in pit of stomach; to back; in vagina; in l. nipple; in clavicle; in big toe; in heels.
Stitching pain: in small of back; in uterus.
Cutting pressive pain: low down in abdomen.
Pinching: in abdomen.
Dragging pain: in back.

Pressing urging pain: in sphincter ani.
Pressing pain: in chest; in forehead; in upper arms.
Tensive pain: in forehead; in middle of sternum; in broad of back through to pubes; in small of back; in joints of r. toes; in extremities.
Contractive pain: in region of uterus.
Aching pain: in r. radius.
Bearing-down pains: from fundus of uterus toward sacrum and along the broad ligaments to each side.
Drawing pain: in teeth; in throat.
Laborlike pains: in abdomen down groins.
Paralytic pain: in small of back.
Lamelike pain: in joints.
Burning sore pain: in the varices; in glans penis.
Circumscribed pain: in each temporal region.
Dragging sensation: in lumbar vertebræ.
Burning: in stomach; in pit of stomach; in anus; of condylomata.
Stinging: in both upper arms; in wrist joint; in hip joints.
Soreness: of abdominal muscles; of thighs.
Painfulness: of thighs.
Painful stricture: over temples.
Throbbing: in all bloodvessels.
Tension: in eyes.
Pressure: in head; in forehead; in metacarpal bones of both feet.
Pressing: on eyes; toward genitals.
Heaviness: of lower extremities.
Dulness: in head; in forehead.
Drawing, twisting and gurgling: in bowels.
Writhing: in abdomen.
Weariness: in lumbar region; of limbs.
Weakness: of head; of limbs.
Dryness: of mouth and œsophagus; of throat.
Tickling: in larynx; in trachea.
Crawling: in larynx
Itching: in anus; of pudenda; of thighs; of condylomata; voluptuous, in nipples.
Coldness: of hands and feet; in r. leg.

44 **Tissues.** Drawing pains through long bones.
Red, shining swelling of affected parts.
▮Gout; arthritic complaints; tearing, stinging in joints after they become swollen; < in heated room; > in cool air or cool room; arthritic nodes.
Chlorosis.
Throbbing in all the bloodvessels.
▮Hemorrhages.

45 **Touch. Passive Motion. Injuries.** Touch: skin around

alæ nasi painful; glans penis sore; pains in upper arms < ; pain in r. radius < ; intense sensibility of great toe.

Pressure: pains in uterus > ; hypogastrium tender; pain in head >.

46 **Skin.** Black pores in skin, especially of face.

▮ Fig-warts, with intolerable itching and burning; exuberant granulations.

Deep ulcers; prickling feeling of tenseness in ulcer; < morning and evening, exertion, touch, warmth of bed; > open air, cold, raising or elevating limbs.

47 **Stages of Life, Constitution.** Chronic ailments of women; arthritic pains; tendency to miscarriage.

Gouty diathesis.

Girl, æt. 12, came into puberty at the age of eleven; dysmenorrhœa.

Girl, æt. 14, tall, thin, scrofulous, has menstruated for more than a year; menorrhagia.

Girl, æt. 16, not yet menstruated, suffered three years ago from intermittents, since then complaining; amenorrhœa.

Girl, æt. 17, strong constitution, menstruated in her thirteenth year; suppressed 18 months ago from immoderate dancing; amenorrhœa.

Girl, æt. 19, sanguine temperament, thin, weakly constitution, menstruated regularly since sixteenth year, seven years ago had hæmoptysis; metrorrhagia.

Woman, æt. 21, delicate, nervous, always aborted at third month after slightest mental disturbance, hemorrhage being profuse; threatened abortion.

Mrs. D., æt. 21, nervous temperament, suffering since her first pregnancy; leucorrhœa.

Miss R. L., æt. 22, nervous temperament, thin, delicate, forsaken and unhappy, seven months pregnant; threatened abortion.

Young lady, æt. 23, in good health; menorrhagia.

J. O, æt. 24, medium height, dark complexion, dark hair, nervous temperament, very fond of music, suffering for years; dysmenorrhœa.

Woman, æt. 24; threatened abortion.

Miss P., æt. 25, ill two years; amenorrhœa and anæmia.

Woman, æt 26, delivered two months ago, since then suffering; uterine hemorrhages.

Mrs. J., æt. 27, mother of two children; retained placenta after abortion.

Mrs. S., æt. 26, brunette, married ten years; uterine hemorrhage.

Servant girl, æt. 30, tall, thin; metrorrhagia.

Mrs. A., æt. 30, in poor health for two years, from living in a damp house in an ague neighborhood, having had chills several times; menorrhagia.

Woman, æt. 30, on ninth day after second labor; uterine hemorrhage.

Woman, æt. 30, strong, sanguine choleric temperament, aborted four times, now three months pregnant; threatened abortion.

Woman, æt. 32, three months pregnant; threatened abortion.

Mrs. N., æt. 38, nine months married; dystocia.

Woman, æt. 40, sanguine temperament, passed through four pregnancies, waters each time escaping eight days before labor; threatened abortion.

Man, æt. 42; chronic rheumatism.

Woman, well built, phlegmatic temperament, delivered five months ago, since then has not menstruated: menorrhagia.

48 **Relations.** Antidoted by: *Pulsat.*

Compatible: *Arsen.*, *Bellad.*, *Pulsat.*, *Rhus tox.*, *Spongia*, *Sulphur.*

Complementary to: *Thuja.*

Compare: *Arnica*, *Calc. ostr.*, *Coccul.*, *Crocus*, *Ipecac.*, *Millef.*, *Ruta*, *Secale*, *Trillium.*

SALICYLICUM ACIDUM.

Salicylic Acid. $H_2 C_7 H_4 O_3$.

Found in nature in Spiræa blossoms, Wintergreen (Gaultheria), etc.

Fragmentary provings by Lewi, H. K., vol. 20, p. 106; Macfarlan (recorded in Thesis of G. W. Shaffer, March, 1877) common symptoms of 20 provings. See Allen's Encyclopedia, vol. 8.

Clinical Authorities.—*Menière's disease*, McClatchey, Hom. Rev., vol. 21, p. 736; Hah. Mo., vol. 13, p. 57; *Deafness*, Claude, B. J. H., vol. 36, p. 356; *Canker of mouth*, Hoffman, M. I., vol. 5, p. 66; *Use in diphtheria*, Grosvenor, Mass. Trans., vol. 4, p. 659; Fontheim, A. H. O., vol. 13, p. 112; *Indigestion*, Goullon, A. H. Z., vol. 94, p. 86; *Dyspepsia*, Hale, N. A. J. H., vol. 25, p. 354; *Flatulent dyspepsia*, Hale, M. I., vol. 2, p. 326; Whitman, M. I., vol. 5, p. 229; *Inflammation of stomach and bowels*, Hoffman; *Flatulence*, Hale, Am. Hom , vol. 1, p. 94; *Diarrhœa*, Œhme, N. E. M. G., vol. 12, p. 412; *Cholera infantum*, Hale, N. A. J. H., vol. 25, p. 354; *Catarrh of bladder*, Hale, M. I., vol. 4, p. 156; *Septicæmia*, Hale, N. A. J. H., vol. 25, p. 354; *Septic fever* (2 cases), Hale, M. I., vol. 5, p. 142; *Sciatica*, Goullon, Hah. Mo., vol. 12, p. 371; *Foot sweats*, Pagi, N. A. J. H., vol. 25, p. 404; *Acute articular rheumatism*, Goullon, Times Ret., 1877, p. 3; H. K., 1876, p. 69; A. H. Z., 1876, p. 76; Times Ret., 1876, p. 118; *Acute rheumatism*, Thompson, Hom. Times, vol. 4, p. 108; *Rheumatism*, Hale, N. A. J. H., vol. 25, p. 355; Griswold, Cal. Med. Times, vol. 1, p. 5; Koeck, N. A. J. H., vol. 26, p. 124; *Arthritis*, Molin, B. J. H., vol. 36, p. 356; *Chronic caries*, Hom. Rev., vol. 22, p. 415.

1 **Mind.** Anxiety; worrying, restless, yet mild.

Melancholic; wants to lie quiet; feels faint.

Excited mood.

Delirium; stupid, can hardly collect his ideas, then he laughed without cause, talked incessantly and disconnectedly, frequently looked about him with apparent hallucinations.

2 **Sensorium.** Stupefaction; dulness of head.

Vertigo; inclines to fall to l. side, while surrounding objects seem falling to right.

▮Menière's disease; vertigo which comes and goes, often from no observable reason; tendency to fall to affected side, while objects seem to fall away to opposite side; headache frequent but not always present; noises in ear; defective or absent perosseous hearing; absence of gastric symptoms, or so slight as not to account for the other symptoms; indeterminate giddiness in horizontal position, but considerable when raising head or sitting up.

3 **Inner Head.** Rush of blood to head.
Severe headache; piercing, in both temples.
Headache, commencing on top or in back of head, running down sterno-mastoid (more r. side), which is tender to touch.

5 **Sight and Eyes.** Diminished acuteness of vision.
⁝Plastic iritis following inflammatory rheumatism, the pupil would contract notwithstanding the local use of a one per cent. solution of Atrop. sulph.; the nightly pain was most agonizing, temporarily > by hot applications.

6 **Hearing and Ears.** ▮Deafness, with noises in ears.
Nervous deafness.
Diminished hearing.
▮Roaring in ears, with difficult hearing.
πDisturbs hearing when given for rheumatism (large doses).
▮Tinnitus dependent upon hyperæmia.
▮Auditory nerve vertigo; a troublesome nausea accompanying head symptoms.
Roaring in ears and difficult hearing; hears music; rush of blood to head; excited mood.
ǁPurulent, fetid otorrhœa.

7 **Smell and Nose.** Wants to sneeze.
▮Incipient catarrh, patients, especially children, sneeze all day.

8 **Upper Face.** Dull, heavy aspect; face flushes quickly on slight excitement.

11 **Taste and Tongue.** Taste: as of something burnt; bitter; food has no taste.

12 **Inner Mouth.** Mouth and throat dry; burning and dryness of mouth and pharynx.
ǁRedness of buccal cavity and fauces. θDiphtheria.
▮Stomatitis, the mouth is hot and dry, tongue covered with burning vesicles.
Foul breath and offensive expectoration.
Mouth dotted with white patches, burning, scalded feeling; ulcers on tip of tongue.
▮Canker sores, with burning soreness and fetid breath.
ǁCanker of mouth, stomach and bowels; patient rapidly sinking.

13 **Throat.** Burning in throat.
▮Tonsils red, swollen, studded white.
Violent efforts to swallow, with difficulty in swallowing, woke him from sleep; the pain and difficulty became confined to r. side, with sticking along Eustachian tube into ear; swelling of r. tonsil noticeable externally, with sensitiveness to touch and increased temperature in

vicinity; mucous membrane of throat and posterior fauces red, swollen, with ulcers size of head of a pin; after a while a small lump of cheesy matter of strong odor was expectorated.

▮Scarlatina anginosa; diphtheritic form.

‖ Little or no fever, but great weakness, difficult deglutition, much inflammation, the exudate soft. θDiphtheria.

▮Diphtheritis; violent fever; entire fauces covered with a white exudate; in two cases hoarseness and barking cough (affection of larynx).

16 **Hiccough, Belching, Nausea and Vomiting.** Nausea, gagging, waterbrash.

Frequent vomiting.

17 **Scrobiculum and Stomach.** Ecchymoses and ulcerations in mucous membrane of stomach and bowels.

Burning in epigastric region.

Weak nervous sensation in stomach.

‖ Flatulent and fermentative dyspepsia.

▮Distension and formation of gases in stomach and bowels after meals.

‖ Excessive accumulation of flatus and acidity of stomach, with much belching of gas, anæmia and great irritability with despondency. θDyspepsia.

▮Dyspepsia with putrid eructations and much accumulation of gas on stomach.

| A young lady of bilious temperament, wasted from a fleshy, strong girl to an emaciated, bony creature; as soon as she would eat, no matter how simple the food, her stomach would bloat up so that it would be necessary to loosen her dress; region of stomach looked like an inflated bladder; after from one to two hours suffering in region of stomach from this extreme distension, was a putrid flatus belched up, accompanied by collapse of stomach and temporary relief; frequent vomiting characterized by putrid fermentation; severe headaches; extremely nervous; sleep fitful and unrefreshing; bowels constipated; urine heavily loaded with sediment; fermentation and decomposition seemed to commence as soon as food reached stomach. θFlatulent dyspepsia.

‖ Woman, æt. 30, of very unhealthy family; always suffering from indigestion; daily, some hours after dinner, has diarrhœa; sometimes looks very badly; least error in diet shows effect in an aggravation of the diarrhœa.

‖ Girl four years old, had relapse from malignant scarlet fever; inflammation of bowels supervened, with immense distension of abdominal region.

20 **Stool and Rectum.** Diarrhœa; stools green; flushes easily as in hectic; acid, sour, or putrid smelling.

Costive; stool dry, hard; then diarrhœa, watery, sour, yellow, with great weakness.

▮Cholera infantum or other diarrhœa in children, when eructations have a peculiarly putrid and offensive odor.

⁝In a case where tænia solium had existed for nine years four doses of 0.5 acid Salicyl. a dose every hour, followed by half an ounce Ol. ricini, caused in half an hour discharge of tænia ten yards long, with head entire.

21 **Urinary Organs.** Diabetes mellitus (two cases).

Albuminuria; rheumatic diathesis.

Urine very offensive, largely composed of mucus; microscope revealed pus, blood and an abundance of mucous epithelium. θCatarrh of bladder.

Urine: scanty, clear, brown; three hours after its passage it has a green tinge and deposits a feathery precipitate, consisting of oblong, six-sided, silvery-white crystals of Salicyluric acid; if these are removed the urine becomes at once putrid; if not the urine remains fresh for above a week.

23 **Female Sexual Organs.** ❘❘Large leuco-phlegmatic woman, æt. 45; constant dull, heavy pain in cerebellum; great forgetfulness, excessive irritability and frequent hot flushes of fever.

24 **Pregnancy. Parturition. Lactation.** ❘❘A primipara, delivered on 9th of May of a large male child; slight lesion of vagina; a piece of membrane as large as finger-nail was torn up; membranes unusully tough and extensive and a small shred was left in utero; on third day chill, followed by fever; pulse 120, temperature 105; lochia offensive. θSeptic fever.

❘❘Confined with second child on May 15th, delivered with forceps owing to the great size of the head; no apparent lesion; lochia not offensive, disappeared on tenth day; considerable hemorrhage after labor, and I suppose a small clot or clots became impacted in uterine blood-vessels and owing to access of air (perhaps) underwent decomposition, and this septic material was absorbed; on eleventh day severe chill, repeated twice next day; pulse 130, temperature 104; chills alternated with febrile heats, and chilliness was excited by slightest touch of anything cold or a swallow of cold water, and she was very thirsty; some pain and swelling of one breast and one knee. θSepticæmia.

26 **Respiration.** Respiration hurried, sometimes deepened, sometimes shallow or sighing and almost panting, as if labored, but no complaint of difficulty of breathing.

27 **Cough.** Dry cough, of a hard, racking, spasmodic character, < at night in old people.

28 **Inner Chest and Lungs.** Spasmodic, flatulent asthma: fetid bronchitis; gangrene of lungs.

29 **Heart, Pulse and Circulation.** Pulse small, rapid, weak.

32 **Upper Limbs.** || Rheumatic gout or rheumatoid arthritis, occurring in some women during climaxis; the pains disappeared, the engorgements and nodosities of fingers subsided, and the hands could again be used.

33 **Lower Limbs.** || Formerly had foot sweats, and since their suppression is more liable to rheumatic pains; attacks especially at night; after an hour's sleep the pains force him to leave bed; he changes to sofa but must soon leave it again, and thus he passes a sleepless night; the seat of pain corresponds exactly to exit of l. ischiatic nerve, goes from behind forward and downward to knees and toes; pain is drawing, shooting, at the toes burning, or as he expresses himself, "as if foot were on an ant-hill" and as if the foot would like to perspire; no fever; can hardly ascend stairs, must look for some support or he might fall. θSciatica.

| Copious foul-smelling foot sweats.

34 **Limbs in General.** | Heat, redness, soreness and swelling about joints; < in knees, with acute piercing pains; < on motion, > from dry heat. θRheumatism.

35 **Rest. Position. Motion.** Lying: indeterminate giddiness.

Wants to be quiet: melancholic

Forced to leave bed: sciatica.

Sitting up: considerable giddiness.

Motion: rheumatism in joints <; exquisitely painful, rheumatism of affected limb causes soreness.

36 **Nerves.** Weakness, faintness.

38 **Time.** Night: dry cough <; attacks of rheumatic pains <.

39 **Temperature and Weather.** Hot applications: rheumatism >.

Dry heat: rheumatism of joints >.

Sitting near open window in a hot room: rheumatism.

Touch of anything cold: excited chilliness.

40 **Fever.** | Slight chill, crawls in spine; yawning; chill in finger tips.

| Fever continuous, burning, then sweat with relief; fever again, with exacerbation of symptoms.

Sweat at times more, at others less profuse.

Profuse but short-lasting sweat.

Weak, faint after fever and sweat.

Flushes easily, as in hectic.

: Rheumatic fever.

41 **Attacks and Periodicity.** Daily: some hours after dinner, has diarrhœa.

Nightly: agonizing rheumatism.

42 **Location and Direction.** Right: difficulty of swallowing; swelling of tonsil; severe pain in several joints; pain in deltoid and gastrocnemius.

Left: inclines to fall to side, vertigo; severe pain in all joints; ankle and knee pains; elbow and wrist enormously swollen; pain in wrist and forearm.

43 **Sensations.** As if foot were on an ant-hill; as if foot wanted to perspire; as if head were squeezed between two beams.

Pain: in shoulder and elbow, then in lumbar region; in r. deltoid and gastrocnemius.

Terrific pain: in knee joint.

Severe pain: in all the joints on l. side and several on r. side.

Acute piercing pain: in joints.

Piercing pain: in head.

Shooting pain: in lower limbs,

Burning pains: in toes.

Sticking: along Eustachian tube into ear.

Drawing pain: in lower limbs.

Rheumatic pains: in hands; exit of l. ischiatic nerves to knees and toes.

Dull, heavy pain: in cerebellum.

Dull, aching distress: in stomach.

Soreness: about joints; in r. deltoid and gastrocnemius.

Burning: of mouth and pharynx; of vesicles in mouth; of canker sores; in throat; in epigastric region.

Painful stiffness: of neck.

Dulness: of head.

Weak, nervous sensations: in stomach.

Dryness: of mouth and pharynx.

44 **Tissues.** Pieces of spongy bone became soft as leather in a few days when placed in a half per cent. solution, while compact bone tissue is very slowly softened; enamel of teeth is very slightly affected by it, but the dentine, when it is exposed by caries, is rapidly destroyed.

The increased amount of the salts of lime in the urine soon after Salicylic acid has been taken shows that the acid deprives living as well as dead bone of its lime salts.

Causes a sort of necrosis, especially of tibia.

▮▮Ulceration of mucous surfaces.

▮▮Acute articular rheumatism.

▮Rheumatism: acute articular; chronic; gonorrhœal; diphtheritic.

▮Acute, inflammatory, articular rheumatism attacking one or more joints, especially elbows or knees, with great swelling and redness, high fever and excessive sensitiveness to least jar; motion impossible.

▮Muscular rheumatism.

▮Severe pain in all the joints on l. and several joints on r. side; large joints on l. side were attacked, except hip and shoulder, while on r. side the wrist and ankle alone suffered.

‖A tall young man, æt. 16, suffered from severe acute articular rheumatism; knee joint especially was seat of terrific pain; painful stiffness of neck; excessive perspiration, followed by miliaria; great lassitude; pulse full, soft, very frequent; went out too early and a relapse set in, with same weakening sweats; patient looked anæmic and emaciated; hurried pulse, reminding one of heart's beat in beginning of phthisis.

‖A teacher suffered from acute articular rheumatism; a relapse followed from carelessness, attack being very severe, with profuse sour-smelling sweats and extensive eruption of miliaria; very nervous, urine showed heavy sediment; desquamation set in just as after scarlet fever in hands and feet; pains first in shoulder and elbow, then in lumbar region, so that the patient could hardly move; during relapse hands greatly swollen, could not be used; sleeplessness or sleep interrupted by frightful dreams, as if his head were squeezed between two beams (stiffness of neck); constipation

:Acute gout.

‖Rheumatism after sitting near an open window in a hot room, so that she felt hot on one side and chilly on the other; l. ankle and knee joint, elbow and wrist enormously swollen, of a pinkish color, very sensitive, every motion exquisitely painful, pulse 120, high temperature, sweat, etc., even in bed, shocks passed from thigh down to foot so that she had to scream.

‖Polyarthritis rheumatica, temperature 105; pain intense, tenderness excessive.

‖Soreness and pain in r. deltoid and r. gastrocnemius, changing next day to l. wrist and forearm; some sensitiveness to touch and great soreness on moving limb; no heat; on following day pain had removed to inside of l. forefinger; when the pain appeared in one part it disappeared in the part which had previously been painful

‖Purpura hemorrhagica, with hemorrhages from all mucous membranes, accompanied by a constant dull aching distress in stomach and occasional vomiting of blood and mucus.

: Has a specific action upon serous membranes and should be very useful in dropsical effusions; should be tried in hydrocephalus, hydropericardium and renal dropsy.

May prove useful in caries and necrosis.

45 **Touch. Passive Motion. Injuries.**

Touch: top or back of head tender; tonsil sensitive; arm sensitive; limbs tender.

46 **Skin.** Skin red; points on skin like flea-bites.

Skin red and sensitive; rheumatism.

▮ Urticaria.

Sprinkled on indolent or inflamed ulcers is said to induce rapid healing.

47 **Stages of Life, Constitution.** Healthy-looking child, æt. 5 weeks, suffering over two weeks; diarrhœa.

Girl, æt. 12; rheumatism.

Young man, æt. 16, tall; rheumatism.

Woman, æt. 30, coming from a very unhealthy family; indigestion and diarrhœa.

Man, æt. 80, robust, formerly had foot sweats, and since their suppression is more liable to rheumatic pains: sciatica.

48 **Relations.** Compare: *Colchic.* (rheumatism, also subsequent weakness); *Kreos.* (piercing in temples; throat; diarrhœa; ulcers, antiseptic properties); *Carb. ac.* (mind; throat; weakness, especially at stomach; hectic; antiseptic properties; topical use; urine); *Salicyl. of Soda* (tinitus aurium, confusion and deafness; rheumatism); *Nitr. ac.; Arsen.; Phosphor.* (bones); *Lac. ac.* (bones, throat): *Cinchona* (preventing sepsis; fever; ringing in ears).

SAMBUCUS NIGRA.

Elder. *Caprifoliaceæ.*

The European elder, Sambucus nigra, differs but slightly from the American, Sambucus canadensis. The tincture is prepared from the fresh leaves and flowers.

Introduced and proved by Hahnemann, assisted by Franz, Gross, Hartmann, Langhammer and Wislicenus, R. A. M. L., vol. 5.

CLINICAL AUTHORITIES.—*Coryza*, Tietze, Gross, Rück. Kl. Erf., vol. 1, p. 391 *Ileus* (3 cases reported cured), Lilienthal, Hah. Mo., vol. 7, p. 116; *Influenza*, Sorge, A. H. Z., vol. 92, p. 110; *Laryngismus*, Wesselhoeft, A. J. H. M. M., vol. 4, p. 19; *Spasmodic croup*, Müller, Rück. Kl. Erf., vol. 5, p. 765; *Croup*, Fielitz, Tietze, B. J. H., vol. 5, p. 308; Hawley, Hom. Phys., vol. 6, p. 441; Pröll, A. H. Z., vol. 112, p. 126; *Cough, Croup, Asthma Millari, suffocative attacks, etc.*, Hartmann, Rummel, Tietze, Hirsch, Hinz, Weber, Fielitz, Rück. Kl. Erf., vol. 3, p. 97; *Asthmatic attacks*, Hirsch, B. J. H., vol. 25, p. 392; *Whooping cough*, Griesselich, Rück. Kl. Erf., vol. 3, p. 84; Arnold, Rück. Kl. Erf., vol. 5, p. 728; *Use in whooping cough*, Wesselhoeft, N. E. M. G., vol. 4, p. 366; *Catarrhal affection of chest*, Boenninghausen, Rück. Kl. Erf., vol. 5, p. 694; *Use in phthisis*, McGeorge, N. E. M. G., vol. 5, p. 131; *Phthisis*, Schüler, Schultz, Rückert, Rück. Kl. Erf., vol. 3, p. 394; *Ague*, Hrg, Herrmann, Baertl, Rück. Kl. Erf., vol. 4, p. 987; Durham, Swan, N. A. J. H. vol. 21, p. 106; *Night sweats*, Müller, A. H. Z., vol. 92, p. 148.

[1] **Mind.** Seeing images when shutting eyes.
Delirium without fever.
Anxiety: with vomiting; with sweat.
Very easily frightened; trembling, anxiety, restlessness.
▮Fright followed by suffocative attacks, with bluish bloated face.
▮Constant fretfulness.

[2] **Sensorium.** Dizziness, cloudiness of head.

[3] **Inner Head.** Dizziness, with tension in head when moving it, sensation as if it were filled with water.
Sudden jerks through head.
Pressive pain on temporal bones.
▮Catarrhal headaches, especially of children.

[4] **Outer Head.** The head is bent backward.
Erysipelas all over l. side of head, ear much swollen, confined to bed, could not move.
Scurfs on head with intolerable itching.
Skull feels as if stretched.

[5] **Sight and Eyes.** ▮▮Child could not open eyes, could not bear light, awoke from sleep screaming.
Eyes and mouth half open in sleep. θAsthma Millari.

6 **Hearing and Ears.** Great swelling, heat, redness and lump just under r. ear, in neck, accompanied by a very sharp pain.

7 **Smell and Nose.** ▮Child starts up suddenly as if suffocating. θAsthma Millaria.

▮▮Sniffles of children.

▮Breathing through nose impeded, with dry coryza, especially in nursing infants.

▮▮Dry coryza of infants; nose dry and completely obstructed, preventing breathing and nursing; constant sniffles.

▮Stoppage of nose with thick tenacious mucus.

8 **Upper Face.** ▮Face: pale, bluish or red; pale, collapsed, covered with cold sweat; appears much older and yellow; bloated, dark blue; red-spotted.

Burning heat: and redness of face; with icy-cold feet.

On waking, face breaks out in a profuse sweat, which gradually extends over body.

Red, burning spots on cheeks; great heat of face; circumscribed redness of face.

Numb tension as from swelling in cheeks and on nose.

10 **Teeth and Gums.** Tearing and stinging in teeth, with sensation of swelling of cheek.

13 **Throat.** Dryness of throat and mouth, with thirstlessness.

14 **Appetite, Thirst. Desires, Aversions.** Thirst, but drink is not palatable.

15 **Eating and Drinking.** Worse after eating fruit.

16 **Hiccough, Belching, Nausea and Vomiting.** Everything makes him feel sick.

Vomiting first of food, later of bile.

19 **Abdomen.** Distended abdomen, with pressure and griping in stomach and umbilical region.

Painful pressure in abdomen, with nausea when leaning against a hard edge.

Great soreness in abdomen.

▮▮Griping in abdomen, with emission of flatus as after taking cold.

▮Ileus.

20 **Stool and Rectum.** Stools: frequent, watery; thin, slimy, with much wind, followed by urging; pressure in stomach and navel; abdomen large.

21 **Urinary Organs.** Nephritis.

Frequent urging to urinate, with profuse discharge of urine.

23 **Female Sexual Organs.** Menses too profuse; menorrhagia.

24 **Pregnancy. Parturition. Lactation.** Mammæ red and swollen.

Milk diminished.

26 **Voice and Larynx. Trachea and Bronchia.** ▮Hoarseness caused by much tenacious, glutinous mucus in larynx.

Voice sounds hollow.

▮Hoarseness, rawness in throat and oppression of chest. θInfluenza.

‖Woke at night with agonizing fits, spasms of glottis, with agony and fear of suffocation; springing up in bed and struggling for breath. θAsthma Millari.

▮Spasm of glottis; breathing is of a wheezing, crowing character, < after midnight and from lying with head low. θCroup.

▮Spasms of larynx occurring frequently during course of acute laryngitis.

‖An infant nine months old has laryngeal spasms several times in day and night; awakes from sleep with suffocation; is able to inspire but not expire; becomes livid in face, gasps in great anguish, and very slowly recovers its breath; had two attacks of this kind in previous night, at 8 P.M. and 11 P.M. θLaryngismus.

‖Sudden disappearance of coryza; on following night very rough, hollow, croupy cough; agitated sleep; following morning fits of hollow, deep cough; whistling respiration; constant crying; burning head; crying or coughing, as if throat were painful. θCroup.

‖Sopor; snoring and whistling, with mouth open and head bent back; starts up, strikes about, is nearly suffocated; becomes blue in face, then cough with rattling breathing; threatening suffocation and paralysis of lungs. θCroup.

‖Much dry heat with restlessness; sudden awaking in fright at night, from 9 P.M. until 2 A.M., grasping its throat; shortly after, perspiration on face, head and neck, going off with sleep; during paroxysms of hoarse, suffocating cough child had purple nails and lips; scanty, tough expectoration, yet tracheal sound was somewhat loose. θCroup.

▮In dangerous cases with excessive weakness, old-looking features and threatening paralysis pulmonum. θCroup.

26 **Respiration.** ▮Breathing: anxious, loud; quick, wheezing, crowing.

Oppression of chest, with pressure in stomach and nausea.

▮Nightly suffocative attacks, with great restlessness; shedding of tears and throwing about of arms.

▮Suffocating attacks after midnight.

▮Child suddenly awakes, nearly suffocated, sits up in bed, turns blue, gasps for breath, which it finally gets; spell passes off; it lies down again, and is aroused sooner or later in the same manner. θAsthma Millari.

‖Drowsiness, breathes with mouth open and with a snoring whistling sound, head bent backward, suddenly springs up, tossing arms about, face becoming blue, suffocation seems inevitable when cough recurs, then with rattling breathing child sinks back exhausted; threatened paralysis of lungs.

||Violent asthmatic attack, respiration rapid and whistling; occasional short but labored coughs; high degree of dyspnœa; constantly pointing to middle of chest; had been suffering twenty-four hours, with intermissions of two or three hours, the free intervals becoming gradually shorter with each attack (which lasted usually from ten to fifteen minutes); threatened suffocation with marked blueness of lips.

||Roused about 2 or 3 A.M. with sense of stoppage of air tubes as by phlegm.

|Asthma thymicum; suppressed perspiration; attack comes on suddenly; awakes from a kind of lethargy with eyes and mouth open; raises himself in bed with great anxiety and dyspnœa; respiration oppressed, with wheezing in chest; head and hands puffed and bloated, with dry heat all over body; no thirst; small, irregular and intermittent pulse; no cough; paroxysms occur principally from midnight until 4 A.M.; difficulty of inspiration but not of expiration.

||Attacks of suffocation, resembling last stage of croup.

27 **Cough.** |Cough: hollow, dry, at night; deep and dry before chill; with regular inhalations, but sighing exhalations; suffocative hollow, deep, whooping, caused by spasm of chest, expectoration of small quantities of tough mucus, only during day; suffocative with crying children; < about midnight, during rest, lying in bed, or with head low, from dry, cold air.

||After suppression of a fluent coryza; rough, hollow, deep, croupy cough; restlessness; frequent desire to nurse; whistling respiration; cries with every cough, as if throat were painful, head hot

|Whooping-cough; suffocative, hollow, deep cough, caused by a spasm in chest, with expectoration only during day of small quantities of tough mucus.

||Dry, hacking cough during chill and heat. θAgue.

Sputa: very yellow, as if colored by bile; taste saltish.

28 **Inner Chest and Lungs.** Oppression and pressure beneath sternum and pressure in pit of stomach and epigastric region, with nausea and sense of weakness.

Oppression and stitches in l. side of chest below nipple.

After catching cold the previous Winter, catarrhal affection of chest; violent hollow, dry cough with hoarseness and accumulation of much tough mucus in larynx, < during night; oppression of chest with stitches in l.

side when lying upon that side; internal heat without thirst; profuse debilitating sweats; great nervousness; great sleepiness, but sleep is restless and he wakes often, when feeling of anxiety prevents him from falling asleep again; face pale, sunken, with circumscribed burning redness of cheeks; pressure in stomach after eating, particularly after milk, frequently with vomiting first of food, then bile; urine watery, increased in quantity; great emaciation; is fond of warmth; feels > when moving about a little than when absolutely at rest; frequent inclination to take a deep inspiration, which he can do without difficulty; dry, burning heat during sleep at once going over into profuse sweat on awaking and continuing until he falls asleep again when the heat returns.

‖After a cold drink while overheated, fever and severe cough and expectoration; the following condition finally developing: pressing pain on chest; constant cough day and night with profuse expectoration of offensive, sweet-tasting mucus; face pale, earthy-colored; great emaciation; pulse rapid, weak; burning heat in palms of hands; great thirst in afternoon; profuse sweats at night; complete loss of appetite. θPhthisis.

‖Constant severe cough, with profuse salty-tasting expectoration; great debility and emaciation; constantly increasing oppression of chest; œdematous swelling of legs, extending up above knees; as the cure progresses profuse urination and severe itching of skin and finally exfoliation of epidermis set in. θPhthisis.

▮Phthisis: hectic flush, night sweats, choking cough, afternoon fevers; wakes up after midnight with feeling of sudden suffocation, without being able to call for help; night sweats only when wide awake, passing over into a dry heat as soon as he falls asleep. θPhthisis.

29 **Heart, Pulse and Circulation.** Orgasm in whole body.

Occasional omission of heart-beat.

▮Angina pectoris where pressure proceeds from spine; in individuals formerly fat and robust and now emaciated on account of mental emotions, sexual indulgence or excessive seminal losses; paroxysms generally come on at midnight, or in middle of night and wake patient up, compelling him to sit up or get up before he can get any relief or summon assistance; in many cases the patient can give no account of what is the matter or how it came on, only sit up in bed and moan and cry, with hand over heart.

Pulse generally very frequent and small; sometimes slow and full, sometimes intermitting.

30 **Outer Chest.** Pressure upon sternum, with a counter-pressure from spine to sternum.
Compression of chest violent, trembling from pain.

31 **Neck and Back.** Sweat on throat and neck; with children.

32 **Upper Limbs.** Paralytic heaviness in elbow joint.
Trembling of hands when writing.
Stitches in wrist.
Dark-blue bloatedness of forearms and hands.
Muscles between little finger and next very sore.

33 **Lower Limbs.** Sharp, deep stitches in tibia.
Œdematous swelling of feet, extending to legs.
Sensation of coldness, numbness and deadness in middle of r. tibia.
Icy-cold feet: with warmth of body; with hot face.

34 **Limbs in General.** Hands and feet bloated, blue.

35 **Rest. Position. Motion.** Rest: cough <.
Lying down: dry heat after falling asleep.
Lying in bed: cough <.
Lying on left side: stitches in chest.
Head low: spasms of glottis <; cough <.
Must sit up in bed to regain breath.
Motion: of head, tension and dizziness.
Writing: trembling of hands.

36 **Nerves.** Great weakness.
General trembling, with anxiety and ebullitions of blood.
Great tendency to start; starts at things to which he is accustomed.

37 **Sleep.** ▮Sleepiness.
Drowsiness with inability to sleep.
▮Frequent awaking, as in a fright, with anxiety, trembling, dyspnœa, as if he would suffocate.
Slumber with eyes and mouth half open.
During sleep, dry heat; after waking profuse sweat.

38 **Time.** 2 or 3 A.M.: roused with sense of stoppage of air tubes.
During day: expectoration of tough mucus.
Afternoon: great thirst; fevers.
Night: spasms of glottis; dry cough; profuse sweat.
7 P.M. to 1 A.M.: profuse sweat without thirst.
About midnight: cough <.
After midnight: spasms of glottis <; suffocative attacks.

39 **Temperature and Weather.** Shunning uncovering during heat.
From dry, cold air: cough <.
After a cold drink while overheated: phthisis.

40 **Fever.** ▮Chill running over whole body, with crawling sensation here and there.
Hands and feet icy cold; rest of body warm.

▮Shaking chills before going to bed. θAgue.

▮Spasmodic deep, dry cough; may occur after chill if absent in prodroma.

▮▮Dry heat: while he sleeps; on falling asleep after lying down; without thirst, dreads uncovering.

▮Hot body with cold hands and feet during sleep; on awaking face breaks out into a profuse sweat which extends over body and continues more or less during waking hours; on going to sleep again dry heat returns.

▮Sensation of burning heat in face, with moderate warmth of body and icy-cold feet, without thirst.

▮Burning heat; dread of uncovering.

▮Hectic flush.

Profuse sweat without thirst, while awake from 7 P.M. to 1 A.M.; drops stood upon face, and there was also perspiration all over, but after sleep he was more hot than sweaty but without thirst.

▮General sweat except on head.

Continued perspiration while awake, changing into dry heat as soon as one goes to sleep.

▮Profuse non-debilitating sweat day and night.

▮Debilitating perspirations which often retard convalescence after delivery.

▮Night sweats except on head, increasing toward morning.

▮Profuse debilitating night sweats. θPhthisis. θAgue.

▮Night sweats in phthisis; sweats come even when awake.

▮Profuse weakening sweats, day and night, last through apyrexia.

▮Prodroma: cough, deep, dry, racking, for half an hour; nausea and thirst.

▮▮Irregular paroxysms occurring every other day (quinine had no effect), cough deep and dry for half an hour, with nausea and thirst; chill for half an hour, without cough, nausea thirst; slight fever with moist skin; profuse sweat at night, not debilitating; apyrexia complete. θAgue.

▮Chills and fever, type quotidian; paroxysms commenced at 3 P.M., with hard dry cough from lower part of chest, racking and shaking whole body and producing a pain over whole head which is > by pressure or having head tightly bound up; no expectoration with cough; great thirst for large quantities of water very often; longing for acids; chills, severe and shaking, lasting for half an hour; lips and nails look blue; nausea and vomiting, < by drinking, substance vomited having a bitter-sour taste; bitter-sour taste in mouth during paroxysm; tongue coated white; skin cool, pulse 90; slight moisture on surface; chills running down back.; back and limbs ache, particularly during chill, and < when they come in contact with bed; cough, headache and thirst continued; fever, great heat with stupor and prostration; thirst and cough continue, but no headache; pains in back and limbs; great difficulty in speaking; with heat, a profuse perspiration; delirium; is distressed because of some one whom she imagines is in bed with her and oppresses her respiration as if she had to breathe for two; continual talking; sense of suffocation, with a quivering or fluttering at heart; great distress in region of heart, whence the cough seems to proceed; hearing painfully acute; great depression of spirits with anxious, vexed, desponding thoughts and weeping; moaning and weeping during sleep; at night a drenching sweat, smelling sour fetid, staining yellow, not debilitating; ineffectual desire to urinate, passing water about once in twenty-four hours, a small quantity of very turbid loam-colored urine; patient suffered for years from chronic dysentery which was cured at same time. θAgue.

▮Dry heat while asleep, profuse sweat while awake, then dry heat again when he sleeps; the profuse sweat is rarely debilitating and never in proportion to its profuseness; always without thirst.

▮No thirst during heat or sweat.

Shunning uncovering during heat; visions when shutting eyes. θTyphus.

41 **Attacks, Periodicity.** Several times in day and night: laryngeal spasms.

Nightly: suffocative attacks.

From 9 until 2 P.M.: sudden awaking in fright.

From midnight until 4 A.M.: suffocative attacks.

Once in twenty-four hours: passes water.

Every other day: paroxysm of ague.

42 **Locality and Direction.** Right: swelling, heat, redness and lumps just under the ear.

Left: erysipelas of whole side of head; stitches in side of chest below nipple.

43 **Sensations.** As if head were filled with water; skull as if stretched; as if suffocating.

Pain: over whole head; in back and limbs.

Great distress: in region of heart.

Sharp pain: under r. ear.

Tearing: in teeth.

Stitches: in l. side of chest below nipple; in wrist; in tibia.

Stinging: in teeth.

Griping: in stomach and umbilical region; in abdomen.

Pressive pain: in temporal bones.

Pressing pain: on chest
Jerks: through head.
Soreness: in abdomen.
Burning heat: in palms of hands.
Rawness: in throat.
Oppression: of chest, beneath sternum; in left side of chest below nipple.
Heat: of face.
Pressure: in stomach; in abdomen beneath sternum and pit of stomach and epigastric region; upon sternum; from spine to sternum.
Tension: in head, in cheeks and nose.
Dryness: of mouth and throat.
Itching: of scurfs on head.
Numbness: in middle of tibia.
Deadness: in middle of tibia.
Coldness: in middle of tibia; of feet.

44 **Tissues.** ‖ Œdematous swellings in various parts of body, especially in instep, legs and feet.
| Œdema; anasarca; general dropsy.
‖ Increased secretion of skin and of respiratory mucous membrane.

45 **Touch. Passive Motion. Injuries.** | Leaning against hard edge: painful pressure in abdomen with nausea.
Pressure: > pain in head.
Tightly bound: > pain in head.
After contusions, tension in dark-red swelling.

46 **Skin.** Bloatedness and dark-red swelling, with tension after contusions.

48 **Relations.** Antidoted by: *Arsen.*, *Camphor.*
Compatible: *Bellad.*, *Conium*, *Nux vom.*, *Phosphor.*, *Rhus tox.*, *Sepia.*
Compare: *Cinchon.*, *Ipecac.*, *Sulphur.*

SANGUINARIA CANADENSIS.

Bloodroot. *Papaveraceæ.*

Introduced by G. Bute.

Experiments by Downey, Inaugural Dissertation, 1803; Tully, Prize Essay, Am. Med. Recorder, 1828; Bute, Freitag, Jeanes, Huseman, Helfrich, Hering's Compilation, N. Archiv für Hom., vol. 2, p. 114; Tinker, Trans. Am. Inst., 1870; Billing, Thesis; also symptoms by Fincke and Macfarlan.

CLINICAL AUTHORITIES.--*Headache*, Smedley, A. J. H. M. M., vol. 8, p. 50; Mills, B. J. H., vol. 36, p. 187; Mills (2 cases), Am. Hom., vol. 1, p. 113; Smith, M. I., vol. 6, p. 344; Leonard, Med. Inv., 1875, p. 441; *Migraine*, Hs., A. H. Z., vol. 109, p. 207; Fulton, A. H. Z., vol. 112, p. 77; *Sick-headache*, Ehrmann, A. H. Z., vol. 113, p. 24; Plimpton, Hah. Mo., vol. 10, p. 212; Raue's Rec., 1875, p. 244; Chamberlin, N. E. M. G., 1873, p. 495; Raue's Rec., 1874, p. 259; Beebe, see Hale's Th., p. 654; *Chronic headaches*, Hansen, A. H. Z., vol. 113, p. 52; *Coryza*, Sanford, N. E. M. G., vol. 2, p. 125; *Nasal polypus*, Price, N. A. J. H., vol. 15, p. 214; Wells, A. H. Z., vol. 109, p. 63; 5 cases reported cured, Thomas, B. J. H., vol. 16, p. 329; *Facial neuralgia*, Drumm, A. J. H. M. M., vol. 3. p. 62; *Œdema of glottis*, Nichol, A. H. O., June, 1874, p. 302; Raue's Rec., 1875, p. 102; *Pharyngitis*, Hedges, Med. Inv., vol. 8, p. 128; Raue's Rec., 1871, p. 77; *Diphtheritis*, Biegler, Hom. Phys., vol. 7, p. 477; *Nausea and vomiting*, Moore, M. I., vol. 6, p. 344; *Neurosis of stomach*, Winterburn, Hah. Mo., vol. 20, p. 533; *Ulceration of os uteri*, Greenleaf, Hah. Mo., vol. 7, p. 527; *Enlargement of breast*, Craig, B. J. H., vol. 32, p. 308; *Use during pregnancy*, Burnett, Hom. Phys., vol. 2, 147; *Laryngitis*, Nichols, A. O., June, 1873, p. 335; Raue's Rec., 1874, p. 120; *Tracheal irritation*, Blake, Hom. Rev., vol. 16, p. 406; *Influenza*, Mossa, Raue's Rec., 1871, p. 79, from Hom. Kl., 1870, p. 98; Kleinert, Rück. Kl. Erf., vol. 5, p. 705; *Croup*, Clark, Hah. Mo., vol. 6, p. 290; Price, A. H. O., vol. 8, p. 235; *Cough*, Hunt, N. A. J. H., vol. 15, p. 211; Sanford, N. E. M. G., vol. 2, p. 125; Bell, N. A. J. H., 1873, p. 380; Clark, Hah. Mo., vol. 6, p. 290; Capen, Mass. Trans., vol. 4, p. 376; Wells, Hom. Recorder, vol. 3, p. 68; *Pulmonary congestion*, Blake, Hom. Rev., vol. 16, p. 406; *Pneumonia*, Hering, Rück. Kl. Erf., vol. 3, p. 333; *Affection of lungs*, Boyce, N. E. M. G., vol. 2, p. 277; *Incipient phthisis pulmonalis*, Parsons, B. J. H., vol. 24, p. 509; *Phthisis*, Bute, Rück. Kl. Erf., vol. 3, p. 396; *Injury to shoulder*, Hom. Phys., vol. 6, p. 294; *Rheumatism of arm*, McClatchey, Hah. Mo., vol. 10, p. 331; *Fungoid growth on hand*, Drury, Hom. Rev., vol. 16, p. 85; *Affection of toe*, Drury, Hom. Rev., vol. 16, p. 85; *Neuralgia*, Fanning, N. A. J. H., 1873, p. 363; *Anæmia*, Parsons, B. J. H., vol. 24, p. 510; *Rheumatism*, Martin, Hah. Mo., vol. 12, p. 473; Berridge, Hom. Phys., vol. 6, p. 411; Goodman, M. I., 1875, p. 300; *Syphilis*, Schlosser, Rück. Kl. Erf., vol. 5, p. 572; *Rhus rad. poisoning*, Hammond, M. I., vol. 11, p. 603; Raue's Rec., 1875, p. 16.

1 **Mind.** Mind confused, relieved by eructations.

Anxiety: and feeling of dread; precedes vomiting and delirium.

Angry irritability; moroseness with nausea; cannot bear a person to walk in room.

Delirium with hot skin.

Mental torpor, stupor, heaviness, sleepiness.

Hopefulness, sanguine of recovery.

Disgusting ideas, and many unpleasant feelings associated with nausea.

|| Sensation as if paralyzed and unable to move while lying on her back, with full consciousness of her surroundings.

|| With open eyes, one dream chases another; her thoughts constantly returning, however, to the one idea, which seems droll to her, "What will become of my condition, shall I have typhoid fever, inflammation of the brain, or shall I remain paralyzed?"

|| It seems to her as if the events that transpired in her dreams were not of hours' but of weeks' and months' duration.

|| It seems to her as if all around her talked very rapidly, and that she is in a railroad car and begs others to hold her.

2 **Sensorium.** | Vertigo: with long-continuing nausea, debility and headache; with singing in ears; with diminished vision, before vomiting; with nausea and headache, followed by spasmodic vomiting; with dull, heavy feeling in stomach, as if caused from some hard substance there; on quickly turning head and looking upward; on lying down at night; on rising from stooping; in cold weather; during sleep; during climaxis.

Head feels dizzy, cannot turn quickly without fear of falling.

3 **Inner Head.** Headache with nausea and chilliness, followed by flushes of heat, extending from head to stomach.

Violent pain over upper portion of whole l. side of head, especially in eye.

| Headache as if forehead would burst, with chill and burning in stomach.

Pressive headache in forehead.

Frontal headache with considerable vertigo, on rising from a sitting posture.

|| Frontal headache extending into cheek bones.

| Pain in forepart of head, shoulders, chest and stomach.

| Headache over r. eye.

| Neuralgia in and over r. eye.

| Head aches as if it would burst; > walking in open air < in temples, especially in r., in afternoon.

| Pains in head in spots; soreness especially in temples.

| Dull headache.

▮Wandering pains in head.

▮Headache with shuddering.

▮Beating headache with throbbing in temporal arteries and bitter vomiting.

▮Pulsations in head, with bitter vomiting, < from motion.

▮Headache, with rheumatic pains and stiffness of limbs and neck.

▮Headache every seventh day.

▮Pains like a flash of lightning in back of head.

▮▮Headache begins in occiput, spreads upward and settles over r. eye.

▮Pain in head in rays, drawing upward from neck.

▮Rheumatic headache, running up posterior auricular region.

Feeling as if head were drawn forward.

▮Severe headache only relieved by pressing back up against something hard, or by pressing back of head.

▮▮Periodical sick-headache; begins in morning, increases during day, lasts until evening; head feels as if it must burst, or as if eyes would be pressed out; throbbing, lancinating pains through brain, < in r. side, especially in forehead and vertex; followed by chills, nausea, vomiting of food or bile; must lie down and remain quiet; relieved by sleep.

A bandlike constriction across forehead just below eyebrows; < by exercise, with violent throbbing of temporal arteries; shooting pains from one temple to other, < in night; < from light, > from sleep.

▮Headache concentrating in a small spot over r. eye; eye becomes red and sore, yet hard pressure upon eye relieves.

‖ Headache especially over r. eye; rheumatic pain in neck and shoulders (more in l.); > when lying perfectly still; patient approaching climacteric period.

‖ Intermittent neuralgia coming in morning and lasting four to six hours; pain at internal superior angle of r. orbit, acute pressing with occasional darts inward and some throbbing; part sore, but he holds his hand there while pain lasts; conjunctiva considerably injected during pain; catarrhal discharge, thick, mostly from r. side of nose; every day for five or six days.

‖ Violent pulsation and tearing in r. temple, < from motion; the slightest shaking is intolerable to her, so that she cannot bear to have any one walk across the floor. θSick-headache.

‖ Headache with distension of temporal veins which are painfully sensitive to touch.

‖ Pressing pains in head, extending from nape of neck

over side of head and settling over l. eye, accompanied by nausea and vomiting of food, bile and mucus; must lie down; > when lying down and vomiting; attacks every eight days for last nine years.

▮Severe pains in head, with nausea and vomiting, frequently with bilious vomiting in weekly attacks or at longer intervals, commonly beginning in morning, increasing in violence through day, only diminished by lying quiet and sleeping.

‖Sick-headache from childhood; eyes weak and sore; photophobia, especially with headache; for last six weeks headache every third day, commencing A.M., pains extend from r. eye through back part of head; she is in dark room and cannot bear least light; if she is quiet all day is usually > in evening; nausea, but does not often vomit unless she goes into bright light, or moves about; catamenia every two weeks, blood dark and clotted; constipation; debility.

‖Sick-headache every two weeks; when overexerted so as to become very tired, she has a great appetite, but satisfying it is followed by sick-headache; is in the habit of eating late in evening; during headache hot flashes and a sensation like that of an electrical current shooting very rapidly from one part of head to the other.

‖Pain commencing in r. occiput, extending to r. temporal bone, a tight drawing, gradually increasing in intensity, like drawing a rope on a windlass as tight as you can get it until it is almost beyond endurance, when it gradually subsides.

‖Sick-headache, commencing in morning on awaking, < during day, > by sleep at night; pain confined chiefly to temples and vertex, so violent as to cause her to cry out; nausea generally in morning, followed by vomiting, first of food, afterward of pure bile, occasionally considerable acid mucus, with severe burning distress in stomach, great weakness and goneness, even worse to bear than headache; least quantity of food or drink is immediately vomited; attacks come on at irregular intervals.

‖Headache and nausea, symptoms increasing hour by hour; patient groaning and writhing in agony, face very red, head hot, injected eyes, sensitive to light; arteries about head and scalp distended like whip cords, blood coursing through them at a furious rate, giving a sensation to head as if temples and scalp were alive with irrepressible pulsation; pain over whole head; paroxysms of violent retching every few minutes; free flow of clear urine as the attack passes off.

|| Distressing sick-headache, for years; in some degree the symptoms were nearly always present; headache commencing in forenoon, gradually increasing in violence until sunset, when it would either quietly subside or confine her to bed for a day or two; the pains originated low in occiput, drawing upward in rays, locating over r., sometimes over l. eye, attended with vomiting, often of bilious matter; subject to sudden flushes of heat, burning of soles of feet and quickly diffused transient thrill felt at remotest extremity; at times sensible throbbing of every pulse in body; urine generally scanty before and during severe headache, but quantities of clear urine pass when getting better.

▮ "American sick-headache;" rush of blood to head, causing faintness and nausea, even continuing until vomiting sets in; violent pains begin in occipital region, spread thence over head and settle over r. eye; pains sharp, lancinating, at times throbbing; can bear neither sounds nor odors; cannot bear any one to walk across floor, the slightest jar annoys her; at height of headache vomiting of food and bile; is forced to remain quiet in a dark room; sleep finally relieves; sometimes pain is so violent that patient goes out of her mind, or seeks relief by pressing head against pillow or pressing head with hands.

|| Neuralgia in r. temple and orbit from getting feet wet.

▮ Pain commences in back of head, rises and spreads over head and settles especially above r. eye, with nausea, vomiting and chilliness; is obliged to seek a dark room and lie perfectly still; flushes of heat; burning of soles of feet; urine at first scanty, later profuse and clear.

|| Frightfully severe headache, the only relief obtained by pressing back of head against headboard of bed.

|| Migraine with bilious vomiting, pains begin in morning, last till evening; eyes feel as if they would be pushed out, < by motion.

▮ Sick headache, with heat and redness.

▮ Headaches: gastric; myalgic; rheumatic; congestive; from suppressed menses; at change of life.

▮ Congestion of blood to head, with ringing in ears; flushes of heat; accumulation of water in mouth.

|| Sanguineous apoplexy with vertigo, dimness of sight, vomiting, burning in stomach, distension of temporal veins.

4 **Outer Head.** Soreness in spots, especially in temporal regions.

Distension of veins in temples; feel sore when touched.

Head very painful to touch.

5 **Sight and Eyes.** Diminished power of vision.

Dimness of eyes, with sensation as if hairs were in them.

Frequent obscuration of vision.

Retinal congestion, with flushed face and congestive headache.

Pupils dilated.

▮Yellowness of sclerotica, with icterus.

Burning dryness in eyes.

▮Pain over eyes.

Redness of eyes in morning.

Superficial injection of eyeball, with feeling of soreness.

Burning and watering of r. eye, which is painful to touch, followed by coryza.

▮▮Acute conjunctivitis, with excessive redness and numerous ecchymoses in conjunctiva, tending toward trachoma, with moderate discharge and some pain in eye.

▮Catarrhal ophthalmia, granular lids.

▮Ophthalmia, followed by ulceration of cornea.

▮Copious lachrymation: following the burning and dryness; tears hot; with coryza.

▮Blepharadenitis: with a feeling of dryness under upper lid and accumulation of mucus in eye in morning; blepharitis and catarrhal conditions of conjunctiva, with burning in edges of lids, < in afternoon; dependent on stricture of lachrymal duct.

▮▮Hard swelling like scirrhus over eyebrows.

▮▮Neuralgia in and over r. eye.

6 **Hearing and Ears.** Beating, humming, with congestion of blood.

▮Hyperexcitation of auditory nerves; painful sensitiveness, especially to sudden sounds; sensation as if she were in a railroad car or in some vehicle which was moving and jarring her, with a feeling as if all about her moved rapidly and confusedly; desires to be held in order to remove this nervous vibratory sensation through body; frequently in women in climaxis.

▮Earache with headache, singing in ears and vertigo.

Beating under ears, at irregular intervals, often only a couple of strokes.

▮Acute internal otitis.

▮Catarrhal affections of inner ear and Eustachian tube.

▮Throat affections causing deafness and otalgia.

▮Increased redness of external ear, with humming and roaring in ears from increased circulation of blood through aural structures.

▮Burning of ears, cheeks red.

7 **Smell and Nose.** ▮Loss of smell and taste.

Dislike to odor of syrup.

▮Fluent coryza, with frequent sneezing; < r. side.

▮Coryza, with dull, heavy pain over root of nose, and stinging sensation in nose; severe pain at root of nose and in frontal sinuses, with dry cough and pain in chest.

‖Severe cold in head; sneezing, severe fluid coryza, irritation and watering of eyes; irritation of throat with severe cough.

‖Severe cold in head; high fever; acrid discharge from r. nostril produced soreness of lips and side of face.

‖Fluid coryza alternating with stoppage; eyes painful to touch; soreness in throat; pain in chest, cough and finally diarrhœa. θInfluenza.

▮Watery, acrid coryza, rendering nose sore, with copious watering of r. eye.

▮Coryza with diarrhœa, worse at night.

‖Smell in nose like roasted onion; wheezing, whistling cough and finally diarrhœa, which relieves the cough. θInfluenza.

▮Rose cold with subsequent asthma; sick and faint from odor of flowers.

▮Acute or chronic coryza, with loss of smell.

‖Severe catarrh in head, following a cold, for some weeks, with some irritation of throat and slight cough.

‖Sensation of stinging and tickling, with irritative swelling of parts, with or without free discharge; yellowish or grayish-white discharge from nose; headache in r. hemisphere of brain, with drawing pain in back into neck; bilious vomiting. θChonic catarrh.

▮Ulcerative ozæna with epistaxis.

▮Chronic nasal catarrh with offensive discharges.

▮▮Nasal polypi.

8 **Upper Face.** Distension of veins of face, with excessive redness, a feeling of stiffness and soreness of veins to touch.

Circumscribed redness of one or both cheeks.

▮▮Red cheeks: with burning in ears; with cough.

▮Cheeks and hands livid. θTyphoid pneumonia.

▮Circumscribed redness of cheeks in afternoon; patient lies on his back; pulse small and quick.

Twitching of cheeks toward eyes.

▮Neuralgia in and over r. eye.

‖Neuralgia in upper jaw running up to nose, eye, ear, neck and side of head; pain shooting and burning, cannot endure pain except by kneeling down and holding head tight to floor.

▮Stitches in l. side of face, with pains in forehead.

‖Neuralgia in face for several years; beginning of pain in upper jaw, running up to nose, eye, ear and side of head; pain shooting and burning, cannot stand pain except by kneeling down and holding head tight to floor.

9 **Lower Face.** Lips feel dry.

Swelling of lips toward evening.

Under lip burns, is swollen, hard and blistered; blisters dry up and form crusts, which drop off.

Stiffness in articulation of jaws.

10 **Teeth and Gums.** ▮Toothache from picking teeth, or in hollow teeth when touched by food.

▮Grumbling toothache with pain in same side of head.

Pain in carious teeth after cold drinks.

Looseness of teeth (with salivation).

▮Spongy, bleeding, fungoid condition of gums.

11 **Taste and Tongue.** ▮Loss of taste, with a burnt feeling on tongue.

Sweet things taste bitter, followed by burning in fauces.

White-coated tongue with slimy, fatty taste.

▮Red streak through middle of tongue.

Top of tongue burns as if scalded.

▮Tongue sore; pains like a boil.

▮Red tongue, burns as if in contact with something hot.

Pricking in point of tongue.

12 **Inner Mouth.** Fetid breath, clammy mouth, sticky teeth.

Sores on gums and roof of mouth.

▮Roof of mouth sore, uvula sore and burning.

‖White patches on mucous membrane of mouth, with salivation; hypertrophy of thymus gland; in a child suffering from hereditary syphilis.

13 **Throat.** In evening after lying down, cough from tickling in throat.

Spasmodic constriction directly beneath lower jaws across throat, very distressing, lasting several hours.

▮Throat very dry, with tickling cough.

▮Burning in throat, especially after eating sweet things.

▮Roof of mouth and uvula sore and burning.

Feeling of swelling in throat on swallowing.

Pain with sensation of swelling, in throat, < r. side, especially on swallowing.

▮Throat feels swollen as if to suffocation; pain when swallowing; aphonia.

▮Tonsillitis; promotes suppuration.

Throat feels raw; some difficulty in swallowing; mouth and throat feel almost denuded of mucous membrane.

▮Heat in throat, better on inspiring cold air; throat so dry it seems as if it would crack.

‖Dryness in throat, with soreness, swelling, and redness as in scarlet fever; in one case of six years' standing, in another with hectic fever and cough.

‖ General feeling of soreness throughout pharynx; sensation as if burned or scalded by hot drinks; dry, constricted feeling; drinking did not moisten throat, mucous membrane felt as if it might crack; pharynx very red and angry looking, highly inflamed.

▮ Putrid sore throat.

▮ Angina; particularly a species of pharyngitis.

▮ Ulcerated sore throat.

▮ Tonsillitis, chronic, recurring frequently.

▮ Suppuration of tonsils; quinsy.

▮▮ Burning in pharynx and œsophagus.

‖ Intense heat and redness of throat, amounting to a burning sensation; choking feeling when swallowing; pearly coating on fauces and tonsils, < on r. side; r. tonsil most inflamed. θDiphtheritis.

▮ Palate and fauces covered with a continuous coating of pearly fibrinous exudation.

14 **Appetite, Thirst. Desires, Aversions.** ▮ Craving for he knows not what, with loss of appetite; wants piquant things.

▮ Loss of appetite with great weakness of digestion.

‖ Aversion to butter.

Sugar tastes bitter and causes burning.

15 **Eating and Drinking.** Sweet things aggravate, produce burning.

Soon after eating: feels empty; difficult breathing, nausea, waterbrash, lassitude almost to fainting, cold sweat until 12 P.M., after a little food.

16 **Hiccough, Belching, Nausea and Vomiting.** ‖ Hiccough whilst smoking.

Spasmodic eructations of flatus.

‖ Frequent flatulent eructations of unpleasant odor, with disposition to vomit and paleness of face.

‖ Pyrosis; a rising of burning, corrosive fluid from stomach, for twenty years.

▮ Nausea: with a burning at stomach; with much spitting; not > by vomiting; with headache, chill and heat; intense, in paroxysms, < when stooping, with flow of saliva; followed by nettlerash; with heartburn; followed by vomiting and sometimes diarrhœa; periodic; followed by sneezing; craves food to quiet nausea.

▮▮ Vomiting: of bitter water; of sour acrid fluids; of ingesta; of worms; preceded by anxiety; with headache and burning in stomach; head > afterward; with prostration.

▮ During vomiting, headache, burning in stomach with craving to eat.

17 **Scrobiculum and Stomach.** ▮ Soreness and pressure in epigastrium < by eating.

▮Sudden attacks of constriction in pit of stomach as if suffocating.

▮Goneness with sick headache.

Sensation of emptiness in stomach : soon after eating; with faint, feverish feeling.

▮Pressure in stomach.

Jerking in stomach as if from something alive.

‖Feeling of warmth and heat in stomach.

▮Burning in stomach; with headache and chill.

▮Gastritis, with nausea, headache, chill and heat; vomiting with severe, painful burning in stomach and intense thirst, red tongue, red and dry lips, hot and dry throat, tickling cough.

Pyrosis; rising of burning, corrosive fluid with flatulence.

▮Great weakness of digestion, loss of appetite. θDyspepsia.

‖Burning sensation accompanied by pressure in epigastrium, coming on soon after lying down and compelling her to rise; pains < at night, but they recurred at any hour when she resumed the recumbent position, though less severe in daytime; > sitting up; appetite voracious; bowels torpid; peculiar drawing pains in shoulders and arms during sleep, so that when she awoke the fists were tightly clenched and flexed upon the sternal end of clavicle; this cramping up of the arms always occurred during sleep and was followed by a sense of lameness and weariness in the affected muscles. θNeurosis of stomach.

‖A chronic inebriate; had been drinking steadily for a couple of weeks, beer and whisky; violent emetocatharsis; *Nux vomica* did not relieve, *Arsenic* checked the bowels and relieved the intense thirst, but had no effect in quieting stomach; very irritable and angry at not being relieved; everything she took in her stomach, even water, was instantly ejected; about once in fifteen or twenty minutes a spasm of stomach, with gagging and coughing and ejection of some frothy mucus; pain in chest and abdomen from the straining; intense burning extending from stomach up œsophagus to pharynx, which felt swollen and dry; lying slightly turned on l. side; impossible for her to lie on r. side, and when rising from lying down was seized with vertigo; cheeks and hands livid; believed she was soon to die and was unwilling to be left alone.

18 **Hypochondria.** Heat, streaming from breast to liver.

▮Liver torpid; skin yellow; colic. θJaundice. θBiliary concretions.

▮Cough from affections of liver.

‖Pain in l. hypochondrium, < from coughing, > from

pressure and when lying on l. side, very copious urination at night.

Violent stitches in splenetic region.

19 **Abdomen.** ‖Flatulent distension of abdomen in evening, with escape of flatus from vagina (os uteri being dilated).

Beating in abdomen.

‖Indurations in abdomen.

Cutting bellyache from r. to l. of iliac fossa, thence to rectum.

❙Soreness in abdomen < by eating.

Colic: followed by diarrhœa; with torpor of liver.

Feeling as from hot water pouring from breast into abdomen, followed by diarrhœa.

20 **Stool and Rectum.** ❙Urging, but no evacuation, with sensation of a mass in lower part of rectum and discharge of offensive flatus only.

Alternate diarrhœa and constipation.

❙Hemorrhoids.

❙Stools: thin, fecal; bright yellow; undigested; watery; watery with much flatus, preceded by cutting pain.

‖Affection of breast always ended with a feeling as if hot water were poured from chest into abdomen which was followed by diarrhœic stool.

‖Diarrhœa following coryza, pains in chest and cough.

Ineffectual urging to stool, then vomiting.

Frequent discharges of very offensive flatus.

Escape of much flatus upward and downward; also with diarrhœa.

21 **Urinary Organs.** ❙Copious and frequent nocturnal urination, clear as water.

‖Very copious urine at night, with pain in l. hypochondrium; < from coughing; > from pressure and lying on l. side.

❙Dark-yellow urine, with icterus.

Urine scanty, high-colored, deposits reddish sediment on standing.

22 **Male Sexual Organs.** Seminal emissions.

❙Gleet; old cases.

‖White oval patches on mucous membrane of mouth, particularly at angles, on mucous membranes of lips, on edge of tongue, on prepuce and glans penis; fetid, cheesy secretions from glans penis, later obstinate inflammatory headache, with constant congestions to head, transient heat, throbbing pain < from motion and stooping, extending upward from nape of neck, with swollen veins in temples. θSyphilis.

23 **Female Sexual Organs.** ❙Os uteri ulcerated; fetid corrosive leucorrhœa.

Uterine polypi, or cancer.

▌Distension of abdomen in evening, and flatulent discharges per vagina, from os uteri, which was constantly open; at same time a pain passing in rays from nape of neck to head.

▌Metrorrhagia occurring at climaxis; blood bright red, clotted and frequently offensive; sick-headache; flushing of face; face becomes scarlet, this high color passes off with faint, weak, sick feeling.

▌Pain in loins, extending through hypogastric and uterine region and down thighs, followed by appearance of menses (in cases of suppression).

▌Abdominal pains (at night) as if menses would appear.

‖ Catamenia preceded by itching in axillæ.

Menses much more profuse than usual, with less pain and weakness in small of back, but with headache in r. side of forehead and side of head, with sensation as if eyes would be forced out of head, < in r. eye.

▌Menses: at right time, offensive smelling, bright red flow; clots, like lumps of flesh; later blood darker and less offensive; scanty, headache from occiput to frontal region, head as if bursting, face red and hot; too early, with a discharge of black blood.

‖ Dysmenorrhœa in feeble, torpid subjects, with tendency to congestion of lungs, liver or head.

‖ Amenorrhœa in consequence of pulmonary disease; hectic flush of face.

▌Climacteric disorders, especially flashes of heat and leucorrhœa.

‖ Burning of palms of hands and soles of feet at climacteric period, compelling her to throw bedclothes off.

‖ Painful enlargement of breasts at climacteric period.

▌Corrosive, fetid leucorrhœa at climacteric period; it continues after menses cease.

Sharp, piercing pain in r. breast, just beneath nipple; very difficult to take a deep inspiration, with some dyspnœa.

Pain in r. breast extends to shoulder and is so severe that it is with difficulty hand can be placed on top of head.

Stitches in mammæ.

The nipples are sore and painful.

24 **Pregnancy. Parturition. Lactation.** ‖ Threatened abortion with nausea, pains in loins, extending through epigastric and iliac regions and down thighs.

Mammæ: stitches in both; sore to touch under r. nipple, and painful soreness of nipples.

25 **Voice and Larynx. Trachia and Bronchia.** Chronic dryness in throat, sensation of swelling in larynx and expectoration of thick mucus.

Aphonia with swelling in throat.

Dryness in throat with soreness, swelling and redness.

Tickling in throat in evening with cough and headache.

▮ Tonsils and pharynx swollen; sawing respiration; expiration easier than inspiration; cough dry and harsh, > sitting, < eating or lying down; difficult expectoration of tough, glairy mucus; inflammation of cervical glands. θŒdema laryngis.

▮ Acute catarrhal laryngitis.

▮▮ Violent dry cough; sensation of burning behind sternum, craves cold water, which soon is vomited; fauces dark-red, not swollen; little or no fever; headache, almost crazy; eyes look inflamed, upper lid swollen; open air relieves pain; vomits as soon as he drinks or eats; sharp pain over r. eye. θInfluenza.

▮ Tracheal irritation secondary to heart disease.

▮▮ Sensation of dryness, soreness and swelling in larynx and expectoration of thick mucus; redness in throat; stoppage of nose with headache across eyebrows. θChronic catarrhal laryngitis.

▮▮ A little girl, æt. 4, who had been subject to bronchial affections since birth; lying on her mother's lap, countenance pale and livid, lips very cold, dyspnœa extreme while cough was muffled as if head had been enveloped in a blanket; no expectoration, sibilant râles remarkably shrill; hands and feet quite cold; half delirium. θLaryngitis.

▮▮ Chronic dryness of throat, sensation of swelling in larynx with expectoration of thin mucus; aphonia, with swelling of larynx; continual severe cough without expectoration, with pain in head and circumscribed redness of cheeks; tormenting cough with sensation of exhaustion. θCroup.

▮▮ Pseudo-membranous croup; hoarse, muffled cough; complete aphonia; pulse 132; soft palate and fauces covered with a continuous coating of pearly fibrinous exudate; hissing sound in larynx; great difficulty in breathing; child stretched back his head and grasped his throat in his agony; features dark and swollen.

▮ Croup: catarrhal, with spasmodic, crowing painful cough and stridulous breathing, with whistling cough; metallic sounding, as if coughing through a metallic tube.

▮ Chronic dryness in throat and sensation of swelling in larynx and expectoration of thick mucus.

▮ Chronic laryngitis, bronchitis and trachitis.

▮ Pulmonary consumption.

36 **Respiration.** ▮ Excessive dyspnœa. θAsthma.

▮ Short, accelerated, constrained breathing; extreme dyspnœa; cheeks and hands livid; compressible pulse. θTyphoid pneumonia.

▮Asthma, especially after "rose cold," < from odors.

Painful, sighing respiration.

Inclination to take deep inspiration, which increases constriction of chest, and causes tearing pains in chest, < r. side.

27 **Cough.** ▮Cough: dry, caused by tickling in throat or stomach; evenings after lying down, from tickling in throat; awakening him and not ceasing until he sits up in bed and passes flatus, upward and downward; dry, with considerable tickling in throat pit, and a crawling extending downward beneath sternum; very severe, causing considerable pain beneath upper part of sternum, with no expectoration; teasing, dry, hacking, with dryness in throat; tormenting, with circumscribed redness of cheeks; with vomiturition; with headache.

ǀǀContinual severe cough, without expectoration, with pain in breast and circumscribed redness of cheeks, with coryza, followed by diarrhœa which relieves.

▮Wheezing, whistling cough; metallic sounding; stridulous breathing. θCroup.

▮▮Severe cough occurring after whooping cough, when patient takes cold, which partakes of the spasmodic nature of whooping cough.

▮Whooping cough; constricted spasmodic action across throat beneath jaws; cough < at night with diarrhœa.

ǀǀSevere cough for six weeks, following a cold; coughed for hours at night, keeping whole house awake.

ǀǀSevere, harassing cough, bloody sputa, with pain in occipital region.

ǀǀAfter exposure, dry hard cough; fever; pain about shoulders and chest; sore throat; headache; < coughing; cough < by eructations of gas from stomach.

▮Distressing, dry, spasmodic, exhaustive coughs, especially in children; < toward night, lying down, going into a cold room to sleep; feeling of rawness and burning in bronchi.

ǀǀFor many years shortness of breath and cough, from taking cold the distress became severe and the attack resembled croup; wheezy, whistling cough, beginning with a wheeze and ending with a whistle; < at night when lying with head low.

ǀǀTroublesome cough for a number of years; excited by an irritation in region of bifurcation of bronchi; coughs a long time to raise a little whitish-yellow phlegm, sometimes streaked with blood, after which she experiences great relief; coughs day and night; is weak and emaciated. (Nitrate of *Sanguinaria*, 2d trit.)

▮Tough, rust-colored sputa in second and third stages of pneumonia.

▮Troublesome, harassing cough, with marked inflammatory action. θChronic bronchitis. θIncipient tuberculosis.

▮Breath and sputa smell badly even to patient.

▮Hæmoptysis during phthisis pulmonalis.

▮Sputa: thick, mucous; rust-colored; offensive, purulent.

28 **Inner Chest and Lungs.** Sharp, piercing pain midway between sternum and nipple, myalgic in character, the surface feels tender on pressure.

Pain beneath sternum and in r. breast.

Intense burning pain between breasts, < in r. side, in afternoon.

Burning sensation under sternum.

Very severe pain in r. side of chest and hypochondriac region.

Hot, burning streaming in r. side of chest commencing below r. arm and clavicle and extending to hepatic region.

Sharp stitches in r. side of chest.

Slowly shooting pain in r. chest about seventh rib; acute stitches in r. breast.

▮Pain in r. chest to shoulder, can only with difficulty place hand on top of head.

▮Stitches in lower part of l. breast to shoulder.

Pain shooting from lower part of l. chest to l. shoulder.

‖Pain in breast with periodic cough.

▮Burning and pressing in breast, then heat through abdomen and diarrhœa.

Constant pressure and heaviness in whole upper part of chest, with difficulty of breathing.

▮Cramps in chest.

▮Pain in breast: with cough and expectoration; with dry periodic cough.

‖Subacute pulmonary congestion in a lady with florid complexion and full habit, æt. 50; was much troubled with general flushings.

▮Dyspnœa, short, accelerated, constrained breathing; speech ceases to be free; sputa becomes tenacious, rust-colored, and is expectorated with much difficulty; position of patient is on his back; not much pain in chest unless pleuræ are involved, then burning stitching pulse quick and small; face and extremities inclined to be cold or hands and feet burning hot, with circumscribed redness and burning heat of cheeks, especially in afternoon. θPulmonary affections. θPneumonia.

▮Pneumonia in second and third stages; with dulness on

percussion; bronchial respiration, with red or gray hepatization and infiltration of parenchyma.

‖ Pneumonia; rust-colored sputum; distressing dyspnœa; hands and feet burning hot or very cold; sometimes, even before amount of hepatization will account for it, there is failure of the heart's action; heart weak and irregular in action; weak, faint feeling about heart; patient is faint; is covered with sweat and suffers from nausea.

‖ Pneumonia, with cold hands and blue nails.

▮Typhoid pneumonia with very difficult respiration cheeks and hands livid; pulse full, soft, vibrating and easily compressed.

▮Pneumonia: l. lung particularly affected; with heart disease.

▮▮Catarrhal irritation in chest; night sweats; after a cold, several months previously.

‖ Sick an indefinite period with lung trouble; complete hepatization of one lung; fever; prostration; night sweats.

‖ Loose, stringy, sometimes flocculent expectoration, attending a severe cough, which seemed to rack whole frame during the paroxysm; darting pains through both lungs, < in apex of l. lung; cough < at night in bed; evening exacerbations of fever, with burning of palms of hands and soles of feet; debilitating night sweats; paroxysms of excruciating frontal headaches; dulness of percussion in l. supra- and infra-clavicular regions; fine whistling and long expiratory sounds in apex of l. lung; bronchial tubes in middle and lower parts of both lungs contained much mucus; pulse 114, easily compressible; anorexia; insomnia; thirst; urine diminished, changeable in color; marked emaciation; cheeks hollow; limbs and body small and bony; eyes sunken, glassy θIncipient phthisis following amenorrhœa.

‖ Great emaciation; bloodless skin; æt. 15, had never menstruated, but twelve months ago there was a slight discharge with pain in loins, at which time she commenced to fail; severe, painful cough, with profuse expectoration of thick, stringy, yellowish-white mucus, < at night; night sweats; chest sore to pressure; respiratory murmur faint and covered in some parts by mucous râles; bronchial tubes seemed filled with mucus; shortness of breath; headache; evening fever; burning in feet; dryness of throat; anorexia; pulse 100, soft and quick; alternate constipation and diarrhœa; high-colored, offensive smelling urine; sleeplessness; shooting, erratic pains through body and especially in chest; great exhaustion. θAnæmia with amenorrhœa.

‖ For several years cough, < in Summer; a year ago had pneumonia which left a suspicious permanent cough; cannot lie down; face bloated; pupils somewhat dilated; pulse very rapid and weak; night sweats; diarrhœa; pain in calves of legs; pain in chest, and with every respiratory effort there is rattling in chest followed by cough; paroxysms of cough with profuse offensive-smelling expectoration; the breath is offensive, even to himself; retching with the cough, throbbing and sensation of tightness in head; spasmodic belching before and after cough; heat continues for a while after the cough, followed by yawning and stretching.

‖ Phthisis florida; hectic; fever usually comes at about 2 or 4 P.M., cheeks having a bright circumscribed flush; cough usually dry at first and seems to be excited by tickling or crawling in larynx and upper portion of chest, probably in trachea and perhaps in beginning of bronchial tubes; great deal of burning fulness in upper part of chest, as if it were too full of blood, which it really is; sharp stitching pains, especially about r. lung and in region of nipple, probably myalgic; muscles of chest are sore with this pain; great dyspnœa.

| Tuberculosis pulmonalis; breath and sputa smell badly, disagreeable to patient himself; before and after coughing, belching of wind; after cough, heat; after heat, gaping and stretching; circumscribed redness of cheeks; diarrhœa; night sweats; pain in lower extremities.

‖ Beginning of galloping consumption, cough and violent fever, with circumscribed redness of cheeks; soreness to touch of veins in temples.

| Hæmoptoe during incipient phthisis, especially in women suffering from amenorrhœa, or during and after climaxis.

‖ Vicarious hemorrhage from lungs from suppressed menstruation in a young consumptive.

| Hæmoptysis during phthisis pulmonalis.

‖ Syphilitic pulmonary inflammation.

| Chronic pneumonia (rivals *Sulphur* and *Phosphor.*).

| Hydrothorax; asthma; pleurisy; intercostal myalgia.

29 **Heart, Pulse and Circulation.** Painful stitches or pressing pain in region of heart.

Palpitation before vomiting, with great weakness.

‖ Surging of blood and racing palpitation, with dry and burning skin.

| Irregularity of heart's action and pulse, with coldness, insensibility, etc.

| Weak feeling about heart.

Pulse: hard, frequent; small and quick; irregular, with great weakness.

▮Extreme reduction of force and frequency of pulse, together with great irregularity of action.

▮Metastasis of rheumatism (or gout) to heart, caused by outward applications in inflammatory rheumatism.

30 **Outer Chest.** Burning in sternum.

Severe soreness under r. nipple, < from touch.

31 **Neck and Back.** Pain in nape of neck.

▮Rheumatic pains in nape of neck, shoulders and arms.

Soreness of nape of neck on being touched.

▮Dull pain along inner edge of l. scapula, worse from breathing.

Rheumatic pains in neck, shoulders and arms, < at night.

Shifting pains in back, < when drawing a long breath.

▮Pain in sacrum, from lifting.

▮Lumbago, from lifting; or, myalgia of great muscles of back.

▮Soreness down muscles of back; pains shifting about; feels pain more when drawing long breath.

32 **Upper Limbs.** Itching in axillæ before catamenia.

▮▮Rheumatic pain in r. arm and shoulder; < at night, on turning in bed; cannot raise arm.

▮▮Pain in r. deltoid muscle of long standing; < from lifting; not felt when swinging arms to and fro; < at night when turning in bed, it wakes him; neither warmth nor weather influences it; it gives him no rest by day or night; is not relieved by motion.

▮Pain in top of r. shoulder.

▮▮Pain in r. shoulder and upper part of r. arm, < at night on turning in bed.

▮▮Pain confined to shoulder, shoulder-cap and cervical region; neck stiff, with great pain on movement; trapezius sore under pressure and painful at every movement of head or shoulder; deltoid and biceps very tender to pressure, and so sensitive by use that it was impossible to raise arm from side. θRheumatism.

▮▮Right arm hung at her side or lay on her lap as helpless as if there had been a fracture of humerus; could not raise it an inch without assistance. θRheumatism.

▮▮A sensation of coldness in body and r. arm, which no amount of clothing could remove; swelling of r. arm between shoulder and elbow joint; complete inability to raise arm from lap, although lateral motion could be made; tenderness and soreness of r. trapezius and deltoid muscles. θRheumatism.

▮▮Aching in ball of r. thumb, which is swollen, pain extending around wrist and back of hand, most severe in ball of thumb; < since hot weather set in; could not use hand properly from pain and weakness in it.

‖ Burning of palms; redness of hands and severe burning; lividity of hands. θPneumonia.

‖ Fungoid growth between second and third metacarpal bones, protruding about a quarter of an inch out of palm.

Stiffness of finger joints.

| Ulceration of roots of finger nails on both hands.

| Panaritium, first r. then l. fingers.

33 **Lower Limbs.** Rheumatic pain in l. hip; also inside of r. thigh.

Bruiselike pain in thigh, alternating with pressure and burning in breast.

Pain through hips, extending down r. limb.

Wandering pains, < at night.

Knees are stiff.

Left leg and foot swelled in evening, with violent burning pain, did not know where to lay limb; limb externally cold; < until 12 P.M.

‖ Indolent ulcer on r. shin, with dirty granulations and dry sharp-cut edges, brownish thin discharge, not sensitive, no pain.

Sharp pain in r. ankle and great toe joint.

| Burning in soles of feet, < in bed.

Cold feet, afternoon.

‖ Ingrowing toe nail, unhealthy granulations, purulent discharge (lotion).

34 **Limbs in General.** | Burning of hands and feet, < at night.

Rheumatic pains < in places least covered with flesh; on touching painful part pain vanishes and appears in some other part.

| Rheumatism in all joints, with swelling and spasmodic pain.

| Rheumatic pains in limbs, with stiffness and rigidity.

| Acute, inflammatory and arthritic rheumatism.

35 **Rest. Position. Motion.** Lying still: > rheumatism.

Lying down: cough from tickling pressure in epigastrium; cough <.

Lying with head low: cough <.

Lies upon back.

Lying on l. side: pain in hypogastrium >.

Slightly turned on l. side: spasm of stomach >.

Cannot lie on r. side: spasm of stomach.

Must lie down: headache.

Sitting up: pain in epigastrium; cough >.

Stooping: nausea <; throbbing pain in head <.

Must kneel down and hold head tight to floor: neuralgia in jaw and face.

Rising from sitting posture: frontal headache with vertigo.

Motion: pulsations <; throbbing pain in head <.

Turning in bed: pain in arm and shoulder.
Turning head quickly: vertigo.
Cannot raise arm from side: rheumatism.
Swinging arm to and fro: pain in arm is not felt.
Exercise: < headache.

36 **Nerves.** ▮Great weakness; palpitation of heart; fainting weakness.

▮▮Lassitude, torpor, languor, not disposed to move or make any mental exertion, < in damp weather.
Limbs weak while walking in open air.
▮▮Lameness of r. arm.
||Chronic paralysis of r. arm.
Convulsive rigidity of limbs.

37 **Sleep.** Sleepless at night, wakes with fright, as if he would fall.

Dreams: of sailing at sea; of business matters; frightful.
Drowsiness causing mental and bodily indolence.

38 **Time.** Morning: headache begins, < during day, lasts until evening; nausea; redness of eyes; accumulation of mucus in eye.

Morning and lasting four to six hours: neuralgia.
Forenoon: headache commences, < until sunset.
Afternoon: headache; burning of eyelids <; circumscribed redness of cheeks; pain in l. breast; cold feet; fever.
2 or 4 P.M.: fever usually comes on.
Evening: cough from tickling; violent distension of abdomen; tickling in throat; l. leg and foot swollen; shivering in back.
Night: pain in temples <; pain in head >; coryza and diarrhœa <; pains in epigastrium <; copious urination; abdominal pains; cough <; shortness of breath <; sweats; expectoration <; pains in neck <; wandering pains <; burning of hands and feet <; sleepless; Rhus poisoning <.
Until 12 P.M.: cold sweat; swelling of l. leg and foot.

39 **Temperature and Weather.** Hot weather: pain in thumb <.

Open air: headache >; pain in chest >; limbs weak while walking.
Damp weather: lassitude <.
Cold room: cough <.
Cold air: inspiring, heat in throat >.
Cold drinks: cause pain in carious teeth.
Cold water: craves.

40 **Fever.** Chill with headache, nausea, pain under scapula on motion; shivering in back, < evening in bed.

||Coldness of feet in afternoon, with painful, sore tongue; stiffness of knee and finger joints.

Shaking chill.

▮Flushes of heat.

▮Slight flushes of heat, followed by chills, then face flushed, hands hot, qualmish feeling all over; lassitude.

▮Heat flying from head to stomach.

▮Burning heat; rapidly alternating with chill and shivering.

▮Afternoon fever with circumscribed red cheeks; fever 2 to 3 P.M., daily.

▮Paroxysms of fever in afternoon, with circumscribed redness of cheeks; cough and expectoration.

▮Burning of palms of hands and soles of feet, compelling him to throw bedclothes off his feet to cool them; these paroxysms generally come on in afternoon or evening.

Slight chill, violent fever, headache and delirium.

▮Copious sweat; cold sweat.

▮Fevers from pulmonary, hepatic or gastric inflammation; nervous fever; marsh fever; hectic fever; scarlet fever (after *Bell.*); typhus, with characteristic headache.

41 **Attacks, Periodicity.** Alternate: diarrhœa and constipation; pain in thigh and pressure in breast; burning heat and chill and shivering.

Periodical headache.

Every few minutes: violent retching.

Every fifteen or twenty minutes: spasm of stomach.

Every day: for five or six days, neuralgia; fever 2 to 3 P.M.

Every third day for six weeks: sick headache.

Every seventh day: headache.

Every eight days for nine years: attacks of headache and vomiting.

Every two weeks: catamenia; sick headache.

For six weeks: severe cough.

For years: distressing sick headache; neuralgia in face.

For many years: shortness of breath and cough.

For six years: dryness in throat.

For twenty years: pyrosis.

42 **Locality and Direction.** Right: headache over eye; neuralgia in and over eye; headache in temple; headache <; neuralgia in orbit; catarrhal discharge from side of nose; tearing in temple; pains from eye through back part of head; pain from occiput to temporal bone; burning and watering of eye; coryza <; headache in hemisphere of brain; pain in throat; diphtheritis <; pain in breast; sharp pain over eye; pain in chest <; burning pain in side of chest; stitches in side of chest; shooting pain in side of chest; stitches in breast; rheumatic pain in arm and shoulder; pain in deltoid muscles; pain in top of shoulder; arm helpless with rheu-

matism; coldness in arm; swelling of arm; aching in ball of thumb; pain in thigh; indolent ulcer on shin; sharp pain in ankle and great toe joint; lameness of arm; chronic paralysis of side.

Left: violent pain over whole side of head; rheumatism in shoulder; pressing pain settling over eye; stitches in side of face; pain in hypochondrium; stitches in lower part of breast; pain from chest to shoulder; pneumonia; darting pain in apex of lung; dulness of percussion in supra- and infra-clavicular regions; pain on inner edge of scapula; rheumatic pain in hip; leg and foot swollen.

From r.: to l.; cutting bellyache in iliac fossa; panaritium.

[a] **Sensations.** As if paralyzed; as if events that transpired in her dreams were not of hours' but of weeks' and months' duration; as of some hard substance in stomach; as if forehead would burst; as if head were drawn forward; as if head must burst; as if eyes would be pressed out; as of a band across forehead; as of an electrical current shooting through head; pain like drawing a rope on a windlass as tight as you can get it; as if temples and scalp were alive with irrepressible pulsation; as if hairs were in eyes; as if she were in a railroad car or in some vehicle which was moving and jarring her, and as if all about her moved rapidly and confusedly; tongue as if burnt; tip of tongue as if scalded; tongue as if in contact with something hot; throat as if swollen; throat so dry it seems as if it would crack; pharynx as if burnt or scalded; constriction in pit of stomach as if suffocating; as of something alive in stomach; as of hot water pouring from breast into abdomen; as of a mass in lower part of rectum; as if menses would appear; cough as if head were enveloped in a blanket; throat and larynx as if swollen; as if upper part of chest were too full of blood.

Pain: in forehead; in forehead and cheek bones; in forepart of head, shoulders, chest and stomach; over r. eye; in head in spots; like a flash of lightning in back part of head; in head in rays; from r. occiput to r. temporal bone; over eyes; in chest; in teeth; in carious teeth; in l. hypochondrium; in loins through hypogastric and uterine region down thighs; in loins; about shoulders and chest; beneath sternum and r. breast; in breast; in calves; in lower extremities; in nape of neck; in back; in sacrum; in r. deltoid muscle; in top of r. shoulder and upper part of arm; from ball of thumb around wrist and back of hand; through hips and down r. limb; under scapula.

Frightfully severe headache.

Violent pain: over upper portion of whole l. side of head; in temple and vertex; from occipital region over head settling over r. eye.

Severe pain: in head; at root of nose and in frontal sinuses; in r. breast, extends to shoulder; in r. side of chest.

Sharp pain: in r. ankle and great toe joint.

Tearing: in r. temple.

Throbbing, lancinating pains: through brain.

Darting pains: through both lungs.

Sharp, piercing pain: in r. breast, midway between sternum and r. nipple.

Cutting pain: from r. to l. iliac fossa, thence to rectum.

Beating pain: in head.

Shooting pains: from one temple to other; from l. chest to l. shoulder.

Wandering pain: in head.

Stitches: in l. side of face; violent, in splenetic region; in mammæ; sharp, in r. chest about seventh rib; in r. breast; in lower part of l. breast to shoulder; about r. lung and nipple; in region of heart.

Burning stitching: in chest.

Violent burning pain: in l. leg and foot.

Intense burning pain: between breasts.

Burning distress: in stomach.

Burning: in stomach; of r. eye; in edges of lids; of ears; of under lip; of uvula; in throat; in œsophagus and pharynx; of palms; behind sternum; under sternum; streaming in r. side of chest extending to hepatic region; in breast; of hands and feet; in soles.

Burning dryness: in eyes.

Stinging sensation: in nose.

Soreness: in spots on head; in throat; of tongue; of roof of mouth; of uvula; throughout pharynx; in epigastrium; in abdomen; of nipples; in larynx; under r. nipple; of nape of neck; down muscles of back; of r. trapezius and deltoid muscles.

Bruiselike pain: in thigh.

Pricking: in point of tongue.

Neuralgia: in and over r. eye; at internal superior angle of r. orbit; in r. temple and orbit; in upper jaw, nose, eye, ear, neck and side of head.

Rheumatic pain: in head; in neck and shoulders; in nape of neck, shoulders and arms; in r. arm and shoulder; in l. hip; in r. thigh; in places least covered with flesh; in all points.

Drawing pain: from back into neck; in shoulders and arms.

Pressive pain: in forehead; from nape of neck over head and eyes; in region of heart.
Dull pain: in head; along inner edge of l. scapula.
Grumbling pain: in teeth.
Aching: in ball of r. thumb.
Dull, heavy feeling: in stomach; over root of nose.
Heaviness: in chest.
Pressure: in epigastrium; in stomach; in breast; in upper part of chest.
Spasmodic constriction: beneath lower jaw, across throat.
Constriction: in pit of stomach.
Tightness: in head.
Stiffness: in articulation of jaw; of finger joints; of knees.
Heat: in throat; in stomach; streaming from head to liver.
Tenderness: of r. trapezius.
Rawness: of throat.
Dryness: under upper lid; of lips; of throat.
Beating: under ears; in abdomen.
Jerking: in stomach.
Throbbing: in temporal arteries; of every pulse in body
Pulsations: in head; in r. temple.
Great weakness and goneness: in stomach.
Faint feeling: about heart.
Weak feeling: about heart.
Itching: in axilla.
Coldness: in body and r. arm.

44 **Tissues.** Languid circulation, limbs cold, skin pallid, sensitive to atmospheric changes.
Veins distended, feel sore.
Surging of blood.
Red or gray hepatization of lungs.
‖ Polypi, nasal and uterine.
‖ Carbuncles; warts; fungous excrescences.
| Roundish or oval, whitish or raised patches of mucous membrane of nose, mouth, prepuce and anus.
| Polypi of larynx and nasal fossæ.
Pains in places where bones are least covered with flesh.

45 **Touch. Passive Motion. Injuries.** Touch: temporal veins painfully sensitive; head very painful; eye painful; nipples sore; soreness of nape of neck; pain vanishes and appears some other part.
Pressure: hard upon eye >; > headache; pain in hypogastrium >; surface of chest tender; chest sore; deltoid and biceps tender.
Pressing back up against something hard: > headache.
Rubbing Rhus poisoning with something rough >.
Slightest jar: < headache.
Lifting: pains in sacrum; lumbago.

46 **Skin.** Heat and dryness of skin.

Itching and nettlerash with nausea.

▮Icterus, eyes yellow, stools white, dark yellow urine, during prevailing intermittent fever.

▮Prickling sensation of warmth spreading over body.

‖Eruption on face of young women, with menstrual troubles, especially deficiency.

▮Rhus poisoning; small pimples coalescing into blisters size of a split pea, filled with yellow watery fluid, with intense itching; < at night after 12 P.M.; the only relief he can get is to rub it with something rough, until blisters are open.

‖Fungous growths.

‖Scaly eruptions; carbuncles.

▮Old indolent ulcers, with callous borders and ichorous discharge; dirty granulations, dry, sharp-cut edges.

47 **Stages of Life, Constitution.** C. P., æt. 15 months; cold in head.

Boy, æt. 1½, of syphilitic parents; patches in mouth.

Girl, æt. 4, subject to bronchial affections since birth; laryngitis.

Boy, æt. 5; croup.

Girl, æt. 10, lively disposition; influenza.

A. R., æt. 12, suffering six weeks; cough.

Girl, æt. 15, of French extraction, nervo-lymphatic temperament; anæmia.

Girl, æt. 16, lymphatic temperament, quiet disposition, menses appeared once, a year ago, since then absent; incipient phthisis.

Boy, æt. 18, scrofulous diathesis; diphtheritis.

Miss F., æt. 25, suffering since childhood; sick headaches.

Officer, æt. 26; syphilis.

Woman, æt. 30; headaches.

A. S., æt. 30; cold in head.

Mrs. M. L. S., æt. 30, a chronic inebriate, after drinking inordinately for several weeks; gastric derangement.

Woman, æt. 34, brunette, single; influenza.

Woman, æt. 35; migraine.

Miss S. C., æt. 38; catarrh in head.

Lady, æt. 47, spare habit, suffering with heart disease; tracheal irritation.

Mrs. F., æt. 48, sanguino-bilious temperament, woman of much energy and refinement; neurosis of stomach.

Mrs. H., æt. 50, fleshy, nearly past the climacteric, suffering for years; sick headache.

Lady, æt. 50, florid complexion, full habit of body; pulmonary congestion.

Mrs. S., æt. 50; cough.

Mrs. P., æt. 55, blue eyes, dark-brown hair, nervo-sanguine temperament, full habit, somewhat corpulent, suffering fifteen years; sick headache.

Mrs. C., æt. 59; œdema of glottis.

Man, æt. 60, full habit, ruddy complexion, full chest, afflicted many years; cough.

Young lady, of rheumatic tendency; rheumatism of arm.

46 **Relations.** It antidotes: *Opium* (dynamic effects).

Compatible: *Bellad.* (scarlatina).

Compare: *Bellad.*, *Iris*, *Paullinia* and *Mellilot.* in headaches; *Ant. tart.*, *Chelid.*, *Phosphor.*, *Sulphur* and *Verat. vir.* in pneumonia.

SARRACENIA PURPUREA.

Pitcher plant. *Sarraceniaceæ.*

Grows in boggy places from Canada southward.

The tincture is prepared from the fresh plant.

Proved by Porcher, Duncan, Thomas, Hale's New Remedies, 1867; Cigliano, Am. Obs., 1871.

Clinical Authorities.—*Visual disorder*, Berridge, N. A. J. H., vol. 22, p. 194; *Phlyctenoid herpes*, Crica, A. J. H. M. M., vol. 3, p. 78; *Variola*, Martiny, Mowremans, Raue's Rec., 1875, p. 287; *Smallpox*, Renshaw, A. H. O., vol. 2, p. 234; *Use in smallpox*, Cigliano, A. H. O., vol. 8, p. 467; Easton, vol. 1, p. 135.

1 **Mind.** Melancholia, anxious about everything.

Great depression of spirits from frontal headache.

Brain clearer, buoyant spirits.

‖Dulness of head, loss of memory, insensibility of r. side; paralysis of hearing and smell.

Want of memory with the headache.

Difficult to concentrate the attention, forgetful; feels dull and heavy; urine sp. gr. 1020; perspires freely.

2 **Sensorium.** Head feels dull and heavy.

Feels light-headed.

Vertigo: with cramps in neck, spreading to forehead; especially at night; sensation as if he received a knock on head, with vertigo, stupor and vacillating gait; he is obliged to support himself or else to lie down; with drowsiness in head and contractions in spinal column.

3 **Inner Head.** Frontal headache, low-spirited.

Head dull and aches at coronal region.

Severe headache in afternoon for two hours.
Full feeling through head just above ears.
Headache with chills, nausea, vomiting; dim sight, surring in ears.
Pulsations and burning heat of head with sensation as if it would split.

4 **Outer Head.** Head is hot and aches.
Head and body warm.
Soreness of frontal bone.
Pruritus and heat of scalp.

5 **Sight and Eyes.** Eyes weak.
Dim sight, headache.
||Gas flame seems a brilliant yellow ring, the two not being distinct; he sees black objects moving with the eye.
Great photophobia.
Soreness of r. optic nerve, just behind eyeball.
Pain in l. eye as if congested, on waking.
Eyes feel swollen and sore.
Eyes and lids inflamed.
Increased mucous secretion.
Cutting, penetrating pains in orbits.

6 **Hearing and Ears.** Surring in ears.
Sticking pains deep in r. ear; transient but recurring often; same in l. ear.
Intense otalgia, fears he will lose his senses.
Swelling of parotids.

7 **Smell and Nose.** Fetid smell.
Epistaxis nearly producing fainting.
Fluent coryza, with cold chills and loss of smell.
Foul-smelling, green-yellowish or bloody discharges.
Nose swollen, red, with pressure and pulsation at root.

8 **Upper Face.** Face flushed.
Heat and redness of face.
Face pale, with heat and chill alternating.
Erysipelatous swelling of face.
Miliary eruption on face with heat as if it were on fire.
Scaly herpes on face and forehead.

9 **Lower Face.** Intense neuralgic pains from temples to jaws.

11 **Taste and Tongue.** Tongue dry.
Tongue coated brownish white.

12 **Inner Mouth.** Mouth dry.
Lips and mouth parched.

13 **Throat.** Dryness of throat not relieved by tea or water, borborygmi.

14 **Appetite, Thirst. Desires, Aversions.** ||Hungry all the time, even after a meal.
||Appetite unusually active, but there was a sense of pain

about stomach like that after inflammation or that in an overtaxed muscle.

But little appetite, yet what is eaten agrees with him; urine 1018; pulse 71; sweats freely.

5 **Eating and Drinking.** Great desire to sleep during eating.

16 **Hiccough, Belching, Nausea and Vomiting.** Copious painful vomiting frequently after meals, with lightness from stomach to back and colicky pains.

Vomiting of bile mixed with blood.

17 **Scrobiculum and Stomach.** Empty, hungry feeling; for he can keep nothing on his stomach.

Burning pains in his stomach, with palpitations and contractions.

Pinching pains in stomach; it feels distended and torn.

19 **Abdomen.** After going to bed, whole abdominal region was in commotion, extending along tract of ascending and descending colon, all in a kind of rolling motion; epigastrium tender on pressure.

Some transient pains in bowels.

Bloated about navel.

Borborygmi and some pain in bowels with constipation; dry throat.

20 **Stool and Rectum.** Much flatus.

First part of stool natural, last diarrhœic.

Much tenesmus; dysenteric diarrhœa.

Stool at first costive, then dark, offensive, soluble.

Costive; stools very hard, covered with mucus and dark.

Stool copious, dark, fetid, evacuated with great straining; morning.

Diarrhœic stools mixed with glairy mucus, bile and blood; anorexia, prostration and painfully strong palpitation.

Rectum and anus swollen and inflamed.

Morning diarrhœa; faint after stool, which is dark, often mixed with blood, foul-smelling or smelling of musk; bloatedness with colic.

Morning diarrhœa; bloatedness with colic; faintness after stool which is dark, often mixed with blood; foul-smelling or of the odor of musk.

21 **Urinary Organs.** Awoke 3 A.M. with urging to urinate; bladder so full it overcame resistance of sphincter and dribbled away.

Voided 27 oz. of urine; sp. gr. 1024; vesical tenesmus.

Urine increased, limpid, colorless, scarcely any sediment even after several hours.

Urine responds to tests for phosphates, earthy phosphates and chloride of sodium.

Urine copious, a little cloudy; sp. gr. 1030 (cloudy from mucus); pale yellow.

Urine scanty, limpid, 1025.

23 **Female Organs.** Watery or milky leucorrhœa, thick, whitish, foul-smelling with spasmodic pains in uterus; pulsative pains in womb with swelling as if from a tumor or dropsy; uterus swollen as if full of cysts, especially on r. side; neck of womb swollen and hot; miliary eruption and heat in vulva; bloody discharge at other times than menstrual period as during climaxis.

28 **Inner Chest and Lungs.** Phthisis pulmonalis and bronchial affections, joined to or depending on a psoric state; hæmoptysis, thick cough; continual tickling in larynx and bronchi; cough, with desire to vomit and vomiting, paroxysms of suffocation and epistaxis; hard cough, shaking chest and bowels and stopping only after expectorating a quantity of compact mucus, tenacious, filamentous with a bitter, putrid, oily taste.

29 **Heart, Pulse and Circulation.** Feeling of congestion about head, with irregularity of heart's action.

Congestion to chest, heavy feeling about heart.

Slight palpitation in morning.

Pulse: full and strong; 68, general malaise; rose to 100 before morning; 61, very small; quick, 80.

30 **Outer Chest.** Slight soreness of whole pectoralis major; pain ran up r. trapezius muscle with a wavelike motion; lumbar heat; pulse 70, full; bloated feeling at navel (probably from flatus).

Pain in angle of ribs for half an hour.

31 **Neck and Back.** Warm sensation passed up back into head.

Weak between and below shoulders.

Back weak, wants to lean on something.

Arms and back tired and sore all over.

Deep-seated pain in back.

Heat in whole r. lumbar region.

Pain and soreness in sacrum.

32 **Upper Limbs.** Paroxysms of pain in r. shoulder joint, pain in l. carpus and tarsus; face flushed.

Arms feel weak.

Bruised feeling from shoulders to hands.

Aching, sore pain in l. humerus.

Bones in both arms pain.

33 **Lower Limbs.** Pain in hip joints < rising to feet from a lying posture.

Paroxysms of weakness in coxo-femoral joint with pains of luxation and fear of falling when trying to walk.

Strange lameness in femur, lower third, < in inner condyle.

Pain in condyles of femur.

Wavelike motion in muscles of femur.

Sensation of fatigue in bones of legs as if they were too thick.

Bruised and luxated feeling in joints.
Pain in r. patella and metatarsal bones.
Knees feel weak.
Bruised pain in knees as after a fall; he falls easily on his knees.
Bone pains in tibia and fibula; intermittent, but bones continually sore.
Bones of feet inflamed; nodes as in gout.

34 **Limbs in General.** Limbs cold when still as from deficient circulation.
Limbs easily benumbed.
Weakness of limbs with paralytic debility.

35 **Rest. Position. Motion.** Wants to lean on something; weakness of back.
Rising to feet from a lying posture: pain in hip joint <.
Trying to walk: fear of falling.

36 **Nerves.** Debility, wants to lie down all the time.
Languid, heavy.

38 **Time.** Morning: stool with great straining; diarrhœa; slight palpitation; feverish, with shaking chills.
Afternoon: severe headache.
Night: cramps in neck <.

39 **Temperature and Weather.** In open air: chilly, hands and feet cold; head hot and sore, feels full.
Cold air: makes him feel chilly and increases bone pains.

40 **Fever.** Feverish, with shaking chills < in morning.
Skin hot and dry.
Hands hot, warm all over; cold air makes him feel chilly and increases bone pains, especially in knees.
Hot, feverish; pulse 80, small and quick.

41 **Attacks, Periodicity.** Alternating: heat and chill.
For half an hour: pain in angle of ribs.
For two hours: headache in forenoon.

42 **Locality and Direction.** Right: insensibility of side; soreness of optic nerve; pain deep in ear; uterus swollen; pain up trapezius muscle; heat in lumbar region; pain in shoulder joint; pain in patella and metatarsal bones.
Left: pain in eye; pain in ear; pain in carpus and tarsus; pain in humerus.

43 **Sensations.** As if he received a knock on head; as if head would split; l. eye as if congested; heat in face as if on fire; swelling in womb as if from a tumor or dropsy; uterus swollen as if full of cysts; as if bones of legs were too thick.
Pain: in l. eye; in bowels; up r. trapezius muscle; in angle of ribs; in sacrum; in r. shoulder joint; in l. carpus and tarsus; in bones of arms; in hip joints; in condyles of femur; in r. patella and metatarsal bones; in tibia and fibula.

Intense neuralgic pains: from temples to jaws.
Severe pain: in head.
Cutting, penetrating pains: in orbits.
Pinching pains: in stomach.
Spasmodic pains: in uterus.
Pulsative pains: in womb.
Deep-seated pain: in back.
Sticking pains: deep in r. ear.
Aching, sore pain: in l. humerus.
Burning pains: in his stomach.
Cramps: in neck to forehead.
Aching: at coronal region.
Soreness: of frontal bone; of r. optic nerve; of pectoralis major; of back and arms; in sacrum.
Bruised feeling: from shoulders to hands; in joints; in knees.
Burning heat: of head.
Pulsations: in head; at root of nose.
Wavelike motion: in muscles of femur.
Pressure: at root of nose.
Heaviness: of head; about heart.
Full feeling: through head.
Dryness: of tongue; of mouth; of throat.
Tickling: in larynx and bronchi.
Dulness: of head.
Luxated feeling: in joints.
Strange lameness: in femur.
Heat: in vulva; in whole r. lumbar region.
Warm sensation: up back into head.
Light feeling: in head.
Weakness: between and below shoulders; of back; in coxo-femoral joint; of knees; of limbs.

44 **Tissues.** Bones feel heavy, sore.
Bones pain, especially cervical and lumbar vertebræ, sacrum and femur, < in inner condyle and great trochanter.
Phlegmonous swelling with a rosy tint on various parts.

46 **Skin.** ‖Phlyctenoid herpes.
|Psoriasis.
|Scrofulous eruptions.
|Variola (decoction taken when eruption is out and beginning to pustulate aborts secondary fever, pitting).
|Fever becomes less, delirium vanishes, pains lessen, eruption develops sooner and matures rapidly, desiccating without leaving pits.
|Eruption out, pustules dissipate, first on face, fever lessens, urine though scanty and dark becomes abundant and pale; strength returns.

▮Arrests pustules, killing as it were the virus from within, preventing pitting.
▮Constitutional symptoms in three or four days subside.
▮Even confluent forms are helped, little or no pitting following.
▮Relieves restlessness, sleeplessness during variola.
▮▮A woman far advanced in pregnancy was cured of smallpox with *Sarrac.* 3, 6th and 9th, her accouchement being happily accomplished during her convalescence, the babe bearing upon its body numerous red blotches, indicating that it had been similarly affected at the same time with the mother.
▮▮An infant a few months old was attacked with a grave form of smallpox, with variolous angina, so severe that it was with difficulty it could take the breast; the mother took *Sarrac.* 3, 6th and 9th, continued to nurse the infant, which promptly recovered from the disease, and the mother did not take the disorder, notwithstanding the immediate and constant contact of the child.
▮▮In an epidemic occurring in the environs of Wavre it was given to more than two thousand persons living in the very middle of the disease and coming in constant intercourse with it, but all who took it escaped the disease; during the same time more than two hundred cases were treated by the same remedy without the loss of a single patient.

47 **Stages of Life, Constitution.** Man, æt. 35, sanguino-bilious temperament, suffering a long time; phlyctenoid herpes.

48 **Relations.** Antidoted by: *Podophyl.* (diarrhœa).

SARSAPARILLA.

Wild Liquorice. *Smilaceæ.*

Proved by Hahnemann, Hermann, Teuthorn, Brunner, Nenning, Schreter, Chronische Krankheiten; Hancock, Krahmer, Pehrson, Hering's Monograph; Berridge, N. Am. J. of Hom., 1872; Am. Obs., 1875; The Organon, vol. 1, p. 107.

Clinical Authorities.—*Melancholia*, Neidhard, Raue's Rec., 1870, p. 366; *Headache*, Neidhard, A. J. H. M. M., vol. 1, p. 106; Farrington, A. J. H. M. M., vol. 2, p. 101; Griggs, A. J. H. M. M., vol. 5, p. 450; *Pains in occiput*, Neidhard, T. H. M. S. Pa., 1884, p. 324; *Bright's disease*, Kent, Med. Adv., Jan., 1889, p. 46; *Urinary difficulty*, Berridge, A. J. H. M. M., vol. 2, p. 101; *Dysuria*, Boyce, Am. Hom., Sept., 1878, p. 99; *Nocturnal enuresis*, W. M. J., Hom. Phys., vol. 6, p. 232; *Affection of bladder*, Lippe, Org., vol. 1, p. 269; Boyce, Org., vol. 2, p. 133; *Cystitis*, Swift, Hom. Phys., vol. 3, p. 354; *Wind from bladder*, Ring, H. M. S. O., 1873, p. 11; Raue's Rec., 1870, p. 217; *Calculi*, Hartm., Gross, Rück. Kl. Erf., vol. 2, p. 31; *Renal calculus*, Knerr, MSS.; *Spermatorrhœa*, Baldwin, N. A. J. H., vol. 22, p. 262; Hunt, Raue's Rec., 1870, p. 243; *Swelling of spermatic cords*, Berridge, Hah. Mo., vol. 10, p. 75; Hom. Phys., vol. 9, p. 147; *Suppressed gonorrhœa*, Rosenberg, Rück. Kl. Erf., vol. 2, p. 98; *Menstrual disorder*, Minton, Med. Inv., vol. 5, p. 19; *Dysmenorrhœa and pain in breast*, Burnett, Org., vol. 3, p. 269; *Leucorrhœa*, Miller, Hah. Mo., vol. 8, p. 43; *Climacteric disorder*, Smith, A. J. H. M. M., vol. 1, p. 146; *Scirrhus of breast*, Hart, Org., vol. 3, p. 107, from A. H. O., 1879; *Use in asthma*, Meyer, Rück. Kl. Erf., vol. 5, p. 801; *Inflammation of knees*, Robert, Org., vol. 3, p. 564; *Ulcer on leg*, Gilchrist, Gilch. Surg., p. 84; *Eczema of leg*, Blake, B. J. H., vol. 30, p. 118; *Faintness*, Hah. Mo., vol. 10, p. 77; *Ague*, Berridge, A. J. H. M. M., vol. 4, p. 38; *Syphilis*, Rummel, Rück. Kl. Erf., vol. 2, p. 167; *Eruptions*, Holcombe, Med. Inv., vol. 9, p. 4; *Chronic eruption*, Hirsch, B. J. H., vol. 25, p. 393.

1 **Mind.** Mental depression caused by the pains.
Anxiety with the pains.
Morose, with inclination to work.
Gloomy, desponding without known cause; debility.
Irritable, impatient or changeable; very easily vexed, cannot forget the cause.
‖ Thinking about the food he has been eating makes him sick.
‖ Desponding, gloomy disposition, amounting to despair, without any known cause; great debility, with acid, raw, slimy taste in mouth, particularly after breakfast.
She thinks she cannot bear the headache.
‖ Child cannot bear the itching, very impatient.

[3] **Sensorium.** Dull, stupid feeling; cannot keep the mind on his study.

‖ Heaviness in head.

Vertigo: while standing at window he suddenly fell backward on floor unconscious, at same time throat was swollen, sour eructations before and afterward, severe perspiration in night; with nausea in morning while gazing long at one object; while sitting and walking, head inclined to drop forward.

‖ Staggers, falls forward, in open air.

[3] **Inner Head.** | Headache, with nausea and sour vomiting.

| Pressure, or pressure with stitches, in l. side of forehead and head.

Headache like pressure of a great weight in head, which is inclined to sink forward.

Pressing and itching deep in r half of head, morning.

| Throbbing in top of head; < from walking, even when sitting down afterward, now and then aching through temples, forehead or occiput.

Violent throbbing in r. side of head, deep in brain.

A kind of buzzing in head, as if a large bell had been struck.

Dull tremor (wuwwern) with a waving in head.

Beating and sounding in r. side of head, deep in brain.

Very warm in head during dinner, with sweat on forehead.

‖ Shooting in r. parietal bone forward to temple or face.

‖ Pressing in vertex, increasing and decreasing slowly.

| Mercurial syphilitic affections of head.

‖ Shooting in r. parietal bone forward to temple or face; staggering and falling forward in open air. θMercurial syphilitic affection.

‖ Shooting back of head to front with violent itching, after syphilis and mercurialization.

‖ Darting from occiput to eyes with nausea, determination of blood to head, feet and hands cold. θNervous headache.

‖ Suffering severely all day, pains becoming more violent as evening approached, causing him to jerk his head to one side and scream with every paroxysm; pains confined to r. side principally, even pulsative and stitching in character, extending from occiput upward and forward over ear, around to temple and across forehead.

‖ Dull aching pain in head, mostly in forehead, < in evening; vertigo, especially in warm room; stupid feeling; prostration; great drowsiness in evening, but unable to sleep quietly through night; nocturnal emissions from one to three times a week, occurring in connection with lascivious dreams; tired feeling in morning with bitter taste in mouth; pain in small of back extending down spermatic cords. θSpermatorrhœa.

‖ Dull, stupid feeling in head, inability to keep his mind on his studies, sometimes a feeling as if something were pressing upon head; at times anguish of mind; unable to read at night on account of a mist or smoky appearance before eyes; great weakness and prostration, render him unfit for work; soft, flabby muscle; least excitement caused ejaculation of semen without sexual feeling; obstinate constipation, seminal losses since puberty from masturbation; emissions with lascivious dreams.

4 **Outer Head.** Sensitiveness of scalp; falling off of hair.

| Moist eruption on scalp, pus from which causes inflammation of any part it touches.

| Crusta lactea, indicated only when it begins with little pimples in face, very itchy, forcing child to scratch; parents subject to tetter.

| Crusta serpiginosa, with widely spread inflammatory affection of skin, child cannot bear it and is very impatient; in open air crusts fall off and new skin cracks.

| Humid scabs on skull.

Falling off of hair, with great sensitiveness of scalp on combing.

| Plica polonica.

| Mercurio-syphilitic affections of head.

5 **Sight and Eyes.** Vertigo while gazing long at one object.

Flickering before eyes, with headache.

Great dimness of l. eye, as if gauze were spread over it.

Mist before eyes, reading becomes difficult.

Reading by candlelight hurts eyes, paper looks red.

| Obscuration before eyes as from a fog; mist when reading; < after seminal emissions.

| Halo around the candle.

Eyes pain from light of day.

Pupils dilated.

Pressure in l. eye, as from a grain of sand.

Pain in l. then in r. eye, with dimness of vision.

On closing eyes stinging in them.

Pressing in eyes alternates with burning.

Stinging frequent in both eyes, as if dust or sand were in them; > outdoors.

‖ Stinging in eyes on closing lids, and violent pain when closed eyes are pressed upon; at same time a broad red stripe extending from cornea to outer canthus.

Internal canthi bluish and bloated; headache from occiput forward; abuse of mercury.

Quivering in r. upper lid.

Lachrymation in daytime; lids agglutinated in morning.
Ophthalmia after checked tetter.
Inflamed, dry eyelids.
I Itchlike eruption on eyelids.

6 **Hearing and Ears.** Words reverberate in ear.
Sound in head when talking as if a bell were striking.
Burning itching scab on ear lobe.

7 **Smell and Nose.** Sneezing and running coryza in morning.
Burning in nose on blowing it, with a dry cough.
Very thick mucus from nose.
II Chronic stoppage of nose.
Coryza and cough.
Itching on r. wing of nose, not > by scratching.
Itching on l. side of nose and around eyes.
Pricking in point of nose as from a needle.
Eruption in l. nostril; sore nose.
II Right nostril stopped up and scurfy.
II Pain in nose; inflamed spots on septum.
Itching eruption under nose, as if caused by acrid discharge.
A suppurating pimple on r. side of nose.
Small boils on nose.
Scabby eruption on and under nose.

8 **Upper Face.** Violent pain in face, as if bruised about both inferior orbital edges on waking in morning, only on pressing them.
Drawing, stinging, tearing in masticatory muscles of r. side, which seem to have spasmodically contracted.
The jaws pain as if being broken.
Fine pricking itching in face and scalp, as well as about neck and shoulders, with feeling of great warmth in these parts; on scratching it begins in another place.
I Face yellow, wrinkled, old-looking.
I Eruption like milk crust.
I Itching eruption on forehead, with burning; becoming humid on scratching.
I Pimples of various sizes on face.
Heat of face; sweat on forehead, in evening in bed.

9 **Lower Face.** Stiffness and tension in muscles and articulation of jaw.
Pressing, stinging pain on lower inner edge of r. lower jaw, but only on handling it and on bending head back.
Herpes on upper lip.

10 **Teeth and Gums.** I Sensitiveness of upper front teeth.
I Tearing in teeth, from cold air and cold drink.
II Toothache in last molars, > from cold air.
Stinging, tearing in gums and root of last r. inferior molar.
Swelling and sore pain of gums of inner side of inferior maxilla.

11 **Taste and Tongue.** Bitter taste: of food; in mouth in morning.
Sweetish taste.
Tongue: coated white; rough several mornings on waking, passing off after eating; red, back of it white.
Mercurial aphthæ on tongue and roof of mouth.
Stitches in tongue.
Acrid sensation on tongue.
|| Blisters on tongue; aphthæ on tongue and palate.
Tasteless water collects in mouth.
Slimy mouth in morning.
Dryness in mouth without thirst.
Dryness in mouth and throat, mornings, in bed.
Pressing drawing pain in soft palate.
In fauces: tickling ulcerative sensation, causing a cough.
Acrid sensation in pharynx.

13 **Throat.** Spasmodic contraction of throat, with dyspnœa, must loosen his cravat.
| Dryness and roughness of throat in morning.
|| Refuses food on account of pain in throat.
|| Sore feeling in throat, r. side.
|| Sore throat, aphthæ on soft palate.
|| Trichotomous ulcers; after plica polonica had been cut off, deep ulcers on tonsils, spreading to soft palate, on back wall of fauces; pale bluish edges; covered with cauliflower excrescences; whitish thin pus, smelling like rancid butter; refuses to take food on account of too much pain; kept alive by injections of milk in rectum.

14 **Appetite, Thirst. Desires, Aversions.** Want of appetite, the thought of food disgusts him.
Want of thirst.

15 **Eating and Drinking.** Burning in stomach, especially after eating bread.
After eating: bitter eructations (also during); feels as if he had eaten nothing; diarrhœa; deep inspirations; heavy, short breathing; asthma; exhaustion and nausea.
Worse from warm diet; > after cold diet.
To drink water sets her to vomiting.

16 **Hiccough, Belching, Nausea and Vomiting.** Hiccough 6 P.M.; after dinner.
Eructation: with taste of food, after dinner; first bitter and sour, then empty; bitter in morning after rising; during dinner; of bitter, sour matter, evenings; continuous, sour; sour after breakfast; of sour water, after noon; with shuddering.
|| Belching with diarrhœa.
| Nausea: when thinking of food eaten; with acrid sen-

sation on tongue and in pharynx; in stomach, less in throat; after breakfast; with constant ineffectual effort to vomit.

17 **Scrobiculum and Stomach.** Burning in stomach, especially after eating bread.

Stomach has no sensation, after eating feels as if he had eaten nothing.

19 **Abdomen.** ▮Rumbling and fermentation in abdomen, with discharge of offensive flatus.

▮Rumbling, with sensation of emptiness in abdomen.

Painful pressure inward and pinching in l. side of abdomen in a small spot, < by deep inspiration.

‖Pressure in abdomen from above downward; pressure on bowels.

Burning, or cold feeling in abdomen.

‖External abdomen very sensitive to touch.

In r. groin severe tension.

Pinching in l. inguinal region.

‖Hernia.

Soreness in bend of r. groin on appearance of menses.

20 **Stool and Rectum.** ‖Motion in bowels as if diarrhœa would follow.

▮Loose stool in evening.

‖Diarrhœa: with discharge of flatus; with bellyache and backache at same time.

▮Very hard stool.

▮Constipation, violent urging to urinate, stool small, with much bearing down.

▮Difficult and painful stool, with fainting attacks; stool retarded, hard and insufficient.

▮Obstinate constipation with violent urging to urinate; urging to stool with contraction of intestines; excessive pressure from above downward, as if bowels were pressed out; during stool violent tearing and cutting in rectum.

▮Diarrhœa after every kind of food that disagrees with his stomach; with belching and rumbling in abdomen.

▮Blood with stool.

21 **Urinary Organs.** ▮Chronic nephritis.

▮▮Neuralgia; attacks of most excruciating pains from r. kidney downward.

▮▮Renal colic and passage of gravel.

▮Small stones are expelled from bladder.

▮Stone in bladder; bloody urine.

▮▮Renal and vesical calculi.

▮Gravel, in children.

Painful constriction of bladder, without urging.

Pain and cramps in bladder, particularly with a painful urging and burning; urine copious and pale.

▮Tenesmus of bladder, with discharge of white acrid pus and mucus.

Tenderness and distension over region of bladder.

||Nocturnal incontinence of urine in a little girl; when awake could pass urine only when standing.

▮Frequent discharge of pale, copious urine.

||Has to get up two or three times at night to urinate and passes a great quantity; he thinks he can never finish, at first with burning, then without.

▮Frequent urination, with hard stool.

▮Frequent inefficient urging to urinate, with diminished secretion.

Frequent desire to urinate with scanty discharge accompanied by burning.

When he sits urine dribbles from him; when he stands it passes freely.

▮The urine passes in a thin, feeble stream, or in drops only, without pain or urging; he has to press much.

||Burning while urine passes, with discharge of elongated flakes.

Strangury, with pressure on bladder, yet the urine will not come, and when it comes there is cutting pain.

▮Painful retention of urine.

▮Urine: bright and clear, but irritating; red, fiery; often and copious, must rise at night; ▮▮scanty, slimy, flaky, sandy; copious, passed without sensation; pale, turbid, immediately after its passage like clay water and scanty, voided in a thin, powerless stream; deposits white sand.

▮Sand in urine or on diaper; child screams before and while passing it.

▮Each time she makes water, air passes out of urethra with a gurgling noise.

▮Urine passes in a thin, feeble stream or in drops without pain.

▮After passage of urine burning and itching, tearing pain from glans to root of penis.

▮▮Much pain at conclusion of passing water, almost unbearable.

▮Jerking sensation along male urethra.

▮Pain at meatus urinarius, with women.

||Great difficulty in urinating, constant ineffectual desire; sometimes urine (which is scanty) becomes turbid on standing; pain in back, at lower part of spine, and from thence across hips and down thighs; lower part of abdomen tender to touch, hard, distended; her symptoms remind her of what she suffered after a confinement.

||A man, æt. 52, addicted to whisky for years; had a copious flow of blood from bowels some four months

ago; the exertion of walking a few blocks causes suffocation; after the loss of blood feet began to swell; both limbs to middle of thighs very œdematous; has had two or three nondescript chills; a few months ago a sudden paralytic weakness of l. arm and leg, passed off in three hours, leaving a numbness in l. hand, and rending pain in l. side of head and face; no appetite; bloody mucous discharges with stools; feels as if in a dream all the time; loss of memory; face covered with varicose veins and very red; general venous stasis; feeling on top of head as if he had been hit with a hammer; must pass urine several times a night; urine thick and cloudy after standing, but clear when first passed; has had much worry from financial losses; cannot pass urine while sitting at stool, but it flows freely when he is standing; albumen in urine.

❙❙After each urination pain at a point near neck of bladder; had to urinate often and had distress more or less all through pelvis; after each urination had chills commencing at region of neck of bladder and spreading upward until he felt them in whole upper part of body.

❙❙After exposure to a draft of cold air while in a profuse perspiration, next morning was unable to move or be moved; felt as if he were bound down to bed by a sort of suction; before he got into this condition had severe sharp pains, principally in back and shoulders, on least motion; but two scanty discharges of urine in the previous twenty-four hours.

❙Mrs. C., æt. 50, took a severe cold, followed by a chill and fever; next morning after chill, awoke with severe pains through bladder, back, hips and down thighs; frequent urination, passing but little and that mostly blood, with a great deal of burning and straining. θCystitis.

❙❙A sickly-looking child, a girl, æt. 3, in bad health several weeks; every time the child urinates, wind comes from bladder with a noise.

❙❙After each urination a pain at a point in vicinity of neck of bladder; after every urination chills commencing at region of neck of bladder and spreading in an upward direction until finally he felt them in whole upper part of body.

22 **Male Sexual Organs.** ❙Seminal emissions, lascivious dreams, with backache, prostration, vertigo.

❙The least excitement causes an emission, even without sexual feeling.

❙❙Painful pollution nearly every night, with lascivious dreams.

❙Lascivious dreams with erections wake him up, with headache, dim sight, prostration and vertigo; inclination to coitus, with restless sleep and frequent emissions; spermatic cords swollen, sexual excitement makes them ache and sensitive; bloody pollutions (*Ledum*); offensive odor about genitals.

▮Swelling of spermatic cords after ungratified sexual excitement.

▮After suppressed gonorrhœal discharge by injections made of a solution of gunpowder, extremely severe rheumatic pains in limbs and extreme emaciation.

▮Gonorrhœa checked by cold, wet weather or by mercury, followed by rheumatism.

▮Herpes on prepuce.

▮Moist eruption about genitals or between scrotum and thighs.

Tearing from glans to root of penis.

Glans red and inflamed.

▮Intolerable odor about genitals.

▮Unbearable itching on scrotum and perineum; after scratching little pimples rise, oozing a moisture, and keep the part sore.

▮Sycosis.

▮▮Old, dry sycotic warts, remaining after mercurial treatment for gouty pains.

▮Syphilis; squamous eruption; bone pain; after abuse of mercury.

23 **Female Sexual Organs.** ▮▮Catamenia very copious, even to hemorrhage, with an old maid.

▮Dysmenorrhœa for twenty years; generally began in morning with bitter vomiting, diarrhœa and fainting fits, with exceedingly cold sweats; dreadful pain in back, thighs and hypogastrium; had to lie down the first day, the second the pain continued very bad, and on the third day it went off; l. nipple considerably retracted, arising from a fall when a child, and she had severe pain in l. breast extending down l. arm, and l. breast was so tender that she would often hold her hand in front of it to avoid contact.

▮Menses: too late and scanty, preceded by urging to urinate; itching eruption on forehead; flow acrid; soreness inside of thighs; griping in pit of stomach in direction of small of back.

▮Leucorrhœa: on walking; pain at meatus urinarius after urinating.

▮▮Leucorrhœa continuing six months after parturition, with severe laborlike pains from sacrum to crest of ilium, or around to uterus; heat and pulsation in sacrum; scanty, white leucorrhœa, when walking or exercising;

scalding micturition; severe pain at close of urination; had had many abortions.

Nipples became retracted and insensible.

❘❘Scirrhus of breast (cured by large doses).

During climacteric period: asthmatic breathing, made < by lying down; pain in back very severe on a line with and immediately to left of sacrum; < from pressure and from turning over in bed; severe and constant nausea, with vomiting, severe frontal headache; great urging to urinate with only slight emissions of urine, accompanied with burning, stinging pain during and after severe rigors over whole body, commencing at feet; rather calm, yet feared she would not recover.

24 **Pregnancy. Parturition. Lactation.** ❚Pregnant women: before and during stool, severe pains in sacral regions, writhing, drawing, radiating upward and downward until fingers, hands, feet and toes are involved and cramped from darting, drawing pains, with anxiety, faintness and palpitation of heart.

❘Suppuration of mammæ.

25 **Voice and Larynx. Trachea and Bronchia.** ❘❘Croup, spasmodic variety; laryngismus stridulus.

Rawness and pain in larynx.

Throat rough, hoarse and dry in morning on waking.

Hoarseness in throat every other day.

Tough slime in throat in morning which cannot be removed by hawking.

Constant hawking of mucus in morning, the slime being reproduced in abundance.

Spasmodic constriction in throat and chest, with difficult breathing.

Loosens clothes from neck in order to get breath; but this is without avail.

26 **Respiration.** Shortness of breath, he must loosen neckcloth and vest.

Stoppage of breath as if by a spasm, with constriction of throat. θSpasmodic asthma.

❚Short breathing on going up stairs.

Rigors over whole body from below upward; asthmatic breathing, < by lying down.

Oppression of chest impeding respiration, mornings.

❘❘Great emphysema; chest barrel-shaped; liver pressed downward; scaleni muscles hypertrophied; constant dyspnœa, < after eating and least motion (relieved).

27 **Cough.** Cough: from tickling in chest or with rattling in chest; with colorless, tasteless expectoration, pain in larynx; with headache; dry, with burning in nose on blowing it; with coryza; with nausea, vomiting of bile, diarrhœa; in morning.

|| Chronic catarrh.

28 **Inner Chest and Lungs.** | Stitches from back through to chest with every motion.

|| Arthritic tubercles in lungs.

29 **Heart, Pulse and Circulation.** Palpitation of heart without fear; mostly during day.

Ebullition of blood and protruding veins.

Pulse accelerated in evening, slow in morning.

30 **Outer Chest.** Breast bone feels as if bruised; sensitive to touch.

On outside of chest, tensive pain, as if it were too short, on straightening up and walking erect.

|| Painful pressure on breast bone, < when touched.

The nipples are wilted, unsensitive and not irritable.

Itching about nipples.

Urticaria on chest.

31 **Neck and Back.** | Neck emaciated; marasmus of children.

|| Had to loosen his necktie; feels narrow-chested.

| Cervical glands indurated; abuse of mercury.

| Stitches in back through into chest from least motion.

Pain down a part of spine, across hips and down thighs; difficult urination.

32 **Upper Limbs.** Stitches in joints of arms, hands and fingers, on motion.

Deep rhagades on fingers, with burning pains.

|| Pain in tips of fingers on pressure, as if ulcerated or as if salt were put on a wound.

| Tips of fingers feel bruised and sore.

|| Sides of fingers burning.

| Fingers burning under nails, with itching.

Urticaria on hands.

| Tetter on hands.

33 **Lower Limbs.** Weakness in thighs and knees.

| Wrenching, excruciating pains in knees, which were hot, swollen and tender to touch, sometimes in l., sometimes in r. and sometimes in both at the same time; motion very painful, especially on going up and down stairs; seat of greatest tenderness on either side of patellæ; frequent attacks brought on by accidentally bruising knees against leg of table (which invariably produces severe inflammation).

Stitches in legs especially from motion.

|| Blue spots on legs, with induration of skin under spots extending deep in, the beginning of long-lasting ulcers.

|| Pains in superficial knots on shin bone.

Red spots on calves.

|| A young man, æt. 30, had been salivated, and in addition to many painful symptoms had a large ulcer on r.

leg, surrounding ankle, as large as hand, invading nearly whole circumference of part and extending down through fascia almost to bone; superficial veins much enlarged, some œdema of foot; constant aching gnawing; parts excessively sensitive to pressure; had been in habit of taking morphia nightly to secure sleep; ulcer irregular in form, ragged edges; dark areola; edges high and rounded; floor of ulcer flat, but uneven; pus profuse, horribly offensive and dark-colored; would frequently partially granulate, then break down again, granulations becoming black and coming away in masses; on l. leg a similar sore not quite so large; a similar ulcer on l. arm, midway between wrist and elbow, not quite as deep as the others; health poor; appetite deficient; sleepless and generally worn out (benefited).

❙❙Eczema of l. leg, with piles, after being relieved by *Hepar* 6x was cured by large doses of *Sarsap.*

❙❙Rheumatic pains at night in feet.

❙❙Icy coldness of feet before going to bed.

❙❙Rhagades on feet.

❙❙Before going to bed swelled feet.

❙❙Burning in sides and tips of toes, with great sensitiveness to pressure of shoes or boots; a similar burning also in fingers, under nails, with itching.

❙Rheumatic pains in joints after gonorrhœa.

❙❙Rheumatism of lower limbs; swelling and induration of glands about upper part of neck. θSyphilis and abuse of mercury.

❙Pain in bones from mercury.

In all joints of body, tearing now here now there for several days, but only of short duration.

❙❙Gout in lower limbs.

❙Arthritis vaga.

❙Exostoses, mercurial bone pain.

34 **Limbs in General.** Limbs immovable as if paralyzed.

Trembling of hands and feet.

❙Hands and feet peculiarly weary.

❙❙Rheumatism, bone pains after mercury or checked gonorrhœa; pains < at night in damp weather or after taking cold in water.

35 **Rest. Position. Motion.** Lying down: asthmatic breathing <.

Lying on back: when sleeping.

Sitting: head inclined to drop forward; urine dribbles from him.

Bending head back: causes pain in jaw.

Standing: girl could only pass urine; urine passes freely.

Stooping: pains in occiput to forehead.

Motion: causes sharp pains in neck and shoulders; dyspnœa <; stitches from back to chest; stitches in joints; of knees painful; stitches in legs <.

Turning over in bed: pain in back <.

Walking: head inclined to drop forward; throbbing in top of head <; causes suffocation: leucorrhœa; erect, chest feels too short; pain from occiput to forehead; pain in small of back.

Going up stairs: short breathing.

36 **Nerves.** Ability to go about all day, fasting; no exertion seemed to tire; numbness of fingers, especially third and fourth on both hands.

Sensation of weakness over whole body; faint feeling.

Fainting attacks, with difficult stool.

Paralysis, muscles atrophied.

37 **Sleep.** Sleeplessness at night; awakens frequently.

Dreams: lascivious, without erections but seminal emissions; of fatal accidents.

Sleeps lying on back.

38 **Time.** Morning: nausea; itching deep in head; tired feeling; bitter taste; lids agglutinated; sneezing and running coryza; tongue coated white; slimy mouth; dryness in mouth and throat; tough slime in mouth and throat; oppression of chest; diarrhœa; pulse slow.

Forenoon: frequent shuddering from feet upward.

Daytime: lachrymation; palpitation of heart.

6 P.M.: hiccough.

Evening: pains increase; headache <; great drowsiness; heat of face; eructations; loose stool; pulse accelerated; heat ebullitions and palpitations; heat and sweat on forehead.

Night: severe perspiration; rheumatic pains in feet; sleeplessness.

39 **Temperature and Weather.** Heat: pimples itch.

Warmth: symptoms >.

Warm diet: symptoms <.

Warm room: vertigo <.

From warm room into cold air: rash appears.

Open air: staggers and falls forward; crusts fall off and new skin cracks.

Cold air: tearing in teeth; pain in molars >; a draft of while in a perspiration, next morning could not move.

Cold drink: tearing in teeth.

Cold diet: symptoms >.

Cold, wet weather: checked gonorrhœa; rheumatism <.

Washing: eruptions <.

Chilliness: symptoms <.

40 **Fever.** Chilliness predominating (day and night).

Frequent shuddering, mostly in forenoon, running from feet upward.

|| Rigor over whole body, from below upward.

▮▮ Worse during chilliness; > as soon as he becomes warm.

Heat in evening, with ebullitions and palpitation of heart.

Ebullition of blood, protruding veins.

|| Heat, evenings in bed, an hour before falling asleep; blood boils, heart beats, and sweat stands on forehead.

▮▮ Sweat on forehead during evening heat.

|| For five days, shooting pain from occiput to forehead, on stooping or walking; for two days, chilliness beginning in legs and going all over body, then general heat, then slight sweat; with heat, thirst, drinking much and often; shooting pain in small of back when walking; feels hot to herself but skin is cool to touch; pulse 120; some days ago exposed to an offensive smell from decomposing substances.

41 **Attacks, Periodicity.** Alternating: pressure and burning in eyes.

Two or three times a night: must get up to pass urine.

Every other day: hoarseness in throat.

For two days: chilliness in legs, thence all over body.

For several days: tearing in joints.

For five days: pain from occiput to forehead.

Two or three times a week: seminal emissions.

Spring: eruptions prone to appear; sycotic eruption <.

For twenty years: dysmenorrhœa.

42 **Locality and Direction.** Right: itching in half of head; throbbing in side of head; beating and sounding in side of head; shooting in parietal bone; quivering in upper eyelid; itching in wing of nose; nostril stopped; pain in masticatory muscles; pain in lower jaw; tearing in root of last inferior molar; sore throat; severe tension in groin; soreness in bend of groin; excruciating pain from kidney downward; large ulcer on leg; boils on side of nose; on dorsal side of foot.

Left: pressure and stitches in side of forehead and head; dimness of eye; pressure in eye; itching on side of nose; eruption in nostril; pinching in side of abdomen; pinching in inguinal region; weakness of arm and leg; numbness of hand; rending pain in side of head and face; nipple retracted; severe pain in breast; ulcer on leg and arm; eczema of leg; boils in gluteal regions.

First l. then r.: pressure in eyes.

Upward: chill passes from bladder.

From above downward: pressure in abdomen.

From below upward: rigors over whole body; shuddering from feet.

Upward and downward: sacral pains radiate.

43 **Sensations.** As of a great weight in head; a buzzing as if a large bell had been struck in head; as if something were pressing upon head; as if gauze were spread over l. eye; as of a grain of sand in eye; as of a needle pricking point of nose; face as if bruised; jaw as if being broken; as if he had eaten nothing; as if diarrhœa would come on; as if bowels were pressed out; as if in a dream; as if he had been hit with a hammer on top of head; as if bound down to bed by a sort of suction; as if breath were stopped by a breath; breast bone as if bruised; as if chest were too short; as if tips of fingers were ulcerated or as if salt were put on a wound; limbs as if paralyzed.

Pain: in small of back and down spermatic cords; in last molars; in throat; in bladder; in lower part of spine, across hips and down thighs; at point near neck of bladder; at meatus urinarius; in larynx; in superficial knots on shin bone; in bones.

Excruciating pains: from r. kidney downward; in knees.

Dreadful pain: in back, thighs and hypogastrium.

Violent pain: in eyes; in face.

Severe, sharp pains: in back and shoulders; through bladder, back, hips and thighs; in l. breast; in back; in head.

Tearing: in masticatory muscles; in teeth; in rectum; from glans to root of penis; in all joints.

Rending pain: in l. side of head.

Cutting: in rectum.

Darting: from occiput to eyes; in sacral regions, thence upward and downward to fingers and toes.

Shooting: in r. parietal bone; back of head to front; from occiput to forehead; in small of back.

Throbbing: in top of head; in r. side of head.

Pulsative pains: in head.

Severe, laborlike pains: from sacrum to crest of ilium, or around to uterus.

Stitches: in l. side of forehead and head; in tongue; from back to chest; in joints of arms, hands and fingers; in legs.

Stitching pains: in head.

Pinching: in abdomen; in l. inguinal region.

Griping: in pit of stomach.

Cramps: in bladder.

Burning pain: in rhagades on fingers.

Aching: through temples, forehead and occiput.

Rheumatic pains: in limbs; in feet; in joints.

Sore pain: of gums.

Stinging: in eyes; in masticatory muscles; in gums and root of molar.
Soreness: in throat; in bend of r. groin; inside of thighs; of tips of fingers.
Burning: in eyes; in nose; in stomach; in abdomen; while urine passes; from glans to root of penis; of sides of fingers; under finger nails; in sides and tips of toes.
Acrid sensation: on tongue; in pharynx; in stomach.
Pricking: in point of nose.
Distress: all through pelvis.
Rawness: in larynx.
Heat: in sacrum.
Tickling, ulcerative sensation: in fauces.
Jerking: along male urethra.
Pulsation: in sacrum.
Beating and sounding: in r. side of head.
Pressure: in l. side of forehead and head; in l. eye; in abdomen; on bowels; on bladder.
Pressing: deep in r. side of head; in vertex; in soft palate; on breast bone
Drawing: in masticatory muscles; in soft palate; in sacral region and upward and downward to fingers and toes.
Tension: in muscles and articulation of jaw; in r. groin.
Heaviness: in head.
Constriction: of bladder; in throat and chest.
Dryness: in mouth; in throat.
Stiffness: in muscles and articulation of jaw.
Numbness: of l. hand; of fingers.
Weakness: in thighs and knees; over whole body.
Dull tremor with waving: in head.
Dull, stupid feeling: in head.
Pricking itching: in face and scalp; in neck and shoulders.
Itching: deep in r. half of head; in head; of scab on ear lobe; in r. wing of nose; on l. side of nose; of eruption on forehead; from glans to root of penis; on scrotum and perineum; about nipples; under finger nails; in spots on scars.
Cold feeling: in abdomen.

" **Tissues.** ▮Great emaciation, skin becomes shrivelled or lies in folds.
▮Scrofulous, sycotic or syphilitic affections.
Chronic abscesses attended by profuse discharge.
▮Rheumatic bone pains after mercury or checked gonorrhœa.
▮Children emaciated; face like old people; big belly; dry, flabby skin; mushy passages. θMarasmus.
▮Eruptions prone to appear in Spring, their bases inflamed, crusts detach readily out of doors and adjoining skin becomes chapped.

Touch. Passive Motion. Injuries. Touch: external abdomen very sensitive; l. breast very sensitive; breast bone sensitive; knees tender; boils sting.

Pressure: upon closed eyes causes violent pain; pain in back <; pain in finger tips; toes sensitive.

Loosens clothes from neck to get breath.

Handling jaw causes pain.

Combing: scalp sensitive.

Scratching: causes itching to begin in another place; eruption on forehead becomes humid.

46 **Skin.** Rash as soon as he goes from warm room into cold air.

Dry, red pimples, only itching when exposed to heat.

▮Rhagades deep and burning.

Base of eruption much inflamed: child cries much and is very uneasy; crusts become detached in open air and adjoining skin chapped.

▮Herpetic ulcers, extending in a circular form, forming no crusts, red, granulated bases, white borders; skin appears as after a warm compress; serous, reddish secretions.

▮▮Ulcers after abuse of mercury.

Shrivelled skin.

▮Tetters appear on all parts of body.

▮Tetters, herpetic ulcers, in syphilis.

▮Ulcers in second stage of syphilis.

Many little warts.

| |Horses lose hair with eruptions.

▮Often returning rash makes the babies chafed.

▮Dry, itchlike eruptions, with emaciation.

▮Pemphigus squamosus.

▮Serpiginous eruptions.

Small pus boils on r. side of nose; on r. dorsal side of foot, l. gluteal region, sometimes with stinging pain on touch.

Pustules which have been scratched open, leaving ulcers suppurating for a long time.

▮Skin does not heal.

▮Red spots, psoriasis-like, after abuse of mercury.

| |An endemic affection occurring in Marienwerder, occasionally with trichoma (plica); patients unwell for a long time; pale-red brownish spots appear on the extremities, rarely on trunk, turn into small, deep ulcers, edges callous, inverted, these heal after a time, but appear on other places; their size is about half an inch, seldom smaller, never larger; they spread in a line like a wreath or garland; the scars elevated, red, winding; later sore throat, pain in nose; inflamed, suppurating spots on soft palate and on septum, soon destroying it; sometimes pains in superficial knots on shin bone and other places; also exostoses.

▮Sycotic eruption consisting of little spots scarcely raised above skin, often scaling a little but looking like the roseola of syphilis and itching intolerably, < in Spring.

||Pustular efflorescence on face, of ichorous character; on rest of body a papular efflorescence; this eruption appeared after violent nocturnal itching, causing scratching sometimes on upper, sometimes on lower extremities, sometimes on body in form of small colorless pimples, containing serum; the latter eruption began a year ago, while that on face appeared a year previously and attacked in varying degrees of intensity and extent the forehead, cheeks and particularly nose.

|Eruption resembling psoriasis in subjects who have taken much mercury. θSyphilis.

|Itching relieved or lessened by scratching.

|Itching in spots on scars after smallpox.

|Blue spots with indurated skin on legs.

|Hardness of skin.

New skin cracks and burns.

||Rhagades: skin cracks on hands and feet; pain and burning, particularly on sides of fingers and toes (after *Hepar*).

|Eruptions following vaccination.

|Boils.

|Eczema.

Eruptions < from washing.

47 **Stages of Life, Constitution.** Dark hair; sycosis.

Girl, æt. 3, sickly looking; wind from bladder.

Young man, æt. 19, nervo-bilious temperament, farmer; spermatorrhœa.

Servant, æt. 20; ague.

Student, æt. 20, nervous temperament, suffering since puberty; spermatorrhœa.

Man, æt. 30, had been salivated; ulcer on leg.

Miss P., maiden lady, light hair and complexion; mental depression.

Mr. ——, syphilis nine years ago, for which he received large doses of mercury; rheumatism in joints; headache.

Mrs. ——, æt. 32; dysmenorrhœa and pain in breast.

Lady, æt. 45, in poor health, passing through climaxis; asthma, etc.

Mrs. C., æt. 50, after taking a severe cold; cystitis.

Man, æt. 50, addicted to stimulants; affection of bladder.

Man, æt. 52, whisky drinker; Bright's disease.

Man, æt. 65, robust, suffering two years; eruption.

Mr. ——, ill for twenty years; affection of bladder.

48 **Relations.** Antidoted by: *Bellad.*, *Mercur.*

It antidotes effects of Mercury.

Compatible: *Cepa, Hepar, Phosphor., Rhus tox., Sepia, Sulph.*

Complementary: *Mercur., Sepia.*

Compare: *Natr. mur.*

SECALE CORNUTUM.

Ergot; Spurred Rye. *A Fungus.*

The alcoholic tincture is prepared from the fresh ergot, gathered shortly before harvest.

This remedy awaits proving.

Toxocological reports and effects of the rye disease are extensive. See Allen's Encyclopedia, vol. 8, p. 551.

Clinical Authorities.—*Asthenopia*, Willebrand, B. J. H., vol. 17, p. 692; *Epistaxis*, Hrg., Gross, Rück. Kl. Erf., vol. 1, p. 414; *Difficult dentition*, Syrbius, Rück. Kl. Erf., vol. 1, p. 476; *Cardialgia*, Hamb., Gueyrand, Rück. Kl. Erf., vol. 1, p. 659; *Hæmatemesis*, Gross, Drescher, Rück. Kl. Erf., vol. 1, p. 575; Rummell, Lobeth, Jean, Syrbius, Gross, Behlert, Weigel, Griessel., Rück. Kl. Erf., vol. 1, p. 847; Von Tagen, A. J. H. M. M., vol. 1, p. 183; *Sinking spells from diarrhœa*, Crow, Hah. Mo., vol. 10, p. 167; *Cholera*, Rummell, Lobeth., Henke, Tietzer, Knorre, Adler, Kurtz, Rück. Kl. Erf., vol. 1, p. 960; *Hæmaturia*, Trinks, Rück. Kl. Erf., vol. 4, p. 63; *Hysteralgia*, Burnett, B. J. H., vol. 35, p. 87; *Prolapsus uteri*, Kallenbach, Rück. Kl. Erf., vol. 2, p. 345; *Uterine prolapsus*, Kallenbach, B. J. H., vol. 1, p. 407; *Uterine hemorrhage*, Hartm., Hirzel, Griessel., Jean, Gross, Ehrhardt, Diez, Nenning, Rupprich, Drescher, Frank, Bernstein, Thorer, Rück. Kl. Erf., vol. 2, p. 332; Stens, A. H. Z., vol. 19, p. 153, Trans. by S. L., A. J. H. M. M., vol. 3, p. 98; Fisher, Bib. Hom., vol. 8, p. 140; Löw, B. J. H., vol. 16, p. 306; *Metrorrhagia*, Hirsch, B. J. H., vol. 26, p. 215; Ruppich, A. J. H. M. M., vol. 4, p. 150; *Menorrhagia*, Linsley, A. J. H. M. M., vol. 1, p. 73; Frank, B. J. H., vol. 1, p. 259; Drysdale, A. J. H. M. M., vol. 1, p. 254; *Menstrual colic*, Syrbius, Hamb, Rück. Kl. Erf., vol. 2, p. 253; *Threatened abortion*, Lembke, Rück. Kl. Erf., vol. 2, p. 386; Hendricks, A. J. H. M. M., vol. 3, p. 98; *Abortion*, Frank, B. J. H., vol. 1, p. 258; *Miscarriage*, Ruhfus, Stens, A. H. Z., vol. 79, p. 152; *Dystocia, premature labor*, Belcher, N. A. J. H., vol. 3, p. 70; *Inertia of uterus*, Searle, A. H. O., vol. 7, p. 513; *Retained placenta*, Fielitz, Bethmann, Rück. Kl. Erf., vol. 2, p. 404; *Violent after-pains and hæmorrhage from irregular contractions*, Beckwith, T. A. I. H., 1871, p. 262; *Post-partum hemorrhage*, J. F. E., Org., vol. 2, p. 239; *Use in labor*, Lobeth., Kurtz, Kallenbach, Diez, Rummell, Ehrhardt, Gross, Nenning, Rück. Kl. Erf., vol. 2, p. 396; *Fetid lochia*, Smith, Med. Inv., vol. 8, p. 116; *Puerperal fever*, M., A. H. Z., vol. 109, p. 76; Gross, Rück. Kl. Erf., vol. 2, p. 454; *Cough*, Goullon, H. Kl. 1872, p. 4; *Hæmoptysis*, Hirsch, B. J. H., vol. 26, p. 216; *Palpitation of heart*, Mossa, Hom. Kl. 1869, p. 118; *Aneurism*, Peare, M. I., 1875, p. 48; *Affection of spine*, Hirsch, B. J. H., vol. 26, p. 218; M. I., vol. 10, p. 633; Raue's Rec., 1874, p. 250; Hah. Mo., vol. 24, p. 390; *Kink in back*, Schüssler; A. H. Z., vol. 78, p. 38; *Cramps in fingers*, Kasemann, Rück. Kl. Erf., vol. 4, p. 613, *Paralysis of legs*, Hale, N. E. M. G., vol. 4, p. 37; *Cramps in legs*, Syrbius, Rück. Kl. Erf., vol. 2, p. 386; *Cramps in calves*, Hirsch, B. J. H., vol. 26, p. 219; *Offensive foot-sweat*, Gallavardin, N. A. J. H., vol. 15, p. 61; *Neuralgia*, Willebrand, Hom. Kl. 1869, p. 117; *Hysteria*, G. B., Rück Kl. Erf., vol. 5, p. 613; *Convulsions*, Helbig,

Anal. Ther., vol. 1. p. 185; *Tetanus*, Navarro, Times Ret., 1876, p. 154; *Chorea*, Hartmann, Rück. Kl. Erf., vol. 4, p. 513; Bodenstab, B. J. H., vol. 6, p. 28; *Epilepsy*, Lobethal, Rück. Kl. Erf., vol. 4, p. 590; *Paralysis*, Laucerosse, Rück. Kl. Erf., vol. 4, p. 484; A. H. Z., vol. 52, p. 112; *Post-diphtheritic paralysis*, Hall, Hom. Phys., vol. 6, p. 407; *Night-sweats*, Goullon, M. I. 1875, p. 125; *Gangrene*, Arnold, Rück. Kl. Erf., vol. 5, p. 861; *Senile gangrene*, Hendricks, A. H. Z., vol. 105, p. 128.

[1] **Mind.** Stupid, half-sleepy state.

Impaired power of thinking.

Delirium: quiet; wandering.

Mania: with inclination to bite; with inclination to drown.

Uncomfortableness and depression.

Fear of death.

Anxiety, sadness, melancholy.

Great anguish; wild with anxiety.

Apathy, indifference.

Constant moaning and fear of death.

Great anxiety and difficult respiration.

Excessive sadness, gradually changes to cheerfulness; talks and acts foolishly; rage, followed by continuous deep sleep.

Paralytic mental diseases; treats his relations contemptuously and sarcastically; wandering talk and hallucinations; apathy and complete disappearance of the senses.

‖ Laughs, claps her hands over her head, seems beside herself. θ After miscarriage.

[2] **Sensorium.** Unconsciousness, with heavy sleep, preceded by tingling in head and limbs.

Diminution and loss of senses, sight, hearing, etc.

All the senses benumbed.

Consciousness seems to continue until the last breath, and just before death it seems as if patient would improve.

Stupefaction; stupor.

Vertigo: constantly increasing; with stupefaction and heaviness of head; reeling, inability to stand erect; peculiar feeling of lightness of head, particularly in occiput; as from intoxication; unsteady gait.

Heaviness of head and tingling in legs.

‖ Sensation of intoxication while undressing.

[3] **Inner Head.** Pulsations in head with giddiness, she cannot walk.

Pain and confusion most in occiput.

Congestion to head and chest.

Headache; hemicrania on l. side.

[4] **Outer Head.** Hair falls out.

Twisting of head to and fro.

‖ Scalp sore.

[5] **Sight and Eyes.** Photophobia.
Dimness of vision; mistiness before eyes. θCataract.
Double or triple vision.
Blue and fiery dots flying before eyes.
Pain in eyes with feeling as if they were spasmodically rotated.
Stitching pain in eyes; pressure on balls.
After an epidemic of the rye disease an unusually large number of cataracts occurred in young people, twenty-three of whom gradually became blind (fifteen men and eight women), associated with headache, vertigo and roaring in ears; of the cataracts two were hard, twelve soft, and nine mixed.
▮Cataracta senilis.
| |Suppuration of cornea; < from warm applications.
| |Retinitis diabetica.
Dilatation of pupils.
Suppressed secretion of tears.
Injection of conjunctiva.
Eyes sunken, surrounded by a blue margin.
Paralysis of upper lids, from coal gas.
Immovable state of eyelids after facial erysipelas.
Eyes look fixed, wild, glazed; staring look.
| |Pustulous conjunctivitis and blepharitis.
| |Exophthalmos with struma.
: Exophthalmic goitre.

[6] **Hearing and Ears.** Undue sensitiveness of hearing, even slightest sound re-echoed in her head and made her shudder.
Confused hearing; deafness. θAfter chorea.
Singing in ears and difficult hearing.
Humming and roaring in ears, with occasional deafness.

[7] **Smell and Nose.** Sneezing.
Nose feels stopped up, yet watery discharge runs from it.
| |Nose stopped up on l. side as with a solid plug.
▮▮Nosebleed: blood dark, runs continuously, with great prostration, small, threadlike pulse; in old people or drunkards; of young women; from debility.

[8] **Upper Face.** Face: pinched, pale, earthy-looking; sunken, hippocratic, ashy; swollen; contracted, discolored, with sunken eyes, blue rings around eyes; risus sardonicus; distorted; wan, anxious.
Tingling in face.
Muscular twitchings usually commence in face and then spread all over body, sometimes increasing to dancing and jumping.
Spasmodic distortion of mouth and lips.
Forehead hot.

9 **Lower Face.** Lockjaw.
Lips deathly pale or bluish.

10 **Teeth and Gums.** Looseness of teeth.
Grinding of teeth.
Bleeding from gums.
‖ Difficult dentition; great weakness; vomiting of everything taken; great thirst; pale face; eyes dim, sunken; dry heat, with rapid pulse; restlessness and sleeplessness.

11 **Taste and Tongue.** Tongue: thickly coated with yellowish-white, dry, tenacious substance; discolored, brown or blackish; deathly pale; cold and livid; clean, with dry, red tip; red tip and edges, centre coated.
Slight but unpleasant warmth on tongue, during day.
Spasm of tongue, projecting it from mouth, forcing it between teeth and rendering speech indistinct.
Feeble, stuttering, indistinct speech, as if tongue were paralyzed.

12 **Inner Mouth.** Bloody or yellowish green foam at mouth.
Increased secretion of saliva; ptyalism.
Much acid fluid in mouth.
Spitting of blood.
Fetid breath.
Speech difficult, slow and weak, with a feeling at every motion as if there were some resistance to be overcome.
Dryness of mouth.

13 **Throat.** Dryness of soft palate, throat and œsophagus, with thirst.
Burning in throat with violent thirst.
Painful tingling in throat and on tongue.
‖ Throat sore on l. side running up into ear.
▮ Follicular pharyngitis; hawking up of little follicular exudates.
▮ Diphtheria: loss of strength; rapid loss of sensibility; numbness of extremities; painful tingling and crawling on tongue; dry gangrene; apathy; dilated pupils; burning pains of affected parts; stammering speech; absence of all reaction.
‖ Severely paralyzed both in swallowing and speaking; could scarcely take food without great danger of choking; speech reduced to a whisper; could not bear heat or covering and would throw all covering off. θPost-diphtheritic paralysis.

14 **Appetite, Thirst. Desires, Aversions.** Ravenous, insatiable appetite, even when dying from exhausting discharges from bowels.
Hunger as from long fasting.
Disgust for food, especially for meat and fatty things.
Thirst: during all stages of fever; unquenchable; for acids.

Great thirst and dryness of mouth and throat, with burning and tingling of tongue.

Desire for: sour things; lemonade.

16 **Hiccough, Belching, Nausea and Vomiting.** Eructations with disagreeable taste; sour, tasteless, but with subjective, disagreeable, empyreumatic odor; empty.

Nausea: inclination to vomit; painful retchings; constant, < after eating.

Excessive nausea and debility, with very little vomiting of a dark brown coffee-grounds fluid.

Vomiting: of food; of bile; of mucus; of green, offensive, watery fluid, painless and without effort, with great weakness; immediately after eating; of lumbrici; of blood; black vomit.

| Hæmatemesis, patient lies still; great weakness but no pain; abdomen soft.

17 **Scrobiculum and Stomach.** | Tenderness of epigastrium.

Anxiety and pressure in pit of stomach, with great sensitiveness to touch.

| Severe anxiety and burning at pit of stomach.

Pain in pit of stomach.

Violent pressure in stomach, as from a heavy weight.

Warmth and feeling of repletion.

Burning in stomach.

Painful constriction of epigastrium.

Great distress and oppression of stomach.

|| Bilious vomiting, with cramping pains in stomach; burning in stomach extending up œsophagus; head sunk upon breast, face pale, yellowish, voice weak, pulse small. θCardialgia.

|| Attacks of severe pressure and constriction in region of stomach extending through to spine, extremely painful and followed in half an hour by vomiting of tasteless fluid or of contents of stomach, thereupon an intermission of several hours occurred; during attack region of stomach felt as if contracted, and on percussion gave a tympanitic note; has three to four attacks daily.

| Hemorrhage from stomach; lies still with great weakness but no pain; face, lips, tongue and hands deadly pale; skin covered with cold sweat, pulse frequent, threadlike; oppression; abdomen soft, without pain. θHæmatemesis.

|| Hæmatemesis; attacks preceded by pains in epigastrium and nausea, pain going to l. side when pressure is made in epigastrium; marked protrusion in l. hypochondrium, with pain; blood red, never containing particles of food, and when collected in a basin appears more like bloody serum than pure blood and is of offensive odor, quantity vomited not very large; frequent chilliness at night,

followed by profuse sweat; strength not much impaired; appetite and sleep good.

[18] **Hypochondria.** Enlargement of liver.

Acute pain in hepatic region,

Inflammation and gangrene of liver; acute pains in hepatic region; tongue thickly coated with a brown tenacious substance, burning in throat, unquenchable thirst; great weakness, but no pain; limbs cold and covered with cold sweat.

Burning in spleen; thrombosis of abdominal vessels.

[19] **Abdomen.** Distension of abdomen; tympanitis; meteorism.

Flatulence with rumbling.

Painful sensitiveness and rumbling, with continued nausea and confusion of head.

Inclination to colic, diarrhœa, and bloatedness of abdomen.

Pain in lower belly, preventing an upright position, even forcing him to lie doubled up in bed.

Colic with convulsions.

▮Pain in abdomen with burning in stomach.

▮Pains in hypogastric region.

Pain in loins as from false labor pains.

Continual bearing down in lower abdomen.

Burning in abdomen.

Cold feeling in abdomen and back.

Srong pulsation in umbilical region.

Lumps and welts in abdomen; in affections of uterus.

▮▮Aneurism of mesenteric artery, in women.

[20] **Stool and Rectum.** ▮▮Diarrhœa: very exhausting; pernicious; very offensive; involuntary, profuse, watery, putrid, brown; discharged with great force; very exhausting; urine suppressed; painful with great prostration; painless with tingling and numbness in limbs; putrid, fetid, colliquative, patient does not want to be covered or to be near the heat, but prefers to be in the air or wishes to be fanned; sudden attacks; of children, discharges whitish, watery; chronic in overfed children, great prostration; during August; great stools undigested, or watery, at times yellowish, also greenish, with forcible expulsion, accompanied by dischare of flatus; paralytic weakness of sphincter ani with involuntary discharges.

Stools: yellowish; greenish; brownish; watery and flocculent; colorless, watery; profuse; frequent; putrid; gushing; involuntary; watery, slimy; thin, olive green; offensive, watery; fetid, dark colored; thin, involuntary; watery, yellowish or greenish, discharged rapidly with great force and even involuntarily; painless, without effort and with great weakness.

Before stool: cutting and rumbling in abdomen.
During stool: cutting; great exhaustion; coldness.
After stool: exhaustion.

‖Five to ten minutes after taking least quantity of food, severe colic which made her bend double and cry out; pain begins between region of stomach and navel, extends thence to sides and rest of abdomen and down to sacral region, accompanied by severe urging and tenesmus, followed by a thin, slimy, yellowish stool with some relief of pain; four to five such attacks follow each other, then relief until she eats again; four to five evacuations during night; she compares pains to labor pains; great thirst; thick mucous coating on tongue; sleep disturbed; prostration. θDiarrhœa.

‖Uncomfortable fulness of abdomen, with transient pinching pains in upper abdomen as from flatus; at night severe cutting pains throughout whole abdomen; restless anxious tossing about, with short unrefreshing naps; during night anus firmly closed, "as if locked up;" in morning frequent short watery evacuations, in gushes, preceded by cutting pains in abdomen.

‖Stools yellowish-white, slimy, undigested, escaping involuntarily, < at break of day. θDiarrhœa.

▮Interminable diarrhœa in Summer, which resists everything, especially in scrofulous children; putrid, fetid and colliquative; choleraic symptoms, with cold, clammy perspiration; sinking spells at 3 A.M. (not the restless anguish of *Arsenicum*).

▮▮Colliquative diarrhœa.

▮Cholerine with more retching than vomiting.

▮Cholera infantum; profuse undigested stools, watery and very offensive, discharged by fits and starts and followed by intense prostration; pale face, sunken eyes, dry heat, quick pulse, restlessness and sleeplessness; great aversion to heat and to being covered. θCholera infantum.

‖Vertigo, cramps or drawing in calves of legs, rumbling in abdomen, nausea, stools in rapid succession, brownish or colorless, rapid prostration, coldness of limbs, tongue but slightly coated.

‖Profuse prostrating evacuations, severe painful cramps in feet, toes, hands and fingers which are spread apart or extended toward back of hands; cramping pressure in stomach; dry, wrinkled, cold skin; cyanotic color θCholera.

▮Cholera infantum; cholera morbus; cholera Asiatica.

‖Patient cold, almost pulseless, with spasmodic twitching of muscles in various parts of body; spreads fingers asunder; eyes sunken, features pinched; much spasmodic retching although not much vomiting; skin harsh, shrivelled, dry, as if there were no moisture left in system; urine suppressed; tingling or formication all over body; stools profuse, watery, ejected with great violence; is cold but cannot bear to be covered. θCholera.

▮▮Aversion to heat or being covered, with icy coldness of extremities. θCholera.

▮Diarrhœa after cholera.

▮Cholera Asiatica, with collapse, sunken, distorted face, particularly mouth; crawling sensation as from ants.

Paralysis of rectum; anus wide open.

▮Hemorrhage from bowels.

▮Constipation.

21 **Urinary Organs.** Retention of urine; urine pale or bloody; discharge of thick black blood from kidneys; obscuration of sight. θScarlatina.

Diabetes; great general lassitude; heaviness of limbs; loss of strength; emaciation; gangrene; skin dry and withered; furuncles; petechiæ; fever, with unquenchable thirst; diminished power of senses; dryness of mouth; morbidly great appetite; cardialgia; costiveness; diarrhœa; watery urine; increased quantity of urine.

▮▮Hæmaturia in a boy suffering from suppuration of glands of neck after scarlet fever; urine also very albuminous; anasarca; great thirst.

▮Passive hemorrhage; blood thin; blood corpuscles wanting in consequence of dissolution; or painless discharge of thick black blood in consequence of kidney disease; coldness of body; cold perspiration on forehead; great weakness. θHæmaturia.

Urine suppressed; on introducing catheter a gill of dark, prune-colored urine passed, which appeared to be full of gritty sediment emitting a very disagreeable odor.

Unsuccessful urging to urinate.

Ischuria paralytica.

▮Paralysis of bladder.

▮Enuresis: of old people; pale, watery or bloody urine.

Urinary deposit looking like white cheese.

▮Bloody, albuminous urine.

▮Discharge of thick black blood from bladder; kidney affections.

22 **Male Sexual Organs.** After lightness in occiput, violent dragging in spermatic cord causing sensation as if testicle were being drawn up to inguinal ring.

After sexual excess palpitation of heart.

▮Weak memory after exhausting coition; impotence.

Clonic spasmodic stricture of urethra.

23 **Female Sexual Organs.** Uterus and r. ovary much congested, very sensitive to touch.

‖ Pain in ovaries and uterus.

‖ Pains of an expulsive character in uterus.

‖ Prolonged bearing down and forcing pain in uterus; thin and scrawny subjects.

Burning pains in greatly distended uterus, which felt hard and was painful to touch.

‖ Putrescence of uterus; abdomen distended, not very painful; discharge from vagina, brownish, offensive; ulcers on external genitals discolored and rapidly spreading; burning hot fever, interrupted by shaking chills; small, sometimes intermittent pulse; great anguish, pain in pit of stomach, vomiting decomposed matter; offensive diarrhœa; suppressed secretion of urine; skin covered with petechial and miliary eruptions or shows discolored, inflamed places, with a tendency to mortification; the patient lies either in quiet delirium or grows wild with great anxiety and a constant desire to get out of bed. θMetritis.

‖ Metritis; tendency to putrescence; inflammation caused by suppression of lochia or menses; discharge of thin black blood, a kind of sanies, with tingling in legs and great debility. θMetritis.

| Cancer and gangrene of uterus.

| Uterine ulcers feel as if burnt, discharge putrid, bloody fluid.

The uterus that had previously been in a normal condition descended so that it almost protruded, was hot and painful; os open as large as middle finger; excessive desire to urinate; labor pains only relieved by wet bandages or pressure upon abdomen; lasted three days, did not miscarry though os remained open during this period; afterward uterus gradually ascended, pains diminished, and after five or six days os contracted; went on to eighth month, when she miscarried.

‖ Uterus about an inch from labia inferiora, membrane around it felt hard, while rest of mucous membrane of vagina was very much relaxed and gathered into a fold at lower part.

| Partial prolapsus of uterus for eight months after a forceps delivery; dysuria; sense of weight over pubes as if contents of abdomen would fall forward.

| Prolapsus of three months' standing; frequent severe cutting pains in abdomen; occasional nausea.

| Dreadful bearing down, dragging out feeling in lower abdomen, so that her life is almost unbearable; every four or five days profuse, thick, yellow discharge from

vagina; hesitation in urinating: rheumatism. θHysteralgia.

Hemorrhage from uterus; apparent death of newborn child.

❙Incessant metrorrhagia.

❙Uterine hemorrhage: when uterus is engorged; with pains in sacrum, extending down thighs and pressing into lower abdomen; after a severe blow upon abdomen of a pregnant woman; profuse protracted flow; tearing, cutting colic, cold extremities and cold sweat, weak, hemorrhage < from slightest motion, blood thin and black, black lumpy or brown fluid, of disgusting smell; black liquid blood.

‖A woman, æt. 45, passed through a normal confinement seven years ago; miscarried about two years ago, hemorrhage kept on for five months under allopathic treatment, with exacerbation during time of menstruation; after ceasing for seven months, hemorrhage set in again with slight intermissions of one or two weeks; excessive anæmia; sunken features; skin cold and dry; pulse small and quick; heavily coated tongue; loss of appetite; headache; since five days, daily ten or twelve painless stools, of mucous, watery, sometimes foul-smelling masses; thin, black, foul-smelling bloody discharges.

‖Feeble and extremely emaciated, skin flaccid, face very pale and sunken, with an expression of suffering, mucous membranes pale and cool, hands and feet deficient of natural warmth, action of heart quickened, breathing short and oppressed, pulse very small, 120; abdomen distended; os uteri very open, with indented and puffy edges, flaccid and soft, vagina tender and cool; manual examination caused much uneasiness and flooding; violent headache limited to one spot, throbbing in temples, roaring in ears, giddiness on slightest movement; enfeebled nervous system showed extraordinary excitability; many times in day, and especially at night, cramps in calves and spasmodic twitchings of limbs, causing exhaustion, remains several hours in bed as if paralyzed; digestion and sleep disturbed to some extent; hemorrhage still continued, even in horizontal position, and elevation of pelvis caused no diminution in large quantity of blackened coagula which were constantly passing, whilst least movement increased discharge in a very great degree. θChronic passive hemorrhage.

❙Uterine hemorrhage, flow passive, dark and may be offensive; tingling or formication all over body, holds her fingers spread asunder, asks to have her limbs rubbed; finally lies unconscious and cold.

‖Metrorrhagia; relaxed condition of body; depressed, anxious state of mind; unusual drowsiness by day; gush of thin black blood on least movement of body; general feeling of prostration; diminished temperature of body; wooden, numb feeling in lower extremities.

Uterine hemorrhage; did not wish to be covered, desired windows to be open, though room was very cold and surface of body like a corpse.

▮Painless flooding in feeble, cachectic, dyscratic women, or such as have long resided in tropical climates.

‖Since last delivery menses too seldom and very irregular, last time rather copious in consequence of unusual exertion; at night dreamed she was ascending the stairs with a heavy load, and suddenly a clot of blood came away and the blood seemed to gush forth; the alarm awakened her and she found that she was bleeding fast; on following morning strength greatly reduced; lips and whole body, even tongue, deathly pale; pulse could not be distinguished; frequent fainting fits; periodic pains with expulsion of clots of blood and between these attacks constant oozing of thin bright blood. θMenorrhagia.

‖An excessive menstrual flow every two weeks, lasting seven to nine days; for last four weeks flow is continuous; very weak and thin; has severe pains in loins and uterine region; bearing down pains as if in labor.

▮Menses: too profuse and lasting too long; with tearing and cutting colic, cold extremities, cold sweat, great weakness and small pulse; or with violent spasms.

▮Menstrual blood: thin and black; black, lumpy or brown fluid and of disgusting smell.

‖Menstrual colic; pains so severe as to frequently cause spasms; uterine region very sensitive to touch; high fever; pains > when flow appears.

‖Menstrual colic; pale face; coldness of limbs; cold sweat; small, suppressed pulse; tearing, cutting pains in abdomen.

▮▮Menses irregular; every four weeks for three to four days, copious dark-red fluid discharge of blood, with pressing, laborlike pains in abdomen; constipation; pressure in occiput; afterward continuous discharge of watery blood, until next period.

Suppression of menses with pain.

‖Gangrene of whole vaginal mucous membrane; on holding apart the labiæ this membrane was found of a dark slate color, emitting the characteristic odor.

Vagina hot or cool.

▮Discharge from vagina almost black, fluid and very fetid

| Leucorrhœa: in thin, scrawny women, with prolapsus uteri; green, brown, offensive; like cream, from weakness and venous congestion.

Ulcers on outer genitals, discolored and rapidly spreading.

24 **Pregnancy. Parturition. Lactation.** Arrested development of fœtus.

Discharge of blood during pregnancy.

| Threatened abortion: more especially at third month; with copious flow of black, liquid blood; false labor pains, with bloody discharge; in feeble, cachectic women, having a wan, anxious countenance, pulse almost extinct, fear of death; convulsive movements.

|| Extremely violent pains, almost without intermission, she seemed to be in the last stage of labor, but on examination os was found about the size of half a dollar, thick and somewhat rigid.

|| Extremely violent pressing labor pains, os, however, being only about as large as a ten cent piece; hysterical convulsions.

|| When advanced about seven and a half months in pregnancy was taken with labor pains, wriggling and not distinctly intermitting; os tincæ open, and about size of a shilling; dulness and slight aching of head; despondent.

|| Prone to abortion in third month; had passed through five although she kept her bed as soon as pregnant; some labor pains with bloody discharge; was able to attend to her household duties and went to full term.

|| After lifting a heavy weight during sixth month of pregnancy severe pains in stomach, abdomen and small of back and a pushing-down sensation; violent movements of fœtus; cold feet; numbness and tingling in feet; small, weak pulse.

| After abortus: difficult contraction of uterus; thin, black, foul-smelling discharge.

| Retained placenta, after miscarriage, especially when occurring during early months of pregnancy; offensive discharges; patient cold and often almost pulseless from loss of blood; uterine contractions very imperfect, or else prolonged tonic contraction.

|| During eighth month of pregnancy violent convulsions with frothing at mouth, etc., followed by variable spasms; insensibility and clonic spasms, < at every pain; on return of consciousness complained of dull frontal and occipital headache and incessant uterine pains. θPremature labor.

|| During pregnancy: frequent and prolonged forcing pains, particularly in thin, ill-conditioned women; cramps in calves.

▮Uterine pains prolonged but ineffectual.

▮A sensation of constant tonic pressure in uterine region; causes great distress; desires fresh air; does not like to be covered.

▮Hour-glass contraction.

▮▮During labor: prolonged bearing-down and forcing pains in uterus; pains irregular; pains too weak; pains feeble, or ceasing; everything seems loose and open, no action; fainting fits.

▮Strength of uterus weakened by too early or perverted efforts.

▮Thin, scrawny women, skin shrivelled, dry and harsh, sallow face, weak in labor; pains seem to be entirely wanting; uterus flabby; bearing down in sacral region, a sort of prolonged urging feeling in abdomen.

‖While the head was passing into lower strait, she was suddenly seized with violent convulsions lasting about three to four minutes, followed by a stupid state with stertorous breathing and uneasy moaning as if from pain.

▮Labor ceases, and twitchings or convulsions begin.

▮Puerperal convulsions with opisthotonos.

▮Retained placenta, with constant, strong bearing down in abdomen, or with relaxed feeling of parts.

‖After labor, pale, weak; uterus distended, burning pains therein, hard, painful to least touch; discharge of black, coagulated or brown, watery, offensive-smelling blood; throbbing, tearing pains in thighs extending down to toes; pain < from motion; strong pulsations in umbilical region, which could be felt by the hand; pulse at wrist weak and rapid; frequent yawning.

‖Post-partum hemorrhage, with relaxation of uterus, only temporarily relieved by compression; after-pains excessive, < when child nursed.

▮▮After-pains: too long and too painful.

‖Violent after-pains with hemorrhage arising from irregular contractions; the longitudinal fibres alone contracting in such a manner as to leave a sulcus in middle, making it appear as if uterus were split open from top to bottom.

‖Cessation of lochia, with fever; inflammation of uterus, subsequently an abscess opened through vagina.

▮▮Lochia: dark, very offensive; scanty or profuse; painless or accompanied by prolonged bearing-down pain; suppressed, followed by metritis; suddenly change character and become of a dirty brown or chocolate color, with fetid odor, grows sad and melancholy and fears death; of too long duration.

▮Fever with frequent watery stools. θPuerperal fever.

▮Strong tendency to putrescence; discharge of sanious blood, with tingling in legs and great prostration; urine suppressed; offensive diarrhœa; voice hollow with difficult breathing, feeble and inaudible; burning fever interrupted by shaking chills, does not care to be covered; cold limbs; cold sweat over whole body; gangrene. θPuerperal fever.

▮Suppression of milk; the milk will not flow from the breast.

▮Lack of milk with much stinging in mammæ.

▮In women who are much exhausted from venous hemorrhage; thin, scrawny women; the breasts do not properly fill with milk.

Thin, scrawny children with shrivelled skin; spasmodic twitchings, sudden cries, feverishness. θCyanosis.

Pendulous abdomen.

25 **Voice and Larynx. Trachea and Bronchia.** ▮Voice: hollow, hoarse, with difficult breathing; feeble and inaudible; weak, unintelligible, stammering.

Thickening of mucous membrane of air passages.

26 **Respiration.** Respiration: slow; labored and anxious; oppressed; moaning; constant sighing; hiccough.

Blood is sometimes expectorated during violent efforts to breathe.

27 **Cough.** Hard, hoarse cough, with but little expectoration.

‖Concussive cough; profuse perspiration; sleepless nights; inclination to colic; diarrhœa; bloatedness of abdomen; emphysema. θBronchitis.

▮Spitting of blood, with or without cough.

28 **Inner Chest and Lungs.** Cramp in chest.

Pains over nearly whole front part of chest, < from coughing and motion.

‖Expectoration of dark, frothy, rather viscid blood, brought up by a slight cough and amounting to a teacupful in four hours; a spot as large as a crown piece on r. side of chest to r. of nipple, dull on percussion, with bronchial respiration and mucous râle over that part.

29 **Heart, Pulse and Circulation.** ‖Palpitation; hot forehead; inclination to sleep; spasmodic shocks from r. half of chest into r. arm and leg; in paroxysms every two or three hours; oftener in night, after each meal; less in open air; coldness and numbness of r. hand, with tingling in fourth and fifth fingers; loss of muscular power and feeling in hand; after sexual excess.

▮Palpitation of heart: with contracted and frequently intermitting pulse.

▌Pulse: often unchanged even during violent attacks; generally slow and contracted, at times intermittent or suppressed; somewhat accelerated during heat, small; empty, weak; threadlike, in hemorrhages.

31 **Neck and Back.** Tumors on neck discharging yellow pus.

Gentle, creeping sensation in back, as if a soft air were blowing through it.

Tingling in back, extending to fingers and toes.

Pain in small of back.

Stitch in back.

▌Sudden "catch" or "kink" in back. θLumbago.

Pains in sacrum with bearing down as if parts would be forced out, < when moving.

‖Hard, hoarse cough, with but little expectoration; pains nearly all over front part of chest, < from coughing and motion; for several years tenderness of lower cervical and upper dorsal spinous processes, with stiffness of neck; < from every exertion or strain upon spine; pressure upon diseased portion of spine produces pain there, as well as all through chest, with irritation to cough. θSpinal irritation.

‖Stitches in upper dorsal vertebræ (between shoulders), constant when sitting, intermittent when standing, at times extending into hands, < by pressure upon vertebræ; frequent formication through all limbs; at times rigidity and spasmodic stretching of fingers so that for several minutes he cannot sew; frequent pressure and swelling beneath epigastrium; pain in back < when sewing.

Violent pain in back, especially in sacral region; anæsthesia and paralysis of limbs, convulsive jerks and shocks in paralyzed limbs; painful contraction of flexor muscles; paralysis of bladder and rectum. θMyelitis.

▌Myelitis diffusa.

Paraplegia preceded by cramps and muscular pains.

Difficult, staggering gait; complete inability to walk, not for want of power but on account of a peculiar unfitness to perform light movements with limbs and hands; contractions of lower limbs on account of which patient staggers; trembling of limbs, sometimes attended with pains; formication of hands and feet; excessive sensation of heat, with aversion to heat or being covered. θTabes dorsalis.

Spine disease with gressus vaccinus.

32 **Upper Limbs.** Arms fall asleep.

Rough rash all over arm.

Spasmodic jerks of hand, with flexion of hand at wrist or of forearm.

▮Numbness and insensibility of hands and arms. θSpinal affection.

Burning in hands.

Hands deathly pale.

Coldness and numbness of r. hand, with tingling of ring and little fingers.

Loss of feeling in backs of fingers.

Loss of muscular power and of feeling in hand.

Fingers convulsively drawn in toward palm, clasping thumb.

▮Contraction of fingers.

Fingers bent backward or spasmodically abducted.

‖Left thumb spasmodically drawn toward dorsum of hand, followed in a few minutes by cramping and flexure of rest of fingers toward palmar surface; hands feel numb, like velvet; next day both hands became affected and after several days felt a tingling and stitches in legs, followed by heaviness of same, > after walking, generally appearing while sitting, while cramps in hands always appear after using them.

Loss of sensation in tips of fingers.

Numbness of tips of fingers.

Crawling in tips of fingers as if something alive were creeping under skin or as if fingers were asleep, as from pressure upon arm.

Peculiar prickling feeling in tips of fingers; they are sensitive to cold.

Painful swelling of fingers.

Violent pains in finger tips.

▮Gangrene of fingers; senile gangrene.

33 **Lower Limbs.** Hammering, tearing pain in both thighs increased by motion.

Legs heavy and tired.

Tingling in legs.

Creeping feeling in anterior femoral and posterior tibial regions.

Shuffling gait as if feet were dragged along.

Rheumatic pains of joints.

▮Cramps in calves of legs and soles of feet, disturbing sleep at night and hindering walking in pregnant women.

‖After an attack of cholera cramps in calves and sensation of numbness and formication in toes.

▮▮Cramp in calves.

▮Burning in feet.

▮The feet seem asleep and stiff.

‖Toes of r. foot spasmodically drawn upward, continuously during day and occasionally at night, causing a peculiar limping gait; this cramp was accompanied by no pain, but by a very tiresome sensation rendering walking, particularly going up and down stairs, very difficult; tendons running along dorsum of foot to toes were tense as wires and the corresponding muscles of leg larger and harder than normal; now and then slight sensation of coldness in back and also a peculiar buzzing (formication) in spine.

Swelling of feet with black spots.

‖ Beginning senile gangrene; swelling and livid coloring of r. foot extending to malleoli; foot cold; severe indescribable pains.

‖ Senile gangrene commenced in great toe of r. foot and slowly extended; foot was livid and swollen; all the symptoms pointed to its complete loss.

‖ Dry gangrene of foot with constant severe, burning tearing pains.

Severe pains in sole of foot and toes; black spot on plantar surface of heel; toes livid, blue, cold; burning pains; foot swollen; walking impossible. θSenile gangrene.

‖ Profuse, stinking and corrosive perspiration of feet, softening and bleaching soles and destroying quickly stockings and shoes; existing two months in a girl eighteen years old.

Tingling in toes.

‖ Gangrene of toes.

34 **Limbs in General.** Lassitude, weakness, heaviness, trembling of limbs.

Limbs cold, covered with cold sweat.

Formication; prickling; tingling; numbness; insensibility of limbs.

Spasmodic pains; drawing and crawling in limbs.

Burning in hands and feet.

| Fuzzy feeling in limbs.

| Cramps in hands and toes.

Painful jerkings in limbs at night.

Most violent convulsive movements of limbs occur several times a day; during intervals fingers are numb and often contracted.

Sudden periodic contractions of limbs, with tensive pain.

Contractions of hands, feet, fingers and toes.

Gangrene of limbs, limbs suddenly became cold, leaden-colored and lost all sensation.

| Paraplegia.

Internal pain greatly < by heat, whether of bed or atmosphere; somewhat > when exposed to a cooler atmosphere, though even then it was scarcely tolerable; the pain extended by degrees from toes to legs and thighs, and from fingers to arms and shoulders, gangrene supervened.

Not the slightest pain in gangrenous limb when pricked or cut, though frequently motion is not entirely lost.
Absolute insensibility of tips of fingers and toes.
▮▮Cold gangrene of limbs.
▮True anthrax, rapidly changing into gangrene.
Hands and feet swollen with a gangrenous black and suppurating eruption.
Pain with some swelling without inflammation, followed by coldness, blue color, cold gangrene and death of limb.
The limbs become cold, pale and wrinkled as if they had been a long time in hot water.

35 **Rest. Position. Motion.** Must lie doubled up in bed: pain in belly.
Sitting: stitches in vertebræ, constant; cannot bend forward or backward without losing his equilibrium.
Holds hands with fingers spread widely apart.
Standing: stitches in vertebræ intermittent.
Inability to stand erect: vertigo.
Every exertion: tenderness of cervical process <.
Motion: hemorrhage <; giddiness; after labor, pains <; pains over chest <; pains in sacrum <; tearing in thighs <.
Walking: heaviness of legs >; impossible from gangrene.
Every attempt to walk knees sink from under him.
Cannot walk: giddiness.

36 **Nerves.** ▮Hyperæsthesia of cutaneous nerves, especially of spine.
ǀǀSensation of soreness in abdomen; formation of large lumps and swellings in abdomen; r. hand very weak, particularly fingers, so that she could hold nothing, nor sew with that hand; when placing open hand to side and taking it away a spasm of hand occurs, the fingers are spread apart and she cannot close the hand; rapid alternations of heat and cold in hands and feet; cramps in legs; icy coldness of knees; trembling of r. arm and hand while eating, must use the left; sensation of coldness in stomach, > for a short time by warm drinks; habitual constipation. θHysteria.
▮▮Burning: in all parts of body as if sparks of fire were falling on them.
▮Neuralgia, caused by pressure of distended veins upon a nerve trunk.
Spasmodic twitchings.
Irregular movements of whole body.
Spasmodic distortion of limbs, relieved by stretching them out.
ǀǀExpression of countenance varied every moment from a constant play of the muscles; eyes rolled about, pupils

dilated, tongue jerked out, head moved about from side to side; arms in constant action with most diverse movements; snatched objects rather than took hold of them, could hold nothing securely; trunk also in constant motion; urine could not be retained; pulse small, weak, quick; heart beat tumultuously; appetite poor; bowels torpid; aching in occiput; sensation of formication in extremities; memory impaired; speech difficult, hurried; no relief at night; staggered about the house almost all night. θChorea.

▮Chorea associated with menstrual irregularities.

▮▮The muscular twitchings usually commence in face and spread thence all over body, sometimes increase to dancing and jumping. θChorea.

Spasms, with fingers spread apart.

Convulsive jerks and starts in paralyzed limbs.

Painful contractions in flexor muscles.

Tetanic spasms, with full consciousness, followed by great exhaustion.

▮▮Convulsions.

Tonic spasms.

Epileptiform spasms; epilepsy.

▮▮Complains of great weakness, constipation, heaviness in epigastrium, formication in legs and cramps; at night while asleep gets epileptiform attacks of which she knows nothing next morning except that she feels greatly prostrated and has a constant heaviness in head.

▮▮After abortus, spasms with full consciousness, afterward great exhaustion; heaviness in head and tingling in legs.

▮▮Convulsions first occurring after a fright when a little girl, returned after each confinement.

▮▮Twitching of single muscles; twisting of head to and fro; contortions of hands and feet; labored and anxious respiration. θSpasms.

▮▮Numbness of extremities; paralysis of some parts; painful tingling (like crawling of ants) on tongue. θPost-diphtheritic paralysis.

▮Paralysis after spasm, and apoplexy, with rapid emaciation of affected parts and involuntary discharges from bowels and bladder.

▮▮Suddenly fell to ground, but without loss of consciousness; on every attempt to walk the knees would sink from under him, especially r.; while sitting cannot bend forward or backward without losing his equilibrium; arms slightly weak, sensation of touch not affected; general dulness; difficult speech; inclination to weep; complains of headache and pain in lumbar region; sleep poor; urine and feces escape involuntarily; no stool for several days; at times oppression of breathing. θParalysis.

|| Paralysis of lower extremities, in a woman past climacteric; a hard, sensitive tumor in one of her breasts had been developing for several years, but for the last year or two had rapidly increased in size and become very painful; by continued application for several months of a yellowish salve the tumor was enucleated; in about a month after ceasing to use the salve a peculiar torpor or deadness was felt in great toes, which extended to whole foot and ankle joint; feet seemed large and heavy and could be moved only by moving whole limb; gait shuffling as if feet were dragged along by lifting legs; slight numbness in hands.

▮ Paralysis, with rapid emaciation, with relaxation of sphincters.

Myelitis and softening of cord.

Trembling; unsteadiness of whole body.

▮▮ Restlessness; extreme debility and prostration.

Loss of power of voluntary motion.

|| Sinking spells from diarrhœa, at 3 A.M.

▮▮ Collapse from choleroid diseases, etc., with cold skin, yet unable to bear warmth.

37 **Sleep.** Frequent yawning.

Inclination to sleep; drowsiness; deep, heavy sleep, stupor.

Sleep at night disturbed by frightful dreams.

Restless and sleepless.

38 **Time.** At 3 A.M.: sinking spells.

At break of day: diarrhœa.

In morning: frequent short evacuations.

During day: warmth on tongue; unusual drowsiness; toes drawn up continuously.

During night: anus firmly closed; cramps in calves and twitchings of limbs; dreamed she was ascending stairs; palpitation; toes drawn up occasionally.

Jerkings in limbs; staggered about house with chorea; ulcers <.

39 **Temperature and Weather.** Open air: palpitation less.

Wants to be in air or be fanned: with diarrhœa.

Warm applications: suppuration of cornea <; ulcers <.

Warm drinks: coldness of stomach <.

Does not wish to be covered; diarrhœa; uterine hemorrhage.

Heat: could not bear it and would throw off all covering, in post-diphtheritic paralysis; with diarrhœa, did not wish to be near; aversion to, with cholera; internal pain much <; gangrene <.

Wet bandages: > labor pains.
Cold: ulcers >; gangrene >.

40 **Fever.** Disagreeable sensation of coldness in back, abdomen and limbs.

Skin cold, with shivering.

Coldness of surface of body, particularly extremities.

▮Violent chill of but short duration; followed soon after by internal burning heat, with great thirst.

▮Chill with thirst.

ǁViolent shaking followed by violent heat, with anxiety, delirium and almost unquenchable thirst.

▮▮Intense, icy coldness of skin, with shivering; pale, sunken face.

▮Cold limbs, cold sweats, great weakness.

Cold stage preceded by vomiting, succeeded by moderate sweating.

▮Severe and long-lasting dry heat, with great restlessness and violent thirst.

ǁHeat with thirst and hot skin.

▮Burning heat, interrupted by shaking chills, then internal burning heat, with great thirst.

▮Sweat: all over body, except face; profuse cold, cold limbs; from head to pit of stomach; especially on upper body; cold, clammy over whole body; colliquative.

ǁExhausting perspiration, accompanied by evening fever and alarming cough.

▮Cold surface; sunken pale face and blue lips; will not be covered; tingling in limbs; holds hands with fingers widely spread apart; cold, clammy sweat; speech feeble, stuttering. θAgue.

▮▮Aversion to heat or to being covered; may feel cold but does not wish to be covered.

▮Great tendency to typhoid. θIntermittent.

41 **Attacks, Periodicity.** Sudden attacks: diarrhœa.

Alternation: of heat and cold, in hands and feet.

Five to ten minutes after taking least quantityof foo d severe colic.

Every two or three hours: paroxysms of palpitation.

Several times a day: convulsive movements of limbs.

For several weeks: formication in tips of fingers.

Every two weeks: excessive menstrual flow; lasting seven to nine days.

For two weeks: profuse corrosive foot sweat.

For four weeks: flow is continuous.

During August: diarrhœa.

In Summer: interminable diarrhœa.

For several years: tenderness of cervical processes.

42 **Locality and Direction.** Right: ovary congested; a spot

on side of chest dull on percussion; spasmodic shocks from half of chest into arm and leg; coldness of hand; toes drawn up; swelling and livid coloring of foot; gangrene in great toe of foot; hand very weak; trembling of hand and arm.

Left: hemicrania; nose stopped up; throat sore; protrusion in hypochondrium; thumb spasmodically drawn toward dorsum of hand.

43 **Sensations.** As if intoxicated while undressing; as if eyes were spasmodically rotated; as of a solid plug in nose; as if tongue were paralyzed; as if there were some resistance to overcome in speech; as of a heavy weight in stomach; region of stomach as if contracted; anus as if locked up; as if testicles were being drawn up to inguinal ring; uterus as if burnt; as if contents of uterus would fall forward; as if soft air were creeping through back; as if sacrum would be forced out; as if something alive were creeping under skin; as if fingers were asleep; as if limbs had been a long time in hot water; as if sparks of fire were falling upon different parts of body; in lumbar region; as if mice were creeping under skin.

Pain: in occiput; in eyes; in pit of stomach; in epigastrium; in lower belly; in abdomen; in hypogastric region; in loins; in ovaries and uterus; in sacrum, down thighs and into lower abdomen; over front part of chest; in small of back; in sacrum.

Excruciating pains: in spine.

Violent pain: in back; in finger tips.

Acute pain: in hepatic region.

Severe pains: in stomach; in abdomen and small of back; in sole of foot and toes.

Cutting: in abdomen.

Tearing pains: in both thighs; in foot.

Throbbing, tearing pains: in thighs.

Tearing, stinging pains: in extremities.

Pinching pains: in abdomen.

Forcing pain: in uterus.

Stitches: in upper dorsal vertebræ.

Stitching pains: in eyes; in legs.

Stitch: in back.

Sudden catch: in back.

Throbbing: in temples.

Cramps: in calves of legs; in feet, toes, hands and fingers; in chest.

Cramping pains: in stomach.

Cramping pressure: in stomach.

Rheumatic pains: in joints.

Tensive pain: in limbs.

Drawing pains: in calves of legs.
Drawing: in limbs.
Dragging: violent in spermatic cord; in abdomen.
Stinging: on mammæ.
Burning: in throat; of tongue; at pit of stomach; in spleen; in abdomen; in uterus; in hands; in feet.
Soreness: of throat; in abdomen.
Tenderness: of epigastrium; of lower cervical and upper dorsal spinous processes.
Distress: of stomach.
Painful constriction: of epigastrium.
Painful jerkings: in limbs.
Jerking: under skin.
Pulsations: in head.
Pressure: on eyeballs; in pit of stomach; in occiput; in uterine region.
Heaviness: of head; in epigastrium.
Lightness: of head.
Peculiar prickling feeling: in tips of fingers.
Tingling: in face; in throat and tongue; of legs; on tongue; in limbs; all over body; in fourth and fifth fingers; in back; in toes.
Crawling: on tongue; in tips of fingers; in limbs; all over body; between skin and flesh; in upper lip; all about mouth.
Formication: in face; in gums; in extremities; in tips of fingers; over whole body.
Gentle creeping sensation: in back.
Fuzzy feeling: in limbs.
Dryness: of soft palate, throat and œsophagus; of mouth.
Numbness: in limbs; of feet; of r. hand; of tips of fingers.
Cold feeling: in abdomen and back; in limbs; of body; of r. hand; in stomach.

Tissues. It destroys the activity of the cord; convulsive twitchings and shocks, painful contractions, tetanic manifestations; perfect paralysis, with increased reflex activity; most excruciating spinal pains, especially in sacral region; paralysis of bladder and rectum; tendency to gangrene; rapid emaciation.

Dissolution of blood corpuscles; blood thin; passive hemorrhages.

Anæmic state, either from exhaustive diseases or artificial depletion; the blood is thin and does not coagulate.

Thrombosis of abdominal vessels.

▮Neuralgia caused by pressure on nerves by a distended vein.

Tumefaction of glands.

▮Lymphatic tumors.

▮▮Collapse from choleroid diseases.

▮Rapid emaciation of paralyzed parts.

Malignant pustule.

Emphysematous swellings.

Passive hemorrhage; blood dark and red, in feeble and cachectic persons, accompanied by tingling in limbs and prostration; desire for air; does not like to be covered; wishes to have limbs extended; skin cold.

Rheumatism (peliosis rheumatica of Schoenlein) generally is found in cachectic individuals, with purpura; affects joints, especially of lower extremities; thrombosis of abdominal vessels.

▮Ulcers: bleeding; becoming black; feeling as if burnt; painless; pricking, producing a prurient sensation; pus putrid; < at night, touch, from external warmth; > from cold.

▮▮Gangrene: from anæmia; external injuries, application of leeches or mustard; > from cold, < from heat; dry, of old people.

▮Dry gangrene of extremities, parts are dry, cold, hard and insensible, of a uniform black color and free from fetor; large ecchymoses, blood blisters on extremities, becoming gangrenous, black suppurating blisters; limbs become pale, cold, shrivelled or lead-colored, losing all sensibility.

45 **Touch. Passive Motion. Injuries.** Touch: pit of stomach very sensitive to; r. ovary sensitive to; uterus painful; ulcers <.

Pressure: upon abdomen > labor pains; upon vertebræ stitches <.

After lifting heavy weight: during sixth month of pregnancy; severe pain in stomach, abdomen and small of back.

External injuries: gangrene.

46 **Skin.** Skin dry and cool.

Cold and dry; dingy, wrinkled, dry and insensible; desquamation.

▮▮Formication: with a sense as if mice were creeping under skin; on face, gums and other parts of body; in extremities with tearing, stinging pains; in tips of fingers, lasting several weeks, with a partial loss of sensibility; over whole body.

▮Crawling: all over body; between skin and flesh; and jerking under skin.

Violent crawling and prickling over whole body, especially in upper lip and at times all about the mouth.

▮Bloody blisters on extremities, becoming gangrenous.

▮▮Boils, small, painful, with green contents, mature very slowly and heal in same manner; very debilitating.

▮Carbuncles; extensive ecchymoses.

▮Petechia and miliary eruptions.

▮▮Purpura hemorrhagica.

▮Cachectic females, with rough skin; pustules showing a tendency to gangrene.

▮Varicose ulcers and enlarged veins in old people.

▮Ulcers turn black, copious vomiting of a mixture of a thick, black, pitchy, bilious or shiny matter.

▮Indolent ulcer, ichorous, offensive pus, > from cold.

General desquamation in scarlatina.

▮Variola pustules of abnormal appearance, either fill with a bloody serum or dry up too soon.

47 **Stages of Life, Constitution.** Irritable plethoric subjects.

Nervous temperament.

Women of very lax muscular fibre.

Feeble, cachectic women; thin, scrawny.

Very old, decrepit persons.

Women of very lax muscular fibre; passive hemorrhages, copious flow of thin, black, watery blood; the corpuscles are destroyed.

Hemorrhagic diathesis; the slightest wound causes bleeding for weeks (*Phos.*); discharge of sanious liquid blood, with a strong tendency to putrescence; tingling in limbs and great debility, when weakness is not caused by previous loss of fluids.

Strumous child, æt. 18 months, suffering three weeks; diarrhœa.

Boy, æt. 5, suffering from suppuration of glands of neck after an attack of scarlet fever; hæmaturia.

Girl, æt. 10, suffering four years; hæmatemesis.

Boy, æt. 13; amaurosis.

Boy, æt. 17, slim, pale and thin, father a weaver; chorea.

Mrs. P., æt. 18, sanguine temperament, healthy, well-developed muscular system, primipara; dystocia.

Man, æt. 18, shoemaker's apprentice, weak, pale face, light hair, flabby muscles, fat cheeks; cramps in fingers.

Girl, æt. 18; offensive foot sweat.

Woman, æt. 20, gentle disposition, lymphatic temperament, gave birth to a child several weeks ago; hæmatemesis.

Man, æt. 20, tailor's apprentice, strong, well nourished; cramps in fingers.

Girl, æt. 22, sanguine temperament, robust; menstrual colic.

Mrs. A., æt. 25; hysteralgia.

Woman, æt. 28; menstrual colic.

Woman, æt. 28, lymphatic-sanguine temperament, pale, leuco-phlegmatic, has had three children and been previously healthy; menorrhagia following an abortion.

Man, æt. 30, strong, well nourished, short neck, addicted to drink; epistaxis, r. side.

Woman, æt. 30; prolapsus of uterus.

Woman, æt. 32, blonde, weak, after labor; uterine hemorrhage.

Woman, æt. 32, well built, married, no children; metrorrhagia.

Man, æt. 32, married; spinal affection.

Mrs. W., æt. 35, mother of three children, very weak and thin; menorrhagia.

Woman, æt. 35, mother of three children; metrorrhagia.

Man, æt. 40, choleric temperament; dark complexion; diarrhœa.

Woman, æt. 40, mother of seven children, weak, cachectic-looking, suffering from prolapsus uteri; hysteria.

Woman, æt. 41, large frame, feeble and emaciated, suffering since her return from the tropics; metrorrhagia.

Woman, æt. 41, had metritis after a forced labor, followed by leucorrhœa, latter cured by *Stannum;* epilepsy.

Architect, æt. 42, robust constitution; spinal affection.

Woman, æt. 45; uterine hemorrhage.

Woman, æt. 45, weak, formerly suffering from hemorrhoids; menorrhagia.

Forester, æt. 50, strong, suffering three months; paralysis.

Man, æt. 53, nervo-bilious temperament, suffering many years with gastric disorder; gastralgia.

Woman, æt. 62, suffering four days; epistaxis.

Woman, æt. 70, gouty; diarrhœa.

Woman, æt. 80; senile gangrene.

Woman, æt. 82; senile gangrene.

Girl, sanguine temperament, healthy but delicate, menses normal, suffering several weeks; cardialgia.

Mrs. E., dark complexion, sickly yellow countenance, nervo-lymphatic temperament; dystocia.

Mrs. ——, nervo-bilious temperament, dark complexion, short, thick-set, has had four children; dystocia.

Woman, just past climacteric, had tumor in breast which was enucleated by applications of a salve, since then suffering; paralysis of legs.

48 **Relations.** Compatible: *Cinchon.*

Compare: *Colchic.* (cholera morbus); *Arsen.*, but cold and heat act opposite; *Cinnam.* (hemorrhage after labor); *Plumbum* (diabetes).

SELENIUM.

Selenium. *The Element.*

The trituration is prepared from the reddish-brown, somewhat translucent metal which resembles sulphur in its chemical relations.

Introduced and proved by Hering, Archiv für Hom., vol. 12, p. 192; proving by Schreter, N. Archiv für Hom., vol. 3, p. 184; Berridge, N. Am. Jour. of Hom., 1873, p. 501.

CLINICAL AUTHORITIES.—*Headache*, Ballard, M. I., vol. 6. p. 182; *Spermatorrhœa*, Greenleaf, A H. O., vol. 10, p. 258; *Prostatitis and atony of sexual organs*, Altschul, Rück. Kl. Erf., vol. 5, p. 586; *Gleet*, Nash, Hom. Phys., vol. 7, p. 289.

1 **Mind.** Great dulness, with complete insensibility and indifference to his surroundings.

Very forgetful, especially in business; during slumber, however, he remembers all he had forgotten.

A kind of stammering; he uses syllables of words in wrong connections, therefore pronounces some words incorrectly.

Difficult comprehension.

Total unfitness for any kind of work.

Great talkativeness when excited, especially in evening.

▮Mental labor fatigues him.

▮Lascivious thoughts with impotency.

Dread of society.

2 **Sensorium.** Vertigo: on lifting head or rising up; on moving about, with nausea, vomiting, faintness; < after breakfast and dinner.

3 **Inner Head.** Violent stinging over l. eye, when walking in sun or from strong odors; with increased secretion of urine, and melancholy.

Headache every afternoon, especially after drinking wine, tea or lemonade.

‖ Violent headache commenced in forehead and gradually involved whole head; heavily coated tongue; nausea; frequent vomiting of bilious-looking matter; her usual cup of tea was followed by an aggravation of all the symptoms.

▮Headache of drunkards; headache after debauchery.

4 **Outer Head.** ▮Hair comes out when combing; also from eyebrows, whiskers and genitals.

▮Tingling itching on scalp in evening, oozing after scratching.

Tension and sensation of contraction of scalp.

5 **Sight and Eyes.** Itching vesicles on edges of eyelids and on eyebrows.

Spasmodic twitching of l. eyeball.

6 **Hearing and Ears.** Ear stopped; hardening of earwax in his deaf ear.

7 **Smell and Nose.** Itching in nose and on edges of nostrils.

Inclination to bore fingers into nose.

Yellow, thick, jellylike mucus in nose.

Discharge of dark blood from nose.

Phlegm in choanæ.

Coryza, ending in diarrhœa.

▮▮Complete obstruction of nose, chronic.

8 **Upper Face.** Twitching of muscles of face.

Great emaciation of face and hands.

Oiliness of skin on face; greasy and shining.

10 **Teeth and Gums.** Picks teeth until they bleed; toothache.

Teeth covered with mucus.

▮Toothache from drinking tea.

11 **Taste and Tongue.** A kind of stammering speech, made mistakes in talking, uttered syllables wrongly, and could not articulate some words.

14 **Appetite, Thirst. Desires, Aversions.** Want of appetite in morning, white-coated tongue.

Aversion to food much salted.

▮Great longing for ardent spirits; an almost maniacal irresistible desire, has to get completely drunk and feels distressed afterward; wants to go to an insane asylum. θChronic alcoholism.

Hungry during night.

15 **Eating and Drinking.** After eating: violent beating all over body, < in abdomen; must lie down.

▮Bad effects: from sugar; from salt food; from drinking tea; from lemonade.

18 **Hypochondrium.** Searching pain in region of liver, < in taking a long breath, with sensitiveness to external pressure; followed by a red, itching rash in region of liver.

Stitches in spleen when walking.

Enlargement of liver with loss of appetite, particularly in morning; white coating on tongue; sharp stitching pains in hepatic region, < from motion and pressure; sensitiveness of liver; peculiar fine rash over hepatic region.

19 **Abdomen.** Pulsation in whole body, especially in abdomen after eating.

20 **Stool and Rectum.** ▮Stool: hard and so impacted that it

requires mechanical aid; mucus or blood passes with last portion; contains threads of fecal matter like hair.

Papescent stool, with tenesmus and feeling in anus as after a hard stool.

|| Stools exceedingly difficult and threaten to tear anus, from their immense size; hours may be spent in an effort at evacuation, stool can be seen through the distended anus as an immense hard, dark-colored ball; the sufferings are great and patient becomes wonderfully agitated.

21 **Urinary Organs.** Sensation in tip of urethra as if a biting drop were forcing its way out.

Twinging pain along urethra from behind forward, with a sensation as if drops were passing out.

▮ Involuntary dribbling of urine while walking, also after urinating, especially after stool.

▮▮ Urine: dark, scanty; red, in evening; sediment coarse, red, sandy.

22 **Male Sexual Organs.** ▮ Erections slow, insufficient; semen emitted too rapidly and with long-continued thrill; weak, ill-humored after an embrace, weakness in loins.

▮ Semen thin, without normal odor.

▮ Lewd thoughts, but physically impotent.

No erection in evening, notwithstanding he was excited; erection in morning without sexual desire.

Diminution of sexual desire.

Impotence with sexual desire.

Lascivious dreams, with seminal emissions, which awaken him, followed by lameness and weakness in small of back.

▮▮ Impotence.

Involuntary dribbling of semen or prostatic fluid during sleep.

|| Seminal emissions about twice a week, lascivious dreams, is always awakened by it; always rises with weakness and lameness in small of back. θSpermatorrhœa.

▮ Prostatic juice oozes while sitting, during sleep, when walking and at stool.

A drop of watery, sticky substance passes from urethra just before stool and soon afterward.

While sitting a drop of prostatic fluid passes from orifice of urethra with a peculiar, disagreeable sensation.

|| Frequent itching in small spots on skin and development of small vesicles on hands and feet; sleep disturbed by confused and lascivious dreams; glowing sensation of skin in various parts of body; severe stitching pain over l. eye, returning every afternoon; belching before eating, particularly after smoking; after eat-

ing desire to lie down with inability to fall asleep; pain in region of r. kidney, < from inspiration; dribbling of urine after stool; while at stool must wait a long while to urinate; discharge of prostatic fluid before and after stool; profuse sweat about abdomen and pubes; dull pain in perineum, < urinating, evacuating bowels and during ejaculation of semen; swelling of prostata, feels hard and causes narrowing of urethra; seminal emissions during sleep; weak erections although sexual desire may be great; premature ejaculation of semen; cough on awaking; expectoration of small lumps of mucus and blood; tearing pains in posterior part of thighs. θProstatitis and atony of sexual organs.

‖ Prostatitis caused by an immense hard stool.

‖ Discharge of slimy mucus from ten to fifteen drops or a tablespoonful looking like milk. θProstatic gleet.

Itching on scrotum.

‖ Gonorrhœa (secondary); gleet.

23 **Female Sexual Organs.** Catamenia copious and dark.

24 **Pregnancy. Parturition. Lactation.** During pregnancy throbbing in abdomen.

25 **Voice and Larynx. Trachea and Bronchia.** | Voice husky when beginning to sing, or from talking long; hawks transparent lumps every morning, sometimes bloody.

| Hoarseness after long use of voice; frequent necessity to clear the throat on account of accumulation of clear starchy mucus.

Increased hoarseness while singing, especially at the beginning.

Is frequently obliged to clear his throat, alternating with hoarseness.

| Tubercular laryngitis; raising of small lumps of blood and mucus; tendency to hoarseness; cervical glands swollen, hard but not sore.

26 **Respiration.** Frequent deep breathing with moaning.

Dyspnœa from accumulation of mucus in windpipe.

27 **Cough.** ‖ Cough in morning though slight and weak affects whole chest, and lumps of mucus with blood are expectorated.

28 **Inner Chest and Lungs.** ‖ Pains in r. side and under last ribs especially on inspiration, extending to kidneys, which are sensitive to external pressure.

29 **Heart, Pulse and Circulation.** Throbbing in vessels throughout whole body, pulsation especially felt in abdomen.

31 **Neck and Back.** Neck stiff on turning head.

Pain as from lameness in small of back, in morning.

32 **Upper Limbs.** Tearing in hands at night, with cracking in wrists.
Emaciation of hands.
▮Itching in palms; vesicles on and between fingers.
▮Dry, scaly eruption on palms of hands with itching, having a syphilitic base.
Painful hangnails.

33 **Lower Limbs.** Cracking of knee joint on bending it.
Flat ulcers on lower legs.
Emaciation of legs.
Itching around ankle, in evening; blisters on toes.
Cramps in calves and soles.
Legs feel weak, with fear of paralysis, after typhus.
Itching about ankles.

35 **Rest. Position. Motion.** Must lie down: after eating.
Lifting head: vertigo.
Turning head: stiff neck.
Bending knee joint: cracking in it.
Sitting: prostatic juice oozes.
Rising up: vertigo.
Any exertion: easy fatigue; sweat.
Motion: vertigo; pains in hepatic region <.
Walking: stitches in spleen; involuntary dribbling of urine; prostatic juice oozes.

36 **Nerves.** ▮Weakness and general debility; easy fatigue from any exertion or labor; especially in hot weather.
▮Irresistible desire to lie down and sleep; strength suddenly leaves him.
▮Easy exhaustion; inability to perform anykind of labor, either mental or physical; sexual desire with debility and relaxation of organs; loss of prostatic juice.
▮Great nervous debility after typhus, particularly when sensations of patient spread from above downward.
After typhoid fever great debility of spine, fears he will be paralyzed.
▮Very great aversion to a draft of air either warm, cold or damp.

37 **Sleep.** Sleepless before 12 P.M.; light sleep, least noise awakens him; starts on falling asleep; sleeps in cat naps.
Dreams of quarrels and cruelties.
Hungry in night.
Awakes early and always at same hour.
Worse after a siesta on hot days; < after sleep.

38 **Time.** Morning: want of appetite in morning; erection without sexual desire; cough; pain in small of back.
Evening: great talkativeness; tingling itching on scalp; urine red; itching around ankle.
Night: tearing in hands; hungry.

12 P.M.: sleepless.

[39] **Temperature and Weather.** Hot weather: weakness and general debility.

Draft of air either warm, cold or damp: great aversion.

[40] **Fever.** Chill alternating with heat.

External heat, burning in skin in single spots.

Sweat: profuse on chest, armpits and genitals; from least exertion; as soon as he sleeps; stains yellow, or white and stiffens linen; staining brownish-yellow.

[41] **Attacks, Periodicity.** Alternation: of chill and heat.

Every morning: hawks transparent lumps.

Every afternoon: headache; pain over l. eye.

About twice a week: seminal emissions.

[42] **Locality and Direction.** Right: pain in region of kidney; pain in side under last ribs.

Left: stinging over eye; twitching of eyeball; pain over eye.

From above downward: sensation's spread.

[43] **Sensations.** As if biting drop were forcing its way out of urethra.

Pain: in region of r. kidney; in r. side under last ribs; in small of back.

Violent pain: in head.

Tearing pains: in thighs; in hands.

Twinging pain: along urethra.

Searching pain: in region of liver.

Sharp stitching pains: in hepatic region.

Stitches: in spleen.

Violent stinging: over l. eye.

Burning: in skin.

Dull pain: in perineum.

Cramps in calves and soles.

Violent beating: all over body.

Throbbing: in abdomen; in vessels throughout whole body.

Sensation of contraction: of scalp.

Tension: of scalp.

Weakness: of loins; in small of back.

Tingling itching: on scalp.

Itching: of vesicles on edges of eyelids and eyebrows; in nose and edges of nostrils; in small spots on skin; on scrotum; in palms; around ankle; in folds of skin between fingers and about joints.

[44] **Tissues.** Great emaciation, especially of face, thighs and hands.

Emaciation and withering of affected parts.

The hair falls out.

[45] **Touch. Passive Motion. Injuries.** Pressure: region of liver sensitive to; kidneys sensitive.

Scratching: oozing on scalp.

46 **Skin.** Red rash on region of liver.

Frequent tingling in small spots of skin, with great irritation to scratch; spots remain humid.

Itch checked by mercury or sulphur.

Flat ulcers.

Itching in folds of skin between fingers and about joints, particularly ankle joint.

▮Hair falls off, on head, eyebrows, whiskers and other parts of body.

48 **Relations.** Incompatible: *Cinchon.*, wine.

Compare: *Phosphor.*, genito-urinary and respiratory symptoms; *Stannum* and *Argent. met.*, cough, transparent, starchy, mucous expectoration; *Alumina*, hard stool.

Antidotes: *Ignat.*, *Pulsat.*

SENECIO.

Golden Ragwort. *Compositæ.*

Proved by Small, U. S. Med. and Surg. Jour., 1866, p. 151; Jones, Hale's New Rem., 1876, p. 971.

Clinical Authorities.—*Dysmenorrhœa*, Blake, Hom. Rev., vol. 16, p. 403; Hale, A. H. O., vol. 1, p. 46; *Hœmoptysis*, Irish, A. H. O., vol. 1, p. 46.

1 **Mind.** ▮▮Low spirits alternating with cheerful mood; ▮sleepless; sensation of a ball rising from stomach to throat. θAmenorrhœa. θHysteria.

▮▮Inability to fix mind on one subject for any length of time.

A feeling like homesickness.

2 **Sensorium.** ▮▮Dizzy feeling while walking in open air like a wave from occiput to sinciput; he feels as if he would pitch forward; nausea.

3 **Inner Head.** ▮▮Dull stupefying headache with fulness of head, as from catarrh.

4 **Outer Head.** ▮▮Sharp lancinating in l. temple, upper part of l. eye and inside of l. lower jaw.

▮▮Sharp stitching pains from within outward in forehead; sharp shooting pains over and in eyes; catarrh; suppressed secretion.

▮Headache preceding leucorrhœa and irritation of bladder.

Forehead hot; sweaty in evening.

5 **Sight and Eyes.** ‖Sharp pains from within outward, l. eye; lachrymation in open air.

‖Catarrhal ophthalmia from suppressed secretions.

7 **Smell and Nose.** ▮Coryza, at first dull headache, dryness of nose and sneezing, burning and fulness in nostrils, later secretion of copious mucus.

▮Coryza with nosebleed.

8 **Upper Face.** |Face pale, depressed appearance; weary, wants to lie down.

9 **Lower Face.** Lips: and gums pale; dry, feverish.

10 **Teeth and Gums.** ‖Teeth tender and sensitive.

11 **Taste and Tongue.** Tongue slightly coated; catarrhal fever.

12 **Inner Mouth.** ▮Mouth and fauces dry, hot. θCatarrh.

13 **Throat.** Tightness in throat, wants to swallow; fauces dry.

16 **Hiccough, Belching, Nausea and Vomiting.** Eructations of sour gas and ingesta.

‖Nausea on rising; morning sickness of pregnancy.

▮Nausea from renal derangements.

18 **Hypochondria.** Stitches in hypochondria; sharp cutting in diaphragm; epigastrium.

19 **Abdomen.** Pains centre about navel, spreading thence in all directions; > by stool; griping pains > bending forward.

Rumbling of wind.

Catarrh of bowels, rumbling colic and watery stools.

‖Abdomen much enlarged and very tense; lower limbs œdematous; urine scanty, high-colored, not more than eight ounces a day; pain in lumbar region and in ovaries; constipation; cervix uteri congested; albuminous leucorrhœa; sense of weight in uterine region. θAscites.

20 **Stool and Rectum.** ‖Stool, thin, watery, bloody; with tenesmus and colic; catarrhal dysentery; evening.

‖Stool copious, with great debility and prostration; flatulence; morning.

Stool in hard lumps mixed with yellow mucus.

21 **Urinary Organs.** Slight pains in region of kidneys.

▮Congestion and inflammation of kidneys.

‖Attacks of renal inflammation, attacking particularly r. kidney, causing intense pain, fever and great prostration; on one occasion suffering intense and bladder seemed implicated; great pain on passing urine, causing him to cry out; constipation; urine reddish, very hot, and acrid; dull headache; dryness of mouth and throat; chilliness, fever and perspiration.

‖Severe renal inflammation with fever, chilliness and pain in lumbar region, particularly in l. kidney; quantity of urine below normal; urine red, depositing a brickdust sediment; considerable arterial excitement;

skin hot and dry; motion caused him to cry out with pain; constipation.

▮Intense pain over r. kidney, severe pain during urination, urine red, hot, acrid; bowels constipated.

▮Renal dropsy.

‖Ascites and œdema of lower extremities in a young woman.

▮Inflammation of kidneys and ureters after passage of gravel.

Tenesmus of bladder; smarting in urethra, dropsy.

Increased urinary secretion; followed by acute inflammation.

▮Hæmaturia; renal pain with nausea.

‖Tenesmus of bladder, with heat and urging.

Urging to urinate following chilliness.

Uncomfortable heat in neck of bladder.

‖Irritation of bladder in children, preceded by heat in head and headache.

‖Renal colic with or without nausea.

▮Chronic inflammation of neck of bladder with bloody urine and tenesmus of bladder.

‖Chronic inflammation of kidneys.

▮Dysuria: of women and children evidently of catarrhal origin; mucous sediment in urine; with uterine displacement.

Smarting in fossa navicularis before urination.

22 **Male Sexual Organs.** Lascivious dreams, emissions.

Prostate gland enlarged, feels hard and swollen to touch.

Dull heavy pain in spermatic cord, moving along cord to testicle.

Gonorrhœa, gleet.

Chronic prostatitis.

23 **Female Sexual Organs.** ‖Menses, every three weeks, very profuse, lasting eight or nine days, accompanied by severe cutting pains in region of sacrum, hypogastrium and groins; she was pale, weak and nervous and had a slight cough, generally at night; after an abortion.

Menses premature and profuse or retarded and scanty.

▮Dysmenorrhœa with urinary symptoms; cutting in sacral and hypogastric regions; flow scanty or profuse or irregular; pale, weak, anæmic; strumous; hacking cough at night.

▮Amenorrhœa: from a cold; nervous irritability, lassitude, dropsy; wandering pains in back and shoulders; sensation of a ball rising from stomach into throat; costive; in young girls with dropsical conditions.

▮Symptoms as if menses would appear, but they fail; nervous, excitable, sleepless: loss of appetite.

‖Suppression of menses from a cold; after venesection.

▮Menstrual irregularities in consumptive patients.

▮Leucorrhœa: preceded by headache, sleeplessness and irritable bladder; in little girls, preceded by headache and sleeplessness.

▮Chlorosis, in scrofulous girls, with dropsy.

25 **Voice and Larynx. Trachea and Bronchia.** Hawking of tough, white mucus.

26 **Respiration.** Respiration as if greatly fatigued.

Labored breathing from mucous accumulation.

27 **Cough.** ▮Hacking night cough.

▮Mucous rattling with suppressed cough.

‖Great debility; loss of appetite; flashes of heat during day; redness of cheeks in afternoon; occasional night sweats; menses very irregular for a year, have now been absent two months; six weeks ago had caught cold, cough, at first dry then loose with copious expectoration of yellowish, thick, sweet mucus, often streaked with blood, with sensation of rawness and soreness in chest; paroxysms of coughing were quite severe and exhausting.

‖Palliated cough and bloody sputa in a woman far gone with consumption and brought back menses which were absent four months.

Cough with bloody expectoration.

28 **Inner Chest and Lungs.** ▮Catarrh of lungs; loose cough and copious mucous expectoration.

▮Hæmoptysis; great emaciation; dry, hacking cough; hectic flush; sleeplessness.

▮Hæmoptysis after venesection or suppressed menstruation.

‖Chronic hemorrhage from lungs with dry, hacking cough, hectic fever, emaciation, sleeplessness.

▮Incipient phthisis, attended with fatiguing cough, result of obstructed menstruation; increased bronchial secretion; loose mucous cough, rattling in chest, labored respiration.

▮Phthisis, with obstructed menstruation; bloody or copious mucous sputa.

31 **Neck and Back.** Pain in back and loins.

Sharp, lancinating pains in lumbar region.

Dull pain in l. lumbar region.

Severe pain in small of back, in morning.

▮Cutting pains in region of sacrum, hypogastrium and groins, with too early or too profuse menses; she is pale, weak and nervous and has a slight cough at night.

‖Wandering pains in back and shoulders; pain in joints.

33 **Lower Limbs.** Lower limbs weary.

34 **Limbs in General.** ‖ Sharp stitches here and there; rheumatic pains in joints.

▮ Œdema.

36 **Nerves.** ▮ Nervousness, sleeplessness and hysterical mood.

▮ Much lassitude and great nervousness.

‖ Hysteria.

‖ Wants to lie down; pale.

Slight exertion produces syncope.

37 **Sleep.** Great sleeplessness, with vivid, unpleasant dreams.

▮ Sleeplessness: of women suffering from uterine irritation, prolapsus and its attendant nervousness (it is the *Coffea* of women); during climacteric period.

▮ At night sleepless, nervous, hysterical; by day drowsy, languid.

‖ Dreams mostly of an intellectual character; memory very active.

38 **Time.** Morning: flatulence; severe pain in small of back; sweat toward.

Forenoon: chilly.

During day: flashes of heat; drowsy, languid; frequent desire to urinate.

Afternoon: redness of cheeks.

Evening: forehead sweaty; stools.

Night: cough; occasional sweats; sleepless; frequent desire to urinate.

39 **Temperature and Weather.** ‖ Sensitive to open air; tendency to catarrhs.

Open air: walking in, dizziness; lachrymation.

40 **Fever.** Chilly forenoon as after taking cold; followed by heat and sweat in evening with moderate thirst.

Chilliness followed by urging to urinate.

Sweat toward morning; catarrh.

Hectic fever.

41 **Attacks, Periodicity.** Alternate: low spirits and cheerful mood; urine profuse and watery or dark colored and scanty.

Every three weeks: menses.

42 **Locality and Direction.** Left: lancinating in temple and eye; pain in lumbar region.

Right: inflammation of kidney; intense pain over kidney.

From within outward: pain in forehead; pain in eye.

43 **Sensations.** As of a ball rising from stomach to throat; as of a wave from occiput to sinciput; as if he would pitch forward; respiration as if greatly fatigued.

Pains: centre about navel; in lumbar region and ovaries; in region of kidneys; in back and loins; in joints.

Intense pain: in r. kidney; over r. kidney.

Severe pain: in small of back.

Sharp pains: in l. eye.

Sharp, lancinating pains: in l. temple, upper part of l. eye and inside of lower jaw; in lumbar region.

Sharp cutting: in diaphragm; in region of sacrum, hypogastrium and groins.

Sharp, shooting pains: over and in eyes.

Sharp, stitching pain: in forehead.

Stitches: in hypochondria; in epigastrium; here and there in limbs.

Griping pains: in abdomen.

Rheumatic pains: in joints.

Wandering pains: in back and shoulders.

Dull pain: in l. lumbar region.

Dull, stupefying pain: in head.

Smarting: in urethra; in fossa navicularis.

Soreness: of chest.

Rawness: of chest.

Burning: in nostrils.

Sensitiveness: of teeth.

Heat: in neck of bladder; in head.

Tightness: in throat.

Fulness: in head; in nostrils.

Dryness: of nose; of mouth and fauces.

Weariness: of lower limbs.

[41] **Tissues.** ▮Catarrhal affections of mucous membranes.

▮▮Face bloated, abdomen enlarged, feet œdematous; urine alternately profuse and watery or dark-colored and scanty; frequent desire to urinate day and night. θDropsy.

▮Hemorrhages from uterus, kidneys, bowels, lungs, etc.

▮Dropsy from amenia; ▮ascites and œdema of lower limbs in a young woman.

▮Anæmia.

[47] **Stages of Life, Constitution.** ▮▮Women and little girls of nervous temperament.

Lady, mother of one child, had an abortion three years ago, another (at second month) four months ago; dysmenorrhœa.

Mrs. H., æt. 30, lymphatic temperament, suffering six years; inflammation of neck of bladder.

Woman, æt. 30; dropsy.

Woman, æt. 40, passing through climacteric period; cough.

Merchant, æt. 45, nervous temperament, inclined to be bilious; renal inflammation.

Woman, æt. 48; amenorrhœa.

Man, æt. 50, nervo-sanguine temperament; attacks of renal inflammation.

[48] **Relations.** Compare: *Aletris*, *Cinchon.* (hemorrhage); *Coffea; Caulophyl.*, *Sepia* (irregular menses); *Actæa racem.*, *Pulsat.*

SENEGA.

Seneca Snake Root. *Polygalaceæ.*

This plant grows wild in all parts of the United States.

The alcoholic tincture is prepared from the powdered, dried root.

For general effects obtained from experiments with the powdered root and tincture see Allen's Encyclopedia, including Seidel's and Lembke's collections, vol. 8, p. 586.

CLINICAL AUTHORITIES.—*Hypopion,* Noack, B. J. H., vol. 23, p. 341; *Paresis of oculo-motor nerve,* Allen, Hah. Mo., vol. 7, p. 106; *Catarrh of pharynx,* Gerstel, A. H. Z., vol. 91, p 150; *Sore throat,* Haynes, Org., vol. 3, p. 97; *Catarrh of bladder,* B. J. H., vol. 27, p. 142; *Influenza,* Hermann, Rück. Kl Erf., vol. 3, p. 50; Trinks, Rück. Kl. Erf., vol. 5, p. 706; Weinke, A. H. Z., vol. 91, p. 150; *Asthma,* Müller, Rück. Kl. Erf., vol. 5, p. 802; *Whooping Cough,* A. R., Rück. Kl. Erf., vol. 5, p. 728; Gerstel, A. H. Z., vol. 92, p. 148; *Soreness in chest,* Ockford, Org., vol. 3, p. 377; *Pleurisy, Pneumonia, Hydrothorax,* Gallavardin, Strecker, Lorbacher, B J. H., vol. 26, p. 338; *Pleuro-pneumonia,* Strecker, Rück. Kl. Erf., vol. 3, p. 335; *Pneumonia,* Kallenbach, Pop. Hom. Ztg., 1867, No. 12; B. J. H., vol. 27, p. 141; *Hydrothorax and Ascites,* Lorbacher, Rück. Kl. Erf., vol. 4, p. 64.

2 **Sensorium.** Confused or reeling sensation in head.

■ Dulness and stupefaction of head, with pressure in eyes and obscuration of sight.

3 **Inner Head.** Aching pain in head, in sinciput and occiput, not increased by pressure, every day when sitting in a warm room, accompanied by pressure in eyes which did not bear touch.

Pressing pain in forehead and orbits after dinner, especially l. side, < in open air.

4 **Outer Head.** Shuddering on hairy scalp.

5 **Sight and Eyes.** Drawing and pressure in eyeballs, with diminution of vision.

Weakness of sight and flickering before eyes when reading, necessitating frequent wiping of eyes, which aggravates.

While reading eyes feel dazzled.

Flickering and running together of letters when reading.

Flickering before eyes and weakness of sight when continuing to read or write.

On walking toward setting sun, another small sun seemed to float beneath it, on turning eyes outward it changed into a compressed oval, disappeared on bending head and closing eyes.

Weakness of eyes with burning and lachrymation.
Obscuration of cornea.
Sensitiveness of eyes to light.
Obscuration of sight, with glistening before eyes, < from rubbing them.
‖ Hypopion in scrofulous subjects.
▮ To promote absorption of lens fragments after cataract operations or injuries to lens.
▮ Paralysis of muscles of eye.
▮ Iritis and specks upon cornea.
‖ Opacities in vitreous.
▮ Paresis of superior oblique.
‖ Oculo-motor paresis; Mr. A., æt. 33, four years ago eyes began to be weak with difficulty in seeing clearly; drooping lids, was obliged to pull them open; began to see double with r. image obliquely above real one; stopped using eyes and improved; this summer visited Mammoth Cave, followed by a return of double vision; walked into room with head thrown backward (occasionally shutting his l. eye and holding his head straight), this position relieving confusion of vision; double vision caused him to make missteps, etc.; paresis of l. oculomotor nerve, with paralysis of superior rectus; upper lid very weak, falling half over eye; difficult convergence; weak back; deficient muscular power; subject to bilious headaches.
▮ Aching over orbits, eyes tremble and water when he looks at an object intently or steadily; eyes weak and watery when reading.
▮ Eyes pain as if they were pressed out, as if eyeballs were being expanded, especially in evening in candlelight.
Congestion of blood to eyes, with pulsation in them on stooping.
Swelling of eyelids, with tingling in them.
Hardened mucus in morning in eyelashes.
Lachrymation in open air when looking intently at an object.
▮ Blepharitis ciliaris, < in morning, much smarting, dry, crusty lashes.
▮ Cilia hang full of hard mucus; smarting of conjunctiva as if soap were in eyes, mornings; blepharitis; sometimes lids stick so after sleep they must be soaked before they can be separated.
Pimple on margin of l. lower lid.
Stye on lower lid.
Hydrophthalmia with intraocular compression.

[6] **Hearing and Ears.** Painful sensitiveness of hearing.

[7] **Smell and Nose.** Sneezing for five minutes, so violent and

long continued that the head became quite heavy and dizzy; afterward a large quantity of thin watery fluid flowed from nose.

Troublesome dryness of Schneiderian membrane.

||Frequent coryza, commencing with feeling as if red pepper were throughout nostrils and air passages, followed by distressing cough. θInfluenza.

Smell of pus before nose.

8 **Upper Face.** ||Paralytic feeling in l. half of face.

Heat in face.

9 **Lower Face.** Burning blisters on upper lip and in corners of mouth.

11 **Taste and Tongue.** Tongue coated white, yellowish-white or slimy in morning, with slimy unpleasant taste.

Taste: metallic; like urine.

12 **Inner Mouth.** Increased secretion of saliva; offensive breath.

Burning in throat, mouth and on tongue.

13 **Throat.** ||Very dry, sore throat; short hacking cough, which tears and scrapes throat; loss of voice, even whispering is very painful to throat and causes cough; < in open air.

Inflammation and swelling of throat and palate.

Dryness in throat and accumulation of tough mucus which is difficult to hawk up.

14 **Appetite, Thirst. Desires, Aversions.** Much thirst, with loss of appetite.

Gnawing hunger with sensation of emptiness in stomach.

16 **Hiccough, Belching, Nausea and Vomiting.** Nausea, vomiting of mucus.

Nausea as from stomach, with vomiturition and straining to vomit.

17 **Scrobiculum and Stomach.** Pressure below pit of stomach; sense of gnawing hunger.

Digging pain in epigastrium, disposition to flatulence; outbursts of ill-humor.

Cramps and burning in stomach.

19 **Abdomen.** Ascites accompanying hepatic diseases, peritonitis or abdominal tumors.

Colic, with pressing pain.

Warmth and oppression in upper part of abdomen when inhaling.

Gnawing in upper part of abdomen.

Griping in bowels.

20 **Stool and Rectum.** Mushy or copious watery stools.

Purging, vomiting and anxiety; watery stools, spurting from anus.

Stools: scanty, hard, dry and large, insufficient.

Watery diarrhœa, with griping pain in bowels; nausea and vomiting.

21 **Urinary Organs.** Urine: diminished; dark and frothy for a long time after passing; passed only night and morning; at first mixed with mucous filaments, afterward thick and cloudy; frequent, with greenish tinge depositing a cloudy sediment; acrid, increased in quantity.

Involuntary micturition at night in bed.

▮Irritability of bladder.

▮▮Urging and scalding before and after micturition; mucous shreds in urine; on cooling becomes thick and cloudy, or deposits a thick sediment, yellowish-red with the upper stratum yellow and flocculent. θCatarrh of bladder.

▮Subacute and chronic catarrh of bladder.

Burning and stinging in urethra during and after micturition.

23 **Female Sexual Organs.** Menses come on too soon; has to press in her l. side at tenth rib to relieve gnawing pain.

25 **Voice and Larynx. Trachea and Bronchia.** Sudden hoarseness when reading aloud.

▮Aphonia from severe cold or excessive use of voice.

Irritation in larynx inducing a short, hacking cough.

Sudden tickling in larynx excites cough.

Tenacious mucus in larynx inducing frequent hawking, which results in discharge of small lumps of mucus.

Constant inclination to clear throat and swallow saliva.

Great dryness of throat impeding speech.

Titillating, scraping feeling in throat.

▮▮Catarrh of pharynx in a tenor lasting six months; not hoarse but when mucus collected in fauces was uncertain of his ability to bring out either high or low tones; voice feeble; throat red, covered with a thin layer of dark green, half-transparent mucus; burning and raw feeling in throat and hawking.

▮Influenza: constant tickling and burning in throat and larynx, leaving patient not a moment's rest and preventing him from lying down; fear of suffocation.

▮Grippe with stitches in r. eye when coughing.

▮Constant burning and tickling in larynx and throat, with danger of suffocation when lying; copious expectoration of tough mucus; relief by outdoor exercise. θInfluenza.

Laryngeal phthisis.

Increased secretion of mucus in trachea, which he is constantly obliged to hawk up.

▮Copious accumulation of tough mucus in air tubes which causes the greatest, often ineffectual, efforts at coughing and hawking for its expulsion. θBronchitis.

26 **Respiration.** ▮Sensation as if chest were too narrow, with tendency to relieve this feeling by taking deep inspirations and respirations. θAsthma.

▮Short breathing and oppression of chest when going up stairs.

Dyspnœa as from stagnation in lungs.

Oppressed breathing, as if chest were not wide enough, especially in open air and when stooping.

Shortness of breath from accumulation of mucus in chest and trachea.

Dyspnœa, especially during rest.

27 **Cough.** Dry cough with oppression of chest and roughness in throat.

Frequent short and hacking cough, occasioned by an increased secretion of mucus in larynx, especially in open air and when walking rather fast.

Dry cough with aphonia; < in cold air and walking, > by warm air and rest.

Irritating cough with secretion of mucus, with much pain about chest.

▮Soreness of chest, dry cough; throat dry; hoarseness, later much mucus in bronchi and trachea.

Cough < in morning, while dressing and before breakfast.

▮Irritating, shaking dry cough, in chronic bronchitis in the aged.

Loose, faint, hacking cough, with expectoration of a little phlegm.

Cough often ends in a sneeze.

Shaking cough like whooping cough, from burning and tickling in larynx, in morning, with copious expectoration of tough, white mucus like white of egg.

▮▮Whistling cough; great oppression of chest; pressing pains when breathing; cough dry or yellow expectoration, at times streaked with blood; inflammatory conditions of chest; useless in convulsive stage. θWhooping cough.

▮Whooping cough: chubby children; tough expectoration clear like white of egg; cough < toward evening; expectoration difficult to raise; crushing weight on chest; < at night with excessive rattling of mucus.

28 **Inner Chest and Lungs.** Congestion to chest, with flushes of heat in face and frequent pulse in afternoon.

Tightness and oppression of chest, especially during rest.

Rattling in chest; loose but feeble cough with little expectoration; hydrothorax

Feeling as if thorax were too narrow, with constant inclination to widen it by deep inhalation; burning in chest.

Certain movements, especially stooping, cause a pain in

chest as if it were too tight; there is a disposition to expand chest by frequent stretching; this leaves considerable soreness in chest.

‖ Soreness through chest, with feeling of oppression when in open air and when reposing; headache > in open air.

Soreness in chest, < by pressure, coughing and sneezing.

Violent aching pain in chest, at night, when waking.

Burning sore pain under sternum, especially during motion and on every deep inspiration.

Stitches in chest when coughing and breathing.

Shooting stitches in chest < during inspiration and rest.

Dull stitches and burning pain in chest when lying on r. side.

| Walls of chest sensitive or painful when touched or when he sneezes (often as a remnant of colds).

Stepping hard, walking fast or running causes pulling, sore pain as if through mediastinum.

Accumulation of mucus in chest.

| Constant accumulation of phlegm in bronchial tubes, with irritation in bowels, tendency to diarrhœa; irritation may alternate from chest to bowels and vice versa.

‖ Profuse secretion of mucus in lungs of old people, with loose, rattling cough.

| Great rattling of mucus in chest, with flying pains in chest.

Great soreness in walls of chest and great accumulation of clear albuminous mucus which is difficult to expectorate; pressure on chest as if lungs were pushed back to spine.

| Profuse expectoration of clear, transparent mucus; whole chest filled with large mucous râles. θGrippe.

| Tough mucus causes the greatest, often ineffectual efforts of coughing and hawking for its expulsion. θBronchitis.

| Bronchitis of old people; irritating, shaking cough.

‖ Twentieth day of pneumonia in a woman, æt. 56, r. side, violent stitches, sinking strength, small, scarcely perceptible pulse, short rare cough without expectoration, great rattling of mucus in chest, somnolence, dejected features.

| Adynamic pneumonia; low fever and much prostration.

‖ Pleuro-pneumonia in l. lung; at first *Bry.*, *Acon.*, *Bell.* had been given; the lancinating pains had completely disappeared, but there was still some oppression; expectoration was without blood, but very difficult, and strength was greatly reduced; in evening covered with cold sweat; pulse very small and wiry; oppression so great he must sit upright constantly; mucus stagnating and rattling in chest.

‖ Pleurisy in a latent form; dulness in lower three-fourths of r. side of chest; ægophony of same side toward upper part of lung; pulse 110; *Seneg.* removed not only the effusion but also the thickening of the pleura consequent on the pleurisy.

‖ Pleurisy; after inflammation has passed; copious mucous secretion with difficult expectoration; tightness and burning in chest.

| Subacute or chronic exudations of pleura; catarrhal pleuro-pneumonia.

Hydrothorax and ascites after scarlatina; anasarca; ascites; hoarse and feeble cough, with little expectoration.

| Phthisis mucosa.

29 **Heart, Pulse and Circulation.** | Boring pain about heart.

Heart's beat shakes the whole body; violent palpitation while walking.

Pulse hard and frequent.

30 **Outer Chest.** General sensitiveness or simple pain of walls of thorax, especially when touching them, it is felt less during a deep inspiration.

| Soreness of walls of chest on moving arms, particularly left.

31 **Neck and Back.** Pressing pain between scapulæ, especially when stepping hard, or on other movements which concuss the chest.

Pulse rather hard and accelerated.

Pain under r. shoulder blade, as if chest would burst, when coughing or drawing a long breath.

32 **Upper Limbs.** Sensation as if wrist were sprained.

33 **Lower Limbs.** Sensation of great weakness or debility in legs; joints feel as if lame.

35 **Rest. Position. Motion.** Most symptoms, especially those of chest, are $<$ when at rest and $>$ when walking in open air.

Rest: dyspnœa; dry cough $>$; tightness of chest; shooting through chest.

Cannot lie down: tickling in larynx; fear of suffocation.

Lying on r. side: pain in chest.

Stooping: oppressed breathing; pain in chest.

Motion: pain under sternum; of arm, soreness of walls of chest.

Going up stairs: shortness of breathing and oppression of chest.

Stepping hard, walking fast or running: causes pulling, sore pain as if through mediastinum; pressing pain between scapulæ.

Walking: fast, causes short, hacking cough; violent palpitation.

36 **Nerves.** Faintness when walking in open air.
Great mental and bodily lassitude.
Lassitude and slight trembling of upper extremities.
▮Sensation of trembling, with no visible trembling.
Legs feel weak, joints feel lame.
Great debility with stretching of limbs, confusion, heaviness and beating in head.
Great weakness which seems to originate in chest.
Mental and physical debility, with dropsical effusions.

37 **Sleep.** In evening, as soon as one lies down, heavy sleep; in morning awakes frequently with dyspnœa.

38 **Time.** Morning: hardened mucus in eyelashes; blepharitis ciliaris <; tongue slimy; cough <; awakes from dyspnœa.
Afternoon: heat in face and frequent pulse.
Evening: pressure in eyes <; toward, whooping cough.
Night and morning: urine passed only.
Night: involuntary micturition; whooping cough <; aching in chest.

39 **Temperature and Weather.** Warm air: dry cough <.
Warm room: pain in head.
Open air: pain in forehead <; lachrymation; sore throat and cough <; oppressed breathing; short, hacking cough; headache >; oppression of chest; faintness when walking; chilliness and chill only in.
Cold air: dry cough <.

40 **Fever.** Shuddering over back, heat in face, weak, burning eyes, beating headache, difficult breathing, body feels bruised.
Flushes of heat; skin hot; skin becomes warmer and moister.
Chilliness and chill almost only in open air, with weakness in legs and dyspnœa.
Shudders over back with heat in face and chest symptoms.
Sudden flushes of heat.
Perspiration wanting.

41 **Attacks, Periodicity.** Alternate: irritation from chest to bowels and vice versa.
For five minutes: sneezing.
For six months: catarrh of pharynx.

42 **Locality and Direction.** Right: stitches in eye; stitches in side; pain under shoulder blade.
Left: pain in forehead <; pimple on margin of lower lid; paralytic feeling on half of face; must press side to relieve pain; pleuro-pneumonia in lung; moving arm causes soreness of walls of chest.

43 **Sensations.** Eyes pain as if they were pressed out; as if eyeballs were being expanded; as if soap were in eyes;

as if red pepper were throughout nostrils and air passages; as if chest were too narrow; dyspnœa as from stagnation in lungs; as if lungs were pushed back to spine; as if chest would burst; as if wrist were sprained; joints as if lame.

Pain: about chest; in walls of thorax; under r. shoulder blade.

Flying pains: in chest.

Boring pain: about heart.

Digging pain: in epigastrium.

Shooting stitches: in chest.

Stitches: in r. eye; in chest.

Dull stitches: in chest.

Cramps: in stomach.

Gnawing: in bowels; under tenth rib l. side.

Pressing pain: in forehead and orbits; in abdomen; between scapulæ.

Drawing: in eyeballs.

Aching pain: in head; over orbits; in chest.

Stinging: in urethra.

Smarting: of conjunctiva.

Burning: of eyes; in throat, mouth and on tongue; in stomach; in urethra; in larynx; in chest; and under sternum.

Soreness: of chest; in walls of chest.

Scraping feeling: in throat.

Heat: in face.

Beating: in head.

Pressure: in eyes; below pit of stomach; on chest.

Tingling: in eyelids.

Titillating feeling: in throat.

Dryness: of Schneiderian membrane of throat.

Oppression: in upper part of chest.

Tightness: of chest.

Dulness: in head.

Emptiness: in stomach.

Weakness: of legs.

Reeling sensation: in head.

Paralytic feeling: in l. half of face.

" **Tissues.** Catarrhs that tend to leave sore and tender places in walls of chest as if there were left circumscribed spots of inflammation.

Diseases of mucous membranes; especially of lining of larynx, trachea and bronchia.

Subacute or chronic exudations of pleura, catarrhal pleuropneumonia (after *Bry.*) in cachectic pleuritis, in hydrothorax, œdema pulmonum, in diseases of heart, primary and secondary anasarca; in dropsies after albuminuria;

hydrophthalmia with intraocular compression; in ascites accompanying hepatic diseases, peritonitis and abdominal tumors; in lymphatic constitutions with tendency to mucous and serous exudations.

Dropsy of internal organs (especially after inflammation).

Inflammation of internal organs.

45 **Touch. Passive Motion. Injuries.** Touch: walls of chest painful; of vesicles causes itching.

Pressure: on l. side >; pain; soreness of chest <.

Rubbing: glistening before eyes <.

Bites of poisonous or enraged animals.

46 **Skin.** Burning vesicles, itching when touched.

47 **Stages of Life, Constitution.** Especially suitable for plethoric, phlegmatic persons.

Girl, æt. 5; after scarlatina; ascites.

Girl, æt. 13, after miliary fever; hydrothorax and anasarca.

Tenor singer, æt. 26, suffering six months; catarrh of pharynx.

Miss X., æt. 30, small stature, poor constitution, pale, thin face; latent pleurisy.

Man, æt. 33; oculo-motor paresis.

Man, æt. 33, slender, leading a sedentary life, first noticed trouble with eyes four years ago; paresis of oculo-motor nerve.

Woman, æt. 56; pneumonia.

Man, æt. 60; pleuro-pneumonia.

48 **Relations.** Compare; *Ammon.* in bronchial affections; *Calc. ost.* in fat and plethoric people predisposed to catarrhs; *Caustic.* in muscular asthenopia, loss of voice, paralytic conditions; *Phosphor.* in laryngeal and pulmonary catarrh; *Spongia* in bronchial catarrh.

SEPIA

Cuttle Fish. *Mollusca.*

Introduced by Hahnemann.

The cuttie fish is an inhabitant of the European seas, particularly the Mediterranean. Its ink bag contains a blackish-brown excretory liquor with which it darkens the water when it wishes to escape its enemies or catch its prey.

The triturations and tincture are made from the pure, dry, genuine Sepia, not from the artificial India ink used in drawing.

Provings by Hahnemann, Gersdorff, Goullon, Hartlaub, Walde, Gross, Archiv für Hom., vol. 19, p. 187; Robinson, Br. Jour. of Hom. vol. 25, p. 331; Berridge, N. Am. Jour. of Hom., 1871, p. 69; Ibid., 1873, p. 193; N. E. Med. Gaz., 1874, p. 402; also provings with the higher dilutions and triturations upon twenty-five individuals under the auspices of the Amer. Institute of Hom., see Transactions, 1875.

Clinical Authorities.—*Mental derangement*, Müller, Rück. Kl. Erf., vol. 1, p. 46; Haynel, Analy. Therap., vol. 1, p. 177; Wilson, Rück. Kl. Erf., vol. 5, p. 11; *Apoplexy*, Gerson, Rück. Kl. Erf., vol .5, p. 32; *Headache*, Hahnemann, Hrg, Kreussler, Tietze, Black, Goullon, Haustein, Hirsch, Schindler, S. in. K., Rück. Kl. Erf., vol. 1, p. 198; Müller, Rück. Kl. Erf., vol. 5, p. 94; Hansen, A. H. Z., vol. 108, p. 93; Berridge, A. J. H. M. M., vol. 4, p. 114; Haynel, A. J. H. M. M., vol. 4, p. 129; Lippe, Hom. Phys., vol. 6, p. 429; Price, Med. Inv., Sept., 1876, p. 194; Ockford, Org., vol. 1, p. 468; *Hemicrania*, Kreussler, A. J. H. M. M., vol. 4, p. 75; *Sick-headache*, Small, U. S. M. and S. J., Oct., 1870; *Matting of the hair*, Lembke, Rück. Kl. Erf., vol. 4, p. 317; *Asthenopia*, Bell, H. M., vol. 6, p. 289; *Short-sight*, Woodyatt, Med. Couns., vol. 1, p. 12; *Incipient cataract*, B. J. H., vol. 33, p. 331; *Cataract*, Goullon, I. Pr., 1875, p. 691; Raue's Rec., 1875, p. 59; *Keratitis*, Norton, N. Y. S. Trans., 1874, p. 432; Raue's Rec.. 1875, p. 54; *Ophthalmia*, Tietze, Schmid, Link, Rück. Kl. Erf., vol. 1, p. 241; Bethmann, Wolf, B. J. H., vol. 6, p. 525; Theobald, Org., vol. 1, p. 109; *Conjunctivitis*, Gerson, Rück. Kl. Erf., vol. 5, p. 109; Norton, T. W. H. C., 1876, pp. 603, 621; *Tarsal tumor*, Reisig, Rück. Kl. Erf., vol. 1, p. 242; *Stitches in ear, etc.*, Schmitt, Hom. Phys., vol. 3, p. 355; *Epistaxis*, Gerner, Rück. Kl. Erf., vol. 1, p. 415; *Nasal catarrh*, Hansen, A. H. Z., vol. 113, p. 61; *Ozæna*, Freytag, Rück. Kl. Erf., vol. 1, p. 399; *Facial neuralgia*, Beckett, Hah. Mo., vol. 11, p. 584; *Warts on face*, Jones, N. A. J. H., vol. 17, p. 11; *Tinea tonsurans*, Burnett, H. W., vol. 8, p. 37; *Fistula of cheek, and cough*, Hesse, Hom. Phys., vol. 3, p. 162; *Scirrhus of lip*, Hartmann, Rück. Kl. Erf., vol. 1, p. 445; *Carcinoma of lip*, Kunkel, A. H. Z., vol. 95, p. 21; *Toothache*, Bœnninghausen, Schindler, Rück. Kl. Erf., vol. 1, p. 477; Bœnninghausen, Hom. Phys., vol. 6, p. 372; Goullon, Bolle, N. A. J. H., vol. 17, p. 224; Goullon, Hom. Recorder, vol. 3, p. 23, from Pop. Zeit., Oct., 1887; *Chronic affections of throat*, Rummel, Diez, Rück. Kl. Erf., vol. 1, p. 540; *Gastralgia*, Boyce, Med. Couns., vol. 1, p 164; Boyce, Org., vol. 3, p. 93; *Pressure in stomach*, Hesse, Hom. Phys., vol. 7, p. 26; *Gastric disturbance*, Emmerich, Kreuss, Rück. Kl. Erf., vol. 1, p. 662; Guernsey, Bib. Hom., vol. 8, p. 30; Guernsey, H. M., vol. 6, p. 18; *Dyspepsia*, Clifton Hom. Rev., vol. 17, p. 159; *Catarrh of stomach*, Hirsch, N. A. J. H., vol. 4, p. 341; A. H. Z., vol. 83, p. 81; Raue's Rec., 1872, p. 131; *Pains in liver*, Hansen, A. H. Z., vol. 113, p. 68; Berridge, Hom. Phys., vol. 9, p. 149; *Functional derangement of liver* (2 cases) Dunham Lectures on Mat. Med., p. 156; *Hepatic disorder*, Hesse, Hom. Phys., vol. 3, p. 160; Berridge, Hom. Phys., vol. 4, p. 288; *Icterus*, Schmidt, Bœnningh., Rück. Kl. Erf., vol. 1, p. 703; *Pain in abdomen*, Berridge, Hom. Phys., vol. 9, p. 195; *Abdominal complaint*, Kreussler, A. J. H. M. M., vol. 4, p. 77; *Chronic diarrhœa*, Tietzer, Rück. Kl. Erf., vol. 1, p. 849; *Diarrhœa*, Kafka, Rück. Kl. Erf., vol. 5, p. 432; Clark, Hom. World, May, 1889; *Chronic constipation*, Nunez, Hom. Phys., vol. 9, p. 323; *Prolapsus of rectum*, Colby, Mass. Trans., vol. 4, p. 185; *Nocturnal enuresis*, Bœnningh., Rück. Kl. Erf., vol. 2, p. 45; Gauwerky, N. A. J. H., vol. 3, p. 342; Warren, N. E. M. G., vol. 9, p. 102; *Incontinence of urine*, Wesselhoeft, A. J. H. M. M., vol. 4, p. 69; *Cystitis and irritability of bladder*, Wesselhoeft, A. J. H. M. M., vol. 4, p. 63; *Irritable bladder*, Swan, N. A. J., vol. 30, p. 105; *Urinary difficulty*, Swan, N. A. J. H., vol. 21, p. 109; *Seminal emissions*, B. in D., Rück. Kl. Erf., vol. 2, p. 63; *Gonorrhœa*, Hansen, A. H. Z., vol. 108, p. 86; Hoyne, M. I., 1876, p. 542; *Gleet*, Lobeth, Seidel, Rück. Kl. Erf., vol. 2, p. 98; *Condylomata*, W. M. J., Hom. Phys., vol. 9, p 228; *Sterility*, Allen, A. J. H. M. M., vol. 3, p. 1; *Ovarian neuralgia*, Gerson, Rück. Kl. Erf., vol. 5, p 618; *Uterine displacement*, Jackson, Hom. Rev., vol. 5, p. 320; Jackson, Med. Inv., July, 1875, p. 74; Pröll, A. H. Z., vol. 94, p. 13; Parsons, T. A. I. H., 1882, p. 180; *Prolapsus uteri*, Tietze, Rück. Kl. Erf., vol. 2, p. 345; Minton, Tr. H. M. S. N. Y., 1870, p. 535; *Partial procidentia*, Goodno, Hah. Mo., vol. 8, p. 63; *Procidentia*, Medley, Med. Adv., Jan., 1889, p. 33; *Metrorrhagia*, Knorr, Kallenbach, Rück. Kl. Erf., vol. 2, p. 334; Terry, N. A. J. H., vol. 25, p. 314; *Hydrometra*, Wells, N. A. J. H., vol. 3, p. 89; *Menstrual disturbance*, Simpson, Hom. Rev., vol. 18, p. 212; Terry, N. A. J. H., vol. 25, p. 314; *Dysmenorrhœa*, Goullon, A. H. Z., vol. 80, p. 7; Polle, Hom. Kl., 1869, p. 125; Kafka, A. H. Z., vol. 78, p. 5; *Amenorrhœa, Dysmenorrhœa*, Bernstein, Diez, Eichhorn, Lembke, Rück. Kl. Erf., vol. 2, p. 254; Hansen, A. H. Z., vol. 108, p. 86; *Pain in vagina and rectum*, Bæthig, A. J. H. M. M., vol. 1, p. 161; *Vaginitis*, Hedenburg, Mass. Trans., vol. 4, p. 295; Gorton, Hah. Mo., vol. 7, p. 514; *Leucorrhœa*, Knorr, Green, Rück. Kl. Erf., vol. 2, p. 365; Gardiner, A. J. H. M. M., vol. 1, p. 79; Minton, Tr. H. M. S. N. Y., 1870, p. 535; Hawley, Hom. Phys., vol. 8, p. 263; *Infantile leucorrhœa*, Sumner, N. Y. S. Trans., 1874, p. 314; *Pruritus vulvæ*, Guernsey, T. H. W. Conv., 1876, p. 984; *Scirrhus mammæ* (2 cases reported cured), Burdick, Org., vol. 2. p. 228; Gambell, N. E. M. G., vol. 5, p. 558; *Disorders of pregnancy*, Tietze, Rück. Kl. Erf., vol. 2, p. 387; Gambell, T. H. M. S. N. Y., 1870, p. 170; *Dystocia*, Schmitt, Hom. Phys., vol. 7, p 260; *Retained placenta and recurring hemorrhages*, Nash, Med. Adv., Feb., 1890, p. 105; *Shortness of breath* (4 cases), Hesse, A. H. Z., vol. 110, p. 148; *Dyspnœa*, Hesse, A. H. Z., vol. 111, p. 44; *Asthma*, Carr, Med Inv., March, 1875, p. 245; *Cough*, Kafka, Rück. Kl. Erf., vol. 5, p. 695; Nithak, Rück. Kl. Erf., vol. 3, p. 198; Analyt. Therap., vol. 1, p. 212; Küsemann, Bethmann, Rück. Kl. Erf., vol. 3, p. 27; Wesselhoeft, A. J. H. M. M., vol. 4, pp. 66, 67; T. A. I. H., 1870, p. 250; Hesse, Hom. Phys., vol. 3, p. 159; *Whooping cough*, Hartmann, Rück. Kl. Erf., vol. 3, p. 84; Wesselhoeft, A. J. H. M. M., vol. 4, p. 3; Goullon, Raue's Rec., 1875, p. 117; *Pain in chest and cough*, Nichols, Hah. Mo., vol. 7, p. 115; *Pleuritis*, Kunkle, Hah. Mo., vol. 15, p. 294; *Phthisis pulmonalis*, Ehrhardt, Gross, Rück.

Kl. Erf., vol. 3, p. 397; *Palpitation of heart*, Hesse, Hom. Phys., vol. 7, p. 27, from A. H. Z., vol. 113, p. 138; *Perimyelitis*, Hirsch, Rück. Kl. Erf., vol. 5, p. 874; *Pain in back*, Hesse, Hom. Phys., vol. 7, p. 27; *Crick in back*, A. F. R., Med. Inv., vol. 6, p. 563; *Whitlow*, Berridge, Org., vol. 1, p. 132; *Sciatica*, Battmann, Rück. Kl. Erf., vol. 5, p. 906; *Aching in legs*, Berridge, Hom. Phys., vol. 9, p. 192; *Eruption on legs*, Hansen, A. H. Z., vol. 113, p. 69; Berridge, Org., vol. 1, p. 113; *Debility*, Dunham, N. Y. S. Trans., 1876, p. 87; *Hysteria*, Hartmann, Lobethal, Rück. Kl. Erf., vol. 2, p. 289; Bartlett, N. A. J. H., vol. 3, p. 530; *Chorea*, Piollet, Rück. Kl. Erf., vol. 4, p. 513; *Morbid sweats*, Gallavardin, N. A. J. H., vol. 15, p. 61; Gorton, U. S. M. and S. J., vol. 9, p. 13; *Gastric fever*, S. in K., Rück. Kl. Erf., vol. 4, p. 649; *Ague*, Schmidt, Rück. Kl. Erf., vol. 4, p. 988; Ring, A. J. H. M. M., vol. 1, p. 261; Morgan, A. J. M. M., vol. 3, p. 131; Kunkel, A. H. Z., vol. 106, p. 189; *Chlorosis*, Rückert, Rück. Kl. Erf., vol. 2, p. 279; Jones, N. A. J. H., vol. 17, p. 8; *Dropsy*, Goullon, I. Pr., 1875, p. 695; *Rheumatism*, Wells, Hom. Rev., vol. 3, p. 259; Berridge, Hom. Rev., vol. 16, p. 495; Hesse, Hom. Phys., vol. 7, p. 26; *Articular rheumatism*, Kunkel, Hah. Mo., vol. 15, pp. 486–9; *Boils and offensive foot sweat*, Morgan, H. W., vol. 12, p. 71; *Brown spots on skin*, Scales, Mass. Trans., vol. 4, p. 185; *Urticaria*, Schwarze, Rück. Kl. Erf., vol. 4, p. 202; *Tetter*, Williamson, T. H. M. S., Pa., 1873; *Psoriasis*, Hesse, A. H. Z., vol. 108, p. 94; Hall, N. E. M. G., vol. 9, p. 53; *Impetigo*, Miller, H. M., vol. 10, p. 162; *Pemphigus*, Moore, Hom. Rev., vol. 12, p. 304; *Warts*, Hartmann, Rück. Kl. Erf., vol. 4, p. 311; *Diseases of skin*, Hahnemann, Knorr, Schmöle, Bethmann, Sommer, Rück. Kl. Erf., vol. 4, p. 260.

[1] **Mind.** ▮▮Weak memory.

▮Heavy flow of ideas; inability for mental activity; it is an exertion to think.

▮Felt all day as if he did not care what happened; no desire to work, inattentive, absent-minded; indolent mood.

▮Language comes very slowly, has to drag out the words to express ideas; forget the chief points.

Uses wrong words when writing.

▮Great indifference to everything; no proper sense of life.

▮Every few minutes inclined to cry, without knowing the cause.

▮Great sadness and frequent attacks of weeping which she can scarcely suppress.

▮Very sad with unusual lassitude.

▮Sad and gloomy mood, mostly when walking in open air and in evening.

▮Sad about her health and domestic affairs, discontented with everything.

▮Gloominess; she feels unfortunate without cause.

▮Dark forebodings about his disease in regard to the future.

▮▮Felt that unless he held on to something he should scream.

▮Depression on awaking in morning.

▮Very nervous; great excitability in company; restless, fidgety; wants to go from one bed to another.

▮Nerves very sensitive to the least noise.

▮Fits of involuntary weeping and laughter.

▮▮Aversion to one's occupation and family.

▮Dread of being alone.

▮▮Anxiety: with fear, flushes of heat over face; about real or imaginary evils; toward evening.

▮▮Great indifference to one's family, to those they love best.

▮Is easily offended and inclined to be vehement.

▮Great irritability alternating with indifference.

▮Greedy, miserly.

▮After overexertion of mind, bookkeepers, etc.

‖Quiet, introspective, rarely speaks a word voluntarily, sits for hours occupied with her knitting, her answers are intelligent but curt.

▮Propensity to suicide from despair about his miserable existence.

▮Fears to starve, is peevish, and feels mortified, easily frightened and full of evil forebodings.

‖After metrorrhagia oversensitive, exalted nervous state; hasty speech accompanied by quick gestures; eyes fiery and glistening; pulse 110; her movements were like those of a passionate person; if she could not talk her friends had to relate stories continually in a quick way: at times in the opposite state, gave short answers and desired to be alone; was then moody and feigned sleep; the nights became more and more anxious and restless; she could not describe how terrible they were.

Contradictory, quarrelsome, complaining about others.

▮Passionate, irritable.

▮Fretful and out of humor for all business.

▮Greatest irritability from slightest causes; very easily offended.

▮Vexed and disposed to scold.

Impatience when sitting, like an uneasiness in bones.

Violent bursts of anger with furious gestures.

‖Great nervous irritability, with sadness, despondency and absentmindedness; everything seems strange to her; least exertion seems a great effort; it seems as if she could not understand anything and would have to learn anew everything she wished to do; greatest indifference to everything, the death of a near relative, or some happy occurrence, leaves her equally unaffected; no trace of her former love for friends or even for her child; aversion for social intercourse amounting to contempt; constant ill-humor; at times headache with anxiety, < lying down; head also hurts externally; confusion and throbbing in head; constant pains in occiput, < lying; oversensitive to noise; frequent pains in back extending down into legs and feet; circulation and action of heart weak, sensation as if heart stood still; menses irregular; at times nervous twitchings; screams on least provocation; strength and general condition good; > in a warm climate, also after nosebleed; < after coffee and opium.

2 **Sensorium.** ▮Stupefaction of head, mental weakness or dulness, can scarcely think.

▮Painful confusion in head, particularly in forehead.

▮Momentary attacks of giddiness when walking in open air or while writing.

▮Vertigo: while walking, as if every object were in motion; with staggering; when drinking; as if objects were moving around one; as if suspended in air, with unconsciousness; when rising from bed in afternoon; after losses of fluids.

▮Congestion of blood to head; heaviness of head.

3 **Inner Head.** Drawing pain seeming to be external on forehead back to occiput, in single drawings.

Single, violent, undulating jerks of pressing headache in forehead.

Tearing in upper part of r. side of forehead.

Tearing in l. frontal eminence.

Violent stitches outward over l. orbit, with complete drawing together of eye, for three successive days, after rising in morning, continuing until noon, somewhat < in open air.

Stitches in forehead with nausea (she cannot eat), > from lying down.

Fulness in temples and forehead and throbbing of carotids.

Tearing in l. temple to upper part of l. side of head.

▮Pressure on vertex, < after mental labor.

Beating, very painful headache in vertex, in morning, soon after rising.

Dull aching frontal headache.

Headache in forehead and vertex, followed by anxiety in pit of stomach with trembling, afterward violent nosebleed.

Heavy pressing pain over l. eye extending toward side of head about 3 30 P.M.; sensation of great fulness deep in l. orbit at 4 P.M.; headache confined to l. side, > in evening and in open air; < by shaking head.

▮Shooting pains from within out, especially over l. eye, extorting cries, with vomiturition.

Occasionally darting pains extending from l. eye over side of head toward occiput.

Headache > after meals, < by mental labor.

Severe pressure in forehead during menses, with discharge of hardened offensive matter from nose.

Stitching, pressive headache continuous in lower part of forehead just over eye,. < from motion, in house, > when walking in open air.

Headache: all day with great mental depression; in forenoon as if brain were crushed; as from pressure from within outward; as if head would burst; also from coughing; in morning, with nausea, until noon; most severe toward evening, especially when shaking head; following perspiration on r. side of head and face, with a surging in forehead, like waves of pain rolling up and beating against frontal bone.

Headache as from commotion of brain when stepping or when shaking head, > when sitting up or from slow exercise.

▮Pressing or bursting headache as if eyes would fall out, or head burst, < from stooping, motion, coughing or shaking head; continued hard motion relieves headache.

▮Pulsating headache in cerebellum, beginning in morning and lasting till noon or sometimes till evening; < from least motion, when turning eyes, when lying on back; > when lying on side, when closing eyes, when at rest and in a dark room.

▮Painful cracking in occiput.

Jerking pain upward like electric shocks in head.

▮Beating: in head; in occiput.

▮Paroxysms of hemicrania, stinging pain from within outward, in one (mostly l.) side of head or forehead, with nausea, vomiting and contraction of pupils; < indoors and when walking fast; > in open air and when lying on painful side.

▮Boring headache from within outward, forenoon till evening, feels as if he would die; < from motion and stooping; > by rest when closing eyes, from external pressure and sufficient sleep.

▮Sensation of coldness on vertex.

▮Headache with aversion to all food.

▮Hemicrania in hysterical women; pains stitching, pressing, tearing or twitching with passive congestion of head; in chronic cases where the nervous system has long been disordered; leucorrhœa between menses; sudor hystericus, peculiar sweet-smelling sweat, particularly in axillæ and about soles of feet; face pale, dirty yellow, slender built.

▮Nervous, rheumatic or gouty pains in head, particularly in delicate, sensitive women.

▮Frequently recurring tearing, stitching pains in r. side of head, during pregnancy.

▮Hemicrania, r. side; drawing, tearing pains and now

and then stitches as if from needles; < morning and evening; menses scanty and of too short duration.

▮Severe pressure in occiput with heat and redness of face; eyes painful; lassitude and tiredness of limbs; inclination to cry; is not disposed to do anything.

▮Sore pain in l. eye and temple; throbbing, tearing and stitching pains in l. temple extending downward; stitching, like in an ulcer, in l. zygoma and teeth; hair of head sensitive to touch; pains < in paroxysms, with fainting; shivering; coldness of feet; transient heat; thirst; anxiety; despair of recovery.

▮Migraine after catching least cold; tearing, boring pains and at times stitches; must lie down and keep very quiet; closes eyes and presses head firmly to painful part; exposure to rough wind brings on an attack; aversion to food; stools pappy; menses too early.

‖Severe headaches, l. side, hysterical in character; tearing, drawing pains beginning at l. parietal region and becoming a pressing, throbbing pain in occiput, accompanied by nausea and vomiting; could not open eyes or move them; photophobia; obstinate constipation; violent desire for an embrace during attack.

‖Subject to headaches for five or six years; the pain is shooting, at a fixed point over eyebrow, generally r., but to-day over l.; pain causes twitching of eyebrow and desire to close eyes; headache is < on moving eyes, also on walking, every step seemed to jar; attacks come on suddenly and are intolerable first day, but always leave him very weak and dreading a return for a day or two; attacks excited by overfatigue, anxiety and vexation or overwork in school; occasionally severe sexual excitement with emission, not always with dreams, during sleep; this precedes but seldom accompanies headache; during headache there is inability to read, think or study; a more frequent attack of bowels, nausea, dislike to any food except toast or biscuits and tea; urine increased, nearly colorless; tenderness of bone of side of head affected and under corresponding supraorbital ridge

‖Vertigo as if intoxicated; tension in forehead and pressure as from a weight over eyes; pressure and burning in eyes and fog before r. eye (is blind in l. eye), lassitude; leucorrhœa, milky white, < during day.

‖Violent stitches in forehead, cries out; they distort his face; stitches return every five minutes during the day and night with unabating force, and extend into l. eye and ear; lachrymation; painfulness of scalp; cannot find an easy position for his head; every noise aggravates his symptoms; talking in the room is unbearable, cannot sleep.

|| Headache every Saturday for several years; boring pain from within outward, accompanied by nausea and vomiting; > binding head up tightly and after a good sleep.

|| Periodical headache coming on at 2 P.M., lasting till bed-time.

| Headache in terrific shocks.

| Dull, stupid headache, with great mental depression; anæmia.

| Shooting from forehead to vertex and both sides of face.

| Chronic congestive headaches with photophobia and impossibility to open eyes on account of weight on upper lid.

| Gouty, or nervous headaches, from abdominal plethora or menstrual disturbances.

| Headache with aversion to all food.

| Chronic paroxysmal headaches in women during climaxis; disorders of digestion, abdominal plethora and leucorrhœa.

| Attacks of sick headache and sudden obscuration of sight with each attack.

| Every time she goes shopping she has a severe nervous headache.

| Attacks of gouty pains in head, boring in character, causing patient to scream with pain, accompanied by vomiting.

| Congestive, gastric, hysteric, nervous and rheumatic headaches.

| Clavus hystericus.

|| Headache with aversion to all kinds of food, a feeling of emptiness and goneness in pit of stomach, very distressing; headache occurring every morning with nausea, vertigo, epistaxis; in women who have moth-patches on their foreheads, of sallow complexion, or who have a yellow streak across bridge of nose and under eyes; smell of food repulsive.

| Hemicrania from an affection of reproductive system; especially in young women in whom the cerebral nerves have excited the sympathetic, producing a long train of hysterical symptoms.

| Boring stinging over r. eye, < in a thunderstorm, in cold air, north wind, taking cold on head, etc.

| Losing hair after chronic headaches.

|| Chronic meningitis, headache < when lying down; > by remaining in a sitting position; when pain increased a sensation like globus hystericus; all coverings

of neck felt too tight; fulness, pulsation and beating in head; had her fingers continually on dress covering neck even when it was wide, the very touch of it distressed her.

▮Meningitis; the child is in a torpid condition, with great depression of vital power: urine has a putrid odor and deposits a clay-colored sediment which adheres to vessel or diaper.

▮Rush of blood to head.

▮Apoplexy: in men addicted to drinking and sexual excesses, with a disposition to gout and hemorrhoids; in women from affections of reproductive system; venous form; headache coming on in terrific shocks; dizziness in walking, with staggering; forgetfulness; coldness of feet; intermitting pulse.

▮Threatening apoplexy in dissipated, middle-aged men who are plethoric, have a large fat abdomen, and are subject to arthritic and hemorrhoidal complaints; they have usually passed through several slight attacks of apoplexy and are frequently visited by the prodromic symptoms.

4 **Outer Head.** ▮Involuntary jerking of head backward and forward, especially forenoons and when sitting.

▮Fontanelles remain open, with jerking of head, pale bloated face, stomacace, green diarrhœic stools.

▮Sensation of coldness on vertex, < when moving head and stooping; > when at rest and in open air.

▮Disposition to take cold from dry, cold wind or getting head wet.

External coldness of head.

Swelling on forehead.

Swelling on one side of head above temple, with itching; sensation of coldness and tearing in it, < when touching it; > when lying on it or after rising from bed.

▮Sweat on head smelling sour, with faintish weakness in evening before sleep or in morning.

▮Scalp pains when touched as if roots of hair were sore.

Itching of scalp.

▮Violent itching, like from insects, on occiput or behind ears.

Small red pimples on forehead, roughness.

▮Eruption on vertex and back part of head dry, offensive, stinging, itching and tingling with cracks; feeling sore when scratching; falling off of hair.

▮Sensitiveness of roots of hair, < in evening, to contact, to cold north winds; burning after scratching.

▮Dandruff comes in circles, like ringworm. θHerpes.

▮▮Great falling out of hair. θClimacteric period.

▮Scurfs very moist, almost constantly discharging puslike fluid.

▮Much scurf on head; moist scalp; tinea tonsurans.

▮Sensitiveness of roots of hair, < in evening, to contact, to cold north winds; burning after scratching.

‖A boy, æt. 9, had a bald spot on front part of head as large as a silver twenty-five cent piece, of glossy smoothness, hair around appeared as if cut short near roots, place covered with dry, crusty scales; soon after a similar spot on r. side of head; finally four bald spots differing in size from a dollar to a quarter.

‖The large coils of hair, for a distance of about two inches from head, became kinky so as to make combing of this part of hair an impossibility; there was no moisture about scalp on these places, nor was the hair itself tangled; the smaller coils at sides of head showed this condition also in the lower third of their length; menses absent; congestion of blood to head and chest; face red; headache.

5 **Sight and Eyes.** ▮Vanishing of sight; vision impeded by fiery zigzags or sparks (whooping cough); flickering before eyes when looking into light; green halo around candlelight; ▮▮black spots

Candlelight fatigues eyes when reading or writing by causing a contractive sensation.

Cannot bear reflected light from bright objects.

▮Gauze, black spots, or stripes before eyes.

▮Dulness of sight; when writing; sees only one-half of object clearly, the other half is obscured.

▮Great sensitiveness to light of day.

▮Prickling of eyes, evening by candlelight.

▮Asthenopia: associated with exhaustion dependent upon loss of semen; dependent upon reflex irritation from uterus (kopiopia hysterica).

‖Mr. B., æt. 32, sick several months; has abused eyes by reading, writing, sewing; trouble began in r. eye, which is the worse; sensation as if eye were gone and a cool wind blew out of socket; severe pains and itching around back of eye, when closing eyes flashes of light; mist like a veil or cloud before eye; < in strong light; using eyes causes intense headache over them; desire to spasmodically close eyes, which gives relief; menses regular, accompanied by severe bearing-down pain, with pain in hips and back and sexual excitement; feeling of weight and heaviness of upper lids as if she could not raise them, < in morning. θAsthenopia.

▮Obscuration of vision dependent upon hepatic derangement.

‖ Astigmatism from granular lids, on reading, black seemed grey; sight > when looking out from under brows, pain on using eyes by artificial light.

‖ A lady, æt. 67, was suddenly attacked after taking cold, with pressing pain around eyes, < in open air; constantly sees dark figures before eyes, like spider-web or lace, of size of a hand; acute pain in orbit of a pressive character, < in open air; r. eye only so affected; sight had been gradually failing for a long time; has been subject to sick headaches all her life. θIncipient cataract.

‖ Keratitis pust.; lashes of l. eye gone and edges of lids raw and sore, considerable purulent discharge from eyes, face covered with an eruption, child cries on washing.

| Very large pustules around cornea with much redness, no pain or photophobia, < in evening, corners of mouth cracked.

| Keratitis parenchymatosa, with uterine troubles.

| Pustules on cornea, also fungus hæmatodes.

| Trachoma, with or without pannus, especially in tea drinkers.

The eyes feel tired and look injected; tendency to keep them closed.

Eyes feel sore as if bruised.

Pressure in r. eye as from a grain of sand, < by rubbing; < when pressing eyelids together.

Pressure in eyes at night.

Great burning of eyes and lachrymation.

Aching over eyes if he goes into bright daylight.

Lids pain on waking as if too heavy to open.

Itching of internal canthus morning after waking; after rubbing, biting and severe lachrymation and sore sensation in external canthus, which is agglutinated.

Biting in r. eye evenings, with inclination of lids to forcibly close.

Sticking in l. eye.

Smarting pain in both eyes.

Burning of eyes mornings with weakness afternoons.

Eyes hot and dry; feel like balls of fire.

Redness of conjunctivæ.

‖ Inflammatory affections of asthenic character, conjunctiva a dull red, some photophobia and swelling of lids, < in mornings.

| Acute catarrhal conjunctivitis, with drawing in external canthus and smarting in eyes, > by bathing in cold water, < morning and evening.

| Conjunctivitis with muco-purulent discharge in morning and great dryness in evening.

| Inflammation of eyes, with stitching and pressure.

‖ Right eye inflamed; heat, vessels much enlarged, with a patch of congestion; sometimes feeling of grit in it; eyeball aches at back, smarts when reading; subject to faceache and indigestion, weight after food and spasmodic flatulent pains.

‖ Right side of face much swollen, deep red, covered with pimples filled with pus and covered with yellow crusts; during day did not open eyes, only raised lids for an instant in the dark; rubbed and scratched cheeks and eyes; lids glued together in morning by thick matter; no appetite; much thirst; little sleep; r. eye seemed much smaller than l.; r. angle of mouth drawn upward.

‖ Stitches in eyes; lids swollen; photophobia, can hardly open eyes; profuse lachrymation; sensation of heat in eyes; stuffiness of l. nostril; head confused, dull.

‖ Coryza with ophthalmia and photophobia recurring often without apparent cause; lids red; spots on cornea. θScrofulous ophthalmia.

‖ Eyes agglutinated in morning; great photophobia and pains in eyes; pustules form on cornea which suppurate and burst, leaving long-lasting maculæ; recurring attacks since a year.

‖ Conjunctivitis; photophobia < in morning; dull redness of conjunctiva; lachrymation; swelling of lids and great heat in them.

‖ Pustular inflammation, dependent on uterine troubles, especially when cornea is affected and inflammation is not confined to conjunctiva; drawing, aching, piercing pains, < rubbing, pressing lids together or pressing upon eye; light of day dazzles and causes head to ache; conjunctiva swollen; eyes agglutinated, morning and evening; considerable purulent discharge; edges of lids raw and sore; feeling as if lids were too tight and did not cover ball; eruption on face. θConjunctivitis.

‖ Conjunctiva palp. injected in morning on awaking; discharge of purulent mucus; toward evening gradually increasing dryness of eye; biting-excoriating sensation in lids; photophobia; later burning pain; blepharospasmus; lachrymation suppressed; pulse hard, rapid; dull pain in forehead; during paroxysm cries aloud, and is greatly agitated; toward midnight spasm of lids ceases, pain decreases and arrested secretions reappear; brown spots in face; sediment in urine like brickdust. θConjunctivitis.

‖ Severe conjunctivitis, every Summer for twenty years, from beginning of warm weather in Spring until its close in the Fall; much enlargement of papillæ; marked aggravation in morning and usually in evening.

▮Phlyctenular conjunctivitis.

▮Follicular conjunctivitis, or a mixed form of follicular and trachomatous conjunctivitis, which is observed only during the Summer, or always < in hot weather.

‖Soreness in internal canthi with entropium, eyes < at night and at any time during day on closing them, the lids feel as if they were too tight and did not cover eye; scratching in eyes.

▮Amaurosis: with contracted pupils; after violent headaches.

▮Yellow color of whites of eyes. θJaundice.

‖Drawing sensation in external canthi, smarting in eyes > by bathing in cold water, < night and morning.

▮Drooping of lids with dull headache; feels as if he had not sense enough left to lift them.

▮Heat and dryness of margins of lids.

Eyelids pain on awaking as if too heavy, and as if he could not hold them open.

▮Lachrymation morning and evening, and in open air.

▮▮Redness of eyelids, with styes.

▮▮Nightly agglutination of eyes or dry scurf on lids on awaking.

Great itching on margins of lids.

Granulated lids, especially in tea drinkers.

‖Chronic ciliary blepharitis; scaly condition of lid margins; small pustules (acne ciliaris) on ciliary border.

▮Tarsal tumors.

‖After repeated styes, hard, indurated tarsal tumor as large as a pea, hindering motion of lid; of two years' standing.

▮Heaviness and falling of under lids as if they were paralyzed.

▮Difficulty of opening eyes in morning; paralyzed condition of lids. θPtosis.

‖Spasmodic entropion, with soreness of internal canthi and scratching in eyes, < at night and at any time during day on closing them; lids feel as if too tight and did not cover eyes.

‖A boy, æt. 12, had many little tumors on lower lids, the result of styes, which impeded movement of lids.

▮Brown-yellowish color of eyelids.

[6] **Hearing and Ears.** ▮Oversensitive to noise, and particularly to music.

▮Loud sounds and humming in ears followed by loss of hearing.

▮Sudden attacks of brief deafness.

Dragging pain or stitches in ears.

‖Chronic otalgia, one-sided, with toothache, returns after every slight cold.

▮Discharge of thin matter from ear.

▮Much itching in affected ear.

▮Swelling of and eruptions on external ear.

▮Tetter on lobes of ear, behind ears and on nape of neck.

▮Stitches in parotid glands, which swell, with tensive pain on turning head.

▮▮Stitches into r. ear, going into brain, commenced several days ago, at 9 A.M., while working in field, l. ear affected first; stitches < at night; small pustules on l. wrist, which, when opened, discharge a milky fluid; before this had panaritia of l. thumb and middle finger; since typhoid fever has been more sensitive to changes of weather, for the last few years bee-stings bother him more than they used to do.

7 **Smell and Nose.** ▮Great sensitiveness to odors.

▮Loss of smell, or fetid, subjective smell.

▮Nosebleed: during menses; during menses, in young girls; during pregnancy and with hemorrhoids; after slightest blow or when becoming overheated in slightest degree.

Nose dry; every symptom of cold in head; stuffed nose.

Dry feeling in nose and fauces.

Frequent sneezing without coryza.

▮Dry coryza, especially of l. nostril.

▮Fluent coryza with sneezing, early morning.

▮Blowing of large lumps of yellow-green mucus, or yellow-green crusts, with blood from nose.

▮▮Dry coryza; nostrils sore, swollen, ulcerated and scabby; discharging large green plugs.

▮Swollen, inflamed nose; nostrils sore, ulcerated and scabby.

▮Tip of nose: inflamed, swelled, scurfy; painful eruption.

▮Extremely offensive smell from nose, profuse greenish-yellow discharge; menses scanty, preceded by yellow, excoriating leucorrhœa, < from motion.

▮▮Large, offensive-smelling plugs from nose, often so large that they had to be drawn back into mouth and expectorated, causing vomiting; offensive-smelling, greenish discharge from l. nostril; severe throbbing pains in forehead (relieved by *Bellad.*); of thirteen years' standing. θOzæna.

▮Catarrh: pressive pain in root of nose; sore feeling in nose on drawing air through; nose swollen and inflamed, nostrils angry and ulcerated; small ulcers in nostrils; scurfy nostrils; discharge of yellow water from nose, with cutting pains in forehead; dryness in nose and throat; dryness in choanæ (though there is much mucus in mouth) with involuntary urging to swallow; catarrhs arising from a retrocession of an eruption.

▮The smell of cooking nauseates.

▮▮Yellow saddle across bridge of nose.

8 **Upper Face.** ▮Face: puffed; pale; yellow, earthy; in morning red, in evening pale; red and flushed.

▮▮Yellow saddle across upper part of cheeks and nose, and yellow spots on face; yellow around mouth.

▮Pale, sallow, puffiness, with margins around eyes.

▮Yellowish face with dyspepsia.

▮Small red pimples on forehead; rough forehead.

ǀǀCircular spots on face and under chin from quarter to half an inch in diameter; several appeared in rapid succession; spots at first bright red, later covered with a white scurf, then returning to original red color; spots are very slightly raised above the skin and attended with but little itching or sensibility; neuralgic pains shifting about in various parts of body, but more persistently located in occipital region, < remaining long in one position, at night in bed, in morning on rising; > changing position, and from slight exertion; constant feeling of languor and weariness, making least exertion disagreeable; complete anorexia. θPsoriasis.

▮Eczema narium.

▮Herpes, scurfs and black pores on face.

▮Tetters around mouth, with itching of face.

▮Swelling of under lip.

ǀǀInflammation and swelling on one side of face, from root of a decayed tooth.

ǀǀIntermittent prosopalgia, with congestion of eyes and head, jerking pains like electric shocks.

▮Faceache: intermittent, with congestion of eyes and head; during pregnancy; jerking, like electric shocks upward; pain appears in morning immediately on awaking, none in daytime but severe at night, spreading over lower and upper maxillæ, radiating to vertex, occiput, neck, arms and fingers; tearing, drawing pains in face and nose, with swelling of cheeks; pains frequently extend through ear, especially l.; < by taking either hot or cold things into mouth; in delicate, sensitive, nervous women, especially when uterine functions are disturbed.

ǀǀParoxysms of facial neuralgia brought on by riding in wind and from excitement; menstrual nisus nearly always attended with neuralgic pains of greater or less severity; when wind is the exciting cause the paroxysm comes on with a chill, and when excitement, it begins with trembling; pains > from pressure, being in a warm room and lying quiet; paroxysms manifest themselves by a slight chill or trembling; cold chills running down spine; neuralgic pains commence in l. temple and run over l. side of face and down ramus of l. jaw; pains are throbbing and digging; noise and odors from cooking make her <; attacks last about a day, usually < in evening; > from sleep; menses last two or three days, are dark, scanty, somewhat stringy; pain and heaviness in r. ovarian region, > by leaning forward; costive; stool alternately hard and soft with straining; emission of urine on coughing, walking or standing on her feet; urine light-colored and frequent; abdomen distended; appetite good; pain running down r. leg; < from northeasterly winds, damp weather and excitement. θFacial neuralgia.

‖ Neuralgic pains in face, l. side, from abuse of tobacco.

Jerking of muscles of face when talking.

9 **Lower Face.** ▮ Yellowness around mouth.

▮ Great dryness of lips.

▮ Moist scaly eruptions on red part of lips and on chin.

▮▮ Swelling and cracking of lower lip. θHerpes.

‖ Fistula in l. cheek in region of lower molars, with ulcerating circumference, size of a ten-cent piece; painless, discharges blood and pus, has lasted about a year; cough, at times with hoarseness, bloody expectoration; has lasted about two years; fine vesicular râles at l. apex; cough < in a dry east wind much more than in damp air or by getting wet; < in morning; is not so well on Sundays, being then at rest and in room, > while at work; < when lying on l. side; appetite good, thirsty in evening, sleeps well; his feet are sweaty and have an offensive odor.

‖ Suspicious tubercle on lower lip as large as a bean, of cartilaginous appearance, with a broad base and frequently bleeding, looking very much like a scirrhus.

‖ An epithelial cancer of lower lip far developed, had been excised; the wound healed kindly; after a few months the patient began to emaciate and to exhibit every sign of cancer cachexy; the decline was alarmingly rapid; eminent surgeons diagnosticated internal cancer; no hope of recovery was entertained.

▮ Swelling and soreness of lower lip, burning pain and a prickling as from a splinter of wood. θEpithelioma of lip.

‖ Carcinoma of lower lip was removed three times in the course of six months; it had again grown and was of size of a walnut, stony hard, etc.; tendency to reappearance every Spring for three years, *i. e.*, painful cracks in scars left by the operations.

‖ Appearance of warts on face, one after another, until

there were twelve about mouth and chin; they were rather long, quite roughed at the top, somewhat pedunculated, and speedily returned after ligation.

▮Swelling of submaxillary glands.

10 **Teeth and Gums.** ▮▮Toothache: drawing in upper molars; in a hollow tooth, extending to ear; throbbing; stitching; all teeth painful, particularly in hollow molar, which pains as if elongated and swollen, with swelling of gums and cheeks, with which the pain ceases; drawing < if anything hot or cold is taken into mouth; during menses drawing from teeth into cheek, which becomes swollen; tearing out through l. ear, during and after eating; sticking, she could have cried; stitches in teeth and jaw extending to ear, she could not sleep at night on account of it and during day had to tie a cloth over it; with rapid decay of teeth; and throbbing in gums during menses; during pregnancy with shortness of breath, worse from every cold draft of air, when touching teeth, when talking; biting teeth together.

▮▮Paroxysmal, beating throbbing toothache; can feel beating of pulse all over body; pains > from cold water, returning as soon as water gets warm; walks about crying; when pain is at its height, tingling in fingers of left hand, becoming a tearing pain as it extends up arm and is ended by a spasmodic attack of asthma; eyelids red, burning; blowing of blood from nose; anxious, despondent, lachrymose; during pregnancy.

▮▮Toothache starts from carious teeth of lower jaw, then spreads over whole left side, with tearing pains; nausea with waterbrash; > in fresh air, < from cold water and at night; no intermissions, difficulty of speaking or chewing; fear of trismus; no swelling or abscess; hot flashes with cold feet; during climaxis.

▮▮Severe pains in teeth for several days, on one side only, extending to r. side of head; great internal heat; obliged to keep her mouth half open to cool the mouth, hence great dryness in it; afraid of tetanus.

▮▮Long-continued severe toothache, caries; l. sided, tearing, drawing pain; waterbrash during pain; < during night, especially before midnight, in bed, by cold and eating; nervousness; migraine; leucorrhœa; climaxis.

▮Chronic throbbing in teeth.

▮The teeth feel dull, are loose, bleed easily and decay rapidly.

▮Swelling of gums, dark red, painful bleeding from slightest touch.

▮Gums painful as if burned.

Swollen dark red gums, with painful throbbing, as if beginning to suppurate, so severe that it was scarcely endurable.

Sore ulcerated gums.

▮Dentition: grinding teeth; dry ringworms make their appearance, or seem to brighten up at evolution of every fresh group of teeth; bad smell from mouth; aggravation of diarrhœa after taking boiled milk; very exhausting diarrhœa.

11 **Taste and Tongue.** ▮Taste: bitter; saltish; putrid or offensive; sour in morning on waking; disagreeably bitter in morning; bitterish sour; unpleasant in morning, mouth dry and slimy; foul, as from an old catarrh; slimy, putrid; food tastes too salt; like manure; metallic; sour after eating.

Tongue and cavity of mouth feel as if scalded.

Tip of tongue feels scalded.

Soreness of tip of tongue, little blisters, sore edges.

▮Tongue painful as if sore.

▮Tongue pale, flabby and indentated. θAtonic dyspepsia.

Blister on tongue and pain as if burned.

▮Vesicles on tongue.

▮Tongue coated: white; with mucus; dirty yellow; brown, with red edges.

Talking is only a stammering.

Tongue stiff.

12 **Inner Mouth.** ▮Offensive smell from mouth.

Sour smell from mouth.

Rinsing mouth sets her to vomiting.

Dryness of mouth, throat and tongue, which in the morning were quite rough.

▮Profuse flow of saliva.

Dryness in fauces; roughness and burning < by hawking.

13 **Throat.** Dryness and soreness in throat at night, it feels quite parched.

Dryness in posterior nares, yet much mucus in mouth with involuntary urging to swallow.

Pressure in throat in region of tonsils, as if neckcloth were tied too tight.

▮During first sleep she often imagines she has swallowed something, which wakes her up in a fright, with a sensation as if it had lodged in her throat, sensation remains after waking.

▮Sensation of a plug in throat.

▮▮Much mucus in throat; hawking of mucus in morning.

Burning of pharynx.

ǀǀSore throat, with swelling of cervical glands.

‖ Soreness and stinging in throat, with swelling of submaxillary glands.

| Pain in throat as if raw, when swallowing; also stitching and scraping from empty deglutition.

| Inflammation of throat: < on l. side; with stitching pain on swallowing; mucous membrane much swollen, but only slightly red; sensation of a lump in throat; secretion of tough, sticky phlegm causing constant hemming, with feeling of dryness in throat.

| Chronic swelling of tonsils; sensation like a plug when swallowing.

| Contraction of throat without swallowing.

‖ Disposition to inflammation of tonsils, usually ending in suppuration.

‖ Chronic pharyngitis; pharynx dark-red; sensation of a plug in throat, particularly when swallowing and frequently accompanied by feeling of constriction in throat; stasis of portal circulation.

14 **Appetite, Thirst. Desires, Aversions.** | Canine hunger, or no appetite, nothing tastes well

| Sudden craving, sudden satiety.

Thirstlessness; or much thirst in morning.

Desire: for vinegar; for wine.

| Aversion to food: particularly meat and fat; to bread, during pregnancy; to milk, which causes diarrhœa; loathing.

15 **Eating and Drinking.** | Disordered stomach after bread, milk, fat food or acids.

| During and immediately after eating, pains are renewed and aggravated.

| After eating: acidity in mouth; eructations, empty or bitter; bloatedness of abdomen.

It creates an aversion to drinking beer.

16 **Hiccough, Belching, Nausea and Vomiting.** Hiccough after a meal, lasting a quarter of an hour.

| Eructations: frequent, with efforts to vomit; bitter; sour; taste like rotten eggs or manure; after eating but little; cause blood to rise in mouth.

| Heartburn extending from stomach to throat.

| Waterbrash after eating or drinking.

‖ Nausea: after eating, also in morning, fasting; from smell of food or cooking; when riding in carriage; with anxiety when exerting eyes; with weakness.

| Morning nausea as if everything in abdomen were turning round.

‖ Morning sickness of pregnancy.

| The thought of food sickens her, with sense of great weight in anus.

▮Nausea as if viscera were turning inside out; inclination to vomit in morning when rinsing mouth.

▮▮Vomiting: of food and bile in morning; of milky fluid; during pregnancy; frequently strains her so that blood comes up; of mucus, caused by taking even simplest food.

17 **Scrobiculum and Stomach.** ▮Sensitiveness of pit of stomach to touch.

▮▮Peculiar faint, sinking emptiness or goneness at pit of stomach.

Pressure in stomach: as from a stone; as if it were sore internally; after a meal and from touch.

▮▮Beating at pit of stomach; sour stomach; fiery zigzag before eyes; metallic taste in mouth; cracking in knee and ankle joints, and painful cracking in occiput.

▮Painful sensation of emptiness in stomach and abdomen.

Uneasy sensation in stomach, cannot describe sensation.

Slight pressure on region of stomach causes great pain.

Painful sensation of hunger in stomach; has to eat something in night or early morning.

Violent pressure under l. ribs passing off when lying down.

▮Pain in stomach after simplest food.

▮Cramp in stomach.

▮Stitches or burning in stomach.

▮Beating in pit of stomach.

▮▮Twisting in stomach and rising in throat, tongue becomes stiff, speechless, body rigid. θHysteria.

▮Pain in stomach < by vomiting; extends to back, with anxiety.

▮Dyspepsia from injury by overlifting.

Cutting, boring, from region of stomach toward spine.

▮Hardness in pyloric region.

▮▮Attacks of a severe cramping pain commencing in pit of stomach, pain goes to r. side, under short ribs, comes in paroxysms and when at its height is almost continuous until she vomits a sour and then a thick fluid substance; generally no nausea, nor does she vomit until she takes something to make her vomit; countenance a dirty-yellow, with distinct eruptions near hair on forehead; dark urine becomes clear as soon as pain leaves; after an attack of pain, is very hungry and eats enormously; the attacks last about six hours or until relieved by vomiting; no day passes without an attack; when at its height pain goes through to back, between shoulders; at times pain commences between shoulders; thirst after spell passes off; breath offensive; constipation; stool in hard, green lumps.

▮Acute catarrh of stomach, especially in young people;

pain in forehead; violent fever heat; inclination to sleep, with restless tossing about; complete anorexia; white or yellow fur on tongue, without lustre; small blisters on edges, sometimes red spots on surface.

|| Vertigo at night with vomiting of bile and food; shivering, heat with great thirst; gums sore behind incisors; pressure in stomach; stitches in r. hypochondrium on touch; constipation, stools hard, difficult, followed by burning in anus; oppression of chest; sleeplessness; itching eruption on hands and thighs. θGastric fever.

|| Since several days fever; drowsiness; vomiting of green slime; lips dry; smell from mouth as of sour milk; urine and perspiration have same smell; perspiration only partial. θCatarrh of stomach.

|| Digestion poor, frequently disordered; loss of appetite; pressure in stomach; diarrhœa alternating with constipation; hemorrhoids bleed profusely; menses too profuse, lasting eight to ten days; tearing pains in head, teeth and limbs on change of temperature; gums swollen, bleeding; frequent pains in throat; at times itching all over body and eruption of small pimples; eyes red, inflamed; earthy-colored face; despondency.

|| Vomits all her food; painful sensation of emptiness in stomach; sleep broken and unrefreshing; costive, stools knotty and difficult, has scarcely been moved for two years without an injection; urine cloudy, offensive, a hard crust difficult to scrape from vessel.

|| For some time pressure in stomach, and drawing from stomach through r. chest into shoulder, one hour after eating; > by loosening her dress and eructating; appetite good; no thirst; hypochondriasis; falls asleep late; dreams constantly and feels unrefreshed in morning; tires easily; feels < in snowy weather.

| Digestion excites heat and palpitation of heart.

|| Beating at pit of stomach; sour stomach; fiery zigzag before eyes; metallic taste in mouth; cracking in knee and ankle joints and painful cracking in occiput.

18 **Hypochondria.** In region of liver: fulness; pressing; sore pain; dull stitches; frequent stitches; stitches when riding.

| Stitches in l. hypochondrium.

| Pain in liver after moving.

|| Sensation in hypochondria as if ribs were broken and sharp points were sticking in flesh.

|| Sensation as of a strap as wide as her hand drawn tightly around her waist, in evening, after supper.

|| Dull, aching pain all around body and feeling of something hard boring through liver; spasms in liver, which catch breath; fulness as if bursting, > by urination.

| Hepatic neuralgia, with great depression of spirits; weight, fulness and tightness in region of liver.

|| Stitching, pressing pains in hepatic region, extending thence to region of r. shoulder; vesical tenesmus; yellow spots on forehead and over bridge of nose; urine reddish-brown, containing a thick, whitish-yellow mucus; heaviness over eyes and in nape of neck; uterus anteflexed.

|| Persistent febrile condition; very weak, keeping his bed; extreme depression of spirits and irritability of temper; occipital headache; sudden excessive desire for food, but eats only a small quantity; two or three stools daily and one or two at night, of normal consistency, but clay-colored and offensive; successive outbreaks of furuncles on nates; on r. side of abdomen, just below arch of ribs, a very tender spot which is the seat of constant pain; whole r. hypochondrium tender and heavy; aching in r. shoulder; restless sleep; urine has a pink deposit; heavy sweats at night. θFunctional derangement of liver.

|| Remittent febrile condition with evening exacerbations, no chills, pulse at 11 A.M. 96; aching weight and soreness in r. hypochondrium, and distress and aching in r. shoulder and scapula; cheeks flushed; forehead and conjunctivæ yellow; irregular yellow patches on forehead; lassitude; limbs and back ache; obstinate constipation; occipital headache; anorexia, loathes fat and milk; thirst; tongue flabby and indented; great flatulence after food; restless sleep; dry, hot skin; urine scanty and loaded with urates. θFunctional derangement of liver.

|| A woman subject to gall-stones, two attacks of shivering, the last at 3 A.M., followed at 7 A.M. by pain in liver, afterward going across to stomach and spleen and around back; liver > by lying on it; pain > by eructations, she feels it would be better if she could pass flatus downward.

| Jaundice, with pain in hepatic region.

|| Jaundice, with stitching pains in forehead, epigastrium and small of back; tearing pains in knees and feet; cannot sleep at night, must constantly change position of legs; lassitude; great thirst; urine stains yellow.

|| Mrs. R., æt. 51, black hair and thin, has had jaundice for three months; has been for some weeks confined to bed; when pregnant seventeen years before had same illness for several months; appetite poor; no thirst; stool every day, whitish; urine like dark tea, with greenish sediment; sleeps badly and has difficulty in

falling asleep; heat, sweat and twitchings, especially in bed; liver much enlarged, smooth and not sensitive; about every two weeks has an attack of gall-stone colic; she lies upon her back; looks wretched, face yellowish-grey, apathetic and silent.

19 **Abdomen.** ❙In abdomen: sensation of emptiness; lax feeling, after stool; soreness and pain as if menses would appear; pain and weight on rising in morning; pain and tenderness; heaviness; sensation of a load, during motion; drawing tensive pressure; bearing down with menses; feeling of crowding and pressing downward; pressure as if everything would issue through vulva; pressing; cutting; stinging; burning; coldness.

❙❙Feeling of bearing down of all pelvic organs.

❙Pelvic distress through night, > by lying on either side, with legs flexed on thighs and thighs on abdomen.

Distress in hypogastric region as of overdistended bladder; < sitting and lying, > on walking about.

Severe pelvic pain, commencing in sacrum, passing forward and down to r. knee.

❙Bearing down in pelvic region, with dragging pain from sacrum; pain extending into loins and down thighs.

Frequent attacks of contractive pain in r. side of abdomen, < in morning; following this, more constrictive pain in stomach; thence the pain extends to chest; > by eructation.

❙In r. side of abdomen: severe stitches; pressing pain.

❙Distension of abdomen; puffed after dinner; loud rumbling noises; distension of lower portion.

Feeling as of something adherent in abdomen, with hiccough.

❙Spasmodic contractions in abdomen, with terrible bearing down.

❙Flatulence from lack of bile; abdomen very much distended after least bit of food; constipation.

❙Colic: with great distension and sensitiveness of abdomen; recurring toward evening; colic and faintness before menses.

❙❙Pot-belliedness of mothers.

❙Soreness of abdomen in pregnant women.

❙❙Many brown spots on abdomen; chloasma.

❙❙Neuralgia of plexus mesogastricus; burning, boring pains; abdomen greatly swollen and very sensitive to touch; terrible anxiety; attacks came on in evening.

❙Pain in abdomen, > by hot flannels; loss of appetite; cannot always swallow solid food, must take it out of mouth; riding causes pain in hypochondria, abdomen and lumbar region, with desire to lie down; full feeling from abdomen to throat; comes on from 11 A.M. to 1 P.M., and then lasts all day; > by resting.

|| Supposed tænia; complains several times a day of rolling in abdomen, as if something alive were there, with spasmodic griping in præcordial region; it then rises upward in her throat; tongue becomes stiff; she loses her voice, and whole body becomes stiff; no appetite; abdomen always tense; stools irregular; menses painful, scanty, irregular.

| Empty, gone feeling in epigastrium, common to patients with tapeworm.

20 **Stool and Rectum.** | Stools: jelly-like, with colic and tenesmus; green mucus; sour-smelling; debilitating; bloody; oozing almost constantly from anus; expelled quickly; frequent; not profuse; fetid; sour; putrid; whitish; grey.

| Diarrhœa, < after drinking milk; rapid exhaustion.

|| Discharge of blood with stool.

| Before loose stool: nausea; colic.

| During loose stool: prolapsus ani; jerking pains from anus upward through rectum.

| After loose stool: exhaustion; debility; prolapsus ani.

|| Feeling as of a weight in anus, during stool and for an hour after.

| Stool has a putrid, sourish, fetid smell, expelled suddenly and the whole of it at once.

|| Summer complaint, sunken eyes and face; emaciation; heat of palms of hands and soles of feet, green stools, but little pain.

|| Painless diarrhœa, of three weeks' standing, four or five stools in twenty-four hours; evacuations dark brown, pappy, very offensive, coming very suddenly; loss of appetite, tongue thickly coated; frequent belching, particularly after eating; meteorism.

|| Painful diarrhœa of several years' duration, extreme emaciation; great disturbance of digestive organs; whole nervous system greatly prostrated.

|| Chronic diarrhœa in women who suffer from leucorrhœa, hysteria, hysterical hemicrania, sudor hystericus, transient flushes of heat, frequent chilliness, particularly when at stool, and whole facial expression indicates uterine disturbance.

| Stool insufficient, retarded, like sheep-dung.

| Pain in rectum during and long after stool; involuntary straining.

|| Constipation: during pregnancy; slow and difficult discharge even of soft stool; stools hard, knotty, insufficient, scanty, like sheep-dung; stools difficult, covered

with mucus; stool retarded with discharge of blood; in pregnant women and in children where manual assistance must be rendered in consequence of excessive straining; with dyspepsia and chronic affections of stomach; chronic or obstinate, especially after failure of *Nux vom.* and *Sulph.;* especially in women, or persons subject to rheumatism; discharge of blood with stools.

▮During constipated stool: pain in rectum extending to perineum and vagina; shooting and tearing in rectum and at anus; prolapse of anus; sense of weight at anus; terrible straining to pass stool, which is covered with mucus; bloody discharge.

▮After constipated stool: sensation of weight at anus; hemorrhoids.

‖Chronic constipation of forty years' standing, in a lady æt. 76, had become so inveterate that she never had a natural evacuation.

‖No stools excepting under influence of purgatives; no movement for several days; abdomen swollen; congestion to head; great torpidity of intestinal canal.

▮Hemorrhoids: painful sensation of emptiness in epigastric region; delicate and sensitive skin; protrusion of varices and of rectum, with difficult micturition; heat, burning and swelling of anus when piles do not protrude, defecation excessively painful, stool being rather small, narrowed by diminished calibre of anus; sometimes fecal mass is triangular and very painful; constant oozing of moisture from anus; stitches and jerkings from anus upward into rectum and abdomen.

▮Pain in rectum: extending to genitals; as from contraction; burning, the entire day; soreness; stitches.

▮Itching in rectum and anus.

▮Prolapse of rectum, < from smoking.

Cancer of rectum.

▮▮Sense of weight or ball in anus, not > by stool.

▮Soreness in anus.

‖Congestion to anus soon after dinner.

▮Heat, burning and swelling of anus.

‖Constrictive pain in rectum extending to perineum and into vagina; pain in rectum on going to stool, persists a long time after sitting down, and finally an imperfect stool is voided, with sore, smarting pain, weight in anus, like a constant drag. θFissure of anus.

‖Anus encircled by a ring of condylomata.

▮Expulsion of ascarides.

▮Oozing of moisture from rectum; soreness between buttocks.

[21] **Urinary Organs.** Feeling as if bladder were full and contents would fall out over pubes, with constant desire to push them back.

Pressure on bladder; with burning after micturition, in evening; in morning, and urging to urinate, urine passing only after waiting several minutes; and frequent micturition with tension of lower abdomen.

Burning in bladder and forepart of urethra.

|| Smarting in urethra.

| Frequent and strong urging to urinate, with painful bearing down in pelvis, in morning; sensation referred to neck of bladder; must rise frequently at night.

|| Urine: clear like water; thick, slimy, offensive, depositing a yellowish, pasty sediment; with much white sediment, fetid; cloudy and dark, as if mixed with mucus; scanty, red deposit; sour-smelling; high-colored, looks like powdered brick; dark-red; deposit of a white, adherent film; turbid, clay-colored, with reddish sediment; blood-red, with white sediment and a cuticle on surface; with dark-brown admixture; lithiasis.

Occasional stitches along urethra.

| Urging to urinate from pressure on bladder.

|| Involuntary discharge of urine at night, especially during first sleep. θEnuresis.

| Mucous discharge periodical, not at each micturition; sometimes pieces of coagulated mucus clog up urethra.

| Smarting in urethra, when urinating.

| Difficulty of urinating especially in morning, a feeling as if drops came out of bladder.

|| Pressure on bladder and frequent micturition with tension in lower abdomen.

| Annoying itching sensation in region of bladder, with urging to urinate, especially in night.

| Only through night a drop or so discharges from urethra, staining linen yellowish.

Stitching pain in female urethra.

Discharge of mucus from urethra, not at each evacuation of urine, but periodically.

| During and after micturition chilliness and heat in head.

| Intense burning and cutting pain when urinating.

| Difficulty of urinating, especially in morning.

|| The bed is wet almost as soon as child goes to sleep, always during first sleep.

|| Urine passed within space of two hours after going to bed, during first sleep.

| Nocturnal enuresis: boys of light complexion; with onanists.

|| Constant pressure on bladder with urgent inclination to

pass water; sensation as if bladder and urinary organs would be pressed out, > by standing or sitting with legs crossed or by lying down; if desire to pass water is not immediately complied with, urine passes involuntarily; urine scanty, sometimes only a few drops, sometimes clear, generally thick and muddy, with a very adhesive brickdust sediment; no pain before or during passage of water, but immediately after, a sharp, shooting pain passes from l. side of urethra to a spot half way between sternum and shoulder on a level with the second rib on l. side, a sore pain constantly remaining in that spot, sensitive to touch or pressure; sleep very much disturbed at night from having to urinate as often as every half hour; dreams of urinating, and finds on waking an urgent desire to do so; weakness and aching in small of back. θIrritable bladder.

‖ Very urgent desire to urinate and difficult discharge throughout day and several times each night, but particularly for some hours after rising in morning, with a feeling of bearing down in region of bladder, above os pubis; constant soreness throughout urethra, bladder and vagina; sore spot to l. of pubis, above Poupart's ligament, near ovarian region, especially tender on pressure; soreness disappears suddenly for a day or two, returns and is most violent during menses, when entire vesical and uterine region burns and aches; constant tickling in bladder; something seems to move in bladder like a worm and causes tickling; sensation of enlargement of bladder (subjective) which seems to fall from side to side; menses appear regularly but very painful, with bearing down; discharge is profuse, blood light-red without clots; pains resemble labor pains, is obliged to brace her feet; this condition lasts two days, after which soreness reappears in l. side mostly; depressed in spirits, owing to tormenting desire to pass water, which prevents her leaving home; sleeps well but has bad dreams; feels bright on awaking till she rises only to be tormented by constant desire to void urine; appetite good but food causes pressure in stomach, with frequent fulness in epigastrium; later, thirst; oppression of respiration, which is sometimes sighing. θChronic cystitis and irritability of bladder.

22 **Male Sexual Organs.** ‖ Increased sexual desire with weakness of genitals; profuse sweat particularly on scrotum; itching around genitals.

Continued erections at night.

‖ After coition: great weakness; weakness in knees; urethra burns.

▮Nightly emissions with sexual dreams; great despondency; sensitive to cold, damp air, it chills him through and through.

▮During coition insufficient erection and but little thrill; after it great weakness.

▮Weak and watery pollutions.

▮After emission burning in forepart of urethra, languid and drowsy.

▮▮Emissions after onanism; despondency, relaxation of body.

▮▮Very debilitating seminal emissions nearly every night; frequent one-sided stitches in forehead; constant offensive sweet taste in mouth, which is always dry, but without much thirst; stools hard; pain in abdomen as soon as inclination is felt for stool; feeling of tiredness and restlessness in legs, particularly calves.

▮Cutting in testes.

Swelling in scrotum.

▮Prepuce ulcerates and itches continually; cracks on foreskin.

Indolent chancres; on glans and prepuce.

Burning, itching, humid or scurfy herpes præputialis; chappy herpes, with a circular desquamation of skin.

Eruption on glans.

Itching and dry eruption on genitals.

▮Profuse yellowish white discharge from urethra. θGonorrhœa.

▮Gonorrhœa after acute symptoms have subsided; urine is loaded with urates, staining everything red and often excoriating and very fetid, associated with prostatitis.

▮▮Gleet: no pain, discharge only during night, a drop or so staining linen yellowish; yellowish discharge, no burning on urinating; painless, of a year and a half's standing, orifice of urethra stuck together in the morning; particularly where sexual organs are debilitated by long continuance of disease or through frequent seminal emissions; of two years' duration.

▮Condylomata completely surrounding head of penis.

[23] **Female Sexual Organs.** ▮Sterility.

▮Sexual intercourse is intolerable.

▮Jerking pains in vagina from below upward in morning on waking.

▮Contractive pain or almost continuous stitches in vagina.

▮Tenderness of sexual parts to touch.

▮Redness, swelling and itching eruption of inner labia.

▮▮Married fourteen years without conceiving, irregular and scanty menses, followed by leucorrhœa; nausea, disgust for food; frequent desire to urinate; a bearing down or drawing pain in lumbar region; pain in l. side of face, disposed to weep and think married life a blank.

Pressure and heavy weight or dull, heavy pain in ovaries.

▮Congestion; stinging in ovary; pain in ovarian region running outward and backward.

▮Neuralgia of ovaries and appendages; stitching or burning pains.

▮Indurated ovaries.

▮Induration of neck of uterus.

▮Dropsy of uterus.

▮Ulceration and congestion of os and cervix uteri.

▮Induration of cervix uteri, with stitching pains extending upward.

❙❙For three or four months previous to last confinement, suffered from great distension of abdomen with pain and soreness; one month previous to confinement labor-like pains with discharge of serous fluid; pains subsided and returned again every three or four days until her confinement; thinks she must have discharged at least three gallons of fluid during four weeks; child was alive, after seven months, great distension of abdomen with pressure and bearing down, especially when standing or sitting a long time, a feeling as if contents would issue through external organs; general soreness through bowels; occasional discharges of serous fluid, similar to those before confinement, gushing out with force; feeling of soreness in uterus and external organs; urine scanty, high-colored, with frequent inclination and involuntary discharge when coughing or sneezing; darting pricking pains through hips and sides, sometimes shooting down to bones of pelvis; pains in back and extremity of sacrum; general debility; easy perspiration from least exercise; night sweats; sometimes flushes of heat at night followed by chill; poor appetite; bowels loose, several thin evacuations daily; neck of uterus low in pelvis, nearly as large as at eighth month of gestation. θHydrometra.

▮Burning, shooting, stitching pains in neck of uterus.

▮Constant sense of pressing into vagina; crossing limbs to prevent prolapsus.

▮Painful stiffness in uterine region.

Pressure in uterus, causing oppression of breath; pressure downward is as if everything would fall out, accompanied by pain in abdomen; she must cross her limbs in order to prevent protrusion of vagina, yet nothing protrudes, increase of gelatinous leucorrhœa.

Prolapsus uteri, with inclination of fundus to l. side, producing a numb feeling in lower half of l. side of body;

dull aching pain; aching in pelvic region somewhat > by recumbent posture, especially when lying on r. side; tenderness of os uteri.

|| Acne on face < before menses; perspires easily, hands moist, perspiration of strong odor, not removed by bathing; urine of very disagreeable odor and depositing sediment adhering to vessel; almost constant severe backache with pains through both ovarian regions, < on l.; frequent headache and stitching pain in vagina. θDisplacement of uterus.

|| Frequent urging to urinate, with scanty discharge; stools tardy although soft; fulness and pressure in pelvis; pressure toward genitals as if everything would fall out; abdomen bloated, as if pregnant; uterus prolapsed, vaginal portion lying between external labia; os uteri open.

|| Vaginal portion of uterus swollen, dry, protruding from between labia; os uteri open, admitting point of index finger, internal os closed; body of uterus fills up pelvis; efforts at manual replacement futile; during twelfth week of pregnancy.

|| Confined two months ago; womb at vulva; unable to sit up, on attempting it violent bearing down; emaciation; loss of appetite; empty, deathly sensation in epigastrium; feeling of weight in anus not > by stool; claylike sediment in urine; fever in afternoon.

|| Face pale; yellow spots on face and saddle across nose; throbbing headache every morning on waking and lasting all day; desire to urinate very frequently; abdomen naturally was very large and she was greatly annoyed by rumbling in abdomen; all kinds of food disagreed, causing bitter eructations; full feeling after eating; complete procidentia with dreadful bearing-down sensation, > crossing limbs.

|| For two years cough and pains in l. lung; discouraged, sad, thinks she will not recover, feels cross and irritable, especially in morning; alternate sensation of burning and coldness (like ice) on vertex; constant dull frontal headaches, has been subject to sick-headaches, usually pain centres over l. eye; empty, gone sensation at pit of stomach; loss of appetite, even smell of cooking disagrees; constipation; cutting and burning during micturition; urine deposits a claylike sediment, which adheres tenaciously to vessel; menses irregular as to time and quantity; leucorrhœa most profuse before and after menses, of a yellowish color; stitches in cervix uteri; bearing-down pain, as if everything would protrude, must lie down or cross her limbs; cough dry and hacking, most in morning, no expectoration; stitches

to l. scapula, < by coughing, inspiration, touch, > by gentle pressure; weakness of back, it gives out in walking; much heat and pain in sacrum; all symptoms < in morning, > in evening. θProlapsus uteri.

❙❙General health much impaired; nerves weakened; constant pain in back and pelvic region; extremely painful menstruation; general depression of spirits; is convinced no one understands her case, and that she cannot be cured; uterus retroverted, os uteri pressed high up against os pubis, fundus low down in hollow of sacrum; slightest attempt to replace organ gave such severe pain as to make all such attempts futile.

▮▮Sensation of weight in rectum not > by an evacuation and a sensation that limbs must be crossed to prevent everything being pressed out of vagina.

▮▮Prolapsus: of uterus; of vagina; with constipation.

▮▮Pain in uterus, bearing down, comes from back to abdomen, causes oppression of breathing; crosses limbs to prevent protrusion of parts.

▮Stitches or shooting, lancinating pains mostly in neck of uterus go up to umbilicus and pit of stomach.

Uterine pains very severe; the uterus feels as if clutched and then suddenly relaxed, causing nausea.

▮▮Metrorrhagia, during climacteric age or during pregnancy, especially fifth and seventh months.

❙❙Menses every four weeks, very profuse for five days, dark, slimy, flowing more profusely at night when in bed and sleeping; preceded two weeks by severe pain in small of back; during catamenia a dull, sickish pain in pubic region, with bearing-down pain and aggravation of that in back, which is > by flow when very abundant; after menses, leucorrhœa, yellow and thick and pain in small of back for two weeks. θMetrorrhagia.

▮Before menses: sadness; acrid leucorrhœa; especially in young women; violent colic, shuddering all over body whole day; sensation as if vulva were enlarged and soreness in perineum.

▮Mania from profuse menstruation.

▮Dysmenorrhœa in women with scanty menses; half-sided headache; weakness of eyes; nausea; constipation.

❙❙Menses regular but accompanied by hemicrania, nausea and vomiting, and great prostration, so that she must lie down.

▮During menses: sadness; toothache; headache; obs uration of sight; violent pressure in forehead, with discharge of plugs from nose; bleeding from nose; soreness of limbs; tearing in tibia; colicky pains.

❙❙Day before menses frequent chilliness and pressure in

abdomen; night previous dry heat in body, restless sleep, with frequent starting and screaming; in morning crampy drawing down along thighs; some hours previous to appearance of menstrual flow pressure in abdomen becomes a violent pain in umbilical region as if intestines were drawn into a lump; frequently faints, and pain continues until menses appear; after menses, mild leucorrhœa. θDysmenorrhœa.

▮▮Menses: too late, scanty; too early, scanty; preceded by violent aching in abdomen; causing faintness, chilliness and shuddering; eight days too early, scanty, appearing only in morning; a week too soon and lasting only one day; five days too late; regular, but scanty and flow dark; only in morning.

▮Insufficient or retarded menses in feeble women of dark complexion with fine, delicate skin and extreme sensitiveness to all impressions.

||Scanty menses preceded by abdominal distress, pain in back and palpitation; constipation with discomfort in rectum; itching papular eruption on chin, cheeks and temples.

||For fifteen months, pain in kidneys, slight leucorrhœa, deficient menses, little appetite, difficult digestion, profuse perspiration of hands and feet, chilliness of lower extremities.

||Great lassitude and tiredness; loss of appetite; belching of wind; disturbed sleep; despondency; pressure in stomach when eating; pinching pains in epigastrium extending to pubes; menses very irregular, scanty, appearing but three times in twelve months; sensation as if something heavy would force itself from vagina; yellow spots on face and forehead; cervix uteri broad and thick but not sensitive to pressure.

▮▮Amenorrhœa: at age of puberty or later; from a cold; in chlorotic women; in feeble women with delicate, thin skin.

||Amenorrhœa: every eight to fourteen days in afternoon and evening, severe burning and stitching pains in centre of chest < from deep inspiration, lasting several hours; lassitude; palpitation of heart, when walking rapidly or ascending steps; bitter taste; loss of appetite; constipation; sensation of fulness and at times cutting pains in abdomen.

▮When menses fail to appear in mothers who do not nurse; abdomen remains very large.

||For three years in place of menses profuse leucorrhœal discharge.

▮Amenorrhœa and profuse yellowish-green leucorrhœa.

▮Between menstrual periods a peculiar offensive perspiration (sudor hystericus), with a pungent, offensive perspiration in axilla and soles of feet.

▮Tenderness of vagina; painful coition; blood from vagina after coition.

|| Leucorrhœa of a yellowish, excoriating character, sometimes attended with a burning sensation; heat and pain in sacrum; menses a dirty-brown color; offensive, mucopurulent sputa; abnormal nasal discharge. θVaginitis.

|| Vaginitis in a blonde child, 5 years old.

|| Burning pain in rectum, could hardly sit on a chair, same pain in vagina and at vulva; constipated, headache, vertigo.

Great dryness of vulva and vagina, causing a very disagreeable sensation when walking, after cessation of menses.

▮Diphtheritic ulcers in vagina and on labia.

▮Brown-reddish color of vagina.

▮Redness, swelling and itching eruption on inner labia.

Soreness and redness of labia, in perineum and between thighs.

▮Pruritus vulva.

▮Troublesome and severe itching of vulva, with pimples all around; painless vesicles in outer parts of vulva.

▮Severe itching of vulva; labia swollen with humid eruption.

▮▮Leucorrhœa: bloody, slimy; yellowish; yellow; like milk; especially profuse after urinating; profuse lumpy, fetid mucus; acrid, with soreness of pudendum; looking like pus; clear as water; green red; during pregnancy; yellow or greenish water; of bad-smelling fluids; at climacteric period; at puberty; with stitches in uterus; with itching of vulva and vagina; < when she has frequent eructations and retchings, face pale; especially profuse after urinating, after making an effort to vomit; only in daytime, with burning pain; pains while walking on account of soreness; with bearing down in pelvis; stinging pain in ovarian region; frequent urging to urinate; itching in genitals; with stitches in neck of uterus; terrible pain during coition; between menses; coming away in starts.

▮Gonorrhœa in women after acute symptoms have subsided.

|| Thick yellow, acrid leucorrhœa during day, none at night; fulness, heaviness and tension in abdomen; constant painful pressure in sides as from a burden.

|| A child, æt. 5, body emaciated, appetite gone, strength rapidly decreasing, afflicted for fifteen months with an

unceasing exhausting leucorrhœa; discharge sometimes thick and of a yellowish-green color, sometimes thin and always very profuse, running through night dress, sheet, and down into mattress on which she lay at night.

▮Induration and sensation of enlargement in mammary gland; stitches; carcinoma.

| |Scirrhous tumor of r. breast, about size of hen's egg, hard, nodulated and tender to touch; stinging pain.

▮Scirrhus mammæ; burning pain.

▮▮Sudden hot flushes at climacteric, with momentary sweat, weakness and great tendency to faint.

24 **Pregnancy. Parturition. Lactation.** ▮Disposition to miscarriages from fifth to seventh month.

| |Retained placenta after miscarriage; discharges offensive, corrosive, with recurrent hemorrhages.

▮Soreness of abdomen; feels the motions of child too sensitively.

▮During pregnancy: yellow-brown spots on face; thought of food sickens her; sensation of emptiness; painful feeling of hunger; vomiting; toothache; colic; diarrhœa; costiveness; congestion to chest; papitation; pain in mammæ; swelling of labia; too quick escape of urine; laborlike pains in seventh month; loose morning cough.

▮Terrible itching of vulva, causing abortion.

▮Labor: os half open, pain insufficient, tenderness of anterior lip of mouth of uterus, pain above pubes, as if everything would come out; shuddering with pains, can bear them > when warmly covered; shooting pains in neck of womb; indurated os uteri, dyspnœa; spasmodic contraction of os; numerous fine needlelike, darting pains, shooting upward from neck of uterus; flushes of heat; cold feet; hour-glass contraction; constant sensation of weight in anus; pain shooting upward in vagina; pain felt mostly in back; severe bearing down or forcing in back, occurring in regular paroxysms.

▮Offensive excoriating lochia; very long lasting.

▮Nipples cracked across crown, bleeding and sore, preceded by itching.

25 **Voice and Larynx. Trachea and Bronchia.** ▮Reflex or sympathetic aphonia from functional or organic disease of uterus.

▮Hoarseness: with tickling in larynx and bronchi; with coryza and dry cough from titillation in throat.

▮Sensation of dryness in larynx.

▮Roughness and soreness of larynx and throat.

26 **Respiration.** ▮Oppression of chest and shortness of breath, when walking.

▮Severe oppression of chest, toward evening.

▮After emotions of mind loses breath and gets palpitation.

Awakes in morning with great dyspnœa, covered with sweat.

Oppression of chest and cold sweat.

Is suddenly aroused from a deep sleep by asthma.

Breathing < after sleep.

‖Shortness of breath, < sitting a long time, particularly in a stooping posture and after motion; walks rapidly without feeling any dyspnœa, but if he is stopped gets so short of breath that he cannot speak and is seized with a feeling of deathly anxiety which disappears when he resumes his walk; sweats very easily on slightest exertion; very sensitive to cold wind; clothing oppressive after eating; very easily irritated.

‖Great shortness of breath, hindering her in her household work, must pause while eating to get breath; after eating pressure in stomach; oppression of breathing > in open air, < in room, morning and evening; dancing and running cause no shortness of breath.

▮Asthma: short, easy inspiration and long, slow, wheezing expiration.

▮Spasmodic asthma.

27 **Cough.** ▮Dry cough: especially in evening, in bed, until midnight, frequently with nausea and bitter vomiting; during sleep without waking; from tickling in larynx or in bronchi, toward morning; whooping and choking, with pain in pit of stomach and scraping sore pain in larynx not felt when swallowing saliva; does not awake from her sleep, but after waking it becomes very severe and continuous; short, seems to come out of stomach; hard, concussive; short evening cough, with intermittent stitches in r. hypochondrium, with eruptions on skin, with women; as if proceeding from stomach and abdomen or from constipation, or as if something remained lodged in stomach that would not pass off; after a meal.

▮Cough: especially evening and morning, with salty expectoration; with rattling of mucus in chest; with expectoration only in morning or only during night; only during day; wakes one at night; with expectoration only before midnight as soon as he gets into bed, not during day; short hacking in evening, after lying down, with much expectoration of pure coagulated blood, once every minute; wakes her at night, with sensation in chest as if hollow, and smarting therein as if sore; most severe in evening after lying down; spasmodic; severe, with little expectoration, with little vomiting, evenings, when lying in bed; day and night, pain therefrom in pit of stomach; affects chest and stomach greatly; from tickling in larynx without expectoration; every evening, not ceasing until he coughs loose a little phlegm; loose in morning, with efforts to vomit; loose especially at night; with expectoration; with taste in mouth as of rotten eggs; with soreness in chest; stitches in chest and back.

Cough < : from repose; standing and sitting; lying in bed, or upon (l.) side; after walking rapidly; going up stairs; getting wet through; taking cold; cold damp air, as in churches and cellars; cold north wind; deep inspiration; eating; sour food and vinegar.

▮Cough and coryza with sneezing commence every morning before getting out of bed and last until 9 A.M.

▮Coughs phlegm loose, but cannot get it up; is obliged to swallow it.

During evening cough after lying down, he can raise > if he turns from l. to r. side.

When she cannot expectorate with the cough her breath almost leaves her.

▮Expectoration: profuse; purulent; offensive; fetid; green; tasting salty; only in morning.

▮Dry, fatiguing cough, provoked by a sensation in region of stomach, and seeming to come therefrom; or the cough comes, as it seems, from the abdomen.

‖Affection of lungs with hæmoptysis and cough for six years; > since appearance in face of a red papular eruption, now existing for two years; hard papulæ on a red base, without suppuration on her cheeks, forehead, nose and chin, burning, itching and smarting intensely, especially in wet, cold weather; appetite good, though food causes pressure in stomach; constipation; menses too often and too profuse; easily exhausted; backache; cough reappeared dry and hard, slight expectoration on rising in morning; constant desire to clear throat, which feels as if filled with phlegm, which it is impossible to raise; oppressed feeling through chest after a hard paroxysm of cough; nausea during and after cough; eruption not very thick on face; cough seemed to come from stomach, which felt as if it were being scraped.

‖Cough and dyspnœa < in dry air, fog, east and north wind; in stormy weather she is almost suffocated; in walking dyspnœa often disappears; lying on l. side is disagreeable to her; she has to lie with her head high, often sitting in bed; a warm room is oppressive; expectoration yellow or green, with salty taste; appetite moderate; no thirst; urine has a blood-red sediment; menses regular but scanty; always < before and during period;

mood depressed and weeping; formerly had cough, bladder trouble, hemorrhoids, weakness of memory and melancholic state.

॥Catarrh every Winter with violent coughing; after being in a draft cough tormenting and dry; severe orthopnœa, had to sit straight up day and night, with horrible anxiety about a rattling in chest, with soreness as if raw on chest; fears to suffocate.

॥Tickling cough in bed at night, particularly before midnight; spasmodic, coming in rapid concussions, till breath is exhausted, then expectoration of mucus, with temporary relief.

▮Paroxysms of spasmodic cough resembling whooping cough, excited by tickling in chest, from larynx to stomach; daytime without, morning with expectoration of yellow, green or grey pus, or of a milk-white, tenacious mucus, generally of saltish taste.

॥Child cries each time it coughs at night; can hardly get its breath, the cough coming in such rapid succession; retching with cough, unless quickly picked up; very cross and cannot be put to sleep as usual during the day; soreness in bends of knees and elbows, on neck and behind ears, rapidly spreading and exuding an offensive-smelling serum, paining when washed.

॥Cough constant whenever child is laid down, particularly violent at night; with spasm of diaphragm and larynx as in whooping cough.

॥Child, 8 months, blonde and fat; teeth developing rapidly; cough day and night, but principally at night, with retching and complete loss of breath; cough comes in rapid succession until the breath is exhausted, then gagging and vomiting of mucus. θWhooping cough.

▮Sudden severe spasmodic cough at night, cannot get enough breath, chest constricted, retching, loud crying; early in second stage. θPertussis.

॥A poor child growing up under most wretched external conditions; characteristic ulcer on frenulum linguæ; complication with bronchitis and later lobular pneumonia. θWhooping cough.

28 **Inner Chest and Lungs.** ▮Oppression of chest.

Severe pressure in chest, evening in bed.

▮Sensation of emptiness in chest.

▮Great pressure on chest, more l. side.

▮Stitch in l. side of chest and scapula, when breathing or coughing.

▮Sensation of soreness in middle of chest.

॥Frequent sensation as if a knife were thrust into top of l. lung, then turned around with pain streaking off through shoulder.

Itching and tickling in chest.
Fulness and pressure in chest.
Constriction of chest with cough.
Rattling in chest with cough.
▮Chest symptoms > by pressing on chest with hand.
||Burning pain in a fixed spot under r. nipple; itching of external chest; dry cough when reflecting; pain < reading and thinking; rarely seminal emissions, which, however, aggravate pains; difficult expectoration of whitish mucus; sweats at night; cold knees at night in bed; slow digestion especially of acids, with sensation of weight in epigastrium; has old pleuritic adhesions in r. chest.
||Pleuritis after a chronic headache had suddenly vanished.
||Severe attack of pleurisy in two old men.
||Pleurisy in a boy, æt. 6; exudation had spread over whole l. chest.
||Severe attack of pleurisy in a young woman where *Phos.*, though apparently indicated, failed.
▮Chronic pleurisy, threatened phthisis.
▮Congestion of blood to lungs, palpitation and great anxiety.
▮Tuberculous and other chronic diseased conditions, of central third of r. lung (*Arsenicum* upper third).
▮Stretching or darting pains through central portion of r. lung.
▮Neglected pneumonia, with copious, very offensive expectoration.
||Short, dry cough, titillation in larynx, sometimes a thick, deep voice, without metallic timbre; sensation of dryness in chest and larynx; dry, screeching, deep, hollow cough, > lying down; difficult expectoration of a little mucus, which is tough, slimy or albuminoid. θPhthisis pulmonum.
||Sharp darting pain through r. side of chest, rather below centre of r. lung; at times very acute, preventing full respiration, then again more dull, but all the time more or less painful; after suppression of a cough some months previously.
||Dulness on percussion in r. lung, posterior to third and fourth ribs; much pain, both dull and sharp, in that region; severe dry cough, < in evening, with expectoration in morning; chills, fever and night sweats; greatly emaciated. θPhthisis pulmonalis.
||Complete anorexia; sleeplessness; cough with a milky-looking expectoration; fever; after a severe paroxysm of cough which lasted two hours coughed up several

cupfuls of blood and a large quantity of offensive-smelling pus; this had occurred once before; next day expectoration was again slimy, milky-looking and very profuse, with almost uninterrupted loose cough, respiration becoming easier. θPhthisis pulmonalis.

|| After relief of a chronic dyspepsia attended with sick-headache he began to suffer with uneasiness and pain just below centre of r. lung; pain increased in severity and he soon began to cough; during a very hot day without unusual effort or exposure was seized with a sense of suffocation, probably from congestion of r. lung; much pressure and sharp pain through central portion of r. chest; cough night and day; an abscess broke in lung, and he expectorated more than a pint of fetid matter; at first discharge greenish, then bloody and yellow, finally grey, excessively fetid, so profuse it came near strangling him; while abscess was gathering, chills, fever and night sweats; abscess broke, continued to cough very severely day and night; great emaciation; very pale; pulse 120; extremely feeble. θPhthisis.

29 **Heart, Pulse and Circulation.** Heart gives an occasional hard thump.

Violent palpitation and beating of arteries in evening in bed.

| Palpitation: after emotions; with stitches in l. side; with anxiety about things which happened years ago; on walking fast.

| Interruption of beating of heart most after dinner, alarmed, quivering motion.

| Wakes up with violent beating of heart.

| Nervous palpitation > by walking fast.

|| A man, about 30, stout, healthy-looking, complains of palpitation and constipation; appetite good; no thirst; after eating, bloatedness of abdomen, anguish and palpitation, especially with alvine discharge; < when sitting down after having had a walk, never during walking or dancing; flatulency in l. side of abdomen rising upward, > by pressure; < in cold wind; cannot lie on l. side, prefers to walk with head uncovered; sweats easily, especially on feet, which often feel cold.

| Affections of heart, with violent intermittent, palpitating and tremulous motion of heart; violent, rather loud and sometimes intermittent sounds of heart, with dulness of percussion over a larger surface; flushes of heat, redness, determination of blood to head and r. temple, with cold hands and feet; scanty urine; costiveness.

Much ebullition of blood in whole body, at night, producing restless sleep.

Orgasm of blood with congestion to head and chest.

She feels pulse beating through body, particularly through whole l. chest.

▮▮Congestion of blood to chest, with violent palpitation of heart.

Pulse: full and quick during night and then intermitting; slow during day; accelerated by motion or being angry; tremulous; intermitting.

Pulsation in all the bloodvessels.

▮▮Dropsy in consequence of valvular insufficiency.

30 **Outer Chest.** ▮▮Brown spots on chest.

▮▮Stitches in breasts.

▮Soreness of nipples.

▮▮Fungus hæmatodes in clavicular region, bleeding profusely.

31 **Neck and Back.** Pain constantly between shoulders and down back.

Great aching between shoulders and under l. scapula, extending into l. lung, < on expiration.

▮Pressure and stitches in r. shoulder blade.

▮Stiffness in small of back and neck.

▮▮In small of back: pain; pain and weakness; at 6 P.M. pain or great weakness; weakness when walking, from uterine troubles; pulsations; aching; pain as if sprained in afternoons and evening in bed; tired pain; pain particularly with stiffness, > by walking.

During whole menstrual period she could not sleep on account of tearing in back, chills and heat with thirst and painful contraction of chest.

Heaviness in back in morning on awaking as if she could not turn or raise herself, or as if she had lain in a wrong position, almost as if parts had gone to sleep.

▮▮When stooping sudden pain in back as if struck by a hammer, > by pressing back against something hard.

▮Stitches in back when coughing.

▮▮Pain in back across hips.

Stitches posteriorly over r. hip, for four days almost continuous; she could not lie on r. side on account of pain, when touching part it pained as from subcutaneous ulceration.

▮Aching pain across loins < on moving.

▮Aching in sacrum in evening, > by pressure.

▮Dull pain in sacrum.

▮Soreness and pain in back in sacral region.

▮Constant dull, heavy pain in sacrum and abdomen extending to thighs and legs.

Pain in sacrum extending through hips and thighs to below knee, with weakness and lassitude when moving, especially when going up stairs, as if limbs would refuse to act before reaching top.

▮Pressing, dragging pain over sacrum and at same time over hips, burning pressure in spine extending across dorsal region and under scapula, like that produced by sewing.

▮Weakness of sacro-iliac region.

▮Belching relieves pain in back.

▮Pains extending from other parts to back.

▮Herpes circinatus r. side of neck, appearing at one time in front, then at back, then at side of neck, at times they extend about ear, swelling of surrounding parts.

‖Throbbing in small of back > by sitting upright, < sitting, leaning back; on turning in bed or stretching out arms a pain catches her there as if something were going to break, stopping breath. θRheumatism.

‖Crick in back; of eight years' standing; caused by a sudden strain when lifting; < when first attempting to move; > by continued motion; leucorrhœa; riding, a jar or a misstep hurts her back severely.

▮Is obliged to walk stooping and gets painful stitches in back by accidentally kicking foot against something.

▮Sudden stitch in back while lifting, cannot move without great pain.

▮Backache causes nausea and faint feeling while standing.

‖Pains in small of back after exposure to wet and cold weather; < in morning, sitting or on beginning to move about; falls asleep late and cannot lie on l. side or upon back; vertigo in morning when rising; feels uncomfortable in a hot room or when sitting too long; perspires easily.

‖After a severe cold, chilliness along back in evening, followed by a severe pain in back, < slightest motion of back, on account of which she must lie very quietly on back; great oppression of chest with shortness of breath and violent beating of heart; pressing pain in region of stomach; > from touch; frequent twitching of arms; pulse tense, 120; loss of appetite; thirst moderate; sweats. θPerimyelitis.

▮The spine is tender to touch on pressure.

32 **Upper Limbs.** ▮Swelling and suppuration of axillary glands.

▮Humid tetter in armpit.

▮Pain as from dislocation in shoulder joint after exertion.

Paralytic drawing and tearing in arm and armpit to fingers.

▮Lameness and falling asleep of arms and fingers.

▮Drawing in arms down to fingers.

▮Bruised pain in arms.

▮Herpes on elbow (scaling off).

▮Stiffness of elbow and wrist joints.

▮Stitches in joints of arm, hands and fingers.

Tensive pain in metacarpal joints of fingers, particularly during flexion.

‖Red, hard spot on skin covering first and second metacarpal bones, rapidly spreading over dorsal surface of hand; scales formed upon the red base falling off in centre and renewed toward periphery.

▮Scaly tetter on backs of hands; < in cold weather.

▮White scaly tetter on back of hand and fingers.

▮Itch and scabs on hands; soldier's itch.

▮Heat in hands during day, with nervous excitement.

▮Cold hands even in warm room, and from hands chill through whole body.

‖Profuse perspiration of hands so that all needles rusted and soiled her work; frequent and severe migraine.

▮▮Hands sweat profusely; cold, sweaty hands.

Things drop from hands.

Burning of palms of hands.

▮Cold perspiration on hands.

▮Skin on palms peels off.

‖Whitlow for six or seven days; last joint of r. thumb inflamed, swollen and itches, with throbbing, shooting and burning in it; redness mostly on dorsal surface of phalanx, throbbing < in palmar surface; the part is dark-red and pus invisible (relieved the pain).

▮Panaritium, with violent beating and stitching pains.

▮Painless ulcers on tips of finger or on joints.

▮Warts on hand and fingers; on sides of fingers; horny.

Many warts of young girls (onanists).

Finger nails yellowish, discolored.

33 **Lower Limbs.** ▮Coxagra with lancinating stitches, must get out of bed for relief; pains < from rising but > from slow walking.

‖Severe tearing pains in l. thigh; along course of sciatic nerve, pain extending to calf of leg and toes; pain 3 to 5 A.M.; during attack veins of affected part are greatly distended, she cannot remain in bed, gets up and walks about room sobbing; lassitude during day; eight months pregnant. θSciatica.

Swelling of limbs and feet; feet swollen and feel as if asleep; feet burn much at night; at the climacteric.

Pains in hips and thighs extending to near the knees.

▮Cramp: in hip joint and thigh; in buttocks at night in bed when stretching out limb; in calves, particularly during latter months of pregnancy; feet mostly in daytime, ankles weak and turn easily when walking.

Pain as if bruised in r. hip joint.
Stiffness of legs to hip joint, after sitting for a short time.
Drawing in thighs.
▮Soreness and burning between nates.
▮Lower limbs go to sleep when walking.
▮Much weakness in lower limbs.
▮Lower limbs pain as if beaten; desires to sit down, when sitting she feels as if she must stand up.
▮Stitches and sticking, drawing pains, with lassitude, coldness of feet or knees; sweat of feet.
▮Restlessness in legs every evening, with formication.
▮Sensation of running as from a mouse in lower limbs.
▮Icy coldness of lower limbs.
▮Swelling of limbs and feet, < when sitting or standing, > when walking.
▮Swelling of knee, soft and painless.
▮Cracking in knee and ankle joints, stiffness.
॥Acute attack of rheumatism in r. knee, which is semi-flexed, stiff, swollen, red and painful; < at night; great sense of weakness in joint; external lateral ligament especially sensitive and painful to touch; extreme sensibility to cold air and to every change of weather.
॥For fifteen years, scaly eruption on legs or a dark, dusky redness of skin; it occasionally improved but never disappeared.
॥Papular, dry, scurfy, ring-shaped eruption, on anterior surface of legs, immediately below knees.
॥Aching in calves, extending to knees, with a feeling almost as if bones were decaying; excitement and occupation of business during morning make him forget his aching limbs; has had much worry lately.
▮Coldness in legs and feet, especially in evening in bed; when feet get warm, hands get cold.
▮Burning or heat of feet at night.
▮Feet swollen, with sensation as if fallen asleep.
॥Feet hot, red, swollen, dorsal surface covered with large pustules, some of which had burst, discharging a thick, yellow greenish pus; severe tensive pains; < in r. foot.
॥Heaviness in feet when walking.
▮Icy coldness of feet. θMetritis.
▮Profuse sweat of feet; or sweat of unbearable odor, causing soreness of toes.
▮Suppressed foot sweat.
▮Tension in tendo-achillis, also swelling of tendon.
Ulcer on heel from a spreading blister.
Stitches in heels and corns during day.
Crumbling misshapen toe nails.

31 **Limbs in General.** ▮Heaviness of limbs.

▮Stiffness and cracking of joints with arthritic pains.
▮Jerking and twitching of limbs and head, during day.
▮Limbs go to sleep easily after manual labor.
▮Weakness of joints, especially of knees.
▮Patient fears joints cannot bear exertion of lifting.
▮Stinging pains in limbs, inner parts, bones.
▮Neuralgia in limbs going up into head.
▮▮Painful indolent little boils in armpits and thighs; irregular catamenia; peculiarly offensive sweaty condition of feet, painful excoriation between toes.
▮Itching in bends of knees, elbows and on hands.
▮Palms of hands and soles of feet burning hot.
▮Ulcers on upper part of joints of fingers and toes.

36 **Rest. Position. Motion.** Rest: pulsating headache >; boring headache >; coldness in vertex <; fistula of cheek <; neuralgia of plexus mesogastricus >; cough worse.

Lying: headache with anxiety <; pain in occiput <; stitches in forehead >; on back, headache <; on painful side, headache >; on it, swelling on side of head >; on painless side, roots of hair more sore; quiet facial neuralgia >; > pressure under ribs; on liver > pain; on back with gallstone colic; distress in hypogastric region <; sensation as if urinary organs would be pressed out >; aching in pelvic region; hacking cough; cough >.

Lying with head high: cough and dyspnœa >.

Lying on side: pulsating pain >; legs flexed on thighs and thighs on abdomen > pelvic distress.

Lying on r. side: aching in pelvic region >.

Lying on l. side: fistula of cheek <; cough <; is disagreeable to her; cannot, pain in back; anxious dreams.

Lying on back: impossible; pain in back; very quietly, compulsory on account of pain; cough with expectoration <.

Must lie down: migraine during menses.

Could not be raised from recumbent position without fainting.

Sitting: impatience; headache >; involuntary jerking of head; distress in hypogastric region <; bearing down a long time shortness of breath <; cough <; palpitation > after a walk; throbbing in small of back, > upright, < leaning back; backache <; too long, feels uncomfortable; a short time, stiffness of legs; swelling of limbs or feet <.

Sitting with legs crossed: sensation as if urinary organs would be pressed out >; to prevent protrusion of vagina; bearing-down sensation >.

Has to sit straight up day and night: orthopnœa.

Stooping: bursting headache <; boring headache <; coldness on vertex <; shortness of breath <; sudden pain in back.

Standing: emission of urine; as if urinary organs would be pressed out; bearing down; cough <; backache causes nausea and faint feeling; swelling of legs and feet <.

Turning in bed: stretching out arms, catching pain in small of back; stitches in back.

Turning from l. to r. side: facilitates raising phlegm.

Could not lie quiet for five minutes: restless sleep.

Rising from bed: pain in swelling on head >.

Rising: pains from coxagra <; very tired in morning.

Leaning forward: heaviness in ovarian region.

Must bend over: pain in stomach.

Kneeling at church: fainting.

Stretching out limb: cramps in buttocks.

Remaining in one position long: neuralgic pains <.

Changing position: neuralgic pains >; of legs imperative.

Desires to sit down, when sitting must stand up again; pain in limbs.

Cannot find easy position for head.

Stepping: headache <.

Motion: pain over eye <; bursting headache <; pain in cerebellum; boring headache <; of eyes < headache; of head < coldness on vertex; leucorrhœa <; fistula of cheek >; pain in liver after; sensation of a load in abdomen; shortness of breath <; pulse accelerated; aching across loins <; weakness and lassitude in sacrum; at first < crick in back, continued >; causes great pain in back; at first < pain in back; chilliness; flushes of heat from least.

Slight exertion: neuralgic pains >; disagreeable from weariness; easy perspiration; fatigues; irritable and faint; sweat.

Slow exercise: headache >.

Exertion: pain in shoulder joint.

Hard motion: continued > headache.

Shaking head: headache <.

Walking: vertigo; hemicrania <; headache <; emission of urine; distress in hypogastric region >; back gives out; after menses a very disagreeable sensation; oppression of chest; rapidly no shortness of breath, only when stopped; cough <; dyspnœa often disappears; fast, palpitation; nervous palpitation >.

Weakness: in small of back; pain and stiffness in small

of back; slowly > coxagra; ankles turn easily; lower limbs go to sleep; swelling of legs and feet >; heaviness of feet; profuse sweat.

A short walk: fatigues much.

Must get up and walk about: sciatica.

Going up stairs: cough <; as if limbs would refuse to act; fatigues.

Dancing and running: cause no shortness of breathing.

36 **Nerves.** Very faint all day.

▮Great exhaustion in morning during menses.

Great exhaustion and indolence; everything seems an exertion; the least exertion fatigues, even going up stairs.

▮Feeling of prostration; general languid feeling of whole body.

▮Feels weary and trembles all over.

▮Very tired in morning, when rising from bed.

▮In morning on waking weak feeling as from nausea.

▮▮A short walk fatigues much.

▮Debility usually characterized by a painful sensation of emptiness at pit of stomach; icy coldness of feet and hands.

▮▮Sudden prostration and sinking faintness.

▮Very irritable and faint from least exertion.

▮▮Great faintness from heat, then coldness; great exhaustion in morning, during menses.

▮Sudden faintness, with profuse sweats and undisturbed consciousness, without being able to speak or stir; rigid like a statue.

▮Fainting: after getting wet; from riding in a carriage; ▮▮while kneeling in church; at trifles.

Frequent trembling of whole body.

▮Extreme nervous restlessness; uneasiness in whole body; fidgety.

▮▮Feels as if she could feel every muscle and fibre of her r. side, from shoulder to feet, an indescribable sensation.

▮Frequent starts of upper part of body.

▮Jerking and twitching of head and limbs.

▮Cramps in buttocks in bed, at night, when stretching out limbs.

▮Twitching of limbs during sleep.

General muscular agitation.

▮Hysterical spasms; sensation of a ball in inner parts.

▮▮Sensation of an icy-cold hand between scapulæ, then coldness over whole body, followed by cramping of chest as if she would suffocate, lasting several minutes; this is followed by clonic spasms of r. leg with twitching therein, and twitching of r. arm when leg is held, finally trembling of legs; sleep frequently disturbed by attacks of anxiety, sudden fainting, profuse sweats, and a condition in which she is conscious and can move about but not speak. θHysteria.

|| In early childhood received a blow upon spine and has ever since complained of tenderness along its course; whole spine very sensitive, could bear no pressure upon it; also a spot in abdomen a little to l. and below umbilicus extremely tender; pain in l. shoulder extending down l. arm and side, at times so severe that she cried out; at times peculiar sensation in l. arm, feels very stiff although flexible as ever; constipation; menses regular; vomiting each meal almost as soon as eaten; continued in this state for two months, sometimes >, at others <; then whole l. side of abdomen became tender, could not bear slightest touch, patient stated that a circumscribed redness appeared over painful spot; paroxysms of great pain and anguish every evening in this spot accompanied by vomiting of bloody water and sometimes of pure blood to the amount of several tablespoonfuls; numbness of l. side and limbs, soon followed by complete paralysis of l. arm; difficulty in urinating, would postpone urinating for two days, then three or four days, each time having terrible paroxysms of suffering; could not be raised from recumbent posture without fainting and aggravation of pains; had several paroxysms of pain during night, summoning whole household to her bedside by her screams; would roll from side to side panting, speaking only in broken words and sentences, then would become unconscious for several minutes, slowly recover and vomit some blood; finally lost all desire to pass urine and during five weeks never passed a drop, suffering no inconvenience therefrom; pulse 72. θHysteria.

Paroxysm of something twisting about in her stomach and rising toward throat; her tongue becomes stiff; she became speechless and rigid like a statue.

| She is very uneasy about the state of her health; constantly worrying, fretting and crying about her real or imaginary illness. θHysteria.

|| Violent spasmodic movement of all the limbs of body, and particularly of head, so that most of hair was rubbed off; talking amounts only to a stutter and is accompanied by twitching of muscles of face; great restlessness, constant desire to change his place and position; red tettery eruption on l. thigh. θChorea.

|| Convulsive motions of head and limbs; when talking (which is only a stammering), jerking of facial muscles; general muscular agitation; desire to constantly change

position and place; ringworm-like eruption on skin every Spring; uterine chorea with menstrual irregularities; > after menses and after a thunderstorm. θChorea.

▮Hysterical paralysis.

▮Paralysis with atrophy.

▮Great sensitiveness to pain (*Coff.*, *Cham.*, *Hep.*).

▮Sensitiveness to cold air.

37 **Sleep.** ▮Sleepiness: in forenoon; during day falls asleep as soon as she sits down; too early in evening.

▮Difficult awaking, no desire to rise, weariness of limbs.

▮Talks aloud during sleep.

▮Restless sleep: confused dreams; felt that she had a weight pressing on her thighs, momentary; on account of anxious dreams and heat; she could not lie quiet for five minutes.

▮Sleep does not refresh, but leaves tired, aching feeling through whole body.

▮Frequent awaking from sleep without cause or because he thinks he has been called.

‖During first sleep, she often imagines she has swallowed something, which wakens her up in a fright, with a sensation as if it had lodged in her throat.

Awakes at night in a fright and screaming.

▮Twitching of limbs.

▮Ebullitions at night, with restlessness.

Nightly delirium.

Awakes in morning at 3 o'clock and cannot go to sleep again.

▮Wakeful, sleepless, from rush of thoughts.

▮Sleeplessness, cannot fall asleep, is nervously oversensitive.

Anxious dreams when lying on l. side.

38 **Time.** 3 A.M.: attack of shivering; awakes and cannot go to sleep again.

3 to 5 A.M.: pains in l. thigh.

Toward morning: tickling in larynx or bronchi.

Morning: depression; beating in vertex; hemicrania; heaviness of eyelids <; itching of inner canthus; burning in eyes; photophobia and swelling of eyelids <; acute conjunctivitis; conjunctivitis with muco-purulent discharge; lids glued together by thick matter; photophobia <; conjunctiva palp. injected on waking; smarting in eyes; lachrymation; difficulty of opening eyes; fluent coryza with sneezing; face red; on rising neuralgic pains <; prosopalgia appears; cough <; sour taste on waking; bitter taste; unpleasant taste; roughness of mouth, throat and tongue; hawking of mucus; much thirst; in morning vomiting of food and bile; on rising pain and weight in abdomen; pain in abdomen <; strong desire to urinate; difficulty of urinating; pain in vagina; cross and irritable <; cough dry and hacking <; prolapsus uteri symptoms <; crampy drawing down along thighs; menses only; loose cough; great dyspnœa; oppression of breathing <; expectoration; cough loose, with effort to vomit; heaviness in back; pain in back <; vertigo when rising; great exhaustion during menses; very tired; on waking weak feeling as from nausea; very cold feet; after waking sweat; sweat with anxiety; paroxysms of ague appear sometimes.

10 A.M.: paroxysm of ague.

From 11 A.M. to 1 P.M.: neuralgia of plexus mesogastricus.

From morning till noon: stitches over orbit; headache with nausea.

Forenoon: as if brain were crushed; till evening boring pain; involuntary jerking of head; weakness of eyes; sleepiness.

During day: milky leucorrhœa <; did not open eyes; on closing eyes; scratching in them <; prosopalgia disappears; leucorrhœa; cough only; no expectoration; pulse slow; heat in hands; cramp in feet; stitches in heels and corns; jerking and twitching of limbs and head <; falls asleep as soon as she sits down; shuddering without chill.

All day: headache; shuddering all over body; very faint; feet damp and cold.

Day and night: pain from cough.

Afternoon: vertigo when rising from bed; pain in small of back; paroxysms of quotidian ague; fever <.

Between 3 and 4 P.M.: paroxysms of ague.

3.30 P.M.: pain over eye.

4 P.M.: fulness deep in orbit.

6 P.M.: pain and weakness in small of back.

Toward evening: increasing dryness of eyes; colic recurring; severe oppression of chest; chilliness with thirst; very cold feet.

8.30 P.M.: flushes of heat all over body.

Evening: sad and gloomy; toward anxiety; headache >; hemicrania <; prickling of eyes by candlelight; pustules around cornea with redness <; biting in r. eye; acute conjunctivitis; great dryness in eyes; agglutination of lids; lachrymation; face pale; thirsty; as of a strap around waist; fever <; attacks of neuralgia; prolapsus uteri symptoms >; oppression of breathing <; dry cough; short cough; hacking cough; pressure in chest;

beating of arteries; pain in small of back; aching in sacrum; chilliness along back; in bed cold feet; early, sleepy; chilliness; very cold feet; face heated; paroxysms of ague; itching of spot on r. hand; acarus-itch itching <.

Night: pressure in eyes; smarting in eyes <; scratching in eyes <; stitches in ears <; neuralgic pains < in bed; very severe prosopalgia; toothache <; throat parched; has to eat something; vertigo; heavy sweat; pelvic distress; involuntary discharge of urine; much disturbed from having to urinate; gleet discharge only; menses more profuse; no leucorrhœa; expectoration; wakes with feeling as if chest were hollow; cough <; spasmodic cough; cold knees; much ebullition of blood in whole body; pulse full and quick; burning of feet; cramp in buttocks; rheumatism in knee <; paroxysms of pain; awakes in a fright and screaming; cold sweat <; itching and burning of skin in bends of elbows and knees.

Before midnight: cough with expectoration; tickling cough.

Toward midnight: spasms of eyelids cease.

39 **Temperature and Weather.** In hot weather: conjunctivitis always <.

Becoming overheated: nosebleed.

Hot flannel: > pains in abdomen.

Warmth: was unbearable during violent headache.

Warm room: facial neuralgia >; oppressive; feels uncomfortable; cold hands; internal chilliness; fine rash over body remains; nettlerash disappears.

Warm climate: nervous irritability >.

Warmly covered: can bear labor pains better.

In room: oppression of breathing <.

In bed: toothache <.

Open air: sad and gloomy; while walking, vertigo; stitches over orbit >; headache >; pain over eye >; in head >; coldness on head >; pressing pain around eyes <; acute pain in orbit <; lachrymation; toothache > in fresh air; oppression of breathing >; chilliness; while walking profuse sweat; urticaria appears.

In dry air, fog, east and north wind: cough and dyspnœa <.

Change of weather: rheumatism of knee very sensitive.

In a thunderstorm: boring stinging over eye <.

After a thunderstorm: ringworm-like eruption >.

Wind: riding in, brings on facial neuralgia.

North wind: boring stinging over eye <.

Northeasterly wind: facial neuralgia <.

Rough wind: exposure to, brings on migraine; walking against, profuse sweat.
Cold north wind: roots of hair sore; cough <; flatulency >.
Dry east wind: cough <.
Stormy weather: she feels almost suffocated.
Snowy weather: feels <.
Damp weather: facial neuralgia; pain in small of back after exposure.
Getting wet through: cough <; fainting.
Cold, damp air: sensitive to; cough <; eruption on face itches and smarts <.
Cold water: acute conjunctivitis >; smarting in eyes >; toothache >; when water gets warm toothache returns.
Cold: toothache <.
In cold air: boring stinging over eye <; scaly tetter on back of hands <; rheumatism of knee very sensitive; sensitiveness; nettlerash breaks out.
Cold room: fine rash disappeared.
Cold draft of air: toothache <.
Hot or cold: things in mouth < prosopalgia.

40 **Fever.** ▮Want of natural bodily warmth.
Very sensitive to cold air.
▮Shuddering during day without chill.
▮Chilliness: evening in open air, and from every motion; with thirst, toward evening, followed by night sweat; for many nights; internal, in warm room; with the pains.
External warmth was unbearable to her during violent headache, yet she was chilly.
▮Coldness: over whole body; between shoulders, followed by general coldness and convulsive twitching of r. side and difficulty of breathing; begins in feet and rises upward.
▮Chill frequently setting in after previous heat.
▮During chill more thirst than during heat.
▮Cold hands and feet, with frequent flushes of heat to head and face.
▮▮Hands generally cold but moist with perspiration.
Icy coldness of both hands, in warm room they send a chilly feeling through whole body.
Very cold feet, particularly in evening, mainly in bed, and afterward, when this passes off, very cold hands.
▮▮Very cold feet with headaches, especially toward evening and in morning.
Feet damp and cold all day, feeling as if they stood in cold water up to ankles.
▮Heat with attacks of chilliness, with thirst.

▮Face much heated: from talking; with heat in evening, in head.

Painful heat in head, frequently, with flushes of heat over body.

Hot flush over face and whole head lasting but a few seconds, followed by slight perspiration.

Flashes of heat all over body about 8.30 P.M.

Attacks of flushes of heat, as if hot water were poured over one, with redness of face, sweat of whole body and anxiety without thirst, yet without dryness of throat.

▮Flushes of heat from least motion.

▮Heat ascends.

▮Sweat: during sleep, particularly on head; profuse, while walking; especially in bends of joints; while walking in open air even against cold wind; over whole body, in morning, after waking, profuse; with anxiety in morning; from least exertion; every morning in bed, after awaking, mostly on lower limbs; of the feet; on upper part of body; continuous, debilitating; pungent, offensive in axillæ, and soles of feet, causing soreness.

▮Night sweat: cold on chest, back and thighs; from above downward to calves, every third night; smelling sour; offensive or like elder blossoms.

▮▮Paroxysms appear 10 A.M.; shaking chill with thirst and vomiting; then severe laborlike pains, > after cold stage, which varies in duration and is followed by profuse sweat with headache in forehead and occiput and palpitation, also night sweats, throbbing in temples, oppression of chest and pain along spine (all during sweat); thirst only during chill, but water is then immediately vomited; falls asleep during night sweat; after paroxysm > although greatly prostrated; mouth full of white mucus; irritable during paroxysm; constipation; urine dark; loss of appetite and irritability of stomach; is three months pregnant. θAgue.

▮▮Paroxysms appear in afternoon, begin with heat in head, redness and stitching pains in temples, pressure in occiput; then shivering and chilliness along back, lasting an hour and a half, with thirst, dry cough, stitches in hypochondria and swelling or r. submaxillary gland; fever; has had six paroxysms. θQuotidian ague.

▮▮Tertian ague; paroxysms appear sometimes in morning, sometimes in evening; chilliness and shivering, followed by heat, then sweat, particularly in face; thirst in all three stages; loss of appetite; bitter taste in mouth; thirst; itching of forehead; vertigo, causing him to fall; stitches in splenic region, also during cough, with expectoration of blood-streaked mucus, epistaxis; stitches in back on turning in bed; rumbling in abdomen.

‖ Paroxysms between 3 and 4 P.M.; chill preceded by thirst; during chill, thirst; severe tearing pains in upper and lower limbs; hands and feet blue, icy-cold, hands seem dead; cough, with scanty expectoration, lasting through hot stage; heat predominates, is of two hours' duration and is followed by sleep and finally cold sweat, particularly at night; during apyrexia, paleness of face; tearing pain in head from ear to ear, also in forearms from elbows into fingers and both knees; cold hands and feet with weakness; no food seems salted enough; cough with scanty expectoration, particularly when lying on back. θQuartan ague.

‖ A girl, æt. 16; every four weeks, to the day, taken in morning with severe chill, lasting two or three hours, followed by very high fever, lasting as long as chill, this is succeeded by profuse sweating; the attack was repeated a second and third time with an intervening well day, after which the ague disappeared until expiration of four weeks from commencement; ague did not return at expected time; instead of it a rather copious menstruation appeared and returned monthly, with entire restoration to health.

‖ Quartan ague chill beginning in legs; preceded by a small, hard lump in l. breast, above nipple, sore to touch; each time (twice) it waked her at 4 A.M.; one hour later, chill; constant cold, damp feeling in front of chest; air seems damp. θAgue.

| Heat ascending, or sensation as if hot water were poured over him.

41 **Attacks, Periodicity.** Alternately: hard and soft stool; diarrhœa and constipation; burning and coldness on vertex.

Periodical: headache from 2 P.M. till bedtime; discharge of mucus from urethra.

Every minute: expectoration of pure blood.

Every five minutes: during day and night, stitches in forehead.

Every half hour: having to urinate at night.

Several times a day: rolling in abdomen.

Several paroxysms during night: of pain.

Every morning: headache with nausea; sweat in bed; cough and coryza with sneezing last till 9 A.M.

Every evening: cough; restlessness in legs; great pain and anguish in spot in abdomen.

Nightly: emissions with sexual dreams; delirium.

Every Saturday for years: headache.

For two days: postponed urinating.

Every third night: night sweat.

Every three or four days: laborlike pains.
For four days: stitches over hip.
For several days: pain in teeth.
Eight or ten days: menses.
Every eight to fourteen days in afternoon and evening; amenorrhœa.
For many nights: chilliness.
Every two weeks: gallstone colic.
Of three weeks' standing: painless diarrhœa.
Every four weeks: to the day taken with severe chill, then fever and sweat.
For five weeks: passed no urine.
For three months: jaundice.
For four months: menses suppressed.
Every Spring: for three years, tendency to reappearance of carcinoma of lip; ringworm-like eruption.
Every Summer: for twenty years, from beginning of warm weather in Spring until its close in the Fall.
Every Winter: catarrh with cough.
Since a year: recurring attacks; agglutination, photophobia, pustules, pain.
A year and a half standing: gleet.
Of several years' duration: painless diarrhœa.
Of two years' standing: hard, indurated tarsal tumor on lid; costiveness; gleet; eruption on face.
For five or six years: headache; affection of lungs.
Eight years' standing; crick in back.
Of thirteen years' standing: ozæna.
For fifteen years: scaly eruption on legs.

43 **Locality and Direction.** Right: tearing in side of forehead; headache follows perspiration on side of head; stitching pains in side of head; hemicrania; boring stinging over eye; as if eye were gone and cool wind blew through socket; pressure in eye; biting in eye; eye inflamed; side of face much swollen, deep red; eye seemed much smaller than left; angle of mouth drawn upward; stitches into ear; heaviness in ovarian region; pain running down leg; stitches in hypochondrium; drawing through chest into shoulder; pain from hepatic region to shoulder; tender spot on side of abdomen; hypochondrium tender and heavy; aching in shoulder; pelvic pain to knee; pain and stitching in side of abdomen; scirrhous tumor of breast; stitches in hypochondrium; pain in spot under nipple; pleuritic adhesions in chest; diseased condition of lung; stitching darting through lung; pressure and pain through chest; determination of blood to temple; stitches in shoulder blade; stitches over hip; could not lie on side,

stitches in hip; herpes circinatus on side of neck; last joint of thumb inflamed; acute rheumatism in knee; as if she could feel every muscle and fibre of her side; clonic spasm of leg; twitching of arm when leg is held; twitching of side; swelling of submaxillary gland; a roundish bright-red spot on ball of hand.

Left: tearing in frontal eminence; stitches over orbit; tearing in temple and side of head; pressing pain over eye; fulness deep in orbit; shooting over eye; sore pain in eye and temple; pain in temple downward; stitching in zygoma; severe pain in head; pain beginning in parietal region becoming throbbing in occiput; violent stitches in forehead; lashes of eye gone, edges raw and sore; sticking in eye; stuffiness of nostril; small pustules on wrist; panaritia of thumb and middle finger; dry coryza in nostril; offensive greenish discharge from nostril; neuralgic pains commence in temple over side of face; fistula in cheek; râles at apex; tearing through ear; tingling then tearing in hand; toothache; inflammation of throat <; violent pressure under ribs; stitches in hypochondrium; pain from side of urethra to a spot between sternum and shoulder; inclination of fundus to side; numb feeling in lower half of side of body; pain in lung; stitches to scapula; pressure on chest; stitch in side of chest and scapula as if knife were thrust into top of lung; flatulency on side of abdomen; cannot lie on side on account of flatulency; feels pulse beat through chest; aching under scapula into lung; severe pains in thigh; of umbilicus, tender spot; pain in shoulder and under arm; peculiar stiffness of arm; numbness of side and limbs; paralysis of arm; tettery eruption on thigh; humid tetter in axilla.

From within out; pains over l. eye; stinging pain in side of head; boring pain in head.

From below upward: pain in vagina; coldness.

From above downward: night sweat.

43 **Sensations.** As if heart stood still; as if every object were in motion; as if suspended in air; as if brain were crushed; as if head would burst; as of waves of pain rolling up and beating against frontal bone; as if eyes would fall out; stitches as from needles in head; vertigo, as if intoxicated; as of a weight over eyes; as if roots of hair were sore, as if cut short near roots; as if eyes were gone and a cool wind blew out of socket; eyes as if bruised; as of a grain of sand in eye; as if lids were too heavy to open; eyes as if balls of fire; as if eyelids were too tight and did not cover eyeballs;

as if eyelids were too heavy; as if lids were paralyzed; hollow molar as if swollen and elongated; gums as if burned; gums as if beginning to suppurate; tongue and cavity of mouth as if scalded; as if something had lodged in her throat; as of a plug in throat; throat as if raw; as if everything in abdomen were turning around; as if viscera were turning inside out; as if stomach were sore internally; as if ribs were broken and sharp points were sticking in flesh; as of a strap as wide as her hand drawn tightly around her waist; liver as if bursting; as if menses would appear; as of a load in abdomen; as if everything would issue through vulva; as of something adherent in abdomen; as if something alive were in abdomen; as of a weight in anus; as if bladder were full and contents would fall out over pubes; as if drops came out of bladder; as if bladder and urinary organs would be pressed out; as if everything would fall out of uterus; uterus as if clutched; as if vulva were enlarged; as if something heavy would force itself from vagina; as from a weight in sides; as if mammary glands were enlarged; as if cough came from stomach and abdomen; as if something remained lodged in stomach; chest as if hollow; chest as if sore; throat as if filled with phlegm; as if stomach were being scraped; as if knife were thrust into top of l. lung, then turned around; as if intestines were drawn into a lump; small of back as if sprained; back as if she could not turn or raise herself, or as if she had lain in a wrong position, almost as if parts had gone to sleep; sudden pain in back as if struck by a hammer; pain in back as from subcutaneous ulceration; as if limbs would refuse to act; as if something were going to break in back; as if shoulder were dislocated; feet as if asleep; r. hip joint as if bruised; lower limbs as if beaten; as of a a mouse running in lower limbs; as if bones of legs were decaying; as if she could feel every muscle and fibre of her r. side from shoulder to feet; as of a ball in inner parts; as of an icy hand between scapulæ; as if she would suffocate; something twisting in stomach and rising to throat; as of a weight pressing on thighs; as if feet stood in cold water up to ankles; as if hot water were poured over one.

Pains: in occiput; in back down to legs and feet; in hips and back; in lids; in r. ovarian region; down r. leg; in stomach; in liver; in tender spot in side of abdomen; in liver going across to stomach and spleen and around back; in abdomen from sacrum; in rectum; in rectum into genitals; in l. side of face; in back and extremity of sacrum, through both ovarian regions; in uterus; in small of back; in kidneys; in mammæ; above pubes; between shoulders and down back; in small of back; in back across hips; in sacrum, through hips and thighs to below knee; from other parts to back; in hips and thighs; in l. shoulder and down l. arm; along spine; in hypogastric region.

Terrific shocks: of pain in head.

Severe pain: in teeth; in pelvis; in small of back; in back; in stomach.

Acute pain: in orbit.

Violent single, undulated jerks of pressing headache: in forehead.

Throbbing pain: in temple; in forehead; in teeth; in head.

Tearing: in upper part of r. side of forehead; in frontal eminence; in l. temple to upper part of l. side of head; stitching in r. side of head; in l. temple; in swelling on side of head; in face and nose; in arm; in teeth; in limbs; in knees and feet; in rectum and anus, in tibia; in back; in arm and armpit to fingers; in l. thigh along sciatic nerve to calf and toes; in upper and lower limbs; from ear to ear; in forearms from elbows into fingers and both knees.

Shooting: over l. eye; from forehead to vertex and sides of face; in rectum and anus; from l. side of urethra to sternum down to bones of pelvis; in neck of uterus; in last joint of r. thumb.

Lancinating stitches: with coxagra.

Stitches: over l. orbit; in forehead; in eyes; in ears; in parotid glands; in ear going into brain; in stomach; in r. hypochondrium; in region of liver; in l. hypochondrium; in abdomen; in rectum; along urethra; in vagina; in cervix uteri; in mammary glands; in chest and back; in l. side of chest and scapula; in breast; in shoulder blade; in back; posteriorly over r. hip; in joints of arms, hands and fingers; in heels and corns; in splenic region; in back; all over body.

Stitching, pressive pain: in lower part of forehead.

Stitching pain: in temple; in l. zygoma and teeth; in throat; in forehead, epigastrium and small of back; in female urethra; in cervix uteri; in neck of uterus; in vagina; in centre of chest; through r. lung.

Cutting pain: in forehead; from stomach to spine; in abdomen; in testes.

Darting pains: from l. eye toward occiput; through hips and sides; through r. lung.

Pressing, throbbing pain: in occiput.

Jerking pain: in head; in vagina.

Pulsating pain: in cerebellum.

Dragging pain: in ears; from sacrum to lumbar region; over sacrum.

Boring pain: in head; over r. eye; from region of stomach to spine; through liver.

Gouty pains: in head.

Laborlike pain: in abdomen.

Pinching pain: in epigastrium.

Griping: in præcordial region.

Severe cramping: in stomach.

Cramps: in stomach; in hip joint and thighs; in buttocks and calves; in feet; of chest.

Neuralgic pains; in l. temple and side of face to ramus of jaw in plexus mesogastricus; in limbs.

Sore pain: in l. eye and temple; in nose; in region of liver; in larynx.

Stinging pain: in one side of head or forehead; in throat; in abdomen; in ovaries; in tumor of breast; in limbs.

Burning: in eyes; of pharynx; in stomach; in anus; in abdomen; at rectum and anus; in bladder and urethra; in forepart of urethra; in neck of uterus; on vertex; in centre of chest; in rectum; in vagina; in vulva; in mammary tumor; in a fixed spot under r. nipple; between nates; of feet; of palms of hand; in last joint of r. thumb.

Smarting pain: in both eyes; in anus; in urethera; in chest.

Pricking pains: through hips and sides.

Bruised pain: in arms.

Soreness: in external canthus; at internal canthi; of lower lip; of gums; of tip of tongue; r. hypochondrium; of abdomen of pregnant women; in rectum; between buttocks; in l. side; in uterus, and external organs; in perineum; of limbs; of nipples; of labia, in perineum and between thighs; of abdomen; of larynx and throat; in bends of knees and elbows; in neck and behind ears; in middle of chest; in sacral region; between nates; of feet.

Tenderness: in abdomen; of sexual parts; of os uteri; of vagina; along spine; of spot below umbilicus.

Sensitiveness: of roots of hair; of abdomen.

Burning pressure: in spine, across dorsal region and under scapula.

Drawing pain: on forehead back to occiput; in l. parietal region; in external canthus; in face and nose; in upper molars; from stomach through chest into shoulder.

Aching: over eyes; in eyeball; in r. shoulder; in small

of back; in pelvic region; between shoulders and under l. scapula; in small of back; across loins; in sacrum; in calves; through whole body.

Dull aching pain: all around body.

Bearing down: in pelvis.

Dull heavy pain: in ovaries; in sacrum and abdomen, into thighs and legs.

Contractive pain: in r. side of abdomen; in rectum; in vagina; in chest.

Constrictive pain: in stomach.

Dull pain: in sacrum.

Heavy pressing pain: over l. eye.

Pressing pain: around eyes; in root of nose; in hepatic region, thence to r. shoulder; in side of abdomen; over sacrum; in region of stomach.

Tensive pain: in metacarpal joints of fingers; in feet.

Violent pressure: under l. ribs.

Beating: headache; at pit of stomach.

Tired pain: in small of back.

Sticking: in l. eye.

Biting: in r. eye.

Painful stiffness: in uterine region.

Painful cracking: in occiput.

Painful confusion: of head.

Tingling: in fingers.

Tickling: in bladder; in larynx and bronchi; from larynx to stomach.

Heat: in eyes; on margins of lids; of palms and soles; in head; in sacrum; in hands.

Painful emptiness: in stomach and abdomen.

Distress: in r. shoulder and scapula; pelvic, in hypogastric region; in abdomen.

Anxiety: in pit of stomach.

Oppression: of chest.

Pressure: on vertex; in forehead; in occiput; over eyes; in eyes; in stomach; in region of liver; drawing, tensive in abdomen; on bladder; in ovaries; into vagina; in pelvis; painful, in sides; in chest; in r. shoulder-blade.

Drawing: in arm and armpit to fingers; in thighs.

Constriction: in throat; of chest.

Paralytic drawing: in arm and armpit to fingers.

Heaviness: of upper lids; in r. ovarian region; over eyes and nape of neck; in back; in feet; of limbs.

Fulness: in temples and forehead; great, deep in l. orbit; in region of liver; in epigastrium; in pelvis; in chest.

Weight: in upper lids; in anus; aching, in r. hypochondrium; in abdomen; at anus; in ovaries; in rectum; in epigastrium; in part from which blood flows.

Tightness: in region of liver.
Tension: in forehead; painful, in parotid glands; in lower abdomen; in tendo-achillis.
Throbbing: in gums; in teeth; in small of back; in last joint of r. thumb; in temples.
Jerking: from anus into rectum and abdomen.
Twisting: in stomach.
Restlessness: in legs.
Discomfort: in rectum.
Uneasiness: in stomach.
Empty, deathly sensation: in epigastrium.
Emptiness; in epigastric region; in chest.
Empty, gone sensation: at pit of stomach.
Goneness: in pit of stomach; in epigastrium.
Weakness: in knees; in small of back; of sacro-iliac region; in lower limbs.
Lameness: of arms and fingers.
Stiffness: in small of back; of elbow and wrist joints; of legs to hip joint; in knee and ankle joints; of tongue.
Dryness: of margin of lids; in nose and fauces; in throat; in choanæ; of lips; of mouth; of tongue; in posterior nares; of vulva and vagina; in larynx.
Numbness: of l. side and limbs.
Numb feeling: in lower half of l. side of body.
Itching: of scalp; on occiput or behind ears; of internal canthus; on margin of lids; in ears; of face; of eruption on hands and thighs; over whole body; in rectum and anus; in region of bladder; around genitals; of prepuce; of eruption on inner labia; of eruption on chin, cheek and temples; of vulva; in chest; of external chest; in bends of knees, elbows and on hands; of forehead; in face; on tip of nose; on arms, hands, back, hips, feet, abdomen, genitals; of pimples on chin; in various parts of body; in ulcer; of nipples; in hands; of elbows; on posterior part of elbow; of ringworm on face; of tetter; of warts.
Coldness: in vertex; of feet; in swelling on side of head; in abdomen; in hands; of lower limbs; in legs and feet; over whole body.

" **Tissues.** ▮▮Uterine troubles.'
▮Bad effects from loss of fluids; bleeding from inner parts.
▮Sensation of weight in part from which blood flows.
▮Considerable swelling of veins of affected limbs.
▮Disposition to gout and hemorrhoids.
▮Painless swelling of lymphatic glands.
▮Erysipelas, generally pustulous.
▮Rheumatism, chronic cases, or obstinate remains of acute.
▮▮Arthritic affections of joints; lithiasis.

▮Crippled nails.

▮Atrophy of children, emaciated, face like old people, big belly, dry, flabby skin, mushy passages.

45 **Touch. Passive Motion. Injuries.** Touch: hair of head sensitive; on swelling on side of head pain < ; roots of hair sore; of teeth, toothache < ; gums bleeding; stitches in hypochondrium; abdomen sensitive; spot on l. side sore; sexual parts tender; tumor of breast tender; of r. hip pain as from subcutaneous ulceration; pain in back >; external lateral ligament of knee sensitive; abdomen very tender.

Pressure: boring headache >; of eyelids together, eyes < ; facial neuralgia > ; slight, on stomach causes great pain; spot on l. side sore; gentle, > symptoms of prolapsus uteri; with hand on chest, > symptoms; flatulency > ; of back against something hard > pain; aching in sacrum > ; spine tender.

Binding head tightly: sick-headache >.

Loosening chothes: > pressure in stomach.

Rubbing: pressure in eye < ; biting of internal canthus and lachrymation; yellowish-brown spots about neck scale off.

Scratching: eruption on vertex feels sore; roots of hair burn; itching changes to burning; does not > itching of spot on r. hand; pimples become dry.

Riding in a carriage: nausea; fainting.

Riding: stitches in region of liver; causes pain in hypochondria; hurts back severely.

▮Seasickness.

Jar: hurts back severely.

Misstep: hurts back severely.

Slightest blow: nosebleed.

From a blow upon spine: tenderness along whole course.

Accidentally kicking foot against something causes painful stitches and must walk stooping.

Injury from overlifting: dyspepsia; crick in back.

46 **Skin.** ▮Delicate skin; least injury tends to ulceration.

▮Itching: on face; on tip of nose; on arms, hands, back, hips, feet, abdomen and genitals; pimples on chin; in various part of body > by scratching, after which there is a pinkish color; in ulcer; of nipples, at times bleed and seem about to suppurate; in bends of elbows; on posterior parts of each elbow.

▮▮Itching often changes to burning, when scratching.

▮▮Soreness of skin; humid places in bends of knees.

▮▮Brown or claret-colored tetterlike spots; chloasma.

Eruption on face, a red roughness of skin.

Painful eruption on tip of nose.

▮▮Herpetic eruption on lips and about mouth.

Red herpetic spots on both sides of neck with much itching.

Yellowish-brown spots about neck that scale off on rubbing.

Red spots on glans penis.

Reddish herpetic spots above hips.

Lentil-sized brown spots on elbows, surrounded with a herpetic-looking skin.

A roundish bright-red spot on ball of r. hand, with violent itching not > by scratching, evening.

Fine rash over body, particularly about bends of elbows and knees; prickling, tingling and itching; in a warm room it remained out and she felt well, if she passed into a cold room it disappeared and she had the most severe rheumatic pains in and about these joints.

Moist pimply eruption at margin of vermilion border of upper lip.

▮Vesicular eruption on back; humid tetter in l. axilla.

Itching eruption followed by desquamation.

▮▮Herpes circinatus.

▮Ringworm-like eruptions every Spring on different parts of body.

▮▮Numerous bullæ, on face near mouth, on wrists and backs of hands; two largest were on wrists, symmetrical in position and size; smaller blebs on arms and below knees; considerable itching and irritation of dermis beneath vesicles; bullæ on wrists were as large as a hen's egg. θPemphigus.

▮▮Urticaria; burning, stitching, itching appearing every time she went out into open air; first appeared on face, neck and forearm, five years ago, gradually spread over whole body, with the exception of back, abdomen and lower legs; attacks preceded by nausea and pressing headache; face swollen as in erysipelas.

▮Nettlerash: most on face, arms and thorax; breaks out during a walk in cold air, disappears in a warm room.

▮Brownish spots on chest.

▮▮Brown-red herpetic spots on skin.

▮▮Brown spots on skin with leucorrhœa.

▮▮Uneasiness in presence of strangers, a slight quivering of whole system when approached; although she strove to appear calm her face flushed up suddenly but soon returned to its usual sallowness; skin disease of long standing; at night an itching and burning of skin in bends of elbows and knees, small pimples would rise up, discharging a small quantity of serous fluid, on scratching they would become dry, leaving skin roughened with brown herpetic spots here and there; chlorotic look; pulse soft; starting at trifles; dreams with good sleep; more fever in afternoon; decayed teeth; tongue coated with thick, slimy fur, dark at root, lighter near edges, clearing off in patches, leaving exposed surface very red; immediately after eating, severe pains in stomach causing her to bend over, with vomiting of food and considerable amount of slimy fluid; even when pain was not so severe, and when she did not vomit she spat a great amount of this fluid, after her meals; lived almost entirely on crackers with as little drink as possible; constipation; menses suppressed for nearly four months; slight pains in hypogastric region most of time; back and limbs very weak. θChlorosis.

▮▮Red spots and papules isolated and in large oval patches covered with shining, white, adhesive scales, looking like stearine, on head, face, chest, back, arms and legs, particularly on extensor surfaces (used sapo viridis locally). θPsoriasis.

▮Large suppurating pustules constantly renewing themselves. θAcarus itch.

▮Acarus itch, after previous abuse of sulphur; itching < evenings; especially in women.

▮Eruptions during pregnancy and nursing.

▮Dry ringworm, especially on face of children; dry offensive eruption on vertex and back of head; itching and tingling, with cracks behind ears.

▮Pruritus, with vesicles on acrid base over all parts of body, face, eyelids, hands, feet, armpits, vulva, anus, ears, hairy scalp, etc.

▮Itching, crusty tetters.

▮▮Tettery eruptions.

▮Stitches all over body, with breaking forth of little pustules.

▮Eruption very moist, almost constantly discharging pus-like matter; the child often jerks its head to and fro.

▮▮Humid tetter with itching and burning.

▮Ringworm; boils; pustules; pemphigus.

▮Ulcers: painless, on joints and tips of fingers, stinging and burning; flat with a bluish-white base.

▮The least injury tends to ulcerate, in thin, delicate skins.

▮Warts: on hands; on neck with horny excrescence in centre; small, itching, flat on hands and face.

▮Large, hard, seed warts; dark color and painless.

▮Varicose veins.

47 **Stages of Life, Constitution.** ▮▮Suited to persons of dark hair, rigid fibre, but mild and easy disposition.

▮Especially suitable for persons with dark hair and for

women, especially during pregnancy, in childbed and while nursing.

▮Children take cold readily when the weather changes.

▮Scrofulous persons.

▮Men who have been addicted to drinking and sexual excesses.

▮Pot-bellied mothers, yellow saddle across nose, irritable, faint from least exertion, leuco-phlegmatic constitutions.

Girl, æt. 5 months; cough.

Child, æt. 8 months, blonde, fat, teeth developing rapidly, had measles three weeks ago, attending cough had never quite subsided; whooping cough.

Infant, æt. 1, suffering several weeks; cough.

J. T. H., æt. 1; cough.

Boy, æt. 2; conjunctivitis.

Girl, æt. 3½, fleshy, leuco-phlegmatic, suffering three years; impetigo.

Child, æt. 4, strong, healthy; ophthalmia.

Child, æt. 5, blonde; vaginitis.

Girl, æt. 5, delicate, face pale, waxen, emaciated, suffering fifteen months; leucorrhœa.

Girl, æt. 5, father scrofulous as a child, suffering three months; eruption on legs.

Boy, æt. 6; catarrh of stomach.

Boy, æt. 7, ill three weeks, said to be suffering from intermittent fever; functional derangement of liver.

Girl, æt. 7, delicate; epistaxis.

Girl, æt. 8, light hair, blue eyes, fair complexion, of scrofulous parents; warts on face.

Girl, æt. 10, strong, well built,. brunette; incontinence of urine.

Girl, æt. 11; scrofulous ophthalmia.

Boy, æt. 12; tarsal tumor.

Girl, æt. 14, blonde, delicate skin, subject to eruptions of skin, not yet menstruated; eruption on hand.

Boy, æt. 14, blonde, lymphatic-nervous temperament, slender, delicate white skin, subject to herpetic eruption every Spring; chorea.

Girl, æt. 16, tall, slender, fair complexion, light hair and eyes, suffering six months; ague.

Girl, æt. 16, sanguine-nervous temperament, tall, slender, fine sensitive skin; chlorosis.

Girl, æt. 16, delicate; hysteria.

Girl, æt. 17, blonde, fair hair, pale, delicate, sensitive skin; displacement of uterus.

Girl, æt. 18, blonde, stout, began menstruating a year ago, menses absent, when a child had tinea capitis; matting of the hair.

Girl, æt. 19, sanguine temperament, brunette, rheumatic; headache.

Miss L. S., æt. 20, dark complexion, hair and eyes, and living in affluent circumstances, suffering six years; cystitis and irritablity of bladder.

Young country-woman, æt. 20; sweating of hands and feet.

Girl, æt. 20, scrofulous, ill several years; nasal catarrh.

Miss P., æt. 20; psoriasis.

Cigarmaker, æt. 21; gonorrhœa.

Woman, æt. 22, single; ophthalmia.

Girl, æt. 22, menses always scanty, suppressed three months after catching cold; chlorosis.

Man, æt. 22, dark-brown hair, short build; quotidian ague.

Man, æt. 22, after catching cold, tertian ague, was given quinine, etc., two years later quartan ague, *China* given, attacks would cease for a time but always reappear; ague.

Man, æt. 22; eruption on feet.

Young lady, sanguine, married; ague.

Mrs. R. L., black hair, moderately well nourished, suffering three years; cough.

Woman, pregnant, blonde, delicate, gentle disposition; toothache.

Woman, æt. 23, four months ago miscarried in her third month; menstrual disturbance.

Man, æt. 23, greatly debilitated by onanism, from which he rid himself two years ago; seminal emissions.

Washerwoman, æt. 23, affected since 3 years old; profuse sweating of hands.

Artilleryman, æt. 24, irritable disposition, blonde; icterus.

Woman, æt. 24, single, brunette, menstruation normal, suffering five years; urticaria.

Man, æt. 24, dark-brown hair, suffering four days; ophthalmia.

Woman, æt. 24; perimyelitis.

Man, æt. 24; gastric fever.

Mrs. M., æt. 25; leucorrhœa.

Man, æt. 25, light hair, rough scurfy skin; tertian ague.

Woman, æt. 25, single, strong, healthy; dysmenorrhœa.

Man, æt. 25, blonde, slender; fistula of neck and cough.

Woman, æt. 25, dark hair, pale sallow face, suffering several years; oppression of breathing.

Girl, æt. 26, after heavy lifting; uterine displacement.

Woman, æt. 26, eight months pregnant; sciatica.

Girl, æt. 27, dark hair; boils and offensive foot sweat.

Woman, æt. 27, nervous temperament; hemicrania.

Woman, æt. 27; headache.

Miss H., æt. 28, dark brunette, sisters died of consumption, six years ago had an affection of the lungs and hæmoptysis, is a nurse; cough.

Woman, æt. 28, of sedentry habits; cardialgia.

Schoolmaster, æt. 29, suffering five or six years; headache.

Woman, æt. 29, single; amenorrhœa.

Mrs. J., æt. 30, scrofulous habit, since two weeks; cough.

Woman, æt. 30, suffering several years from loose cough, a few days ago delivered of her first child which died, had pneumonia during pregnancy; phthisis pulmonalis.

Woman, æt, 30, blonde, sanguine temperament, mother of several children, twelve weeks pregnant; prolapsus uteri.

Woman, æt. 30, brunette, choleric temperament, married several years, three weeks ago delivered of a child, after exertion; prolapsus uteri.

Man, æt. 30; scirrhus of lip.

Woman, æt. 30, single, three years ago lifted a heavy article, since then suffering more or less; uterine displacement.

Man, æt. 30, dark-brown hair, after being rapidly cured of an ulcer on leg; headaches.

Man, æt. 30, suffering four weeks; pains in back.

Man, æt. 30, palpitations of heart.

Lady, æt. 30, ill ten days, her disease is said to have been pronounced remittent fever and prescribed for as such; functional derangement of liver.

Mrs. B., æt. 32, sick several months; asthenopia.

Woman, æt. 32; headache.

Woman, æt. 32, mother of several children, now three months pregnant, first attack of ague when twelve years old, since then frequently recurring, and always suppressed by quinine; ague.

Woman, æt. 33, brunette, suffering several weeks; leucorrhœa.

Mrs. S., æt. 35, nervous temperament, has had three children, the youngest seven months old, suffering since last pregnancy; hydrometra

Woman, æt. 36, blonde, sanguine temperament, no child for last ten years, now seven months pregnant; disorders of pregnancy.

Woman, æt. 36, small stature, suffering many years; gastric disorder.

Man, æt. 36, gunner on ship; psoriasis.

Miss E., æt. 37, lymphatic temperament; vaginitis.

Woman, æt. 37, mother of five children, last one still-born four years ago; amenorrhœa.

Woman, æt. 37, dark hair, pale face, mother of four children; pemphigus.

Tailor, æt. 37, dark hair, pale, lean; rheumatism.

Mrs. P., æt. 38, black hair and eyes, married, mother of three children, says she has been under treatment most of the time for the last four years. θFalling of the womb.

Woman, æt. 38, tall, slim, dark hair and eyes, bilio-nervous temperament, married fourteen years, has never conceived; sterility.

Jewess, æt. 38, blonde, plethoric, in poor circumstances, suffering since last childbirth three years ago; amenorrhœa.

Mrs. H., æt. 40, suffering nine years; facial neuralgia.

Miss St., æt. 40, suffering several days; toothache.

Woman, æt. 40, single, tall, slim, mild disposition, first noticed growth six months ago; scirrhus of breast.

Farmer, æt. 40, hardworking, robust man, dark complexion, jovial temperament; stitches in ear, etc.

Woman, æt. 40, suffering since fourteen years old; headaches.

Woman, æt. 41, married, no children; pain in liver.

Mrs. H., æt. 43; gastralgia.

Mrs. R., æt. 45, large, fat, light complexion; urinary difficulty.

Man, æt. 45, dark hair, muscular; dyspnœa.

Woman, æt. 48, is said to have passed through four attacks of meningitis since fifteen years old; since last attack, mental disturbance.

Lady, æt. 49, stout and fleshy; cough.

Woman, æt. 49, corpulent, when five years old had scarlet fever, since then hoarse, and in Winter afflicted with a loose cough, after repeated exposure to drafts cough became dry; severe cough and orthopnœa.

Woman, æt. 50, single, good health until five years ago, when she ceased menstruating; headache.

Mrs. R., æt. 51, black hair, thin, jaundiced for three months; hepatic disorder.

Mrs. M., æt. 52; pain in vagina and rectum.

Mrs. W., æt. 55, caught cold six or eight weeks ago, since then ill; pain in abdomen.

Mrs. W., æt. 56; procidentia.

Lady, æt. 67; cataract.

Man, æt. 75, afflicted fifteen or sixteen years; eruption on legs.

Lady, æt. 76, suffering forty years; constipation.

48 **Relations.** Antidoted by: Vegetable acids, *Nitri spir. dulc.*, *Acon.*, *Ant. crud.*, *Ant. tart.*, *Rhus tox.*

It antidotes: *Calc. ost.*, *Cinchon.*, *Mercur.*, *Natr. mur.*, *Natr. phos.*, *Phosphor.*, *Sarsap.*, *Sulphur.*

Incompatible: *Lachesis.*
Complementary: *Natr. mur.*
Compare: *Borax, Mezer.*, in vesicular eruptions and ulcers about joints; *Arsen., Ars. jod.*, in psoriasis; *Lycop., Nux vom., Sulphur, Curare*, in chloasma; *Calc. ost., Tellur.*, in ringworm; *Caustic., Pulsat.*, in sadness; *Bellad., Iris, Nux vom., Pulsat., Sanguin., Therid.*, in hemicrania; *Natr. mur., Lilium, Kali carb., Jaborandi, Cyclam., Pulsat., Graphit., Thuja, Alumina*, in eye troubles; *Aloes, Lycop., Sulphur*, in abdominal troubles; *Murex, Kreos., Stannum, Podoph., Pulsat., Secale, Cauloph., Natr. carb., Natr. mur., Actæa rac., Aletris, Helon.*, in diseases peculiar to women.

SILICA.

Pure Silica triturated.

Introduced by Hahnemann.

Provings by Hahnemann, Froissac, Goullon, Gross, Hering, Stapf, Wahle, Knorre, Ruoff, Baker, Robinson (with high dilutions), see Allen's Encyclopedia, vol. 9, p. 1.

Clinical Authorities.—*Mental disturbance*, Jahr, B. J. H., vol. 12, p. 476; *Vertigo*, Martin, T. H. M. S. Pa, 1880, p. 241; Berridge, Hom. Phys., vol. 3, p. 198; *Headache*, Tietze, Rück. Kl. Erf., vol. 1, p. 203; Stens, B. J. H., vol. 34, p. 723; A. H. Z., vol. 91, p. 188; (with Calc.), Weber, p. 156; Allen, Hom. Cl., vol. 4, p. 61; Cochran, H. M., vol. 6, p. 396; Berridge, Org., vol. 1, p. 264; Farley, Med. Adv., Apr., 1890, p. 212; *Neuralgic headache*, Hirsch, N. A. J. H., vol. 22, p. 243; *Chronic headache*, Goullon, A. H. Z., vol. 83, p. 41; *Meningeal sclerosis*, Baldwin, A. H. O., Sept., 1877; B. J. H., vol. 36, p. 196; *Tenderness of scalp*, Martin, Org., vol. 3, p. 364; *Eruption of occiput*, Becker, Rück. Kl. Erf., vol. 4, p. 261; *Eczema capitis* (3 cases), Arcularius, N. A. J. H., vol. 20, p. 285; *Impetigo capitis*, Small, B. J. H., vol. 24, p. 314; *Abscesses on head*, Richards, Hom. World, Apr., 1870, p. 84; *Cephalhæmatoma*, Goullon, A. H. Z., vol. 83, p. 151; (locally), Goullon, Raue's Rec., 1870, p. 18; *Enchondrosis on head*, Grauvogl, A. H. Z., vol. 92, p. 29; *Keloid on temporal region*, Clarke, Med. Adv., vol. 20, p. 108; *Parenchymatous iritis*, Schlosser, N. A. J. H., vol. 7, p. 515; *Ulcer on cornea*, Skinner, Hom. Phys., vol. 6, p. 113; *Lead particles in cornea*, Shuldham, Org., vol. 2, p. 107; *Use in opacity of cornea*, Jonez, Med. Art. Jour., 1876, p. 227; *Ophthalmia*, Stens, A. H. Z., vol. 91, p. 188; Miller, H. M., vol. 12, p. 309; Stens, B. J. H., vol. 34, p. 724; *Scrofulous ophthalmia*, Becker, Rück. Kl. Erf., vol. 1, p. 279; Schlosser, N. A. J. H., vol. 7, p. 514; *Recurrent phlyctenular conjunctivitis, Corneal ulceration*, Foster, Amer. Hom., Aug., 1878, p. 67; *Blepharitis*, Norton, N. A. J. H., vol. 23, p. 355; *Swelling of lids*, Hirsch, Rück. Kl. Erf., vol. 5, p. 109; *Tumor on lid*, Stens, A. H. Z., vol. 89, p. 156; *Inflammation of lachrymal sac*, Dudgeon, B. J. H., vol. 13, p. 135; *Fistula lachrymalis*, Payr, N. Z. H. Kl., vol. 14, p. 124; Raue's Rec., 1870, p. 101;

Caries of the orbit, Norton (see Ophth. Therap., p. 166); *Dysecoia*, Goullon, A. H. Z., vol. 81, p. 29; *Affection of ear*, Goullon, Hom. Recorder, vol. 3, p. 73, from Pop. Zeit. f. Hom., Jan., 1888; *Use in suppurative inflammation of labyrinth*, Searle, A. H. O., Dec., 1872, p. 368; *Otorrhœa*, Chamberlin, N. E. M. G., vol. 8, p. 497; Nankivell, H. W., 1871, p. 136; *Chronic sinus in front of ear*, Nankivell, H. W., vol. 7, p. 106; *Loss of smell and taste*, Hirsch, I. Pr., 1873, p. 348; *Inflammation of nasal duct*, Chapusot, Hom. Cl., vol. 3, p. 26; *Coryza*, Kafka, Raue's Rec., 1870, p. 129; *Chronic coryza*, Rosenberg, Rück. Kl. Erf., vol. 5, p. 168; *Ozœna*, Guernsey, A. H. Z, vol. 110, p. 143, from Med. Adv., Oct., 1884; *Itching of nose*, Hale, H. M., vol. 9, p. 265; *Hard swelling of face*, Goullon, Hom. Cl., vol. 1, p. 197; *Eruption on face*, Kämpfer, Rück. Kl. Erf., vol. 4, p. 261; *Rhagades around lids and lips*, Goullon, N. A. J. H., vol. 22, p 379; *Induration of cheek*, Kretschmar, Rück. Kl. Erf., vol. 1, p. 446; *Tumor of lip*, Petroz, N. A. J. H., vol. 2, p. 312; *Cancer of lip*, Pancin, (de Corveirac), Bib. Hom., p. 150; Raue's Rec., 1875, p. 81; *Mastoid periostitis*, Sherman, Boericke and Dewey's Tissue Remedies, p. 135; *Toothache*, Bönningh., Alts., T., Rück. Kl. Erf., vol. 1, p. 478; *Cancer of tongue*, K. in L., Rück. Kl. Erf., vol. 1, p. 499; *Tumor of mouth*, Slocomb, N. E. M. G., vol. 5, p. 485; *Angina*, Goullon, Rück. Kl. Erf., vol. 1, p. 541; *Affection of throat*, Berridge, Hom. Rev., vol. 16, p. 499; *Anorexia*, Krummacher, A. H. Z., vol. 95, p. 164; *Pressure in stomach*, Payne, Hah. Mo., vol. 5, p. 199; *Gastric disorder*, ——— Rück. Kl. Erf., vol. 1, p. 663; *Hepatic disorder*, T., Rück. Kl. Erf., vol. 1, p. 703; *Ascites*, Brewster, H. M., vol. 4, p. 571; *Inguinal abscess and hernia*, Slocomb, N. E. M. G., vol. 5, p. 486; *Use in enteritis*, Bauer, Hom. Times, vol. 5, p. 177; *Summer complaint*, Moore, U. S. M. and S. Jour., Jan., 1871; *Chronic diarrhœa*, Maischler, N. A. J. H., vol. 19, p. 415; *Constipation*, Bowie, T. H. M. S. Pa., 1885, p. 184; Nichols, Org., vol. 3, p. 345; Johnson (see Hemple and Arndt's Mat. Med.); *Hemorrhoids and constipation*, Miller, H. M., vol. 7, p. 372; *Anal abscess*, Clements, Hom. World, vol. 6, p. 81; *Fistula in ano*, Stow, Hah. Mo., vol. 8, p. 353; Stow, Raue's Rec., 1874, p. 202; (6 cases), Hendricks, A. H. Z., vol. 103, p. 175; *Enuresis*, Gause, Hom. Cl., vol., 4, p. 132; *Incontinence of urine*, Metcalf, N. A. J. H., vol. 3, p. 342; *Seminal emissions*, Wesselhoeft, N. E. M. G., vol. 8, p. 53; *Masturbation*, Gallavardin, N. A. J. H., vol. 22, p. 242; *Hydrocele*, Hartm., Rück. Kl. Erf., vol. 2, p. 215; Guernsey, Raue's Rec., 1870, p. 242; Richardson, Med. Inv., Oct., 1868, p. 2; *Removed putrid odor in uterine cancer*, James, Hom. Phys., vol. 7, p. 179; *Peri-uterine cellulitis*, Carr, Times Ret., 1877, p. 110; *Metrorrhagia*, Teste, Boericke and Dewey's Tissue Remedies, p. 171; *Vaginismus*, Skinner, Org., vol. 1, p. 76; *Leucorrhœa*, Hahnemann, Rück. Kl. Erf., vol. 2, p. 366; Gross, H. M., vol. 10, p. 409; *Tumor in breast*, Bell, N. E. M. G., vol. 4, p. 242; *Scirrhus mammæ*, Schneider, Hom. Cl., vol. 3, p. 94; Bell, N. E. M. G., vol. 4, p. 243; Thompson, Hom. Cl., vol. 4, p. 80; *Mammary fistula*, Gross, Rück. Kl. Erf., vol. 2, p. 425; *Suppressed lochia*, Miller, H. M., vol. 8, p. 43; *Asthma*, Stens, A. H. Z., vol. 91, p. 156; B. J. H., vol. 34, p. 719; *Cough*, Williamson, Hom. Cl., vol. 1, p. 205; Temple, Hom. Cl., vol. 3, p. 101; Boyce, Hom. Phys., vol. 5, p. 167; *Pertussis*, Pomeroy, Med. Inv., vol. 8, p. 168; *Pain in r. lung*, Durand, Med. Adv., 1890, p. 179; *Lung affection*, Stens, I. H. Pr., vol. 1, p. 357; *Compression of lung after pleuritic exudation and curvature of spine*, Schmitt, Hom. Phys., vol. 3, p. 132; *Phthisis*, Hartm., Gauwerky, Rück. Kl. Erf., vol. 3, p. 398; Brigham, Boericke and Dewey's Tissue Remedies, p. 180, from Brigham's Phthisis; Pomeroy, Med. Inv., Jan., 1871, p. 169; Brigham, Cin. Med. Adv., vol. 6, p. 97; *Palpitation of heart*, Brauns, Hom. Cl., vol. 3, p. 95; *Swelling on chest*, Nunez, Hom. Phys., vol. 9, p. 324; *Abscess on chest*, Fornias, Hom. Phys., vol. 7, p. 169; *Necrosis of acromio-clavicular articulation*, Mass. Trans., vol. 4, p. 94; *Swelling of neck*, Berridge, Hom. Rev., vol. 16, p. 496; *Goitre*, Beebe, Tr. World's Hom. Conv., 1876, p. 768; *Carbuncle on neck*, Gross, Rück. Kl. Erf., vol. 4, p. 195; *Recurrent fibroid on neck*, Kent, Hom. Phys., vol. 4, p. 193; *Pain and swelling in cicatricial tissue about neck*, Strong, Org., vol. 3, p. 368; *Disease of cervical vertebræ*, Nankivell, B. J. H., vol. 29, p. 209; *Psoas abscess*, O. M. and S. R., vol. 7, No. 5; *Affection of sacrum and spine*, Pope, B. J. H., vol. 29, p. 549; *Coxitis*, Eidherr, B. J. H., vol. 27, p. 52; *Bone disease of upper limbs*, Seidel, Hartlaub, Heichelheim, Goullon, Chargé, Kämpfer, Gauwerky, Kirsch, Theuerkauf, Battmann, Schindler, Rück. Kl. Erf., vol. 4, p. 441; *Inflammation of arm*, Berridge, H. M., vol. 10, p. 108; *Fungous growth on stump of arm*, Preston, Hah. Mo., vol. 8, p. 83; *Caries of ulna*, Biegler, Hom. Phys., vol. 7, p. 472; *Swelling on wrist*, Swan, N. A. J. H., vol. 19, p. 254; *Contraction of fingers*, Holcombe, Rück. Kl. Erf., vol. 4, p. 615, from Phil. Jour. of Hom., vol. 1, p. 548; *Swelling and suppuration of thumb*, Theuerkauf, Hom. Cl., vol. 1, p. 19; *Caries of metacarpal bones*, Grauvogl, from text-book; *Caries of bone of forefinger*, C. T. M., Boericke and Dewey's Tissue Remedies, p. 107; *Enchondroma on finger*, Knickerbocker, M. I., vol. 4, p. 193; *Swelling of finger*, Sager, A. H. Z., vol. 90, p. 203; B. J. H., vol. 34, p. 155; *Injury to fingers*, Berridge, N. A. J. H., vol. 22, p. 191; *Glass in finger*, Turrill, Hom. Phys., vol. 4, p. 102; *Panaritium*, Hg., Sommer, Holeczek, Rück. Kl. Erf., vol. 3, p. 566; McClatchey, Hah. Mo., vol. 10, p. 179, from Bib. Hom., May 1874; *Felon on finger*, Gallupe, Org., vol. 1, p. 482; *Whitlow*, Stow, Hah. Mo., vol. 8, p. 353; Eidherr, B. J. H., vol. 27, p. 53; *Abscess in buttocks*, Goullon, H. M., vol. 13, p. 443; *Sciatica*, Willard, T. H. M. S. Pa., 1882, p. 159; *Luxation of femur*, Schnapfauf, Rück. Kl. Erf., vol. 5, p. 917; *Necrosis of femur*, Gilchrist, Med. Inv., vol. 8, p. 8; Gilchrist, Med. Inv., 1870, p. 7; *Fistulæ of thigh*, Cigliano, Hom. Cl., vol. 4, p. 133; *Swelling of knee*, Gross, Rück. Kl. Erf., vol. 3, p. 589; Billig, Rück, Kl. Erf., vol. 5, p. 926; Bell, A. H. O., vol. 10, p. 327; *White swelling of knee*, Billig, Rück. Kl. Erf., vol. 5, p. 927; *Housemaid's knee*, Newton, Hom. World, vol. 4, p. 100; *Swelling and suppuration at knee*, Schmitt, Hom. Phys., vol. 7, p. 472; *Hygroma of patella*, Swan, N. A. J. H., vol. 19, p. 254; *Enlarged patella bursa*, Newton, Hom. Rev., vol. 15, p. 474; *Chronic bursitis*, Newton, Hom. Rev., vol. 14, p. 539; *Gonitis*, Terry, N. A. J. H., vol. 25, p. 317; *Periostitis of tibia*, Eidherr, B. J. H., vol. 27, p. 52; *Injury of tibia*, Lippe, Org., vol. 3, p. 26; *Boil over tibia*, Berridge, H. M., vol. 10, p. 108; *Pain in leg*, Löw, Rück. Kl. Erf., vol. 5, p. 916; *Suppuration of leg*, Davis, Med. Inv., 1875, p. 155; *Chronic suppuration of leg*, Gallupe, Org., vol. 1, p. 482; *Pain in feet*, Guernsey, Org., vol. 3, p. 92; Guernsey, Med. Couns., vol. 1, p. 62; *Traumatic inflammation of foot*, Sircar, Calcut. M. J., vol. 1, p. 416; *Abscess of foot*, McClatchey, Hah. Mo., vol. 10, p. 180; *Abscess of foot and caries*, McClelland, Hah. Mo., vol. 8, p. 358; *Suppuration of foot*, Sircar, Calcut. Jour., vol. 1, p. 416; *Ulcer on foot*, McClatchey, H. M., vol. 10, p. 180, from Bib. Hom., May, 1874; *Enchondroma of toe*, Knickerbocker, T. W. H. Conv., 1876, p. 864; *Suppressed foot sweats*, Goullon, A. H. Z., vol. 81, p. 47; *Abnormal foot sweats*, Gallavardin, N. A. J. H., vol. 14, p. 137; vol. 15, p. 60; *Hysteria*, Knorre, Rück. Kl. Erf., vol. 2, p. 289; *Spasms*, Schönfeld, Rück. Kl. Erf., vol. 4, p. 591; *Spasms after vaccination*, H., Hah. Mo., vol. 7, p. 374; *Convulsions*, C. Hg., Raue's Rec., 1870, p. 18; *Epilepsy*, Hartm., Bönningh., Weber, Rück. Kl. Erf., vol. 4, p. 590; Lindsay, Org., vol. 1, p. 471; Hoyne, Boericke and Dewey's Tissue Remedies, p. 137; *Somnambulism*, Lindsay, Org., vol. 1, p. 471; *Night sweats of phthisis*, Holcombe, N. E. M. G., vol. 4, p. 9; *Ill effects of vaccination*, Hering, Hah. Mo., vol. 7, p. 374; *Scrofulosis*, Knorre, Griessel., Sollier, Rück. Kl. Erf., vol. 4, p. 410; *Ulcerations*, Knorre, Gross, Billig, Rück. Kl. Erf., vol. 4, p. 289; *Use in suppura-*

tion, Noack, B. J. H., vol. 23, p. 424; Marwick, Hom. Rev., vol. 12, p. 552; *Chronic suppurations*, Armstrong, Med. Inv., 1875, p. 228; *Use in caries*, Radcliff, N. E. M. G., vol. 11, p. 251; *Areolar hyperplasia*, Yeomans, Hom. Times, vol. 4, 225; *Threatened cancer*, McClatchey, H. M., vol. 10, p. 180; *Multiple cheloid*, Clarke, Hom. World, Aug., 1885; *Enchondroma*, Laird, H. M., vol. 15, p. 193; *Furuncle*, Neumann, Rück. Kl. Erf., vol. 4, p. 182; *Acne simplex*, Cooper, Hom. Rev., vol. 14, p. 33; *Eczema squamosum*, Cooper, Hom. Rev., vol. 14, p. 36; *Herpetic eruption and hydrocele*, Williamson, Hom. Cl., vol. 1, p. 205; *Lupus*, Eidherr, B. J. H., vol. 34, p. 724; McClatchey, H. M., vol. 10, p. 180, from Bib. Hom., May, 1876; *Elephantiasis Arabum*, Sana, N. A. J. H., vol. 22, p. 443.

1 **Mind.** Indifferent, apathetic.

▮Confusion of mind; difficulty in fixing the attention.

▮Mental labor is very difficult.

▮Reading and writing fatigue, cannot bear to think.

Becomes confused, makes mistakes; she is unable to control herself.

Affections from egotism.

▮Compunction of conscience about trifles.

▮Overanxious about himself; low-spirited; weeps every evening.

Longing for his relations and home.

▮Very irritable, low-spirited, peevish mood.

‖Sensitiveness to noise and anxiety therefrom.

▮Very sensitive, weeping mood.

▮Desponding, melancholy, tired of life. θSpermatorrhœa.

▮Gloomy, feels as if she would die.

▮Wishes to drown herself.

▮Yielding, faint-hearted, anxious mood.

▮Restless, fidgety, starts at least noise.

▮Child becomes obstinate, headstrong; cries when kindly spoken to.

‖When crossed has to restrain himself to keep from doing violence. θMegrim.

‖Screaming violently, groaning. θEpilepsy.

‖She screams during increase of moon. θSomnambulism.

Imagines to be in two places at the same time.

‖Complains of pain in throat on swallowing; although there is no indication of any inflammation, the condition of her throat is the sole thing occupying her mind; believes she has swallowed pins, and asks those about her whether she has not done so; seeks for hours for lost pins; will take no sewing into her hand, and carefully examines her food for fear of pins; very indifferent to friends and former amusements; restlessness; anxiety; vertigo, < stooping; headache daily, < mornings; loss of appetite; constipation; emaciation; entire absence of menses; < during increase of moon. θHysteria.

2 **Sensorium.** ▮Vertigo: as if one would fall forward; ascend-

ing from dorsal region, through nape of neck into head; inclining to fall backward; < from motion or looking upward; accompanied by nausea; with rachitis; from excessive use of eyes; when riding; with sleepiness; all day, while stooping at work; during sleep; when rising from a recumbent position; is obliged to walk to the r. side; commencing in cerebellum; in neurasthenia and epilepsy; as if drunk; is obliged to sit down; when closing eyes; from lying on l. side.

The brain feels muddled and thick.

ǀǀHeaviness in head. θParalysis.

Disagreeable feeling, as if head were teeming with live things whirling around it.

▮Fainting; when taking cold; from suppressed foot sweat.

[3] **Inner Head.** ▮Headache or cold feeling rising from nape of neck to vertex; extreme heaviness of head.

▮Congestion to head; cheeks hot; slight burning in soles of feet.

▮Burning in head, with pulsation and sweat of head; < at night from mental exertion, talking; > by wrapping head up warmly.

▮Shooting from nape to vertex.

▮Violent periodic headache, in vertex, occiput or forehead; one-sided, as if beaten; throbbing in forehead; coming in night, with nausea, vomiting.

▮Violent headache, with loss of consciousness or reason.

▮Loud cries, nausea to fainting; subsequent obscuration of sight. θMegrim.

▮Obstinate morning headaches, with chilliness and nausea.

▮Headaches, with or followed by severe pain in small of back; heaviness and uncomfortable feeling in limbs.

▮Tearing, frequently one-sided, with stitches through eyes and in cheek bones.

▮Pulsating, beating, most violent in forehead and vertex, with chilliness.

▮Headache worse: from mental exertion; excessive study; noise; motion, even jarring of room by footstep; light; stooping; pressing at stool; talking; cold air; touch.

▮Headache better: from wrapping head up warmly; hot compresses; in warm room; lying down in dark.

▮Headache every seventh day.

▮Vibratory shaking sensation in head when stepping hard, with tension in forehead and eyes.

▮Headache caused by hunger.

▮Headache as if everything would press out and burst skull; as if brain and eyes were forced forward.

▮Headache wakes him at night.

Tearing in whole-head starting from occipital protuberances and extending upward and forward over both sides.

Tearing pain as if head would burst, with throbbing in it, commencing at crown as if internal and external at same time, with chilliness; was obliged to lie down and tossed about in bed for four hours; > by binding head tightly.
Violent tearing in head as if forehead would be torn asunder.
Violent headache above eyes so that he could scarcely open them.
Stitches in temples.
Hard jerklike pressure in top of head, extending deep into brain, in paroxysms lasting one or two minutes.
The hat causes acute pain in occipital protuberance.
Pressive headache in occiput as if in bone.
Pressure in occiput, followed by stitches in forehead, with chilliness in nape of neck and back.
Pressure in both sides of occiput.
Bruised pain above eyes, could scarcely open them; first affected l. side of forehead, a sticking extending to r. side, pressive, < by opening eyes.
Pressive jerking in middle of forehead renewed by suddenly turning around, stooping or talking.
Pressure as from a heavy weight in forehead over eyes.
Tearing in frontal region.
Acute sticking pain in forehead.
Roaring and shattering in brain when stepping hard or knocking foot.
Tension and pressing in head as if pressed or forced asunder.
Pressive headache at night; could not remember where she was; everything turned around, with throbbing at heart.
Violent pressive headache in morning, extending into eyes, with violent chill in afternoon, nausea and weakness, thought she would faint; eyes painful on turning them sideways or closing them, and when closed are still more painful to touch.
Constant pressive headache from above downrward over whole head, with intermittent itching at vulva.
Pressure at occiput and nape of neck in morning.
▮Headache with small lumps or nodules or scalp.
▮Diseases of brain, spinal marrow and nerves of a paralytic nature.
Fluttering feeling in both temples and aching at occiput.
‖Frontal sinus affected; pounding and throbbing in forehead and up into head. θChronic coryza.
Feeling like water pipes bursting in head.
▮Headache from organic causes, excessive study, nervous prostration with vertigo and weak memory.
Sickening pain in l. side of head, < from pressure or least movement.
When coming into dark she feels a pressure on vertex as if a tremendous weight were falling on it.

Strange coldness about breadth of two fingers across vertex in a line with forepart of ears; rush of blood to forehead.

▮Extreme heaviness of head; she cannot hold it up, it feels so weighty.

▮Rushes of blood to forehead.

❙❙Congestion to head, hot cheeks and burning in soles of feet. θChronic hepatitis.

▮Heat in head. θSpermatorrhœa.

❙❙For years terrible headaches coming on in evening in bed, with shivering and coldness over body; the pain began in cervical vertebræ, extending to cerebellum and from there went to forehead where it was most severe; pain > wrapping head warmly; feeling in neck as if some one pulled downward on cords of neck.

❙❙Chronic headache; never entirely free, at times fearful; when it reaches its height scalp becomes covered with papules and is then so sensitive that she cannot comb her hair; these violent spells are caused by draft and scrubbing; cannot bear cold or heat; during headache she has violent roaring in ears, as if something alive were in them; chronic sweat of feet; habitual constipation.

❙❙Head felt constantly as if it were in a cushion and some one were pressing his two fingers in it at occiput, as if feeling for pins in side; with occasional lightning-like flashes in eyes and feeling as if something obscured vision; < in cold weather or in a draft; > wrapping head up warmly.

❙❙Cephalalgia from spinal irritation; pain began in spine and neck, coming up and over r. temple and thence to l. temple; scalding feeling in vertex; burning pain in head; feeling of internal soreness as if sore brain collided with skull; pain very hard to bear; < from light, noise, least jar and odors; sore aching in nape, < by moving head, > from wrapping head in pillow and from contact of any warm hand.

❙❙Pain at one time in vertex and occiput, at another in forehead; sometimes affects only one side, head then paining as if bruised and being very sensitive to touch; throbbing in forehead, with weakness of sight, is awakened from sleep by the pain and has then nausea and vomiting; pain < from touch, motion, open air; food tastes like clay; discharge of particles of tapeworm; trembling of limb and general feeling of weakness with the pains. θHeadache.

❙❙Severe headache, every two or three weeks, lasting from thirty-six to forty-eight hours; pain commences in nape of neck and base of brain and extends up and over whole head in paroxysms; pain so severe that she calls for some one to hold her head tightly to keep it from bursting.

II Feeling of waves of water from occiput over vertex to forehead, making her feel with each wave as if she would gradually lose her senses, > from warm wraps around head; vomiting of bitter yellow substance on moving, > when perfectly quiet.

II Chronic sick headaches since some severe disease in youth; rising from nape of neck to vertex, as if coming from spine and locating in one eye, especially r; > by pressure and wrapping up warmly.

I Congestive, gastric, nervous and rheumatic headaches.

I Headaches from excessive mental exertion, from overheating, from nervous exhaustion.

I Cerebral apoplexy, preceded by deep-seated stitches in r. parietal region and dull, heavy, crampy pain in arms.

I Child grasps at its gums continually, as if they were painful; profuse sweat about head at night, scrofulous diathesis. θMeningitis. θHydrocephalus.

4 **Outer Head.** II Open fontanelles; head too large and rest of body emaciated, with pale face; abdomen swollen, hot.

I Rolling of head from side to side.

I Head feels as if too large.

Head feels as if falling off, causing straining pains at back of neck as if head were hanging by a piece of skin at nape.

I Head falls forward. θSpinal disease.

Strange coldness, about breadth of two fingers, across vertex, in a line with forepart of ears.

II Tendency to take cold in head, which cannot be uncovered.

I Tearing in scalp, < from pressure and at night.

II Tenderness of scalp in region of coronal suture; brushing or combing hair causes violent attacks of sneezing.

II Head sore to touch externally; sensibility of pericranium; scalp sensitive to pressure of hat and to contact; she cannot brush her hair, the scalp is so tender.

I Much itching on scalp.

II Itching spots on head painful, as if sore, after scratching.

II Itching on occiput.

Pricking and itching of scalp.

Burning and itching, mostly on back part of head; < from scratching, which causes burning and soreness; < when undressing in evening and on getting warm in bed.

II Lumps rise on head, hair falls out, scalp sensitive to touch; tearing pains.

II Profuse head sweat; body dry; likes wrapping up; sweat sour; face pale; emaciated; large abdomen; weak ankles.

▮Profuse sweat of head, body being dry or nearly so.

▮▮Head wet from sweating, particularly at night, likes wrapping up.

▮Profuse perspiration on head, sour-smelling and offensive, in first sleep.

▮Patches of eruption on scalp, exfoliated thin, dry, furfuraceous scales.

▮▮Eruption on back of head, moist or dry, offensive, scabby, burning, itching, discharging pus.

| |Impetigo capitis; entire head covered; eruption humid, discharging a greenish fluid of somewhat putrid odor.

▮Eczema capitis; patch of eruption on scalp, over occipital protuberance, dry, furfuraceous scales, with some itching; enlarged cervical glands; headache with shooting pains from nape of neck to vertex; leucorrhœa; backache.

▮Scaly eruption on scalp; > in Summer, but < upon approach of Winter; cervical glands enlarged.

▮Itching pimples on head and nape of neck.

▮Itching pustules on scalp and neck very sensitive, > wrapping up warmly.

▮▮Moist eruption on occiput.

▮Scalp becomes covered with papulæ and is then so sensitive that she cannot comb her hair. θChronic headache.

▮Itching pustules and bulbous swellings on hairy scalp and on neck.

▮Hair falls out; premature baldness.

▮Suppurating wound of scalp.

▮Phagedenic ulcer on forehead painful and discharging offensive pus.

| |Keloid on temporal region; frontal headache.

| |Cephalhæmatoma; almost the whole l. parietal bone is covered with a large, soft, elastic swelling; the characteristic ring of the bone can be traced by the finger.

▮Cephalatoma neonatorum.

| |Enchondrosis; large, hard swelling, but soft in some places, on a child's head, beginning above ears and extending to larynx; whistling, breathing and suffocative attacks.

▮Painful distension of frontal bone; periostitis.

5 **Sight and Eyes.** ▮Long-lasting photophobia; daylight dazzles the eye.

▮▮Letters run together, appear pale.

▮Dim vision after suppressed foot sweat.

▮Occasional lightning-like flashes in eyes and a feeling as if something obscured vision; nervous sensation in head.

▮Black spots, or sparks, before eyes; a persistent speck before r. eye.

▮Momentary loss of sight, with uterine affections; pregnancy.

Eyes weak; vision indistinct, misty, with flickering before eyes.

Dimness of vision; could neither read nor write; everything ran together; as if looking through a grey cover.

▮Amblyopia: from checked foot sweat; from abuse of stimulants; nervous, sensitive persons; after diphtheria.

ǁMomentary attacks of sudden blindness.

▮Day blindness, with sudden appearance of furuncles.

Slight fluttering before eyes.

ǁCataract; a decided, greyish cloudiness of lens of r. eye was reduced to a small spot size of head of pin; smoke or vapor before eyes, cannot discern objects; eyes red, inflamed, watering.

ǁSclero-choroiditis ant. relieved by this remedy; conjunctiva and sclera injected and a bluish irregular bulging around cornea; retina hazy, no vitreous opacities; severe pains extending from eyes into head on one side, >by warmth; severe aching in back of head on one side, corresponding to eye which is worse; symptoms alternate from one eye to the other.

ǁChoroiditis in a myope, in whom upon any exertion of eye excessive pain extended to head and ears.

▮Irido-choroiditis and other forms of inflammation of uveal tract.

ǁIrido-choroiditis and other forms of inflammation.

ǁIrido-choroiditis, great tenderness of eye to touch, deep ciliary injection, contraction of pupils, posterior synechiæ, excessive sensitiveness to a draft of air.

ǁParenchymatous iritis with abscess in upper part of iris, violent supraorbital pain, night and day.

▮Ciliary neuralgia.

▮Iritis, with hypopion and corneitis.

▮Fungus medullaris.

ǁFormation of abscess size of a lentil in upper portion of iris, having appearance of a yellowish-red swelling, coloring the pupil; the pus of which a small portion had entered the anterior chamber was absorbed.

▮Cataract: after suppressed foot sweat; preceding worms.

ǁCataract of right eye (diagnosis confirmed by two physicians) cured in one year by repeating *Silica* once a month. θCataract.

ǁCataract of r. eye in a man, æt. 61.

▮Perforating or sloughing ulcer of cornea.

▮Small round ulcers, with a tendency to perforate, especially if situated near centre of cornea and having no bloodvessels running to them.

▮Deep or crescentic ulcers of cornea.

‖Sloughing ulcer with hypopion in a syphilitic patient; iris inflamed; ulcer quite deep with profuse purulent discharge, small flakes on cornea, chemosis of conjunctiva.

▮Ulcus corneæ sloughed through; sticking pains night and morning.

▮Pustular keratitis after psoriasis.

▮Opaque cornea after smallpox.

▮Spots and cicatrices on cornea.

▮Corneal fistula.

‖Total pannus in a boy æt. 9; both corneæ completely opaque, presenting a wholly whitened appearance.

‖Cornea thick, rough, warty as if it were a mass of hypertrophied tissue loosened up little by little and scaled off from cornea leaving it clear and healthy.

‖Ulceration of cornea; painless tumefaction of lids.

▮Fungus hæmatodes.

‖*Silica* 3x caused the discharge of lead particles (arising from lead lotion) from cornea.

▮Eyes painful as if too dry and full of sand in morning.

Tension in eyes and forehead, with weakness of body.

Piercing stinging pain in l. eye.

▮Tearing, shooting, or at times throbbing, stinging pains in eyes, in paroxysms.

▮Smarting of eyes.

Aching in upper lid, with severe stitches in it as from a splinter, with vanishing of sight.

▮Pressure and soreness in orbits.

▮Ciliary neuralgia: especially over r. eye; darting pains through eyes and head upon exposure to any draft of air or just before a storm.

‖Every day about 1 o'clock, severe burning pains in r. eye and flow of tears over cheek, which feel scalding; these symptoms last for several hours; r. conjunctiva injected; pain on pressure in r. lachrymal sac, which feels somewhat swelled; mucous secretion in eye in morning; finally great swelling of lachrymal sac, forming a little lump at corner of eye exquisitely painful to touch, the seat of throbbing pains, the skin over it being red; hot tears run over cheek; nasal duct quite obstructed.

A feeling as if both her eyes were dragged back into head with strings.

▮Pain over eyes from wearing steel spectacles.

Pressive pain over l. eye about size of a sixpence.

Pain from occiput to eyeball, mostly r., sharp darting and a steady ache; eyeball sore and painful when revolved.

Smarting and pricking in l. eye.

Redness at first around eyes then also of conjunctivæ, with inflammation and lachrymation.

▮Redness of whites of eyes with pressive pain.

▮▮Trachoma of conjunctiva of r. eye, hyperæmia and swelling of conjunctiva and copious secretion of tears and mucus, after exposure to a storm the inflammation increased and there was also cloudiness of lenticular capsule; horizontal oval dilatation of pupil; violent supraorbital pain day and night; urine strongly ammoniacal, deposited a yellowish sediment and contained a large amount of albumen; sight very much diminished; copious muco-serous secretion from conjunctiva; after some time there was an abscess arising from upper part of iris, having a yellowish-red coloration, and covering whole pupil. θParenchymatous iritis.

▮▮Pain and photophobia and inability to open eyes even in dark; ulceration of r. cornea, with a deep, transparent base, threatening perforation; great hyperæmia of lids, of conjunctiva, and of epithelial layer of cornea; engorgement of submaxillary gland; moist vesicular eruption on back of head. θScrofulous ophthalmia.

▮▮Woman, æt. 28, has suffered for two months with recurrent phlyctenular conjunctivitis; phlyctenules have varied both in size and location, being at times very large and isolated, appearing almost like pustules and coming on any part of ocular conjunctiva; again they are smaller, like minute vesicles but more numerous, and sometimes form almost a complete circle at sclero-corneal junction; conjunctival redness, profuse lachrymation, intense photophobia, at times very severe pain; pain neuralgic, < at exit of supraorbital nerve; duration of attacks from eight to twelve days.

▮▮Eye inflamed from traumatic causes; foreign particles have lodged in the eye· abscesses.

▮▮Hypopion.

▮Blennorrhœa with suppuration; sensitive to cold air, wishes to keep warmly covered.

▮▮Twitching of eyelids.

▮Blepharitis: with agglutination in morning; caused or aggravated by working in a damp place or from being in cold air; objects seem as if in a fog, > by wiping eyes, fluent coryza, corners of mouth cracked, with psoriasis on arm.

▮▮For four months, constant discharge and ulceration under r. lower lid, the result of a severe inflammation; over r. inferior orbital ridge, cicatrices which everted the lid and three openings as found over dead bone, discharging a yellow white pus, on probing caries of lower orbital arch was found extending over malar and superior maxillary bones and connected by sinuses with the upper jaw opening over first molar tooth, through which opening the discharge escaped into mouth.

▮Boils around eye and lids.

▮Cystic tumors of lids.

▮Tarsal tumors; styes.

‖Cystic tumor of lower lid existing one year.

▮Styes, nodules and indurations on eyelids.

▮Affections appearing in angles of eyes.

▮Swelling in region of r. lachrymal gland and sac.

▮Lachrymation in open air.

▮▮Fistula lachrymalis; bone affected.

‖Swelling of r. lachrymal sac, skin over it inflamed; glistening; throbbing pain; tears hot; < evening.

‖Obstruction of canaliculi attending an attack of ophthalmia of six weeks' standing and affecting both eyes; acrid tears overflowed lower lids.

‖A completely established fistula of sac, with disorganization of walls of sac, denudation of internal horny wall and closure of nasal canal.

▮Stricture of lachrymal duct.

▮Blennorrhœa of lachrymal sac.

‖Swelling of r. tear bag forming a perceptible protrusion, skin covering it inflamed and glistening; throbbing in it; the flowing tears are hot, particularly in evening. θSwelling of lachrymal sac.

Soreness and smarting of eyelids, she cannot close them.

6 **Hearing and Ears.** ▮Oversensitive to noises; ears painfully sensitive to loud sounds.

▮Ringing or roaring in ears.

The ears seemed stopped.

▮Stoppage of ears, which open at times with a loud report.

▮Difficult hearing, especially of human voice and during full moon.

▮Diminished hearing from roaring in head.

‖Hardness of hearing, of long standing; < from washing and changing of linen; > from application of electricity.

Dulness of hearing with swelling and catarrh of Eustachian tubes and tympanic cavity.

▮Deafness without noise in ear, disappearing on blowing nose and coughing.

▮Hardness of hearing: of nervous origin; suddenly after a faint; ringing in ears and deafness with paralysis.

▮During headache roaring in ears as if something alive were in them.

‖ Deafness in a hemorrhoidal patient of twelve years' standing.

| Menière's disease.

| Itching: in Eustachian tubes, chronic coryza; in both ears, in ear, especially on swallowing.

Drawing pain in meatus auditorius, like otalgia.

| Stitches in ears.

| Otalgia; with stitches from within outward.

Shooting pain in l. ear, with a feeling as if humor were flowing from it.

Pricking, aching and itching in ears, l. chiefly.

‖ Sleep disturbed by pain in ears. θScarlatina.

‖ Boring pain. θOtorrhœa.

| Inflammation of labyrinth after cerebro-spinal meningitis.

‖ After overexertion, heaviness of head, earache and difficulty of hearing; hypersensitiveness to sounds, even sound of voices in speaking; catarrhal cough, pain in stomach and severe pain in back; between the shoulder blades any pressure on spinal column produced a violent and long-continued pain, so that she had a well-marked spinal irritation.

| Constant, watery, curdy and ichorous discharge without pain except after a fresh cold; pain drawing, shooting < at night and from change of weather or movement, also after being long seated.

| External meatus dry at outer portion, ulcerated farther in and at drumhead.

| Child bores into its ears with fingers when asleep, causing a discharge of blood and pus; it enjoys having the ear cleansed.

| Feeling of sudden stoppage in ear, > by gaping or swallowing.

| Hissing sounds in perforated ear.

| Increased secretion of thin cerumen.

‖ Otorrhœa: offensive, watery, curdy; with soreness of inner nose and crusts on upper lip, after abuse of mercury; with caries.

‖ Constant discharge, usually thin and watery, sometimes ichorous and curdy, from r. ear; quite deaf on affected side; after scarlatina, six years ago. θOtorrhœa.

| Purulent discharges from ears.

| Swelling of external ear, with discharge of pus from ear.

‖ Discharge of bloody mucus. θSuppuration of middle ear.

‖ Offensive discharge from ears, of several years' standing, with soreness of inner nose and crusts on upper lip. θOtorrhœa scrofulosa.

▮Discharge from ear after abuse of mercury.

‖Chronic sinus in front of l. ear; an ill-conditioned fistulous wound, had existed three years.

‖For six days pain in mastoid region; membrana tympani highly injected; tuning fork heard indifferently on either side when pressed against parietal bones; temperature 102; very weak and nervous; complete muscular paralysis of r. side of face; found some relief and sleep by placing head in a warm poultice of Indian meal. θMastoid periostitis.

‖Child puts hand behind ears. θScarlatina.

▮▮Caries of mastoid process.

▮▮Scabs behind ears.

▮Itching of outer ears.

▮Hard swelling of parotid; suppuration, especially if slow, painless.

7 **Smell and Nose.** ▮▮Loss of smell.

‖Smell of blood or of recently slaughtered animals. θChronic coryza.

▮Fetor from nose. θNasal catarrh.

▮Nosebleed.

Complete stoppage of nose, could scarcely speak.

Soreness on back of nose as if nasal bone had been beaten.

Drawing in root of nose and in r. malar bone.

▮Itching in nose.

▮Much sneezing, sometimes ineffectual; with acrid coryza.

▮Painful dryness of nose.

▮Troublesome itching, feeling of dryness in nose extending to forehead and antrum; periosteum is affected.

▮Dryness and stoppage after checked foot sweat.

▮Long-continued stoppage of nose from hardened mucus.

▮Coryza: fluent; violent for several weeks; dry, could not get air through nose; long-lasting, oft-returning; acrid, corroding; chronic, with swelling of mucous membrane; constant.

▮Nose stuffed up, or alternately dry and fluent; obstructed mornings, fluent during day.

▮With every fresh cold, stoppage and acrid discharge; makes inner nose sore and bloody.

▮Obstruction of nose in morning, followed by coryza during day.

▮Discharge of acrid water from nose, making inner nose and nostrils sore and bloody. θChronic coryza.

▮Food and drink rise into choanæ.

▮Nose inwardly dry, excoriated, covered with crusts.

▮Swelling of nasal mucous membrane. θChronic coryza.

A smarting, painful scab deep in r. nostril.

▮▮Gnawing and ulcers high up in nose, with great sensitiveness of place to contact.

▮Sore, painful scabs below septum of nose, with sticking pain when touched.

▮▮Ozæna with fetid, offensive discharge when the affection is seated in submucous connective tissue or in periosteum.

▮▮Offensive smelling nasal catarrh; every morning blows from nose hard, dry masses of mucus, followed by a quantity of offensive-smelling pus; headache; lassitude; loss of appetite; miserable appearance; profuse, offensive-smelling foot sweat; excoriation between toes when walking much.

▮▮Chronic catarrh: with stoppage of nose, loss of smell and taste; slimy, tough, purulent secretion stopping frequently in morning; swelling of nasal membrane; chronic inflammation of tonsils and painless swelling of submaxillary glands; tough slime in fauces, with hoarseness and rough cough; stoppage in morning followed by thick, green-yellow fetid masses after getting up; frontal sinuses inflamed, with pounding and throbbing pain in forehead; fauces dry and painful; uvula swollen; Eustachian tubes itching; chronic inflammation of tonsils and swelling of submaxillary glands.

ǁ Miss A., æt. 26, lymphatic and delicate, suffers since two years from inflammation of nasal duct, discharging large clots of blood mixed with dry mucus of a very foul smell; corner of eye red, oculo-palpebral mucous membrane slightly inflamed and itching, sac on l. side swollen so that the sore appears larger; frontal headache.

▮Caries of nasal bones from syphilis or scrofulosis.

▮Intolerable itching of tip of nose.

ǁ Man, æt. 48, ten years ago was much shocked on seeing tip of a friend's nose destroyed by cancer; since then his own has itched intolerably, < when thinking of it, and often keeping him awake at night.

Voluptuous itching about nose obliges constant rubbing in evening.

Tip of nose red.

▮Nose cold.

Herpetic eruption around nostrils and lips.

Burning, shooting pains in tip of nose flying up to forehead.

▮Tetters on nose (after *Calc. ostr.*).

8 **Upper Face.** ▮Face: pale; cachectic, body cool, sweaty; earthy; yellow, distorted; waxy; white and red spots.

Paleness of face before fainting.

▮Pale, cachectic appearance. θEczema capitis. θCancer of lip. θPanaritium. θCoxalgia. θMastitis. θTumor of eye. θCaries of tibia.

‖ Yellowish color of face. θGastralgia. θPerforating ulcer of stomach.

‖ Face emaciated, pale, yellowish. θAbscess of l. arm after dissecting wound.

❚ Rhagades about lids and lips.

❚ Skin of face cracks.

❚ Acne on forehead and back of hands.

Face distorted, eyes closed.

❚ Neuralgia of face, head, eyes, teeth and ears; pains < after being in bed a short time.

‖ Boring, tearing pains day and night, < during night, spreading over whole chest, also in bones of face.

❚ Prosopalgia; with hemorrhoids; with affection of periosteum; itching, with sensation of dryness in inner nose, extends into frontal cavities and antrum; with small lumps and nodules on scalp and face.

‖ Large hives on face and body before appearance of caries on lower jaw; after caries got well, vesicles appeared on whole body, with fever.

‖ A thick crop of papules on forehead, face and back of both hands. θAcne.

‖ Slight papular eruption upon forehead, similar to varicella. θPertussis.

‖ An induration extending from l. corner of mouth to a great portion of cheek.

‖ Induration of cellular tissue on one side of face, after parulis.

❚ Lupus; serrated ulcers, with greyish purulent surfaces; corroding, threatening to perforate cheek.

‖ Lupus; whole face corroded; tubercles on face, with ulceration of their apices; suppressed perspiration of feet (improved).

‖ Lupus in face, at interior extremity of cicatrix a deep ulcer threatening to perforate cheek, border of ulcer serrated, its surface greyish, bathed in a purulent sanies.

‖ Lupus in face, began on r. ear lobe, healing one side, corroding on other, advancing downward and forward, leaving irregular cicatrix (after *Bellad.*).

❚ Comedones.

‖ Swelling on r. cheek, made its appearance after scratching a pustule; burning pain on centre of swelling formed a black vesicle which broke and discharged burning ichor.

❚ Red spots on cheeks with burning heat.

❚ Blood-boils on cheeks.

Sycosis menti.

❚ Herpes on chin.

9 **Lower Face.** ❚ Articulation of jaw spasmodically closed.

Rheumatic pains in jaw and decayed teeth extending to temple.

Aching of both jaws.

‖Pricking and lancinating pains in region of r. inferior maxillary, with cancerous diathesis.

‖Pains more in jawbone than in teeth, swelling of jaw.

‖Bony swelling of the inferior maxillary, size of half a walnut.

▮Swelling and caries on lower jaw.

‖Caries of l. lower jaw.

▮Necrosis of lower jaw.

Boil on chin, with stinging pain when touched.

Ulceration of corners of mouth.

Painful ulcer in corner of mouth.

Corner of mouth ulcerated with an itching sensation with scabs for many days.

▮Nose and lips large, swollen and distorted.

▮Dry and parched feeling of lips.

‖Foam at mouth. θEpilepsy.

Swelling of lower lip.

‖Blisters on margins of lips.

▮Scabby eruption on lips, which smarts.

▮Large, hard, brownish crusts on lips, especially about corners of mouth.

‖Woman, æt. 61, cancer of lower lip after having picked lip. θCancer of lip.

‖External third of lower lip on r. side swollen and congested with an induration size of an apricot-stone in centre of swelling, on red border superficial ulceration with greyish base; excrutiacing pain. θCancer of lower lip.

‖For more than a month, felt an itching, sometimes burning, in a very circumscribed spot in a part of lower lip, finally succeeded by intolerable shooting pains; a hard spot became perceptible in thickness of lip which soon made its appearance externally in shape of a conical pimple; tumor soon became black, wrinkled and as large as a good-sized hazelnut.

▮Cancer of lower lip; ulcer greyish, superficial, excruciatingly painful.

▮▮Painful or painless swelling of submaxillary glands.

10 **Teeth and Gums.** ▮▮Difficult dentition: teething delayed; gums sensitive, blistered; frequently grasping at gums; scrofulous children having worms, with profuse salivation; fever toward evening and all night with heat in head; difficult stools; stool recedes before child can effect its passage; feet smell badly, notwithstanding every effort to prevent it; profuse sour-smelling perspi-

ration upon head in evening; fontanelles large, head larger in proportion than rest of body; protruding gum seems blistered and is sensitive; stools when loose are usually dark and sometimes offensive.

▮Teeth feel too large and too long for the mouth.

▮Looseness of teeth.

Teeth loose and gum painful to slightest pressure.

▮Caries of teeth, pains < at night and on inhaling cold air.

▮Throbbing toothache, swelling of periosteum.

▮Stinging toothache, preventing sleep.

Constant aching in all the teeth.

|| Neuralgia in all the teeth, with heat and tearing pain in head; constant spitting of tenacious slimy saliva; raging at night; not affected by cold or warmth.

In scrofulous and rachitic subjects with carious teeth toothache is particularly < at night from inhaling cold air.

▮Throbbing toothache with swelling of periosteum or lower jaw, where the pain is more severe than in teeth; unable to sleep on account of general heat; every hurt festers and is slow to heal.

|| Erysipelatous swelling on gums and roof of mouth after extraction of teeth.

▮Tedious, boring, tearing pains day and night, < during night, spreading over whole cheek, and into bones of face; discharge of offensive matter from openings near roots of teeth or from gums; swelling of jaw.

▮Burning stitching in several teeth, < at night, < by cold air in mouth, with heat in head and burning in chest; pain in submaxillary glands, with or without swelling.

Gum is painfully sensitive on taking cold water into mouth.

▮▮Gums very sore, inflamed; gum-boils.

Cool feeling in upper gums, soreness of palate, lips feel much parched.

|| Tumor, size of a walnut, in place of two bicuspid teeth.

11 **Taste and Tongue.** ▮Taste: of blood, morning; of soapsuds; bitter, morning, with thick mucus in throat; of rotten eggs.

▮Loss of taste and appetite.

▮Water tastes badly; vomits after drinking.

▮Tongue feels sore.

Sensation as if a hair were on tip of tongue extending into trachea, where it causes a crawling so that he is frequently obliged to cough and hack.

|| Whitish, trembling tongue. θAbscess of l. arm.

Soreness of tongue.

▮Tongue coated with brownish mucus.

▮Glossitis.

▮Indurations in tongue.

‖Ulcer on r. border of tongue eating into it and discharging a great deal of pus. θCarcinoma.

▮One-sided swelling of tongue.

12 **Inner Mouth.** ‖Acidity in mouth, after eating.

▮Bad odor from mouth in morning.

▮Constant dryness in mouth ; without thirst.

▮Accumulation of mucus in mouth.

▮Saliva runs out of mouth.

▮▮Inflammation and suppuration of salivary glands.

‖Irritable condition of mucous membrane of mouth; skin of body pale and flabby. θNeuralgia.

▮Stomacace ; mouth gangrenous, with perforating ulcer of palate.

13 **Throat.** Soreness of palate, which assumed a pale yellow color.

▮Swelling in palate; swelling of uvula. θChronic coryza.

‖Fauces affected, dry painful throat. θChronic coryza.

▮Tough slime in fauces.

▮Hawking up of thick, green, yellow, fetid mucus, or yellow, very offensive balls.

‖Swelling in front of throat, region of thyroid body extending around to parotids, commencing on l., extending to r. side, cannot move, holds neck stiffly.

Sensation as of a lump in r. side of throat; she could only swallow with great difficulty.

▮Pricking in throat, as from a pin, causing cough, l. side.

▮Tonsils swollen, each effort to swallow distorts face.

▮▮Tonsillitis when suppurating gland will not heal; pus continues to flow, but gets thinner, less laudable, darker and more fetid.

▮Periodical quinsy.

▮▮Inflammation of tonsils when too late for absorption.

▮Chronic inflammation of tonsils.

▮Throat feels as if filled up, as if he could not swallow; frequent cough bringing up white, frothy, saltish mucus; < toward evening.

▮Swallowing painful, no inflammation. θHysteria.

Sore throat, as from a lump in l. side, on swallowing.

Burning in throat.

Dryness of throat as from a cold.

Soreness of throat, as if he swallowed over a sore spot, at times stitches in it.

Pressive soreness on l. side of throat when swallowing.

Sticking sore throat only on swallowing, with pain in throat even to touch.

▮Feeling as if throat were filled up, as if he could not swallow. θChronic sore throat.

▮When swallowing, soreness and stitches in throat.
▮When swallowing food easily gets into choanæ.
▮Sequelæ of diphtheria; amaurosis.
▮Swallowing difficult as from paralysis.
▮Paralysis of velum pendulum palati.
▮Chronic pharyngitis with constipation.
▮Mouth gangrenous with perforating ulcer of palate.
▮Swelling of submaxillary and cervical glands.
▮Submaxillary glands painful to touch but not swollen.
▮Enlarged thyroid gland.

14 **Appetite, Thirst. Desires, Aversions.** ▮Excessive hunger.
▮Canine hunger, but on attempting to eat has sudden disgust for food.
▮Canine hunger, with nervous, irritable persons.
▮Want of appetite; excessive thirst.
No desire for anything but small quantities of preserves.
▮▮Thirst.
▮Averse to warm, cooked food; desires only cold things, disgust for meat.
▮▮Aversion to mother's milk and vomiting whenever taking it.

15 **Eating and Drinking.** ▮▮While eating, pain in head much better.
In evening, while eating, an acute pain extending from abdomen to testes.
▮After eating: sour eructations, fulness and pressure in stomach; waterbrash and vomiting; sleepiness, vomits large masses of water.
▮▮Painfulness of epigastrium upon pressure, griping pain also after eating. θGastralgia.
▮▮Regularly after eating chilliness on back; icy-cold feet in evening. θChronic hepatitis.
▮▮Pyrosis and vomiting after eating. θPerforating ulcer.
▮Hectic fever in debilitated persons, < after meals.
Small quantities of wine cause ebullitions and thirst.
Vomits after drinking.
▮▮Screwing, pressing, twisting pain in stomach after drinking. θPerforating ulcer.
▮Dry cough after drinking cold water.
Diarrhœa after milk.

16 **Hiccough, Belching, Nausea and Vomiting.** ▮Eructations: sour; tasting of food; loud, uncontrollable, with pain in stomach.
▮Intense heartburn, sensation of a load in epigastrium.
▮Waterbrash: with chilliness; with a brownish tongue.
Ineffectual retching, waterbrash with nausea.
▮Nausea: with violent palpitation; after every exercise that raises bodily temperature; after eating a little; and

vomiting of tenacious mucus, hiccough; sense of emptiness at stomach; after stools.

▮Nausea and vomiting of what is drunk < in morning.

▮Vomiting while drinking, especially if drinking be hasty.

▮Water tastes badly; vomits after drinking.

▮Child vomits as soon as it nurses.

▮Vomits: ingesta, at night.

Morning vomiting, with nausea, much exhaustion.

▮Nausea and vomiting during pregnancy.

▮▮Nausea and vomiting of mucus in morning, much exhausting a young and vigorous man. θSuppressed foot sweat.

17 **Scrobiculum and Stomach.** ▮Anguish in pit of stomach, attacks of melancholy.

▮Burning or throbbing in pit of stomach.

▮Sensitiveness of pit of stomach to pressure.

▮Pressure as after eating too much.

▮Heaviness like lead in stomach.

▮Cutting feeling, at other times weight, crampy sensation, tightness at pit of stomach.

Felt as if knives were running into her stomach.

Cold pain at epigastrium as if a cold stone were in stomach.

▮▮Nearly every morning after partaking of any kind of drink a digging and twisting, followed by retching and vomiting of bitter, salty water, coming with such force as to make him sweat and tremble all over. θGastralgia.

▮Gastralgia: with pyrosis, hiccough or nausea and glairy vomiting; heat, weight, sensitiveness and a feeling of constriction; flatulency, eructations, somnolency, languor, coldness of extremities, loss of appetite, slow and painful digestion, often hunger which cannot be satisfied.

▮▮After a meal, load as of a stone or lead in stomach, particularly after eating raw vegetables.

▮▮Yellowish complexion; screwing, pressing, twisting pain after drinking, pyrosis and vomiting after eating. θUlcer of stomach.

▮Induration of pylorus.

18 **Hypochondria.** Pressure or aching pain in hypochondrium.

▮Beating soreness in liver; < on motion, when walking, when lying on r. side.

▮▮Sore, ulcerative pain and frequent throbbing, two fingers' breadth below r. floating ribs; cannot tolerate least pressure; cannot step upon r. foot without greatly aggravating pain to an intolerable degree; confusion of head; dull pain in occiput; pressing pain in forehead; vertigo on stooping; loss of appetite; pressure in stomach after eating; stool delayed two or three days; constant severe cough all day, awakening her at night, < from motion; scanty, slimy expectoration; sensation as if sternum were grasped; tearing in limbs, stitches, and a dropping or running sensation; muscles weak, flabby; emaciation; after eating, chilliness along back, congestion to head, heat in face, slight burning in soles of feet; feet icy-cold in evening; sweat on slight motion, profuse and debilitating in morning in bed; pulse small, weak, rapid, irregular; lassitude, desire to sleep, restless sleep, at night suddenly starts from sleep, trembling and frightened; despondency. θHepatic disorder.

▮Liver complaint with obstinate constipation; want of expulsive power in rectum; hardness and distension in region of liver; abscesses; throbbing, ulcerative pain < from touch and motion; < at night and during new and full moon; scrofulous diathesis.

‖Neurosis of chest with pain in region of spleen and indescribably quick breathing.

Morbus maculosis Werlhofii, with disorganization of spleen.

19 **Abdomen.** ▮Pressure in abdomen, especially after eating, clothing feels too tight.

▮Tightness transversely across abdomen.

Abdomen constantly hard, greatly distended, making him very uncomfortable.

▮Hard, hot, distended abdomen, especially in children.

▮▮Large abdomen in children.

Abdomen feels thick and heavy like a weight.

Abdomen hot, tense, constant rumbling and grumbling in it, diarrhœa.

▮▮Flatulence: much rumbling; incarcerated; very offensive; shifting; difficult to discharge; with costiveness; with distended abdomen; rumbling and gurgling in abdomen; fetid, smelling like wet brass.

Violent cutting in lower abdomen with incarcerated flatus; every step is painfully felt.

Colicky pains in lower abdomen, with straining and increased pain during stool.

▮Tenderness about hernial tumor.

▮Colic: from worms; with constipation or difficult stool; with yellow hands, blue nails; with reddish, bloody stools; > by warmth.

Momentary pinching pain at navel.

Cutting pain in region of navel going through to back and coming on at intervals.

▮▮Abdominal pains relieved by warmth.

‖Abdominal dropsy; effusion so great that his weight was thirty-six pounds in excess; frequent attacks of watery diarrhœa, lasting several days, leaving him exhausted, emaciated and unable to leave his bed; would then rally and filling-up process recommence.

▌Rhagades and cracks on surface of abdomen.

▌▌Discharge of pus, intestinal gases and fecal matter through abdominal fistula.

▌Inflamed inguinal glands, painful to touch.

▌Inguinal hernia.

▌▌Mr. D., æt. 67; abscess in r. groin, hernia both sides; irritation of truss the supposed cause; syphilitic taint; tumor increased till it contained as much as two gills of matter; got well without breaking; both hernia got well without further treatment.

20 **Stool and Rectum.** ▌Stools: frequent, scanty, liquid, offensive as carrion; pasty; paplike; offensive; contain undigested food, with great exhaustion, but painless; mucous, followed by itching in anus; watery, weakening; liquid, slimy, frothy, mucous or bloody; mushy, horribly offensive; purulent; cadaverous-smelling; putrid; sour (during dentition).

▌Diarrhœa: from exposure to cold air; after vaccination; with griping pains in bowels; in morning before rising, from 6 to 8 A.M.; watery, weakening; chronic, from ulceration of bowels; in thin, scrawny children with sweaty head and sweaty, offensive-smelling feet; child very much emaciated, nurses well but food passes through undigested, open fontanelles; much perspiration about head; great thirst; emaciation; cold hands and feet with cold sweat on them; rolling of head; suppressed secretion of urine.

Before stool: pain in bowels.

During stool: chilliness and nausea in throat; colic; itching and stinging in rectum; piles; succus prostaticus.

After stool: burning and smarting in anus; remission of abdominal pains; pressing and burning in anus; burning in prepuce; eructation.

▌▌Child, 1 year old; on mother's side dyscrasia, scrofula, softening of brain, tuberculosis; teething process delayed; relapsing summer complaint; feet very dry and smelled like an old person's.

▌Natural stool, evacuated with much pressure and straining.

▌▌Constipation: very hard, unsatisfactory stools, with very great effort; constant but ineffectual desire for stool in evening; stool dry, hard and light-colored; stool very hard, followed by burning in anus; very hard, nodular, like clay stools, evacuated only with great effort; stool scanty, difficult, after great urging and straining until abdominal walls are sore, the stool that has alredy protruded slips back again; stool remains a long time in rectum as if there were no power to expel it; from inactivity in rectum, with pain and ineffectual desire for stool; prolonged efforts during stool render muscles of abdomen sore; before and during menses; stool comes to verge of anus then slips back into rectum; with spinal affections, as if rectum were paralyzed.

▮Loss of expulsive power with a large but soft stool.

❘❘Constipation; large slime-covered feces; stools five to seven days apart and occurred then only upon use of injections or cathartics; copious sweat on head and face directly upon falling asleep; child, æt. 8 mos., suffering since birth.

▮In rectum: sharp stitches when walking; jerking, almost dull sticking pain; cutting; stinging; burning, stinging, itching during stool.

▮Hemorrhoids; intensely painful, boring cramping from anus to rectum or testicles; protrude during stool, become incarcerated; suppuration; discharge of bloody mucus from rectum; intense pain with slight protrusion.

▮In anus: tension; boring cramplike pain extending into rectum and testicles; pain as if constricted, during stool; sticking; burning after a dry hard stool; itching; stitches and shooting pains; moisture.

▮Fissura ani, great pain half an hour after stool, lasting several hours.

▮▮Fissura ani and fistula in ano.

❘❘Aching, beating throbbing pain in lumbo-sacral region, with occasional perineal tumefaction which discharged blood and pus; constipation, stools slipping back after much effort; great anxiety.

▮▮Fistula in ano; also with chest symptoms.

21 **Urinary Organs.** ▮Suppuration of kidneys; abscesses.

▮Diabetes mellitus.

▮Purulent blennorrhœa of bladder.

▮Tenesmus of bladder and anus.

▮Paralysis of bladder.

Obliged to rise nearly every night to urinate.

Desire to urinate without emission.

▮Continuous urging, with scanty discharge; also at night.

▮Weakness in urinary organs; constant desire to urinate.

▮Profuse urination relieves headache.

▮Involuntary micturition at night; also in children, with worms and in chorea.

❘❘Nightly incontinence of urine, after a blow upon head, when three years old, in a girl æt. 7.

|| A boy, æt. 15, troubled ever since his recollection with nocturnal enuresis nearly every night, until he was thirteen, when he left home; by a strong effort of will and care it was not so frequent, but still quite beyond his control.

▮ Enuresis nocturna, complicated with worms or chorea.

▮ Urine: light-colored; suppressed; turbid; sediment of red or yellow sand.

During urination: burning and soreness in urethra; pressure in bladder; itching of vulva; cutting pain.

Strangury.

After urination: involuntary discharge of urine.

Suppression of urine.

▮ Renal and vesical calculus.

22 **Male Sexual Organs.** ▮ Sexual desire increased, or decreased.

▮ Painful erections, before rising in morning; frequent violent erections.

▮ Sexual erethism, with spinal or paralytic disease.

▮ After an embrace, sensation on r. side of head as if paralyzed with soreness of limbs.

▮ Lascivious thoughts and dreams; nocturnal emissions, followed by great exhaustion; prostatitis.

Violent erections without sexual desire.

▮ Sexual desire very weak.

|| After masturbation seminal emissions twice a week, between 3 and 5 A.M.; great depression of spirits; aching in sacrum; sweat of scrotum; heat in head; burning of feet with sweat; weakness and heaviness of arms; melancholy; < A.M. and before an emission; > after an emission.

▮▮ Discharge of prostatic fluid while straining at stool.

|| Prostate gland enlarged, without pain, but irregularly indurated, one point being hard, another soft.

▮ Prostatitis; suppuration, thick fetid pus from urethra.

|| Gonorrhœa, with thick fetid pus; < after exertion to the extent of sweating.

▮ Gonorrhœa; pus or puslike bloody discharge; slight shreddy discharge.

▮ Chronic syphilis; suppurations and indurations.

▮ Chancres: with raised edges; inflamed, painful, irritable, discolored; thin bloody discharge; granulations indistinct or absent.

▮ Red spots and itching on corona glandis.

▮ Painful eruptions on mons veneris; itching, moist or dry eruptions of red pimples or spots on genitals. θSyphilis.

▮ Slight swelling of penis and testicles.

▮ Squeezing pain in testicles.

At the height of chill penis and testicles are hot.
Sharp pricking pains in penis.
Prepuce red and itching; swollen and itching humid pimples on it.
▮Itching moist spots on genitals, mostly on scrotum; sweat on scrotum.
❙❙Pale-red, sensitive swelling hard as a stone extending from l. inguinal region across mons veneris, with burning stinging tearing pain in swelling, sacrum, and l. thigh, preventing sleep; slimy fluid discharges from two fistulous openings.
▮▮Hydrocele; men and scrofulous children.

23 **Female Sexual Organs.** ▮Sterility.
▮Increased sexual desire, with paralytic or spinal affections.
❙❙She feels nauseated during coition. θUterine cancer.
▮Nymphomania due to plethora or spinal irritation.
▮Prolapsus uteri in consequence of myelitis.
▮Serous cysts in vagina.
▮Pressing-down feeling in vagina.
▮Indurations of cervix uteri.
▮Ulceration of neck of womb and os.
▮Periuterine cellulitis; areolar hyperplasia.
❙❙Metrorrhagia of six weeks' duration in a washerwoman who attributes her sickness to constantly standing in cold water.
▮Metrorrhagia: offensive foot sweat; icy-cold body; painful hemorrhoids.
▮Bloody discharge between periods.
▮Menses: too early and scanty; too late and profuse; irregular, every two or three months; during lactation; strong-smelling, acrid; repeated paroxysms of icy coldness over whole body.
▮Before menses: pressing pain in forehead; violent colic, shuddering all over body whole day, acrid leucorrhœa; sensation as if vulva were enlarged, with soreness in perineum.
▮During menses: pain in abdomen; tearing pain in tibia; toothache and obscuration of sight; violent pressure in forehead, with discharge of plugs from nose; constipation; sensation as of a heavy lump in anus; cold feet; burning and soreness about vulva; eruption on inside of thighs; drawing between shoulders; melancholy, anxiety and weariness of life.
▮Discharge of a quantity of white water from uterus instead of menses.
▮▮Amenorrhœa with suppressed foot sweat; pain in abdomen.

‖ Mucous surfaces of external genitals red, vascular, moist and exquisitely sensitive to touch; married six months, but there was no possibility of sexual intercourse; examination of internal surfaces impossible without inducing anæsthesia artificially; chronic headache of a pressing, pulsating or tearing character, < by mental exertion, stooping, talking, or cold air; > by warmth and warm wraps; frequently profuse, sour perspiration on head in evening; tendency to take cold in head from slight causes, especially if head is uncovered; weight or pressure in vagina, with painful bearing down, vagina being tender to touch. θVaginismus.

Discharge of a quantity of white watery fluid from vagina.

▮▮ Serous cysts of vagina; vaginal fistula.

▮▮ Itching of pudenda.

▮ Violent burning and soreness of pudenda, with eruption on inner sides of thighs, during menses.

▮ Itching of vulva; acrid leucorrhœa.

▮ Ascarides of vulva.

▮▮ Leucorrhœa: profuse, acrid, corroding; milky, preceded by cutting around navel; causes biting pain, especially after acrid food; during urinating; in gushes; with cancer of uterus.

‖ Profuse, yellow, excoriating leucorrhœa; discharge tenacious; astringent injections produced a peculiar sensation at pit of stomach; continual headache; feels > with head covered up warmly.

▮▮ Inflammation, induration, and suppuration of breasts; fistulous ulcers, discharge thin and watery or thick and offensive; substance of mamma seems to be discharged in pus; one lobe after another ulcerates and discharges into one common ulcer, often with pain, or there may be several orifices, one for each lobe.

▮ Inflammation of nipples; they crack and ulcerate.

‖ Hard nodular tumor of breast.

‖ Scirrhus of r. breast in an old lady, æt. 70; great itching of swollen gland.

‖ Scirrhus mammæ, in a woman æt. 40, weakly constitution; since frequent catarrhal affections, somewhat asthmatic; for some time observed a lump in r. mamma; near nipple toward right, a scirrhus as hard as cartilage, of uneven surface, movable, and size of a hazelnut.

‖ A lady, æt. 65, thin; for six months a tumor of r. breast, making it twice natural size; had itch twenty years ago; palpation showed fluctuation; trochar detected pus; further examination showed carious rib.

21 **Parturition. Pregnancy. Lactation.** ▮ Threatened abortion; hemorrhage after abortion.

▮▮Hemorrhage after abortion, < from least motion, mental or sexual excitement; painful hemorrhoids and obstinate constipation.

▮Promotes expulsion of moles; shooting pains.

▮Nausea and vomiting of pregnancy; menses had been accompanied by palpitation.

Soreness and lameness of feet from instep to sole, during pregnancy.

▮Too violent motion of fœtus.

▮After-pains felt in hips.

Suppressed lochia followed by boring pain in l. temple, l. supraorbital nerve, and orbit of eye; < by talking, or mental exertion; before suppression, nursing produced a venous metrorrhagia.

▮▮While nursing: sharp pain in breast or uterus, pain in back, increase of lochia; pure blood flows every time child nurses; complains every time she puts child to breast.

▮▮Aversion to mother's milk; child refuses to nurse, or if it does nurse, it vomits.

▮Milk suppressed.

▮Mammæ swollen, dark red, sensitive, burning pains prevent rest at night.

▮▮Hard lumps in mammæ.

▮Great itching of swollen mammæ. θScirrhus.

▮Inflammation of nipples.

▮Darting, burning in l. nipple.

▮Nipple is drawn in, like a funnel.

▮▮Scirrhus near r. nipple, hard as gristle, uneven surface.

▮Nipple ulcerates; is very sore and tender.

▮Hard-edged fistulous ulcers remaining after mammary abscesses.

▮Fistula of mammæ discharging serum or milk.

▮Rhagades of mammæ, or other parts covered with delicate skin, or on parts affected by tettery eruptions.

▮▮Pain in nodular swelling of l. breast, cutting pains in abdomen.

▮Inflamed breast, deep-red in centre, rose-colored toward periphery, swollen, hard and sensitive to touch; constant burning pain prevents her from resting at night; high fever, face sunken, but excited. θMastitis.

25 **Voice and Larnyx. Trachea and Bronchia.** ▮Hoarseness, roughness of larynx.

▮Husky voice; < in morning; chronic coryza.

▮▮Fibrous, painless swelling of larynx, connected with thyroid cartilage.

▮Foreign bodies in larynx.

▮Laryngeal morning cough commencing immediately on

rising, with tough, gelatinous and very tenacious expectoration.

▮Bronchial affections of rachitic children; copious purulent or transparent expectoration.

Tickling in larynx with slight cough and hoarseness.

Roughness and soreness in trachea and bronchia.

26 **Respiration.** Deep sighing breathing.

▮Shortness of breath and panting from walking fast, or from manual labor.

▮Dyspnœa: when lying on back; when stooping; when running; also after running; when coughing.

▮Oppression of chest, cannot take a long breath.

▮Asthma: < when lying down; spasmodic cough; spasm of larnyx; pulsations in chest; often with profuse, purulent sputa; cannot bear a draft of air on back of neck.

❙❙Nervous asthma, dry spasmodic cough; oppression does not permit him to lie down or stoop; spasm of larynx and pulsations in chest.

❙❙Breathing so difficult that eyes seemed to protrude from their sockets and the doors and windows had to be thrown open; attacks came only during a thunderstorm.

▮Hay asthma coming on about the last of August.

27 **Cough.** ▮Cough: dry, with hoarseness; with soreness in chest; excited by tickling in throat pit; hollow, spasmodic; loose, day and night; with profuse expectoration vomiting of tenacious mucus in morning; with thick purulent sputa; awakens him at night; < from motion; scanty mucous expectoration; especially troublesome after lying down in evening and after waking in morning; hacking caused by nightly tickling in pharynx; at first caused by tickling in throat, gradually seeming to come from lower down in throat until it came from chest and shook the abdomen, during day consisting of sudden explosive coughs without expectoration, < in evening.

▮Cough and sore throat with expectoration of small badly smelling granules.

❙❙Cough with purulent expectoration; prevented the ulcers in lungs from spreading.

▮Phthisis; cough with profuse expectoration, vomiting of tenacious mucus in morning, during attack of cough; dyspnœa; blood-spitting; night sweats.

❙❙Child 3 years old, strongly marked scrofulous constitution; suffocative cough; obstructed, difficult, rattling respiration; profuse expectoration of purulent matter; great emaciation; frequent, copious, fetid, papescent stools, with great exhaustion; slight pustular eruption, (similar to varicella) upon forehead.

▮Cough < from cold, > from warm drinks. θChronic bronchitis.

▮Influenza with difficulty of hearing, at times ringing in ears.

▮▮Stonecutters' pulmonary affections, copious fetid expectoration.

||After artificial evacuation of an empyema continuing suppuration, hectic fever, emaciation, night sweats and diarrhœa. θPhthisis.

▮▮Expectoration: profuse, fetid, purulent, green; only during day; of viscid, milky, acrid mucus; at times pale frothy blood; tastes greasy; makes water turbid, that which sinks to bottom has an offensive odor; when thrown into water falls to bottom and spreads like a heavy sediment.

28 **Inner Chest and Lungs.** ▮Lungs feel sore.

▮Stitches in chest and sides through to back.

▮Excruciating deep-seated pains in chest.

▮Pain under sternum.

▮Painless throbbing and beating in breast bone.

▮Sticking pains in chest on inspiration.

Pressive pain in sternum toward pit of stomach.

▮Pressing pain, stitches; general sensation of weakness in chest; can hardly speak, is so weak. θPhthisis.

||Severe stitching pain in r. lung two inches below nipple, extending through to back; < on motion of any kind and deep breathing.

Painful stitches in chest, shooting from sternum around to back.

Tensive pain across chest lasting for some hours.

Tight feeling around chest, as if she were tied in with a tape.

Pressure at lower sternum as from a stone; pain under sternum.

▮▮Inflammation of lungs resulting in suppuration.

▮Dropsy of chest, or empyema; motion produces severe palpitation of heart; from anæmia and lack of nutrition; also in stonecutters.

▮Empyema after pleurisy.

▮Congestion to chest; body chilly.

▮Chronic neglected pneumonia, passing over into suppuration.

▮▮Chronic bronchitis and phthisis.

▮Phthisical abscess of lungs; formation of cavities.

||Several attacks of hæmoptysis, after which he gradually declined; about eight months afterward large cavity in r. lung at second intercostal space about three inches to r. of sternum; heavy rales in l. bronchus with decided in-

dications of breaking down of parenchymatous structure and cavernous lesions there, also sputa very heavy and largely purulent; cadaverous odor present, musty and offensive; no appetite; could hardly sit up long enough to have bed made; skin cold, clammy; drenching night sweats; marked absence of vital warmth. θPhthisis.

❙❙Hemorrhage from lungs for nine months; cavities in both lungs; symptoms of septicæmia from absorption of pus from cavities; clammy, cadaverous sweat covering whole body, which had the feeling as if mould was forming; no appetite; large quantities of thick, heavy mucopus, largely purulent. θConsumption.

❙Stonecutters' consumption.

29 **Heart, Pulse and Circulation.** ❙Palpitation: while sitting, the hand in which he is holding something trembles; violent hammering after every quick or violent motion; and throbbing over whole body while sitting.

Awoke with rapid pulse, palpitation and sensation of heat.

Orgasm of blood at night; throbbing in all the vessels.

The circulation is easily agitated.

❙Heart troubles from nervous exhaustion.

❙Pulse: small, hard, rapid; frequently irregular and then slow; imperceptible, with earthy complexion (carbuncle).

30 **Outer Chest.** ❙Painless throbbing in sternum.

❙Tightness across chest; after suppressed foot sweat.

❙❙Sensation as if a hand had grasped her breast bone. θChronic hepatitis.

❙❙A scrofulous child æt. 11, swelling size of a plum, occasioned by closing of an issue; between fifth and sixth ribs on r. side, below nipple.

A man, æt. about 60, had a tumor in l. breast, one and a quarter inches in diameter, and a half inch in depth, the nipple occupying the centre; it slowly increased and became painful, pain sharp, stinging and twinging; almost intolerable itching of whole breast, had an ulcer about three inches long and one inch wide on r. leg, over upper end of fibula, which had been carious and a part of it removed, but the ulcer did not heal. θCancerous tumor.

❙❙When convalescing from a severe attack of typhoid fever, a tumor appeared in one of the right intercostal spaces, which, after being frequently poulticed, broke open and commenced to discharge first a thick, creamy pus, mixed with some blood, but becoming thinner and more offensive every day; was pale and weak, and the discharge, which, by its long duration, was causing decided harm to the organism, consisted of thin, dirty, fetid ichorous fluid, and the surrounding parts were hard, swollen and bluish; pain in ribs < in a warm room, but as soon as he would go out into cold air (being Winter) his sufferings became unbearable.

|| Necrosis of acromio-clavicular articulation with complete anchylosis of l. shoulder joint.

|| Malignant scrofulous ulcers and fistulous openings of lymphatic glands of neck, with caries of clavicle.

|| Fistulous opening near sixth rib from an abscess, with gnawing pain; a spongy growth size of a nut, broken by fistulous openings, protrudes; fistulous openings have a scarlet border, discharge ichorous, stinking pus.

|| Small tumor in l. breast of a man, æt. 60, with sharp, stinging, twinging pain and intolerable itching.

▮ Eruption like varicella, covering breast and itching violently.

An eruption like chicken pox covering the breast, with vehement itching, which obliges one to scratch and rub the affected parts with force.

31 **Neck and Back.** || Pain in nape of neck follows lumbar pain. θSpinal disease.

▮ Rheumatism of lower cervical vertebræ.

Stiffness and chilliness at nape of neck, and chilliness all down back.

▮ Stiffness: of nape of neck; of one side of neck, cannot turn head on account of pain; of nape of neck, with headache.

▮ A recurrent fibroid tumor the size of a hen's egg and very hard in l. side of neck, not connected with parotid, though growing a little below it, he was > by wraping up, even head; timid about going into a new enterprise; lacks confidence in his own ability.

|| Purulent infiltration of tissues of neck, following carbuncle.

▮▮ Cervical glands and parotids swollen, indurated.

▮▮ Glandular swellings of neck and in armpits, with suppuration.

▮ Scrofulous swelling and induration of cervical and parotid glands, coming gradually, of long duration, often attaining an enormous size; hot skin, without pain or redness.

▮▮ Boils or carbuncles on nape of neck; anthrax; want of vital warmth; slow progress of disease.

|| Swelling hard, discolored, purplish-red, discharging from an opening near edge, acrid, corroding, stinking, yellowish-green ichor. θCarbuncle.

|| Large dusky patch on front of neck, and another on

nape of neck, extending to scalp, covered with minute scales. θEczema.

Itching pimples, like nettlerash, on nape of neck.

▮▮Swelling and soreness in old cicatricial tissues about neck and breast, the result of scrofulous abscesses.

▮▮Right lobe of thyroid gland swollen, having the appearance of an elastic cyst.

▮Struma, with suppurating fistula.

▮Rheumatism of lower cervical vertebræ; violent tearing pain between scapulæ.

Tearing pain beneath scapulæ while walking.

Frequent sticking in r. scapula.

▮In small of back: violent pain; pain after stooping; pain as if beaten, at night; pain when getting out of bed in morning; feeling as if dead after suppressed foot sweat; spasmodic pain does not allow him to rise; stiffness and pain on rising from a seat; spasmodic drawing compelling him to lie still.

Weakness of back and a paralyzed feeling in lower extremities, could scarcely walk.

▮▮Pain in curved spine.

Burning in back while walking in open air and becoming warm.

Violent shooting pain in back between hips.

▮Aching, beating, throbbing in back.

Stiff, sore feeling down r. side of spine, then across loins and over r. hip joint.

▮Constant aching in centre of spine.

▮▮Spinal irritation, paralytic symptoms; cold feet; constipation.

▮Aching in loins, shooting down legs.

▮Spinal curvature to the right, painful to touch and motion.

▮▮H., æt. 16, eighteen months ago fell; after first shock felt well until nine months, when pain appeared in sacrum and hip; applied *Rhus* liniment; now suffers from pain from sacrum upward to lumbar region, and across l. ilium to superior spinal process; pain throbbing, < on pressure over lumbar vertebræ, and this, when severe, gives rise to a pain in nape of neck and a sense of loss of power in lower extremities; stooping causes severe pain darting up spine. θTraumatic periostitis of sacrum and lower vertebræ.

▮▮Disease of cervical vertebræ in a boy, æt. 3; when sixteen months old head would fall forward, chin resting on sternum, and he began instinctively to support head by placing hands under chin, and when lifted up, especially if hands were not supporting chin, opened his mouth in a gaping manner; by-and-by had no longer any power to hold things in hands, soon after the power of walking and then of standing ceased, nor could he even sit up; bowels costive; urine free; intellect precocious; memory excellent; emaciation.

|| Bony structure of spine affected; chronic gouty nodosities. θMyelitis.

▮ Caries of lumbar vertebræ.

▮ Spina bifida.

▮ Psoas abscess.

▮ Diseases brought on by exposure of back to draft of air.

▮ Aching in sacrum. θSpermatorrhœa.

▮▮ Lame feeling in region of sacrum.

|| Aching, beating, throbbing pain in lumbo-sacral region.

|| Coccyx hurts after riding; coccygodynia.

Elevated scabby spots on coccyx above fissure of nates.

Stinging in os coccygis, which is painful to pressure.

32 **Upper Limbs.** Pain in shoulder and arm at night, > by warm wrappings.

Momentary sharp pain in r. shoulder joint.

Acute pain in r. shoulder blade.

|| Swelling on l. scapula seven inches broad, five inches long, of thickness of a finger, raised in middle and inflamed, after two weeks it opened in several places and discharged profuse matter.

▮▮ Swelling, induration and suppuration of axillary glands.

▮▮ Offensive axillary sweat.

▮ Bones of arm feel bruised.

|| Shaking of l. arm; before epilepsy.

Arms and hands feel heavy, paralyzed; as if filled with lead.

▮ Right arm and wrist weak; cannot raise anything heavy.

▮ Arms go to sleep when resting on them; pricking in them.

|| Limbs tremble; forearm jerks so could not feel pulse; after bleeding.

Numb feeling in r. arm, like pins and needles.

|| Arms cold after the fever. θIntermittent.

|| A child, æt. 2, vaccinated three weeks ago; about ninth or tenth day, arm was inflamed and swollen; in a few days an ulcer as large as a half-penny, excavated, laying bare the muscles, occurred in the spot where the operation had been performed.

▮▮ After vaccination, red and inflamed swellings sometimes extending over whole arm; fever; sickness at stomach; headache; backache; abscess in axilla, etc.

▮ Blood-boils and warts on arms.

|| Abscess and œdematous swelling of arm after dissection wound.

▮Caries or necrosis of humerus.

▮▮Inflammation of elbow joint, with considerable swelling, a fistulous opening led to rough bone discharging thin, greenish pus; hectic fever and great emaciation. θCaries of elbow joint.

▮▮Anchylosis of elbow joint, with swelling and pain at every attempt to move, almost complete stiffness of fingers.

▮▮Stinging, drawing, tearing pain in bones of elbows day and night, < from slightest touch or motion.

▮▮Suppuration of cellular tissue of whole r. forearm.

▮▮Caries of ulna.

▮▮Fungous growth involving stump of arm after amputation for cancer.

▮▮A large fleshy wart on l. forearm.

▮Furuncle on arms.

Tearing pain in wrist and ball of hand.

Stitches in wrist at night, extending to arm.

▮Caries of wrist joint.

▮▮Exudation of synovial fluid in wrist resulting from a strain.

▮▮A ganglion or elastic cyst on extensor side of l. wrist.

Cramplike pain and lameness of hand after slight exertion.

Sense of numbness in hands and pricking in both arms.

Falling asleep of hands at night.

Frequently obliged to lay down the pen while writing on account of lameness in r. hand.

Tonic spasm of hand while writing.

▮Paralysis of hands. θLeprosy.

▮▮Enchodroma on r. hand, metacarpal bones enlarged, all the joints stiff, exposed in many places by ulceration of skin, bones carious.

▮▮Wen on tendons of extensors of middle finger; hygroma.

A pustule on back of hand.

Cracking of skin on arms and hands.

A bursa on back of hand.

▮Moist tetter on hand.

▮▮Profuse sweat on hands.

▮Contraction of flexor tendons; painful when moving fingers.

Left middle finger flexed and stiffened, on bending it out great pain along whole extensor tendon in back of hand.

Pain as from a splinter in flexor surface of one finger.

Pain in l. index finger as if a panaritium would form.

Sensation as if tips of fingers were suppurating.

Feeling of numbness of one finger, as if it were thick and the bone enlarged.

Paralytic drawing in fingers.

Tearing in fingers and in joints of fingers and thumbs.

Sticking pain as if asleep, now in one now in another finger, also in arms.

Stitches in ball of thumb.

Drawing feeling in joints of r. finger as if they were being pulled out of their sockets.

▮Atrophy and numbness of fingers.

▮Burning in finger tips.

▮Gouty deposits in large joints of fingers.

||A corroding blister with violent itching on first joint of index finger.

||A robust middle-aged man was bitten in l. thumb by a man, four weeks previous; the thumb was swollen to double its size; the whole length was hot, red; a small opening on the inside of the middle of the first phalanx surrounded by a red elevated margin; the probe could be introduced to ball of thumb; there was great pain on pressure with a very copious discharge of a very offensive fluid, appearing like the yeast of wine; burning, shooting pain, < on pressure, from motion and at night.

A small crack in index finger began to burn and pain, a lymphatic becomes inflamed, extending thence over wrist, and in the sore spot a corroding vesicle forms with burning, pressing, stinging pains.

||Mrs. H., æt. about 50, called to have r. index finger amputated; one year ago she ran a fine splinter of glass into apex of index finger and did not succeed in removing all the glass, as it became finely comminuted; gave no trouble until early last Summer, when end of finger became painful and very sensitive; pain extended up r. arm to axilla, thence to r. side of thorax; some lymphatic swellings and loss of power in r. arm, threatening paralysis; was unable to perform household duties without pain; pain no longer durable; worn out in body and mind; face pale, cachectic; scrofulous diathesis; restless, fidgety; r. arm and wrist weak; felt as if she could not lift or do anything; nails yellow and brittle; insomnia from pain; feels unrefreshed in morning; after *Silica* fine splinters of glass came out; general health improved and she resumed her duties, which are arduous, and has had no more pain or trouble in side, arm or finger.

▮▮Whitlow; panaritium; lancinating pains; inflammation extends deep to tendons and cartilages and bones.

||Burning, itching, stinging, aching in r. forefinger. θWhitlow.

▮Caries on fingers.

||After a bite thumb swollen to double its size, hot, inflamed, painful to pressure.

||After cutting one finger and grazing the skin off another the wounds would not heal; they suppurated, pus being a dirty white color; throbbing pain in abraded surface.

||Painful hard swelling on middle joint of little finger, with reddened skin over swelling.

||Disease of bone of forefinger midway between knuckle and next joint; slight whitish discharge from a minute opening and flesh much swollen and discolored at the place.

||Metacarpal bones of first four fingers of r. hand swollen to such a degree that oval, hard, knobby masses of uniform surface were formed; joints obliterated and immovable; in places ulcerated surfaces under which the bones gave a rough sound to the probe; formation of sinuses; no appetite; great pain; drowsiness during day; lassitude and depression.

▮▮Bone felons; deep-seated pains; < from warm bed; burning stinging, aching in superficial parts.

||Felon on lower third of second phalangeal bone of r. middle finger, from the first very painful and much swollen, preventing sleep; a free opening had been made (lengthwise) an inch long and was now widely spread out in centre, but this had only relieved for two or three hours and it had been much more painful since; it was much swollen and highly inflamed nearly to wrist with a red streak extending nearly to elbow; pain felt up to shoulder, severe throbbing, twinging; ichorous discharge; felt exhausted from pain.

||Whitlow on r. forefinger where matter had already formed; the whole finger was swollen, bluish-red and painful to touch; palm of hand also much swollen; in a few days four separate deposits of pus were formed, one in each of the three phalanges, the fourth on metacarpal bone of r. forefinger; the destruction of soft parts was so great that in some places the bone was visible; small necrosed osseous splinters came away from metacarpal bone and the first phalanx.

▮Run-arounds; ulceration about nails; hang-nails.

||Subcutaneous whitlow of r. forefinger; finger swollen, red, on its dorsum a large collection of pus beneath skin; burning, itching, stinging, aching; every little injury caused ulceration.

▮▮Nails: rough, yellow, crippled, brittle; white spots; blue, in fever; stimulates growth of new ones.

Great dryness in tips of fingers, in afternoon.

33 **Lower Limbs.** ▮Hip joint inflammation.

▮Hip disease with fistulous openings.

Tearing pain in hips.

Violent bruised sensation in hips and small of back, painful on stooping.

▮▮Suppuration and caries of hip joint; fistulous openings very tender to touch.

‖Spontaneous luxation of head of femur backward, in a babe eight days old; shortening of limb half an inch.

‖Severe pain extending from hip to foot; > at night so that she moans and cries and cannot sleep; slightest pressure causes trembling of whole body and at times spasms; cannot move foot; temperature elevated; loss of appetite; great thirst; stool difficult; emaciation.

‖Sciatica of seven years' standing.

Weakness of lower extremities; great weariness from a short walk.

Heaviness of lower extremities.

Limbs and feet feel very tired and as if paralyzed.

▮Trembling of legs with extreme nervousness.

▮Sensation of loss of power in legs.

‖Left thigh affected below trochanter. θNecrosis.

Aching pains in loins, shooting down both legs.

Pricking and shooting pain in left thigh.

Dragging feeling from r. hip down to toes.

The femur pains as if beaten while walking, sitting, and lying, even in morning on waking.

Frequent pain in thigh, drawing and sticking.

Drawing in thighs, extending to feet.

Tearing or sticking pain in thighs.

Pulsative sensation in r. thigh.

▮▮Gressus gallinaceus.

▮Phlegmasia with contraction of tissues and sheaths of tendons.

‖Inflammation of cellular tissue of thigh which has reached double its size, rest of body emaciated; motion and touch cause violent pain.

‖Abscess on inside of r. thigh; l. ankle and foot swollen.

▮Furuncles on thighs.

‖Two fistulæ at inferior third of femur. θCaries.

‖Pains and fistula in upper third of r. leg. θCaries.

‖Necrosis of femur of two years' standing.

‖Swollen and necrosed femur with sequesters.

‖Two fistulæ at inferior third of femur, which (in spite of caustics) refused to close; whole foot swollen and red, and caries easily demonstrated.

‖Boy, æt. 15, two years ago had a painless soft swelling on outer side of l. femur, just below trochanter, as large as a hen's egg, which in a few days opened and discharged thin, excoriating, watery pus; soon spiculæ of bone of a dark color were thrown out, some almost black and occasionally in form of scales; there were three openings about size of a wheat straw, with elevated rounded edges; limb flexed, walked with the aid of a cane; occasional attacks of constipation, when, after much straining, feces were brought to verge of anus, they seemed to slip back. θNecrosis of femur.

▮Blood-boils on thighs and calves.

▮Weakness of knees.

Knee is painful as if too tightly bound.

Tearing in knees, while sitting, disappearing on motion.

Weakness of legs particularly on descending steps, trembling of knees.

❙❙Violent stinging or lacinating pains in knees. θGonorthrocace.

❙❙Inflammation of knee joint with considerable swelling and lacinating pain deep in joints. θTumor albus of l. knee.

❙❙Left knee joint double size of healthy one, white shiny doughy swelling, temperature but slightly raised, motion limited, leg contracted, moderately emaciated.

❙❙For years inflammation of r. knee; unable to get about at times; joint fully one-half larger than its mate, œdematous and painful on pressure, or from exercise.

▮▮Enlarged bursa over patella.

❙❙Large cyst on r. patella, not inflamed but extremely sensitive to contact, interfering with walking, or working on sewing machine; cold feet, especially at night, and cramps in calves; feet always cold during menstruation. θHygroma of patella.

▮▮Gonocace, pains stinging, lancinating; swelling doughy; fistulous openings with hard edges, discharging greenish-yellow pus.

▮Chronic synovitis of knee with great swelling and anchylosis.

❙❙Gonitis after suppression of gonorrhœa; pale swelling, great stiffness; $<$ at night; sensation of heat in affected part; painful to touch; sweaty skin; restlessness in bed; $>$ from warmth.

❙❙Incipient anchylosis of knee. θCaries.

❙❙In bend of l. knee, thin crusty eruption eating its way and discharging thin, corroding ichor.

❙❙Elephantiasis Arabum; both feet, legs and lower part of thighs affected; back of hand also affected; now and then erysipelatous manifestations.

Red, smarting spot on r. tibia.

Ulcers on lower leg on tibia.

▮▮Caries of tibia.

❙❙A boy, æt. 18 months, injury of tibia after a fall about

nine months ago; almost entirely deprived of use of leg, walked with apparently great pain; upper part of tibia much inflamed, pus discharged from two openings.

ııPeriostitis on inside and anterior ridge of tibia from its upper third to within two inches of ankle.

ııBoy, æt. 16, lymphatic temperament, from a bruise eighteen months ago, the leg sore, discharging a thin excoriating watery pus; spiculæ of bone were thrown out.

ııAnterior border of tibia hypertrophied. θCaries.

▮▮Caries of tibia and fibula.

Pressive-stinging pain in ulcerating part of leg.

Sticking and burning in and about an ulcer on leg.

Nightly pains in ulcer.

ııA swelling size of a walnut in r. popliteal space.

Furuncle on calves.

Lameness of legs, < in morning with heaviness in head and buzzing in ears.

When one leg is in great pain the other is quite numb.

▮Ulcers on lower leg with pale face.

▮Cold legs and feet after suppressed foot sweat.

When walking sensation as if calves were too short, immediately disappearing on sitting.

▮Tension in calves as from cramp when walking.

▮▮Cramps: in calves; in soles.

Calves tense and contracted.

ııFour months after cutting r. calf of leg with an axe; wound was about three and a half inches long and middle spread out a full inch and filled up with soft fungoid granulations, discharging a thin serous secretion like meat-washings, of fetid odor, which had also traversed down fascia, covering muscles to ankle so as to fill space just above and beside ankle, it got quite full during day, had to raise foot above knee to let it discharge by the opening; cavity was about nine inches deep; whole calf swollen and in hard, knotted bunches, tender to pressure, with dull, heavy aching.

▮Boils on calves.

▮Weak ankles.

Spasmodic pain in ankle.

ııJohn D., æt. 34, sat with his feet in water; next day glands of neck swollen; a large abscess then formed on inside of r. thigh, and at same time l. ankle and foot swelled up, with formation of pus; seven weeks later abscess in thigh still discharging, and from five to six fistulous openings in ankle and foot a large quantity of unhealthy pus is being discharged; foot enormously swollen; general health greatly impaired; hectic fever;

pulse 130; appetite poor; amputation probable result; openings were enlarged by free incisions; internal malleolus was found to be carious and tarsal bones similarly affected; after *Silica* 2c., one dose a day and warm poultices of linseed meal, there was marked improvement in two weeks; abscess in thigh had closed; after *Silica* 6m., in four weeks more, swelling was almost gone and discharge had ceased; there was slight motion in ankle joint, this gradually improved, and when the man left the hospital several weeks later he could walk with a cane.

▌Weakness of feet.

▌▌Cannot walk on account of a lameness or soreness in feet, from instep down through foot to sole, and all through that part of foot. θPregnancy.

Painful tonic spasm in feet and toes during a long walk.

Pains through foot from ankle to sole.

Feet insufferably tender.

Burning of feet.

Feet give way under her when walking.

Swelling of feet as far as ankles.

Swelling of feet with redness in which pressure caused a white spot in a short time; with pains extending from toes to malleoli.

▌▌Man, æt. 55, from wearing tight boots, a blister size of silver quarter on dorsum of r. foot which peeled leaving an ulcer which did not heal, increasing in depth.

▌▌Woman, æt. 80, sprained toes of r. foot by slipping; signs of abscess here and there; on opening one of them, blood and fluid oozed out; blisters formed; gangrene threatened.

▌▌Mme. P., æt. 25, in delicate health, had been afflicted for three years with a malady which annually began at commencement of Winter and caused intense suffering for two or three months, during which time she was obliged to remain in bed; there appeared on dorsum of foot, pains, redness and swelling; this became an abscess and suppurated for two or three months with much violent pain; discharge ichorous and sometimes brought away fragments of bone.

▌Caries of tarsus.

Pricking and stitches in l. heel.

▌▌Cramps in soles.

▌Voluptuous tingling in soles, driving to despair.

▌Caries in bones of heel.

▌Icy-coldness of feet.

▌Hot feet in evening, at other times extremities are cold.

▌▌Feet very dry, smelled like an old person's. θDiarrhœa of dentition.

▮Burning of soles of feet.

Intolerably bad, sour or carrion-like odor of feet, without perspiration, every evening.

▮▮Foot sweat: offensive, making feet sore; rawness between toes; fetid, suppression causes other ailments; excessive.

❘❘Extreme perspiration of feet which were cold in Winter and sore in Summer.

❘❘Feet perspire constantly but get easily cold, then follows fainting, afterward great exhaustion; before fainting fit, paleness of face and trembling; must sit down; formerly had nosebleed almost every week.

❘❘A young vigorous farmer, who had never been sick, caused a suppression of sweat of his feet by getting them wet; from that time on, two months since, he cannot get his feet warm; feels prostrated and as if beaten all over; has pressure and tightness over chest; small of back and whole of back feel as if dead; in morning nausea and vomiting of slimy substances, whereby he becomes much exhausted.

▮▮Suppressed foot sweat: mist before eyes; cataract; continual toothache; loss of appetite; icy-cold feet evenings in bed.

A large corrosive ulcer with violent itching on heel.

Constant violent pain in great toe so that he can scarcely step.

▮Pains beneath nail of great toe and stitches in it.

Frequent boring pain in great toe.

Tearing in great toe in evening.

Violent stitches in corns.

Stitches in corn, jerking up the feet.

Itching cutting pain beneath toe nail.

Itching, suppurating scabs upon toes that had been frozen.

▮▮Ingrowing toe nails.

❘❘Ulceration of big toe, with stinging pain.

❘❘Enchondroma in a little boy began in index finger, this was amputated; soon the other had the same history and the toe became affected.

▮▮Offensive toe sweat.

Drawing feeling in joints of toes as if being pulled out of their sockets.

▮▮Caries of l. great toe and metatarsal bone discharging watery fluid through fistulous openings.

❘❘Abscess after spraining toes of r. foot.

34 **Limbs in General.** Trembling of limbs, especially arms.

▮Weakness in limbs.

▮Twitching of limbs day and night.

▮Limbs: go to sleep easily; sore and lame, evenings.

▮Stinging in limbs at night.
▮Limbs cold; transient local sweats of feet and armpits.
▮Rheumatic pains in limbs.
▮Obstinate pains in limbs, < when weather changes; after a cold.
ǀǀTearing pain in limbs, dropping and running sensation. θChronic hepatitis.
▮Sweat on hands and feet after fever.
▮Frequent ulceration about nails.
▮Nails grey, dirty as if decayed, when cut scattering like powder and splitting into layers.
▮▮Crippled nails on fingers and toes.

35 **Rest. Position. Motion.** Rest: feeling of waves of water over head >.
Lying down: asthma <; compulsory drawing in back; femur pains.
Lying on side: fainting.
Lying on r. side: pains in liver <.
Lying on l. side: vertigo.
Lying on back: dyspnœa.
Wants to lie down: sense of great weariness; debility.
Must lie down: headache.
Cannot lie down: oppression.
Resting on arms: they go to sleep.
Sitting: long, earache <; palpitation; throbbing over whole body; femur pains; tearing in knees; sensation as if calves were too short disappears; long, great restlessness of body.
Gaping or swallowing: stoppage in ear >.
Must sit down: vertigo.
Stooping: vertigo; headache; renews jerking in forehead; headache <; dyspnœa; pain in small of back; severe pain up spine; bruised sensation <.
Rising from recumbent position: vertigo; impossible; pain in back.
Rising from a seat: pain in small of back.
Motion: vertigo <; headache <; pains in head <; vomiting of bitter, yellow substance; pain in ears <; beating soreness in liver <; cough <; sweat; pain in region of liver <; least, < hemorrhage; pain in lungs; curvature of spine painful; pain in stiff fingers; pain in elbows <; of fingers, flexor tendons painful; of sore swollen thumb pain <; of foot impossible from pain; tearing in knees disappears; of leg limited, swelled knee; muscles painful; causes chilliness.
Opening eyes: pressive pain <.
Writing: tonic spasms of hand.
Sudden turning around: renews jerking in forehead.

Walking: excoriation between toes; beating soreness of liver <; sharp stitches in rectum; shortness of breath and panting; difficult, weakness and paralyzed feeling in back, burning in back; causes great weariness; femur pains; as if calves were too short; tension in calves; long, tonic spasms in feet and toes; feet give way.

Stepping hard: vibratory shaking sensation in head.

Every step is painfully felt; incarcerated flatus.

Cannot step upon r. foot without greatly aggravating pain in liver.

Descending stairs: weakness of legs and trembling of knees.

Exercise: after every, nausea; to sweating gonorrhœa <; inflamed knee painful; want of vital warmth.

Exertion: slight pain and lameness of hand; least, sweat.

Running: dyspnœa.

36 **Nerves.** ▮▮Strong desire to be mesmerized.

▮▮Sense of great weariness and debility, wants to lie down.

Great weakness, in morning.

Very weak and tremulous, after walking in evening.

▮▮Excessive debility. θTyphus.

▮▮Protracted convalescence. θCerebro-spinal meningitis.

Sensation of great debility and sleepiness during a thunder-storm.

Great nervous debility; emaciation; fainting when lying on side.

The child is slow in learning to walk.

▮▮Cannot hold things. θSpine disease.

▮▮Feels prostrated and as if beaten all over. θSuppressed foot sweat.

▮▮Great nervous debility; exhaustion with erethism; depression may be overcome by will force.

▮▮Dissipation, hard work, with close confinement, cause obstinate neuralgias, hysterical attacks or paralysis.

▮Oversensitive persons imperfectly nourished, not from want of food but from imperfect assimilation, they are usually constipated and are subject to sudden neuralgias, erethism and melancholy.

Dreadful trembling in limbs, hands in particular at times quite unable to lift a cup of tea.

▮Tremulousness when working.

▮Great restlessness in body when sitting long.

Internal restlessness and excitement.

▮Restless; fidgety; starts at least noise.

▮▮Sensitiveness to cold air; takes cold very easily.

▮Takes cold easily, especially when uncovering head or feet.

▮Want of vital warmth, even when taking exercise.

▮The limbs go to sleep easily, especially the parts on which one lies.

Easy orgasm of blood, and constant excitement.

▮Ebullition with thirst from drinking small quantities of wine.

Easily overstrained by lifting.

Bruised pain over whole body, as if he had lain in an uncomfortable position.

Bruised feeling over whole body, after coition.

All the muscles are painful on motion.

▮Progressive sclerosis of posterior column.

Great coldness of whole l. side of body, followed by frequent slumbering and starting up, as if she would go away without knowing whither, then she begins to lose consciousness, speaks unintelligibly, recognizes no one, and becomes so weak that she cannot turn over alone; after this violent convulsion, with staring look, distortion of eyes, twitching of lips, lolling of tongue, stretching and distortion of head and limbs, lasting quarter of an hour.

▮Epilepsy: spasms spread from solar plexus to brain; come at night or at new moon; attacks preceded by coldness of l. side, shaking and twisting of l. arm.

▮▮Convulsions after vaccination.

||Spasms (probably due to worms) in a child, æt. 1½, within three weeks gradually increasing in number until there were fifteen attacks daily, and finally paralysis of r. side.

▮Spasms or paralysis from checked foot sweat.

▮Spasms or paralysis depending on alterations in connective tissue in brain or spinal cord.

▮Spasms; aura, like a mouse running through limbs or from solar plexus to brain; l. side cold; l. arm twists; starts in sleep; moaning, loud groaning.

▮Spasms from slight provocation.

||Woman, æt. 30, epileptic convulsions occurring monthly at exact full of the moon.

▮Paralysis from tabes dorsalis.

▮Progressive locomotor ataxia.

37 **Sleep.** Excessive gaping.

Drowsiness with lassitude and depression.

Sleepiness: after eating; in evening.

Restless sleep: frequent waking with chilliness; dreams crowding one upon another; starting with trembling of whole body.

Woke at 2 A.M. and could not fall asleep again on account of rush of thoughts.

▮During sleep: whining and laughing; loud talking;

starts, jerkings of limbs, snoring; night sweats; **night-mare.**

| Night walking; gets up while asleep, walks about and lies down again; somnambulism.

|| Child wakes and throws arms about and screams. θScarlatina.

|| Sleep walking at new and full moon. θLumbricoid worms.

| Sleepy but cannot sleep.

| Sleepless; from ebullitions, orgasm of blood.

Sleeplessness or sleep broken by lascivious or frightening dreams; heat and congestions.

|| Sleeplessness with tuberculosis.

| Dreams: pleasant; lascivious; anxious, of murders, horrid things; vivid of past events; with violent weeping; of some one choking her.

| Night sweats; obstinate morning headache; chilly, nauseated.

Erections and urging to urinate awake him.

| Feels unrefreshed, wishes to remain in bed.

38 **Time.** Between 1 and 7 A.M.: violent chill.

2 A.M.: woke and could not go to sleep again from rush of thoughts.

6 A.M.: sweat.

From 6 to 8 A.M.: diarrhœa.

Morning: headaches; violent headache; pressure at occiput and nape of neck; sticking pains in cornea; mucous secretion in eye; agglutination of eyes; nose obstructed; taste of blood; bitter taste; bad odor from mouth; nausea and vomiting; profuse debilitating sweat; diarrhœa; painful erections before rising; husky voice <; vomiting of tenacious mucus; cough after waking; pain in small of back when getting out of bed; unrefreshed; femur pains; lameness of legs <; great weakness; obstinate headache; sweat.

Day: supraorbital pain; coryza; tearing pains in chest and bones of face; sudden explosive cough; expectoration only; drowsiness; chilliness; acne eruption itching only.

Afternoon: violent chill; dryness of finger tips; chilliness; violent heat and thirst.

3 to 5 P.M.: sweat.

5 P.M.: shaking chill.

Evening: terrible headaches; pain in swelling of lachrymal sac <; the flowing tears are hot; itching of nose causes constant rubbing; fever; toward, throat <; acute pain from abdomen to testes; icy-cold feet; constant desire for stool; perspiration on head; cough after lying down; cough <; hot feet; cold feet; tearing in great toe; limbs sore and lame; very weak and tremulous after walking; sleepiness; chill in bed; legs icy-cold; violent heat and thirst; sweat on scrotum.

Day and night: toothache; trembling of limbs.

11 P.M.: sweat.

Night: burning in head <; headache wakes him; sweat about head; tearing in scalp <; head wet from sweating; supraorbital pain; sticking pains in cornea; shooting in ears <; tearing pains over whole chest <; fever; pain in teeth <; neuralgia in teeth raging; toothache <; vomiting of ingesta; pain in region of liver <; urging to urinate, involuntary micturition; burning pain prevents rest; cough wakes him; orgasm of blood; pain in small of back; pain in shoulder and arm; stitches in wrist; falling asleep of hands; pain in thumb <; pain from hip to foot <; cold feet; gonitis <; stinging in limbs; epilepsy; sweats; chilliness; violent heat and thirst; fever <; profuse sweat; itching and pricking in various parts of body <.

59 **Temperature and Weather.** Hot compresses: headache >.

Overheating: headaches.

Sitting near fire: shivering; a cold, starved feeling.

Warmth: pains in eyes >; colic >; abdominal pains >; headache >; burning in back; gonitis >.

Wrapping up warmly: burning of head >; feeling of waves of water over head >; chronic sick-headache >; desires it; itching pustules on scalp >; headache >; feels > if head is wrapped; tumor on neck >; pain in shoulder >.

Wishes to keep warmly covered: blennorrhœa.

Warm poultice: > pain in mastoid region.

Warm room: headache >; pain in ribs >; chilliness.

Getting warm in bed: burning and itching of head <; pain in felons <.

After being in bed a short time: neuralgia <.

Contact of warm hand: cephalalgia >.

Warm food: averse to.

Warm drinks: cough >.

Uncovering head or feet: takes cold.

Cannot uncover head: tendency to take cold.

Undressing: burning and itching on back part of head <.

Changing linen: hardness of hearing <.

Open air: headache <; lachrymation; burning in back.

Draft: causes headache; eyes sensitive; cannot bear it on back of neck; on back causes trouble.

Cannot bear cold or heat: headache.

Cold air: headache <; sensitive to, blennorrhœa; blepharitis <; inhaling, toothache <; diarrhœa from exposure; headache <; sufferings unbearable; sensitiveness to.

Change of weather: pain in ears <; pains in limbs <.

Washing: < hardness of hearing.

Cold water: gum is painfully sensitive; dry cough; standing in, causes metrorrhagia.

Cold drinks: desire for; cough <.

Getting feet wet: suppressed foot sweat.

After sitting with feet in water: abscess on thigh.

Just before a storm: ciliary neuralgia.

During a thunderstorm: attacks of difficult breathing come only; great debility and sleepiness.

After exposure to storm: inflammation in eye <.

40 **Fever.** ▮▮Want of animal heat; always chilly, even when exercising.

▮Suffering parts feel cold.

▮Left side suddenly cold; before epilepsy.

▮Chill, in evening in bed.

▮Frequent chilliness, with occasional feverishness.

▮▮Chilliness: constant, internal; on every movement, all day; at night, while half awake; in evening; in afternoon, especially in arms, in a warm room; in evening in bed so that he shivered.

Did not dare to put her hands out of bed.

Shaking chill at 5 P.M.

Icy-cold shivering, frequent creeps over whole body.

The legs so far as knees and feet are icy-cold in evening.

Shivering all over, a cold, starved feeling, if he sat ever so near the fire he could not get warm.

Violent chills between 1 and 7 A.M.

▮Frequently short flushes of heat, principally in face and head.

▮Violent general heat, violent thirst in afternoon, evening and all night.

▮Fever < at night.

▮Periodical returning heat during day, no previous chill; followed by slight sweat.

▮▮Sweat: on head; of a strong odor; running from face; wetting pillow; on scrotum, in evening; profuse sweat on hands; only on head and face; from least exertion; warm, after epilepsy; profuse in typhus; periodically 11 P.M., 6 A.M. or 3 to 5 P.M.; profuse at night; on loins; in morning.

▮Night sweats; sour and offensive; debilitating; mostly after midnight; profuse from suppuration or in phthisis.

▮Fever during dentition.

▮▮In a child, æt. 21 months, every day on awaking

after morning sleep, about 12 or 1 P.M., fever lasting till 4 or 5 P.M., followed by sweat on hands and feet; with the fever short, quick breathing, cold feet, no appetite; lies still; arms cold and has cutis anserina.

▮Worm fevers assume a slow chronic form in scrofulous children with large bellies and much perspiration about head.

▮▮Hectic fever, particularly during long suppurative processes.

▮Intermittent fever, heat predominating.

▮Typhoid forms of fever, great debility, profuse sweat; desire to be magnetized.

▮Spotted fever; also in slow convalescence.

41 **Attacks, Periodicity.** Paroxysms: one or two minutes, jerklike pressure in head; pains in eyes.

Attacks: of whistling breathing and suffocation.

Periodic: headache; heat during day; sweats.

Alternation; symptoms from one eye to the other; dry and fluent nose.

Lasting several hours: pain after stool; pain across chest.

For four hours: tossed in bed with headache.

Every morning: blows from nose hard, dry masses of mucus followed by pus.

Every day; about 1 o'clock, severe burning pains in r. eye; on waking, about 12 or 1 P.M., fever lasting till 4 or 5 P.M.

Daily: fifteen attacks of spasms.

Every evening: intolerable odor of feet without perspiration.

Nightly: incontinence of urine; tickling in pharynx.

Nearly every night: obliged to rise to urinate; nocturnal enuresis.

For several days: attacks of watery diarrhœa.

Twice a week: seminal emissions.

Five to seven days: stools apart.

For six days: pain in mastoid region.

Every seventh day: headache.

Almost every week: nosebleed.

For several weeks: violent coryza.

Every two weeks: menses.

Every two or three weeks: severe headaches lasting thirty-eight to forty-eight hours.

Of six weeks' standing: ophthalmia.

For six weeks: metrorrhagia.

During new and full moon: pains in region of liver <.

At new moon: epilepsy; sleep walking.

At full moon: epileptic convulsions; sleep walking.

For two months: phlyctenular conjunctivitis.

Every two or three months: menses.

For four months: discharge and ulceration under r. lower lid.

For nine months: hemorrhages from lungs.

Last of August: hay asthma.

Summer: scaly eruption on scalp >; sore feet.

Approach of Winter: scaly eruption of scalp <; pain, swelling and suppuration of foot.

Winter: cold feet.

For one year: cystic tumor of lower lid.

For two years: suffered from inflammation of nasal duct; necrosis of femur.

For three years: pain, redness and swelling on dorsum of foot, then abscess.

For years: terrible headaches; inflammation of knee.

Of several years' standing: offensive discharge from ears.

Seven years' standing: sciatica.

Of twelve years' standing: deafness.

42 **Locality and Direction.** Right: must walk to side, vertigo; stitches in parietal region; persistent speck before eye; cloudiness of lens of eye; cataract; neuralgia over eye; burning pains in eye; conjunctiva injected; pains in lachrymal sac; trachoma of conjunctiva of eye; ulceration of cornea; discharge and ulceration under lower lid; cicatrices over inferior orbital ridge; swelling in region of lachrymal gland and sac; swelling of tear-bag; ichorous discharge from ear; muscular paralysis of side of face; drawing in malar bone; painful scab deep in nostril; lupus on ear lobe; swelling on cheek; pain in region of inferior maxillary; side of lower lip swollen; ulcer on border of tongue; as of a lump in side of throat; lying on side soreness of liver <; below floating ribs ulcerative pain; cannot step upon foot without < pain in liver; abscess in groin; as if side of hand were paralyzed; scirrhus in breast; lump in mamma; tumor of breast; scirrhus near nipple; great itching of swollen mamma; stitching pain in lung; large cavity in lung; swelling below nipple; ulcer on leg; lobe of thyroid gland swollen; sticking in scapula; sore feeling side of spine over hip joint; pain in shoulder joint; acute pain in shoulder blade; weakness of arm and wrist; numb feeling in arm; suppuration of cellular tissue of forearm; lameness in hand; enchondroma on hand; drawing in joints of finger; index finger injured by splinter of glass, pain extending to arm, thence to thorax; loss of power of arm; weakness of arm and wrist; aching in forefinger; bones of fingers swollen; felon on middle finger; whitlow on forefinger; dragging from hip to toes; pulsative sensation in thigh;

abscess on inside of thigh; pains and fistula on leg; inflammation of knee; large cyst on patella; smarting spot on tibia; swelling in popliteal space; wound in calf of leg; abscess on thigh; blister on dorsum of foot; abscess after spraining toes; paralysis.

Left: lying on side, vertigo; sickening pain in side of head; parietal bone is covered with a large, soft, elastic swelling; piercing stinging in eye; pressive pain over eye; shooting pain in ear; pricking, aching, itching in ear; chronic sinus in front of ear; sac swollen and itching; abscess of arm; induration from corner of mouth to cheek; caries of lower jaw; abscess of arm; pricking in throat as of a lump in side of throat; soreness, swelling from inguinal region across mons veneris; tearing in thigh; boring pain in temple, supraorbital nerve and orbit of eye; darting in nipple; pain in nodular swelling of breast; heavy râles in bronchus; tumor in breast; anchylosis of shoulder joint; small tumor in breast; tumor side of neck; swelling of scapula; shaking of arm; a large fleshy wart on forearm; a ganglion on wrist; middle fingers flexed and stiffened; pain in index finger; thumb swollen from a bite; necrosis of thigh; shooting in thigh; ankle and foot swollen; painless soft swelling on femur; knee joint double size of healthy one; eruption in bend of knee; pricking and stitches in heel; caries of great toe; coldness of side; shaking and twisting of arm.

From r. to l.: pain in temples.

First l. then r.: bruised pain above eyes; swelling in front of throat.

From above downward: pressive headache.

From within outward: stitches in ears.

Sensations. Susceptible to nervous stimuli, to magnetism; as if she were divided into halves and that the l. side did not belong to her; as if one would fall forward; vertigo as if drunk; as if head were teeming with live things whirling round in it; headache as if beaten; as if everything would press out and burst skull; as if brain and eyes were forced forward; as if head would burst with throbbing in it, internal and external at same time; as if forehead would be torn asunder; as from a heavy weight over eyes; as if head were forced asunder; as of water pipes bursting in head; as if tremendous weight were falling on vertex; as if some one pulled downward on cords of neck; as if something alive were in ears; head as if in a cushion and some one were pressing two fingers into it at occiput; as if feeling for pins; as if something obscured vision; as if brain collided with skull; head as if bruised; as of waves of water from occiput over vertex to forehead; as if gradually losing senses; sick-headaches as if coming from spine and locating in one eye; head as if too large; as if head were falling off; as if head were hanging by a piece of skin at nape; as if looking through a grey cover; as if cornea were a mass of hypertrophied tissue; eyes as if too dry and full of sand; as of a splinter in upper lid; as if both eyes were dragged back into head by strings; objects as if in a fog; as if nasal bone had been beaten; as if a hair were on tip of tongue extending into trachea; as of a lump on r. side of throat; as of a pin in throat; throat as if filled up; as if he could not swallow; as if he swallowed over a sore spot; as of a load in epigastrium; as if knives were running into her stomach; as if a cold stone were in stomach; as of lead in stomach; as if sternum were grasped; as if there were no power in rectum to expel stool; as if rectum were paralyzed; as if anus were constricted; r. side of head as if paralyzed; as if vulva were enlarged; as of a heavy lump in anus; as if she were tied around chest with a tape; as of a stone under sternum; as if mould were forming over whole body; as if a hand had grasped her breast bone; small of back as if beaten; small of back as if dead; arms and hands as if filled with lead; as of a splinter in finger; as if a panaritium would form in index finger; as if tips of fingers were suppurating; as if finger were thick and bone enlarged; as if joints of fingers were being pulled out of sockets; limbs and feet as if paralyzed; as of loss of power in legs; femur as if beaten; knee as if too tightly bound; as if calves were too short; as if spasms in ankles; whole of back feels as if dead; as if joints of toes were being pulled out of their sockets; nails as if decayed; as if beaten all over; as if he had lain in an uncomfortable position; feels as if she would die.

Pain: in spine and neck up and over r. temple, thence to l.; in vertex and occiput, at another time in forehead; first in nape and base of brain, then up and over whole head; in r. lachrymal sac; over eyes; in stomach; in mastoid region; in jaw bones; in submaxillary glands; in throat; in stomach; in region of spleen; in bowels; in abdomen; in back; in nodular swelling of l. breast; under sternum; in ribs; in nape of neck; in curved spine; from sacrum up to lumbar region, across l. ilium to superior spinal process; in shoulder and arm; in flexor surface of one finger; up r. arm to axilla, thence to r. side of thorax; in ulcer; through foot from ankle to sole; from toes to malleoli; beneath nail of great toe; in limbs.

Excruciating pain: in cancer of lower lip; deep-seated pain in chest.

Terrible pain: from cervical vertebræ to cerebellum, thence to forehead.

Excessive pain: from eye to head and ears.

Violent pain: vertex, occiput or forehead; above eyes; in small of back; in abscess on foot; in great toe; in joints.

Severe pain: in small of back; from eyes into head on one side; in back; from hip to foot.

Great pain: along extensor tendon on back of hand.

Acute pain: in occipital protuberances; from abdomen to testes; in r. shoulder blade.

Sharp pain: in breast or uterus; in r. shoulder joint.

Anguish: in pit of stomach.

Sickening pain: in l. side of head.

Lancinating pains: in region of r. inferior maxillary; whitlow; in knees; deep in joints of knees; gonocace.

Tearing: one-sided in head; in whole head in frontal region; in lumps on head; in eyes; over whole chest and bones of face; in teeth and cheeks; in limbs; in swelling; in sacrum and l. thigh; in tibia; between scapulæ; beneath scapulæ; in bones of elbows; in wrist and ball of hand; fingers, joints, thumbs; in thighs; in knees; in great toe; in limbs.

Cutting: at pit of stomach; violent, in lower abdomen; in region of navel to back; in rectum; around navel; beneath toe nail.

Pounding pain: in forehead and into head.

Beating: in lumbo-sacral region; in breast bone; in back.

Throbbing pain: in forehead and into head; in eyes; in lump in corner of eye; in teeth; in lumbo-sacral region; in abraded surface of finger.

Darting pains: through eyes and head; sharp, from occiput to eyeball; in l. nipple; up spine.

Spasmodic pain: in small of back.

Shooting: from nape to vertex; in eyes; in l. ear; in tip of nose; in anus; from sternum around to back; in back between hips; down both legs; in l. thigh.

Piercing, stinging pain: in l. eye.

Stitches: through eyes and in cheek bones; in temples; in forehead; deep-seated in r. parietal region; in upper lid; in ears; in throat; in rectum; in anus; in sides and chest to back; in wrist; in ball of thumb; in l. heel; in great toe; violent, in corns.

Acute sticking pain: in forehead.

Burning stitching: in several teeth.

Stitching pain: in r. lung.

Sticking pain: in ulcer on cornea; below septum of nose; in rectum; in anus; in chest; in r. scapulæ; in fingers; in thighs; in ulcer on leg.

Ulcerative pain: below r. floating ribs.

Screwing pain: in stomach.

Pinching pain: at navel.

Twinging pain: in tumor of breast.

Squeezing pain: in testicles.

Twisting pains: in stomach.

Boring pains: in ears; over whole chest and bones of face; in teeth and cheek; in l. temple, l. supraorbital nerve and orbit of eye; in great toe.

Boring cramping: from anus to rectum or testicles.

Crampy pain: dull, heavy, in arms; at pit of stomach; in hand.

Griping pain: after eating; in bowels.

Digging: in stomach.

Gnawing: high up in nose; in fistulous opening near sixth rib.

Colicky pains: in lower abdomen.

Cramps: in calves; in soles.

Pressive, stinging pain: in ulcerating part of leg.

Pressive pain: in occiput; in head; over l. eye; in eyes; in stomach; in forehead; in sternum; in chest.

Neuralgic pains: at exit of supraorbital nerve; of face, head, eyes, teeth and ears; in all the teeth.

Rheumatic pains: in jaws and teeth to temple; of lower cervical vertebræ; in limbs.

Drawing pain: in meatus auditorius; in ears; in thigh.

Tensive pain: across chest.

Pressive jerking: in middle of forehead.

Aching: at occiput; sore, in nape; severe, in back of head, one side; in upper lid; from occiput to r. eyeball; in ears; of both jaws; in all the teeth; in hypochondrium; in lumbo-sacral region; of sacrum; in back; in centre of spine; in loins; in sacrum; in r. forefinger; in wound in calf.

Dull pain: in occiput.

Burning pain: in r. eye; in tip of nose in centre; in breast.

Stinging pains: in eyes; in boil on chin; in teeth; in rectum; in tumor of breast; in os coccygis; in bones of elbows; in sore spot on finger; in r. forefinger; in felon; in whitlow; in knees; in ulcerated big toe; in limbs.

Pricking: of scalp; of l. eye; in ears; in region of r. inferior maxillary; in throat; sharp, in penis; in arms; in l. thigh; in l. heel.

Smarting: in eyes; of l. eye; of eyelids; of scab deep in r. nostril; of eruption on lips; in anus; spot on tibia.
Scalding feeling: in vertex.
Bruised pain: above eyes; in hips and back; all over body.
Beating soreness: in liver.
Soreness: in limbs; in perineum; about vulva; of pudenda; of feet; in trachea and bronchia; in chest; in lungs; in feet.
Soreness: internal, in head; in orbits; of eyelids; of inner nose; on back of nose; of palate; of tongue; of throat; in urethra.
Stiff, sore feeling: down r. side of spine.
Burning: in soles; in head; on back of head; in chest; in throat; in pit of stomach; in anus; in prepuce; during stool in rectum; in urethra; of feet; of swelling; sacrum and l. thigh; about vulva; of pudenda; in l. nipple; in back and finger tips; in sore spot on finger; in r. forefinger; in felon; in whitlow; in and about ulcer on leg; of feet; of soles of feet.
Painfulness: of epigastrium.
Tenderness: about hernial tumor.
Peculiar sensation: at pit of stomach.
Running sensation: in limbs.
Dropping sensation: in limbs.
Shattering; in brain.
Vibratory shaking: in head.
Violent tearing: in head.
Dragging: from r. hip to toes.
Fulness: in stomach.
Heaviness: in head; in all the limbs; in stomach; of arms; of lower extremities.
Hard, jerklike pressure: in top of head deep into brain.
Pressure: in occiput; in both sides of occiput; in forehead; nape of neck; on vertex; in orbits; in stomach; in hypochondrium; in abdomen; in bladder; downward in vagina; at lower sternum; over chest.
Pressing: in head: in sore spot on finger.
Drawing: in root of nose and in r. malar bone; between shoulders; in fingers; in joints of r. finger; from thighs to feet; in joints of toes.
Tension: in forehead and eyes; in eyes and forehead; in anus; in calves.
Tightness: at pit of stomach; transversely across abdomen; around chest; over chest.
Throbbing: in forehead; at heart; in pit of stomach; in breast bone; over whole body; in all the vessels; in back; in lumbo-sacral region.
Pulsative sensation: in r. thigh.

Pulsations: in chest.
Lameness: of feet; of hand; of legs.
Lame feeling: in region of sacrum.
Stiffness: at nape of neck in small of back; of fingers.
Heat: in head; in penis and testicles; in affected parts; in feet.
Painful dryness: of nose.
Dryness: in inner nose into frontal cavities and antrum; of lips; in mouth; of throat; in finger tips.
Roughness: of trachea and bronchia.
Tingling: voluptuous in soles.
Fluttering feeling: in both temples.
Tickling: in larynx; in throat pit; in pharynx.
Emptiness: at stomach.
Trembling: of limbs.
Weakness: of body; of arms; in chest; in back; arm and wrist; of lower extremities; of legs; of feet; of limbs.
Paralyzed feeling: in lower extremities.
Itching: at vulva; on scalp; spot on head; on occiput; on back part of head; of eruption on back of head; of eczema capitis; of pimples on head and nape; pustules on scalp and neck; in Eustachian tubes; of outer ears; in nose; of tip of nose; in ulcerated corner of mouth; in anus; in rectum; in rectum during stool; of vulva; on corona glandis; of eruptions on genitals; of prepuce; of pudenda; of breast; of swollen mammæ; of whole breast; of eruption covering breast; of pimples on nape of neck; on first joint of index fingers; in r. forefinger; in whitlow; on heel; beneath toe nail; of scabs on toes; of face, arms and back.
Voluptuous itching: about nose.
Numb feeling: in r. arm; in hands; in one finger
Chilliness: in nape of neck and back.
Cool feeling: in upper gums.
Cold feeling: rising from nape of neck to vertex; about breadth of two fingers, across vertex.
Coldness: of nose; of feet; over whole body; icy, of feet; of extremities; of l. side; in ulcers.
Cold pain: at epigastrium.

41 **Tissues.** ▮▮Emaciation with pale, suffering expression.
▮Fungi easily bleeding.
▮Discharges and excretions offensive: pus, stools, sweat of feet, etc.
▮Hemorrhages from nose, stomach, bowels and lungs.
▮▮Swelling, inflammation and suppuration of glands, cervical, parotid, axillary, inguinal, mammary, sebaceous.
▮Inflammation of lymphatic vessels.
▮▮Hard lumps on neck, not of glands, extending to l. side, in a gouty subject.

ǁ Painless swelling of glands, very unpleasant itching.
ǁ Inflammation, swelling, caries and necrosis of bones.
ǁ Exostoses; curvatures.
ǁ Inflammation of fibrous portions of joints, particularly knee.
| Children or young people suffering during growth with fever, violent pains in joints, swelling of limbs and congestions.
| Gout.
ǁ Multiple cheloid, which appeared after excision of a tumor, but rapidly returned and increased in size.
ǁ Rachitis; open fontanelles; head too large, rest of body emaciated; head sweats and body dry.
| Cellular tissues inflamed; deep-seated suppurations, including tendons, ligaments and bone.
| Suppuration: pus copious or scanty; brown and watery; gelatinous; thin and watery; very putrid.
| Suppurating chilblains.
| Neglected cases of injury if suppuration threatens.
| Inflammation followed by suppuration or gangrene.
| Suppurative conditions after protracted disease.
ǁ Proud flesh.
| Chronic gouty nodosities.
| Mercurio-syphilitic ulceration of skin and bones.
| Swellings which became hard after threatening to suppurate.
| Indurations hardening as of a stye on eyelid, hardening of tissues around a part formerly acutely diseased.
| Anasarca. θStonecutters.
| Old ulcers with burning and lancinating pains.
| Boils, carbuncles, felons, and malignant pustule, during suppurative stage.
| Boils, little lumps, not mattering; blood-boils.
| Carbuncles, if intractable and very hard, or with very profuse discharge of matter.
| During process of ulceration it seems to clear wound of its decayed masses and to promote healthy granulations. θCarbuncle.
ǁ Ailments following vaccination, abscesses, etc., even convulsions.
| Ulceration constantly extending in depth; edges irregular.
ǁ Malignant and gangrenous inflammations.
| Tumors in persons with herpetic dyscrasia; wens smooth and shining on scalp; sebaceous cysts, particularly when atheromatous; pus scanty and smelling like herring-brine.
ǁ Palpebral cyst.

▮Synovial cysts.
▮Fibrous tumor.
▮Epulis.
▮Encephaloma oculi.
▮Scirrhus mammæ; cancer.
▮▮Uterine cancer, strong putrescent odor.
▮Enchondroma.
▮Tumor albus.
▮▮Fistulous openings, discharge offensive, parts around hard, swollen, bluish-red.
▮▮Disease caused by suppressed foot sweat: exposing back to any slight draft of air, from vaccination; chest complaints of stonecutters, with total loss of strength.
Suffering parts feel cold.

45 **Touch. Passive Motion. Injuries.** Touch: headache <; eyes painful; scalp sensitive; head very sensitive; < pain in head; scalp tender; eye very tender; sticking pains in scabs below septum of nose; stinging in boil on chin; submaxillary gland painful; pains in region of liver <; inflamed inguinal glands painful; vagina tender; curvature of spine painful; pain in elbows <; whitlow painful; fistulous openings on hip joint tender; gonitis painful.
Contact: ulcerated place in nose sensitive; cyst on patella very sensitive.
Combing hair: causes violent attacks of sneezing; impossible, scalp covered with papulæ.
Wiping eyes: blepharitis >; wants head tightly held.
Binding tightly: headache.
Pressure: of hat causes pain; pain in head <; chronic sick-headache >; tearing in scalp <; of hat, scalp sensitive; pains in lachrymal sac; gum painful; epigastrium painful; sensitiveness of pit of stomach; cannot tolerate, below floating ribs; over lumbar vertebræ pain <; os coccygis painful; pain in swollen thumb; slightest on hip causes trembling of whole body; inflamed knee painful; whole wounded calf tender; causes white spots in swelled feet; the parts upon which he lies go to sleep.
Riding: vertigo; coccyx hurts.
Scratching: itching spots on head painful.
Irritation of truss: supposed cause of abscesses.
From tight boot; blister on dorsum of r. foot.
From a bruise: sore leg.
Strain: caused exudation of synovial fluid in wrist.
Sprain of r. foot: signs of abscess.
Every little injury causes ulceration; every hurt **festers**.

Pricked lip with a sharp point: cancer.
Splinter of glass: in r. index finger, pain and swelling.
From a bite: thumb swollen and painful.
After a cut: wound would not heal.
After a fall: pain in sacrum and hip; injury of tibia.
After a blow upon head: nightly incontinence of urine.
Ailments following vaccination, abscesses, etc., even convulsions.
‖Small foreign bodies under skin or in larynx; fishbones; needles in hands or elsewhere; to promote expulsion of bone splinters.

46 **Skin.** ‖Skin waxlike: tuberculosis, caries, etc.
‖Icterus.
‖Cutis anserina.
‖Earthy, yellowish, dry, relaxed skin sometimes covered with pityriasis.
‖Skin painful and sensitive.
‖Itching over whole body.
Itching and pricking of skin of arms, face and back.
Itching and sticking in various parts of body, especially at night.
‖Itching exanthema; small pustules filled with lymph, drying quickly.
‖Acne: eruption, itches and burns only by day; solaris and rosacea.
‖Eczema of scalp, hands and forearms.
‖Small wounds in skin heal with difficulty and easily suppurate.
‖Small wounds suppurate profusely.
‖Suppuration of skin and cellular tissues beneath it.
‖Intertrigo; impetigo; psoriasis inveterata; scabies maligna; herpes exedens; pemphigus; zona; zoster; ecthyma.
‖Eczematous, impetiginous, or herpetic eruptions.
‖Rhagages around eyelids, lips, etc.
‖Rose-colored blotches; brownish-white spots.
‖Small blisters.
‖Phlegmonous erysipelas; excessive, ichorous, offensive suppuration; tendency to extend in depth rather than superficially.
‖Large dusky patch on front of neck as large as a medium-sized orange, first appearing about a year ago as a very small discoloration after some boils on back had healed; similar one on nape of neck rapidly extending up scalp; spots covered with minute scales, place being redder and darker than surrounding skin; menses too profuse, every two weeks. θEczema.
‖Variola-like pustules on forehead, occiput, sternum and spine, extremely painful and at last suppurate.

▮Crusta lactea.

▮Small foreign bodies under skin or in larynx.

▮Papulous psoric impetiginous forms of eruption with dry relaxed skin, furuncle.

▮Boils come in crops; tendency to boils; leave indurations.

▮Abscesses speedily point, but secretion of pus is too scanty.

▮Malignant pustule.

▮▮Ulcers: form suppuration of membranous parts; phagedenic; extend in depth; after abuse of mercury; flat, with bluish-white base; offensive, with ichor, proud flesh, stinging, burning, itching; edges hard, high or spongy; readily bleeding; carcinomatous.

▮Sensation of coldness in ulcers.

▮Large fleshy warts, suppurating.

▮Variola; suppuration exhausts patient and desiccation delays; bone diseases as sequelæ.

▮▮Elephantiasis of lower limbs in a negro.

47 **Stages of Life, Constitution.** ▮▮Especially suitable for children, large heads, open sutures; much sweat about head; large bellies.

▮Nervous, irritable persons, with dry skin, profuse saliva, diarrhœa, night sweats.

▮Weakly persons, fine skin, pale face; light complexion; lax muscles.

▮Scrofulous diathesis.

▮Rachitic, anæmic conditions; caries.

▮Oversensitive, imperfectly nourished, not from want of food but from imperfect assimilation.

▮Stonecutters; chest affections and total loss of strength.

▮Scrofulous children, who have worm diseases, during dentition.

Baby, æt. 4 days; hydrocele.

Child, æt. 8 months, fair and vigorous, suffering since birth; constipation.

Boy, æt. 18 months, after a fall; injury of tibia.

Child, æt. 21 months, suffering six days; ague.

Child, æt. 1, scrofulous; summer complaint.

Boy, æt. 2; enchondroma of toe.

Child, æt. 2; ulceration after vaccination.

Boy, æt. 3, strumous constitution, after scarlet fever three weeks ago; abscesses on head.

Child, æt. 3 months; pertussis.

Boy, æt. 4; light hair and complexion, lymphatic temperament; psoas abscess.

Boy, æt. 4, swelling and suppuration of knee.

W. B., æt. 5, after scarlet fever; otorrhœa and cough.

Boy, æt. 7, affected since birth; impetigo capitis.

Girl, æt. 7, scrofulous, frequently troubled with cutaneous

eruptions and inflammation of eye, since her vaccination; scrofulous ophthalmia.

Boy, æt. 7, suffering three years; sinus before l. ear.

Girl, æt. 7, after a blow upon head when three years old; incontinence of urine.

Girl, æt. 7, blonde, blue eyes, four weeks ago had pleurisy; compression of lung after exudation and curvature of spine.

Boy, æt. 8; eczema capitis.

Girl, æt. 8, had scarlatina six years ago, since then affected; otorrhœa.

Boy, æt. 10, after vaccination; spasms.

Boy, æt. 11, tall; phthisis.

Scrofulous child, æt. 11; swelling on chest.

Girl, æt. 11; swelling of knee.

Boy, æt. 12; caries of mastoid process.

Boy, æt. 12; palpitation of heart.

G. N., æt. 12, cachectic and anæmic; fistulæ of thigh.

Girl, æt. 13, scrofulous; caries of bones of leg.

Girl, æt. 14, blonde, pale, phlegmatic, short in stature, corpulent: keloid on temporal region.

Girl, æt. 14, suffering four months; caries of orbit.

Boy, æt. 14; caries of metacarpal bones.

Boy, æt. 15, suffering ever since his recollection; nocturnal enuresis.

Boy, æt. 15, suffering two years; necrosis of femur.

Boy, æt. 15, laborer; acne.

Girl, æt. 16; eruption on occiput.

Girl, æt. 16, servant, after a fall eleven months previously; affection of spine and sacrum.

Boy, æt. 16 lymphatic temperament, from a bruise, eighteen months since; suppuration of leg.

Boy, æt. 16, after revaccination; convulsions.

Boy, æt. 17, farmer, light complexion, blue eyes, scrofulous during childhood, about nine months ago had typhoid pneumonia, has been suffering four months; abdominal dropsy.

Girl, æt. 17; goitre.

Girl, æt. 17, after some boils on back had healed, a year ago; eczema squamosum.

Girl, æt. 18; mental disturbance.

Miss B., æt. 18, suffering many months; headache.

Negro, æt. 18; contraction of fingers.

Girl, æt. 18, strong; caries of tibia.

Girl, æt. 18, phlegmatic, torpid disposition, mind poorly developed, subject to skin eruptions; hysteria.

Girl, æt. 20, suffering for weeks; hard swelling of cheek.

Girl, æt. 20; epilepsy.

Girl, æt. 21, nine months ago had nephritis, since then suffering; hepatic disorder.

Man, æt. 21, pale, transparent skin, suffering eight months; fistula in leg.

Man, æt. 23, light complexion; seminal emissions.

Woman, æt. 23, single, suffering five years; epilepsy.

Woman, æt. 24, married six months; vaginismus.

Man, æt. 24; phthisis.

Governess, æt. 24; housemaid's knee.

Woman, æt. 25, brunette; swelling of eyelid.

Miss A., æt. 26, lymphatic and delicate, suffering two years; inflammation of nasal duct.

Mrs. H., æt. 26, mother of three children, suffering since birth of last child, three months ago; constipation.

Mrs. C., æt. 26, has had two children; periuterine cellulitis.

Woman, æt. 26, single; pain in leg.

Housemaid, æt. 26, suffering eighteen months; bursitis.

Mme. P., æt. 26, delicate health, suffering three years; abscess of foot.

Country-woman, æt. 26; elephantiasis.

Woman, æt. 28, single, brunette, suffering a long time, headache.

Mrs. K., æt. 28, suffering four months; recurrent phlyctenular conjunctivitis.

Woman, æt. 29; chronic headache.

Mrs. T., æt. 29; ulceration of cornea.

Man, æt. 30, sanguine bilious temperament, five feet ten inches high, weight in health 160, family consumptive, two sisters and a brother having died of this disease; phthisis.

Woman, æt. 30, suffering since death of her husband, six years ago; epilepsy.

Woman, æt. 30; epilepsy.

Woman, æt. 32, blonde, sanguine temperament, formerly had scrofulous ophthalmia; eruption about mouth.

Man, æt. 32, in good health, a little pale, habitually sad and anxious, having lost his father at the age of 60 from cancer of face; threatened cancer.

Woman, æt. 33, single; tumor albus.

Man, æt. 34; abscess of ankle and foot with caries.

Man, æt. 36, four months ago cut leg with an axe, since then suffering; chronic suppuration.

Man, æt. 37, cigarmaker, after attack of typhoid fever; abscess.

Lady, æt. 40, school-teacher, single; vertigo.

Woman, æt. 40; swelling of lachrymal sac.

Mrs. M., æt. 40; inflammation of lachrymal sac.

Woman, æt. 40, suffering seven months; cancer of tongue.

Man, æt. 40, face somewhat yellowish, with red cheeks, suffering six years; gastric disorder.

Woman, æt. 40, weakly constitution, subject to catarrhal affections, somewhat asthmatic; scirrhus mammæ.

Mrs. B., æt. 42, strong, well nourished; headache.

Woman, æt. 44, married, medium stature, weak constitution, light complexion, still menstruates regularly, has been cured of catarrh of stomach, and psoriasis diffusa; parenchymatous iritis.

Green-grocer, æt. 45; enlarged bursa over l. knee.

Mrs. H., æt. 47; scirrhus mammæ.

Man, æt. 48, ten years ago saw a cancer of nose, since then affected; itching of nose.

Woman, æt. 50, married, Irish; eczema capitis.

Man, æt. 50, large, apparently good constitution; pain in lung.

Miss M., æt. 55, suffering for a year; tumor in mouth.

Man, æt. 55, suffering five days; felon on finger.

Mrs. G., æt. 55; glass in finger.

Man, æt. 55, in good health, after wearing tight boots; ulcer on foot.

Man, æt. 60, formerly suffering from glandular swellings; induration of cheek.

Man, æt. 60; tumor in breast.

Mrs. P., æt. 60, tall, dark complexion, dark hair, rather masculine appearance, predisposed to lung disease; cough for several weeks.

Woman, æt. 60; carbuncle on neck.

Woman, over 60, in moderately good health; elephantiasis.

Madam X. de Cerveirac, æt. 61, enjoying good health, never been seriously sick, melancholic disposition; cancer of lip.

Mme. C., æt. 63, apparently in good health but having a leaden-hued, earthy complexion, for about twenty years; lupus.

Man, æt. 67, syphilitic; inguinal abscess and hernia.

Lady, æt. 70; scirrhus mammæ.

Woman, æt. 80, after a sprain; inflammation of foot.

Young lady; tumor of lip.

Young woman, delicate health, pale, earthy complexion, suffering a month; panaritium.

Washerwoman, fat, robust, brown complexion, standing much in cold water; metrorrhagia.

Mrs. J., mother of four children, apparently healthy, suffering several months; constipation.

Robust, middle-aged man, bitten in thumb by a man four weeks ago; swelling and suppuration of thumb.

Lady, ten years past climacteric; leucorrhœa.

48 **Relations.** Antidoted by: *Camphor*, *Hepar*, *Fluor. ac.*
It antidotes: *Merc. cor.*, *Sulphur.*
Compatible: After *Bellad.*, *Bryon.*, *Calc. ost.*, *Cina*, *Graphit.*, *Hepar*, *Ignatia*, *Nitr. ac.*, *Phosphor.*; before *Hepar*, *Fluor. ac.*, *Laches.*, *Lycop.*, *Sepia.*
Incompatible: *Mercur.*
Compare: *Phos. ac.*, *Picric ac.*, *Mur. ac.*, *Sulphur*, *Kali carb.*, *Nux vom.*, *Opium*, *Arnica*, *Hypericum*, *Ruta.*

SINAPIS NIGRA ET ALBA.

Black and White Mustard. *Cruciferæ.*

Provings by Butler, N. Am. Jour. of Hom., 1872, p. 541; some symptoms by Cattel, Brit. J. of Hom., vol. 11, p. 524.

The symptoms belonging to Sinapis alba are designated *a.*

Clinical Authorities.—*Coryza*, *Hay fever*, Butler, Med. Adv., vol. 21, p. 353; *Sore mouth*, Ellis, Hah. Mo., vol. 24, p. 61, from Hom. Jour. Obstet., Nov., 1888; *Cough*, Walser, A. J. H. M. M., vol. 4, p. 134; *Variola*, Rockwith, Med. Union, vol. 1, p. 59.

Note.—Found of use in Philadelphia with potassium cyanide as a means of prevention in the epidemic of smallpox, 1870–71, by Hering, Korndoerfer, Farrington, Knerr, and others.

1 **Mind.** Irritable disposition.
Cross, dissatisfied without cause; must guard himself constantly or be uncivil and pettish.
|| From fright during coition, impotence.
Cannot keep his attention fixed.
From least mental exertion: sweat.

2 **Sensorium.** | Vertigo of old people.
| Violent attacks of vertigo, with hard hearing after eating heavy food; mostly after fat.
Every evening while conversing sudden headache and loss of consciousness of surrounding objects. *a.*

3 **Inner Head.** Dull pain across forehead commencing at outer angle of each eye, more severe around edges of orbits and across bridge of nose.
Dull, dragging-down sensation in anterior part of head, not amounting to decided pain.
Heavy headache in top and sides of head.

Dull headache, with qualmishness about pit of stomach.

Dull headache, replaced (at 11 A.M.) by burning prickling in face, moderately full pulse, dull feeling in top of head, as if empty.

Headache does not interfere with mental exertion, in fact, is forgotten during it; < when attention is drawn to it; in warm room; better in open air, eating and lying down.

Pains are < on one side, r.; sometimes on the other, l.; mostly anterior part of head and less often vertex is involved (no prover had it in occiput).

Headache as if she had taken cold, with tired feeling all over.

Dull, heavy, drawing or pressing pain in head.

▮Apoplexy.

4 **Outer Head.** Sensation as if scalp were adherent to bones.

Forehead hot and dry.

5 **Sight and Eyes.** When pressing on eyeballs, sensation as of pins sticking.

Eyeballs as if pressed on from above, with tired feeling of eyes and some dull pain in them, > closing eyes and by eating.

Sudden feeling of warmth, with stitching in l. eye; it fills with tears, which relieve.

Sticking or smarting in l. eye.

Eyes sore, weak.

Eyes feel tired.

Pain over eye, sometimes r., sometimes l.; sometimes passing from outer angle to root of nose.

Eyes smart with profuse lachrymation.

Hard work to keep eyes open.

Headache and confusion, especially over eyes, < on moving about. *a.*

6 **Hearing and Ears.** Hard hearing, with vertigo.

7 **Smell and Nose.** ▮Dryness of anterior nares.

▮Nostrils dry; l. < with discharge of some dried mucus; tender to pressure.

Dryness of posterior nares and pharynx, > swallowing and clearing throat of small white lumps of tenacious mucus with slight hacking.

Scanty acrid discharge from anterior nares, makes skin red.

▮Left nostril stopped up all day; scanty acrid discharge from nose.

▮▮Mucous membrane of nose dry and hot; no discharge; symptoms < in afternoon and evening; either nostril may be affected alone or alternately with the other. θHay fever.

Dryness in posterior nares and pharynx > by swallowing and attempts to clear throat, which brings up small lumps of white tenacious mucus with slight hawking.

Much discharge of mucus from posterior nares, it accumulates there and requires an effort to dislodge; tasteless, cold and in quite large, tenacious white masses.

Accumulation of mucus, usually white, at times yellow, drops from posterior nares, causing nausea and even vomiting.

|Scurvy, with copious and frequent nosebleed.

‖Profuse, thin, watery discharge from anterior nares, excoriating and acrid; wings of nose red and sore; draws considerable mucus into throat from posterior nares; voice thick, nasal; frequent short, hacking cough, painless, < during day; > by lying down. θAcute coryza.

‖A man of nervous temperament was caught in a thunder-shower and wet through; nasal passages feel stopped up while a thin acrid mucus is discharged profusely from anterior nares; wings of nose red; eyelids smart and itch.

‖For some years subject to severe colds; severe acrid nasal discharge with much lachrymation and irritation of eyelids; sneezes frequently, with coryza; hacking cough harder and more paroxysmal, lasts for weeks; nose feels stopped up, especially at bridge, although he has considerable nasal discharge which irritates and reddens skin; voice very nasal; partial loss of taste and smell.

‖Feeling as if nostrils were stopped up although they discharge profusely a thin mucus, which excoriates nose and lip; itching and smarting of eyelids; post-nasal discharge; continually clearing throat; infrequent hacking cough; dull frontal headache; voice nasal. θAcute coryza.

‖Hay fever; eyes suffused, itched and smarted; nose swollen and discharging continually a thin acrid mucus; oppression of chest, as if movement were impeded all around her chest, not a contraction, but as if something heavy oppressed her in all sides from her neck to diaphragm; < at night lying down.

‖Subject to hay fever for eight years; comes on July 28th of each year and stays until after first hard frost; two weeks after commencement of attack, smarting and itching of eyelids, < toward inner canthi; margins of lids reddened; eyes filled with tears; nasal discharge profuse, watery and excoriating; much sneezing, < in morning for a while, and on lying down at night, but continuing more or less all day long; itching, burning, tickling in nostrils high up; frequent hacking cough during day, but none at night; dull frontal headache; mentally irritable.

|| Has been for two weeks suffering from her annual attack of hay fever, which came on, as usual, about middle of August; nose swollen, alæ nasi excoriated, while lips were but little reddened; eyes watery, must keep wiping them; eyelids itch; voice nasal; nose feels stopped up at bridge and posterior nares; post-nasal discharge, which she draws down in considerable quantities and expectorates; it is thick, of brownish color and tastes cold; breathing much oppressed all the time, but < at night; every night she has attacks of asthmatic breathing, which last an hour or more; during attacks must sit upright and has a dull pain from upper part of chest through to shoulder blades, and dull, hard aching in temples; can never lie with head low because it brings on attacks; attacks more frequent in damp weather, and < on lying down and moving, > by sitting up in bed with shoulders drawn forward (round-shouldered position) and by perfect quiet.

|| Mrs. D., æt. 71, small, dark, dried-up old woman, bronchial asthma; sat in one chair, leaning her head upon back of another; breathing labored and noisy, wheezing and rattling of mucus in chest plainly audible all over room; anxious for death that she might be relieved; intensely despondent and sure that she would not recover; acrid nasal discharge reddened skin about nose and slightly on upper lip.

8 **Upper Face.** Sensation as if cheeks were bulged out by a bubble of air just below malar bone.

9 **Lower Face.** Lips dry, skin as if stiff; smarting of lips; red around mouth.

10 **Teeth and Gums.** Teeth, especially such as have been filled, sensitive to warm drinks or cold air.

Gums sore, tender to touch, can hardly eat hard food.

| Swollen, bleeding gums.

Convulsions during dentition.

11 **Taste and Tongue.** Tingling, scalded feeling of tongue.

Tongue can hardly bear weight of teeth; raw, sore.

Tongue feels dry, sticky, sense of blisters on tip.

Tongue dirty white in middle, edges and tip hot.

Fissure down median line.

Tongue yellow at base, on waking. *a.*

| Black tongue.

12 **Inner Mouth.** Breath offensive, smelling like onions.

Mouth dry.

Burning in mouth to stomach; with nausea, > by eating.

Saliva increased; alkaline.

▮Sore mouth, accompanied by hot, burning, sour eructations; burning started in stomach and would come up throat to mouth, with sour eructations; mouth very sore all over, with little white points surrounded by red mucous membrane.

▮Ulcers in mouth, especially on tongue, with violent burning pain, where whole buccal cavity is so sensitive that even blandest food or drink is unbearable.

▮A woman eight months pregnant, constantly suffering with burning in stomach extending up œsophagus to throat and mouth; mouth full of canker sores; < from food or drink.

13 **Throat.** Left side sore, felt only on swallowing saliva and forcing mucus from choanæ; very slight when eating or drinking.

Throat behind uvula injected light red.

Sore throat r. to left.

▮Burning along œsophagus. *a.*

▮Angina œdematosa; pale swelling with much phlegm.

14 **Appetite, Thirst. Desires, Aversions.** ‖Appetite good.

▮Averse to sweets.

Toward evening, thirst.

15 **Eating and Drinking.** While eating: headache >; nausea >; pain in eyes >.

After eating: vertigo <; desire for stool; fulness after a little, must loosen garments.

After eating or drinking: fulness and heaviness; distension, clothing must be loosened.

16 **Hiccough, Belching, Nausea and Vomiting.** ▮Obstinate hiccough.

▮Heartburn.

‖Frequent belching: tasteless, or tasting like horseradish or of ingesta; of hot air which increases heartburn.

Nausea: > in repose, < from motion. *a.*

Copious vomiting, much straining; it relieves nausea.

Vomit contains pieces of mucus mixed with dark lines like coagulated blood. *a.*

17 **Scrobiculum and Stomach.** Sensation of a load in stomach.

Burning, later sharp and intermittent with faintness, > bending forward in sitting posture.

Burning in stomach and umbilical region.

Burning, nausea and waterbrash. *a.*

After a moderate meal, aching and pressure in stomach, as if a hard body lay there, < from touch and pressure, extending to both sides under false ribs. *a.*

Burning pressure under ensiform cartilage, frequent itching, abundant salivation. *a.*

Burning pressure in cardiac region, with frequent inodorous, tasteless belching. *a.*

Ulceration of stomach and intestines.

▮Chronic catarrh of stomach.

18 **Hypochondria.** Pressure in epigastric region.

Dull pain across epigastrium on bending forward, > sitting erect.

Dull pain in l. hypochondrium.

19 **Abdomen.** Abdomen and epigastrium sensitive to pressure. *a.*

After a scanty breakfast, weight and distension of abdomen, with tenderness on respiration and touch. *a.*

All day fulness and tension in abdomen, with qualmishness and an occasional pain in stomach and epigastrium. *a.*

Pains < about navel; sometimes in lumbar region.

Pains from navel down to l. inguina.

Rumbling of flatus.

Heavy, dull pain below navel as from a weight.

Fulness and tension in abdomen, with qualmishness and occasional pain in stomach and epigastrium. *a.*

Continuous dull pain in r. groin, > by pressure.

Sharp pain in r. groin.

Dull, heavy pain in l. groin, at times sharp and sticking.

Gland in l. groin swollen, painful.

▮Chronic catarrh of intestines.

20 **Stool and Rectum.** Stool once in three days.

Stool large in amount and rather hard, with no difficulty in passing; or loose, scanty, expelled with difficulty.

Frequent desire without any passage, passage small, in balls or lumps, at first large then tapering.

After stool feeling as if all had not passed; sharp smarting pain in lower rectum and anus.

Dark blackish-green, not copious stool, of normal consistency. *a.*

A small, friable, hard, dark-green stool in evening. *a.*

A dark green stool, of which one-half is normal in consisttency, and the other pappy, after 8 A.M. *a.*

Scanty, pappy, dirty brown stool, with much undigested food. *a.*

Copious pappy stools of dirty, grey yellow color. *a.*

Copious, half hard, half soft, pappy stool, preceded by urging desire; first part dark brown, second part yellow, with many worms and covered with dark-red blood. *a.*

A dark, blackish green, not copious stool, of normal consistency. *a.*

Pappy, dark brown stool, with burning in anus; much undigested food with mucus and dead worms.

Copious, half hard, half pappy stool, preceded by urging; first part dark brown, later dark yellow, with many worms and covered with dark red blood. *a.*

Stitching in anus while sitting, so severe he nearly screamed out. *a.*

In evening small, blackish stool covered with mucus, followed by pricking and burning in anus. *a.*

: Cholera, with cyanosis.

21 **Urinary Organs.** Urine frequent but normal in quantity; of a pale straw-color; sometimes increased; sp. gr. 1025.

Large quantities of urine are passed during night, passage preceded by a violent erection.

After urinating: sensation as if more would be voided and a little later dribbling of a few drops.

Urine: darker; golden, acid; clear yellow; a cloud suspended in it with little granules like frog spawn.

▮Catarrh of bladder.

22 **Male Sexual Organs.** Sexual desire excited.

Violent erections during the day with lascivious thoughts.

Obstinate and violent erections at night, usually with lascivious dreams and even emission of semen.

|| Impotence, from a fright during coition.

23 **Female Sexual Organs.** Menses appeared in a few hours, long before period.

▮Amenorrhœa and chlorosis.

▮Cessation of catamenia.

25 **Voice and Larynx. Trachea and Bronchia.** ▮Hoarseness; toward night and in evening, with frequent attempts to clear throat.

Rough scraping sensation in throat extending to trachea, with a continual desire to clear throat and a slight hacking cough, < in evening.

Continual desire to clear throat, with difficult dislodgment of small lumps of tenacious white mucus, freer in forenoon, scanty at night.

26 **Respiration.** ▮Asphyxia.

▮Pituitous asthma.

27 **Cough.** Short, hacking cough in evening, leaves on retiring; usually dry, but sometimes sputa in small tenacious lumps of white mucus; excited by laughing; < in cold air; > on lying down and while eating; sensation of an obstruction low down in trachea.

|| Neurosis of nerves of respiration since two years; loud coughing spells, lasting about ten minutes at a time; loud barking respirations could be heard at a distance.

28 **Inner Chest and Lungs.** Pain in r. side as if heart were there and one could feel its beating.

Sharp, severe pain in l. side of chest in cardiac region, passing off soon.

Wandering pains in chest.

▮Catarrh of lungs.

29 **Heart, Pulse and Circulation.** Uneasiness and occasional dull pains in region of heart, unaltered by pressure, deep inspiration or motion.

Occasional sensation of oppression and pricking in region of heart, soon passing off.

Quite persistent dull, circumscribed pain in heart toward apex.

Pains about heart recur daily about 10 A.M., and from 4 to 6 P.M., lasting a short time only, sometimes quite persistent, with a feeling of dread and oppression.

Pulse grows less frequent and later rises until it is a little too frequent.

31 **Neck and Back.** Dull but quite severe pulsating pain under lower angle of l. scapula.

Cannot sleep on account of pain in small of back and hips; > by motion.

Pain in small of back, becoming intolerable near bedtime.

32 **Upper Limbs.** Drawing pain at insertion of r. biceps brachialis on flexing and extending arm.

Occasional dull pains in l. shoulder joint.

33 **Lower Limbs.** Weakness of muscles of calves.

Cramps in calves.

Dull, heavy aching in legs, calves and ankles.

Œdema of feet.

▮Ulcers on legs.

35 **Rest. Position. Motion.** Rest: oppressed breathing; nausea >.

Lying down: headache >; hay fever <; oppressed breathing >; short, hacking cough <.

Sitting: burning in stomach >; erect, pain across epigastrium >; stitches in anus.

Sitting up in bed with shoulders drawn forward: hay fever and oppressed breathing >.

Must sit upright: oppressed breathing.

Bending forward: pain across epigastrium.

Movement: hay fever <; oppressed breathing <; nausea <; pain in back and hips >; sweats easily.

Flexing and extending arm: pain at biceps.

36 **Nerves.** Weak, languid, with desire to sleep during day.

▮Chorea.

37 **Sleep.** ▮▮Sleepless at night, but no inconvenience from loss of sleep.

Sleepy during day, vivid or lascivious dreams.

Sleep after dinner with anxious dreams.

Dreams of the dead and of thieves.

38 **Time.** Forenoon: desire to clear throat >.

11 A.M.: headache replaced by prickling and burning in face.

Day: acute coryza <; frequent hacking cough; desire to sleep.

Evening: toward, thirst; dark green stool; small blackish stool; hoarseness <; short, hacking cough.

Night: hacking cough <; oppressed breathing <; large quantities of urine passed; hoarseness; desire to clear throat.

39 **Temperature and Weather.** In warm room: headache <.

Warm drinks: teeth sensitive to.

In open air: headache >.

Damp weather: attacks of oppressed breathing <.

After getting wet through: nose feels stopped while thin mucus is discharged.

Cold air: teeth sensitive; short, hacking cough <.

40 **Fever.** Chilly all over, with cold hands and feet, after vomiting.

Heat through whole body, < down spine.

Sweat, with feeling of hot water in bloodvessels, disappearing when nausea comes on.

Sweat general; more on forehead and upper lip.

Sweats easily from least exertion, mental or physical.

■Quartan ague and inflammatory fever.

■Typhoid and putrid fevers; delirious; great prostration; petechia.

■Febris mucosa.

41 **Attacks, Periodicity.** Daily: return of pains about heart about 10 A.M., and from 4 to 6 P.M.

Every evening: sudden headache while conversing.

Every night: attacks of asthma.

Middle of August: hay fever.

Since two years: neurosis of nerves of respiration lasting ten minutes.

For eight years: subject to hay fever; comes on July 28th and lasts until after first hard frost.

42 **Locality and Direction.** Right: dull pain in groin; sharp pain in groin; pain in side as if heart were there; drawing pain at insertion of biceps brachialis.

Left: nostril stopped; pain in hypochondrium; dull, heavy pain in groin; gland in groin swollen, painful; severe pain in side of chest; pain under lower angle of scapula; dull pain in shoulder joint.

43 **Sensations.** Head as if empty; as if she had taken cold; as if scalp were adherent to bones; as of pins sticking in eyeballs; eyeball as if pressed on from above; as if nostrils were stopped up; as if movements were impeded all around her chest; as if something heavy oppressed

her on all sides from neck to diaphragm; as if cheeks were bulged out by a bubble of air below malar bone; skin of lips as if stiff; as of blisters on tip of tongue; as of a load in stomach; as of a hard body lying there; as if more urine could be voided; pain, as if heart were on r. side; as of hot water in bloodvessels.

Pain: over eyes; in eyes; about navel; from navel down to l. inguina; in stomach and epigastrium; in r. side; about heart; in small of back and hips.

Sharp pain: in r. groin; in lower rectum and anus; in l. side of chest.

Dull but quite severe pulsating pain: under angle of l. scapula.

Stitching: in l. eye.

Wandering pains: in chest.

Aching: in stomach.

Dull pain: across forehead; in eyes; upper part of chest through to shoulder blades; across epigastrium; in l. hypochondrium; in r. groin; in region of heart; in heart toward apex; in l. shoulder joint.

Heavy pain: in top and sides of head; below navel; in l. groin.

Dull, hard aching: in temples.

Dull, heavy aching: in legs; in calves; in ankles.

Dull, heavy, drawing or pressing pain: in head.

Drawing pain: at insertion of r. biceps brachialis.

Dull feeling: in top of head.

Dull, dragging-down sensation: in anterior part of head.

Burning pressure: under ensiform cartilage; in cardiac region.

Pressure: in stomach; in epigastric region.

Tension: in abdomen.

Heaviness: in stomach.

Fulness: in stomach; in abdomen.

Tired feeling: all over.

Violent burning pain: in ulcers in mouth.

Sticking: in l. eye.

Burning: in nostrils; in mouth to stomach; from stomach up to throat and into mouth; along œsophagus; in stomach and umbilical region; in anus.

Burning prickling: in face.

Smarting: in l. eye; of eyelids; of lips.

Soreness: in eyes; of tongue; of mouth; of throat.

Sudden feeling of warmth: in l. eye.

Tingling scalded feeling: of tongue.

Pricking: in region of heart.

Rough, scraping sensation: in throat.

Tickling: in nostrils.

Dryness: of anterior nares; of nostrils; of posterior nares and pharynx; of lips; of tongue; of mouth.

Itching: of eyelids; in nostrils.

44 **Tissues.** Great muscular weakness.

Mucous secretion increased, tenacious, lumpy.

Anasarca after intermittents.

Rheumatalgia.

Pituitous dyspepsia.

Constipation from want of action of bowels.

Flatulency.

Disposition to nervous apoplexy.

Epilepsy.

Hypochondriasis.

Chlorosis.

Asthma.

Intermittent fever in swampy districts.

Autumnal intermittent, quartan septimana.

Pleurisy.

Smallpox.

45 **Touch. Passive Motion. Injuries.** Touch: gums sore; pressure in stomach < ; abdomen tender.

Pressure: nostrils tender; abdomen and epigastrium sensitive; pain in r. groin > ; pain in region of heart unaltered.

46 **Skin.** ▮▮General ecchymosis.

▮Eczema chronica.

▮▮Smallpox; to be given until sulphocyanides reappear in saliva.

Ulcers on legs.

47 **Stages of Life, Constitution.** Vertigo of old people.

Convulsions of teething children.

Girl, æt. 13, tall, slender, dark complexion; hay fever.

Mr. H. B., dark complexion, grey eyes; acute coryza.

Mrs. K., æt. 28, small, dark complexion, slender figure, nervous temperament; hay fever.

Lawyer, æt. 36, dark complexion, nervo-bilious temperament; coryza.

Mrs. D., widow, short, stout, florid, light complexion; acute coryza.

Mr. A., light complexion, nervous temperament, after exposure; coryza.

48 **Relations.** Antidoted by: *Sapo sodæ* for blisters from external application; *Nux vom.* when abused as a condiment.

SPIGELIA.

Pinkroot. *Loganiaceæ.*

An annual, growing in the West Indies and South America.

The alcoholic tincture is prepared from the dried herb.

Provings by Hahnemann, Becher, Franz, Gross, Gutmann, Hartmann, Herrmann, Hornburg, Kummer, Langhammer, Meyer, Stapf, Walther, Wislicenus and others, Hahnemann's Mat. Med., vol. 5.

Clinical Authorities.—*Headache*, Tietze, Nehrer, Hrg., Rück. Kl. Erf., vol. 1, p. 203; Meyer, B. J. H., vol. 24, p. 353; Stens, B. J. H., vol. 33, p. 318; *Cephalalgia*, Lehmann, A. J. H. M. M., vol. 1, p. 171; *Iritis*, Woodyatt, U. S. M. and S. Jour., vol. 8, p. 201; *Ophthalmia*, Angell, A. H. Z., vol. 108, p. 23; *Conjunctivitis*, Rummel, Lobethal, Lorbacher, Rück. Kl. Erf., vol. 1, pp. 294, 302; Lippe, Tülff, Rück. Kl. Erf., vol. 5, pp. 138, 140; *Supraorbital neuralgia*, Pitcher, A. J. H. M. M., vol. 1, p. 77; Dinsmore, Hah. Mo., vol. 14, p. 748; *Ciliary neuralgia*, Norton, N. Y. S. T., 1877, p. 68; Allen, A. J. H. M. M., vol. 1, p. 211; Stapf, A. H. Z., vol. 89; p. 94; Norton, Org., vol. 2, p. 119; *Nasal catarrh*, Rosenberg, Rück. Kl. Erf., vol. 5, p. 168; Korndœrfer, T. H. M. S. Pa., 1879; *Eruption on nose*, Rosenberg, Rück. Kl. Erf., vol. 5, p. 174; *Facial neuralgia*, Gross, Bönningh., Hrg., Rück. Kl. Erf., vol. 1, p. 432; Schrön, B. J. H., vol. 11, p. 297; Hah. Mo., vol. 24, p. 254; Small, U. S. M. and S. Jour., vol. 7, p. 158; Greenleaf, A. H. O., vol. 10, p. 257; Payr, Hom. Kl. 1869, p. 4; Stens, Hendrichs, A. H. Z., vol. 83, p. 136; Hinks, Mass. Trans., vol. 4, p. 366; Berridge, Hom. Phys., vol. 9, p. 148; Birdsall, Hom. Phys., vol. 9, p. 190; *Prosopalgia*, Hirsch, A. H. Z., vol. 95, p. 108; Heyberger, H. K., vol. 12, p. 126; Hughes, B. J. H., vol. 22, p. 235; Smith, M. I., vol. 4, p. 267; *Toothache*, Hirzel, Knorr, Hrg., Rück. Kl. Erf., vol 1, p. 478; Kunkel, A. H. Z., vol. 110, p. 29; Stens, A. H. Z., vol. 83, p. 136; Stens, B. J. H., vol. 33, p. 318; Morgan, H. W., vol. 12, p. 70; *Neuralgia of tongue*, Leboucher, Rück. Kl. Erf., vol. 1, p. 502; *Stuttering speech*, Hirsch, Rück. Kl. Erf., vol 5, p. 18; *Gastric disorder*, E. W., Rück. Kl. Erf., vol. 5, p. 391; *Worm affections*, Hartm., Maly, Rück. Kl. Erf., vol. 1, p. 808; *Rheumatic pain in chest*, Lehmann, A. J. H. M. M., vol. 3, p. 106; *Palpitation of heart*, A. H. Z., vol. 94, p. 36; *Angina pectoris*, Jousset, A. H. Z., vol. 107, p. 127; Kendall, B. J. H., vol. 26, p. 157; *Pericarditis*, Hansen, A. H. Z., vol. 113, p. 4; *Rheumatic pericarditis*, Hansen, Hom. World, Feb., 1889; *Endocarditis*, Weber, A. H. Z., vol. 85, p. 181; *Rheumatic carditis*, Wesselhœft, N. E. M. G., vol. 1, p. 257; *Carditis* (probably peri or endo) 56 cases reported cured, Fleischmann, B. J. H., vol. 14, p. 28; *Insufficiency of mitral valve*, Schneider, N. A. J. H., vol. 22, p. 83; *Cardiac disorder*, Bethmann, Weber, Rück. Kl. Erf., vol. 3, p. 456; *Use in aneurism*, Nichol, N. E. M. G., vol. 8, p. 106.

1 **Mind.** ▮ Weak memory.
▮ Disinclined to work.
▮ Restless and anxious; solicitude about the future.

▮Gloomy suicidal mood.

▮Afraid of pointed things, pins, etc.

▮Easily irritated or offended.

2 **Sensorium.** ▮Vertigo: as if he would fall, < in morning on rising, with headache, depriving him of his senses; when looking down or turning eyes; with nausea; with heart disease.

Vertigo while sitting, standing or walking (most tolerable while lying); head sinks backward with nausea at palate and discomfort in abdomen and thorax; in abdomen a pinching pain, with a sensation as if he would be obliged to go to stool, whereupon he loses all consciousness.

▮▮Stumbling and falling as if intoxicated; pressing pain in top of head, < from stooping, walking and talking; > when lying; feeling of fainting. θHypertrophy of heart.

3 **Inner Head.** ▮Nervous headache, < from thinking, from noise or jarring; face pale; anxious palpitation; nausea and vomiting.

▮Boring from within outward, in forehead, vertex or cerebellum.

▮Pulsating stitches in frontal protuberances.

▮Stitches in l. side of head and out of l. eye.

▮Pressing headache, mostly in r. temple; < from stooping, least motion or noise; > at rest and lying with head high.

▮Headache beginning at cerebellum (in morning), spreading over l. side of head, causing violent and pulsating pain in l. temple and over l. eye, periodical.

▮Dull stitches from within outward, on top of head; < from touch and after washing, but > while washing.

▮Feels as if head would burst.

▮Painfulness of cerebellum, with stiff neck.

▮Headache when stooping, as from a band around head.

Sensation in brain as if head were tightly bound.

Headache like a heaviness; on drawing facial muscles it seems as if skull would burst, upward and asunder.

Does not dare to shake head; it hurts in brain and he becomes dizzy.

Swashing in brain when walking; he feels every step.

Fine burning, tearing pain in brain; violent pain in l. parietal bone on motion or walking, or making a misstep; toward evening.

Violent pressure and pressing outward in forehead; < on stooping; < by pressure with hand.

Tensive, tearing pain in forehead, especially beneath frontal eminence extending toward orbits.

Thrustlike tearing pain in forehead, < in r. frontal eminence, causes an involuntary fixing of eyes on object on which he is looking, while standing and sitting.

▮Very violent tearing in forehead, occiput and temple.

▮Shooting pain through forehead.

▮Sharp sticking just behind and above frontal eminence.

▮Burning pain in r. side of forehead, extending to eye, could not move it without pain.

Burning pain in l. side of frontal bone.

Violent pressure from without inward, in both temples, especially in right.

Jerking tearing in r. zygoma.

Violent, fine stitches, as from electric sparks, in l. temple.

Pressive drawing in r. side of vertex and occiput.

Pressive pain in r. side of head, involving r. eye, in morning in bed, but still more after rising; pain deeply seated, unaffected by pressure, very acute on motion; on suddenly turning head brain seemed to be loose; < from every jar, step or straining at stool.

Burrowing and tearing pain in occiput, in l. side of vertex and in forehead, < on motion, from loud noise and when he speaks loudly or even on opening mouth slightly; > when lying down.

Pain darting from behind forward through eyeball, causing violent pulsating pain in l. temple and over l. eye.

Pulsating headache, mostly in r. temple; < from least motion or noise; > at rest and lying with head high.

Painfulness of cerebellum with stiff neck.

Headache every morning at sunrise, at its height at noon, gradually declines till sun sets, appearing even in cloudy weather.

▮When moving muscles of face, sensation as if skull would burst.

▮Sensation as of a band around head.

▮Severe stitches in l. temple.

▮▮Supraorbital neuralgia, especially on l. side; pain recurs at regular intervals, tends to spread to face or neck and to involve eyes; < from least concussion or motion, but especially by stooping; pale face; restlessness; palpitation.

▮▮Neuralgia, pain centres in, above or below eye, from cold, in damp rainy weather; hyperæsthesia of filaments of fifth pair.

▮▮Violent throbbing shooting pains over l. eye; moderate fever; attack followed by general perspiration; urine dark but without sediment; after confinement.

▮▮Excruciating, burning, stitching pains, that seemed to come from deep in head, affecting l. eye, and seemed to follow supraorbital nerve of same side; attacks every morning at 4 o'clock, growing < each succeeding morning; at time of attack eye slightly congested with profuse acrid lachrymation; nausea, vomiting and no thirst, tongue clean; > by being bolstered up in bed. θSuppressed intermittent.

|| Headache several times a week, begins soon after rising, generally lasts whole day; tearing, rooting up pain, < from motion, especially walking in open air, when every step is attended by a violent jerk in head, but especially severe when lying down; > sitting still, or walking about room a long time; head confused, often a feeling of emptiness, almost destroying power of thought; any concussion, even loud speaking, aggravates headache; feeling as if brain were shaking in skull on quickly moving head. θChlorosis.

▮ Migraine, affecting either supraorbital region during cold rainy weather; severe throbbing or tearing stitching pains, with redness and lachrymation of eye of affected side; attacks last twenty-four hours.

|| Severe uninterrupted twitching, tearing, at times sawing pains, as if nerves were being torn out by a fine instrument, in r. side of forehead and temple, extending over eye and into malar bone; r. eye inflamed, profuse lachrymation, sensation as if eye would be pushed out of head, photophobia; burning heat in affected parts of face; distension and violent pulsation of temporal arteries; coryza; disturbed sleep.

|| Frequent headaches, sometimes on r., sometimes on l. side, then in forehead, vertex or occiput, often spreading to face and shoulder; throbbing, shooting, drawing, pressing; weak digestion and catarrh of stomach after eating fat food; after catamenial period, attacks of pain in upper and lower jaw, tearing lightning-like twitches, with palpitation and fluttering of heart; < from cold water, cold air, and chewing.

▮ Any quick movement converts the dull aching pains into acute stabbing.

▮ Headache < : from thinking; by a bright light; by noise; by sneezing; by motion of eyes or facial muscles; by opening mouth; by speaking aloud; by cough; from stooping; shaking or jarring head; making a misstep; from least motion; by touch; by warmth.

▮ Headache > : when lying with head high; from pressure, and laying hand on it; from washing head with cold water; while at rest.

Outer Head. ▮ Shaking in brain, < when moving head or stepping hard.

▮Tension of scalp; feels sore externally and is sore to touch.

▮Head feels as if too large.

5 **Sight and Eyes.** Illusion as if hairs or feathers were on lashes; < on wiping them.

▮Weakness and dimness of vision; sparks before eyes.

Farsighted.

▮Photophobia: oversensitive retina.

▮Accommodative asthenopia with slight retinitis, neuralgia, anæmia of optic nerve from excessive tea-drinking.

Sparks before eyes.

On shutting eyes a sea of fire appears.

Vanishing of sight; all things appear as if through a mist; dimness of lens.

▮▮Rheumatic cataract of l. eye.

▮Dilated pupils. θHelminthiasis.

▮Eyes look dim and faint; upper lid hangs down as if paralyzed.

▮▮Sharp, stabbing, sticking pains through eyeball back into head, or radiating; < from moving eyes and at night.

▮Eyeballs feel too large

Violent burrowing stitch in middle of eye and in inner canthus, does not prevent vision but presses upper lid downward.

▮Intolerable pressive pain in eyeball, < on turning eyes, dizzy on attempting to move eyes, is obliged to turn whole head to see.

Pressive pain in eyeballs.

Contractive burning pain in r. eyeball.

Tensive pain in l. eyeball.

Constant sticking pain in r. eyeball.

Itching stitch in r. eyeball, returns after rubbing.

▮Eyes hurt on motion, as if too large for their orbits.

Pain as if sand were in eyes.

▮▮Shooting pain through r. eye going back into head, causing eye to fill with hot water.

▮Pains as if needles were thrust into r. eyeball.

▮Stabbing pains through eye and around it, often commencing at one point and then seeming to radiate in every direction. θChoroiditis.

▮Dry heat and burning in eyes; is compelled to close them.

▮Excruciating pains as if eye would be pressed out of socket.

▮▮Eyeball sensitive to touch. θIritis.

▮Eyes < when thinking about them.

▮▮Pain in eye < at night.

Eyes pain in open air.

▮▮Pain spreads from eye to frontal sinuses and head.

Eyeball painful when moved, feels tense.

▮▮Sensation as if eyes were too large for their orbits.

||Muscles of eyeball stiff on movement. θIritis.

||Squinting; convergent strabismus. θHelminthiasis.

▮Severe neuralgic pains, particularly in rheumatic arthritic inflammations.

||Pterygium, from inner canthus of r. eye some distance over cornea, beginning after a severe pain two years ago; pain in l. eye as if it would fly into pieces, < on stooping and in morning, continuing till noon, then suddenly disappearing.

▮Pains of glaucoma and sclero-choroiditis.

||Rheumatic iritis in l. eye with excessive ciliary neuralgia, for three weeks; much redness, deep ciliary injection and posterior synechiæ, with violent pain from 3 A.M., for two or three hours, continuing more or less until 3 P.M. (*Atropine* was used externally and *Sulphur* internally), the adhesions were torn and pain relieved the first night; on second night, although pupil was widely dilated, pain returned more severely than ever; pain as if eye were being pulled forward and backward, with numb pain through head, which woke him at 2 A.M., and continued the remainder of the night and all the forenoon; it seemed as if it would drive him crazy; each attack of pain was accompanied by a chill.

Redness of conjunctiva; vessels strongly injected.

Inflammation of cornea.

||Inflammation of l. eye of four weeks' standing; lachrymation; photophobia; high degree of injection; severe stitching pains in eye, and l. temple; sleeplessness.

▮Scrofulous conjunctivitis and keratitis, if accompanied by sharp pains.

▮Rheumatic ophthalmia, profuse lachrymation with or without pain; ptosis.

▮Gonorrhœal ophthalmia, nocturnal pains in eye extremely severe and extend to bones of cavity of eye.

Bluish ring around cornea; iris discolored.

||Ten years ago was struck over l. eye with a brick, leaving a large scar and considerable depression over supraorbital nerve; at irregular intervals extreme pain over site of wound, at times so severe that he feared he would lose his mind; pain came about 10 A.M. and reached its height about 3 P.M., sharp and cutting, extending over temple and forehead, with profuse flow of water from eyes; > in a dark room, when quiet, and almost entirely relieved at night.

▮Upper lids feel hard and immovable.
▮Lids inflamed and ulcerated.
▮Great inclination to wink.
▮Lids lax and paralyzed, they hang low down and must be raised.
▮Lachrymation; tears acrid.
▮Pricking in lids.
Agglutination of eyelids by a viscous gum.
▮▮Everted eyelids.

6 **Hearing and Ears.** ▮Oversensitive hearing, in neuralgia and headache.
▮▮Sensation of distant ringing in both ears, with a sensation as if ear were loosely stopped or a thick mist were in front of it.
▮Periodical deafness; ears feel as if stuffed.
▮Otalgia, pressing pain as from a plug.
▮Neuralgia of ear, sudden stitch extending to eye, zygoma, jaw, teeth, throat.
▮Pinching, drawing, itching pain in external ear; loud noises painful, when speaking the sound of one's voice resounds like a bell through brain.
▮▮Itching in r. concha.

7 **Smell and Nose.** ▮Tickling and itching in nose.
▮▮Tickling on back of nose, as if lightly touched by hairs, or as if a gentle wind were blowing across it, lasting a long time.
▮▮Smarting in nose. θHelminthiasis.
▮▮Violent nosebleed. θEndocarditis.
▮Coryza: fluent or dry; with dry heat, no thirst; eyes water; headache, with hoarseness; anxiety about heart; discharge so profuse that it causes coughing and suffocating fits as soon as patient lies down.
Stoppage of anterior part of nose, with profuse discharge of mucus through posterior nares.
▮▮Flow of water from nose. θProsopalgia.
▮▮Discharge of large quantities of mucus through choanæ, nose being dry. θNasal catarrh.
▮▮Mucus from choanæ tastes and smells badly. θNasal catarrh.
▮Copious offensive mucus flows through posterior nares, causing choking at night.
▮Chronic nasal catarrh.
▮Herpetic eruption on nose.

8 **Upper Face.** ▮Face: bloated, distorted, < morning on awaking; pale, sickly; yellow around eyes; red; sweaty; anxious, in rheumatism.
▮▮Prosopalgia: mostly l. sided, with tearing, shooting, burning into eye, malar bone and teeth; periodical;

from morning till sunset, < at noon; < from motion or noise; with lachrymation, ciliary neuralgia, palpitation; cheek dark red.

▮Neuralgia affecting infraorbital and maxillary branches of fifth pair of nerves.

▮Periodical faceache; pains burning and tensive, especially in cheek bones, above eyebrows, in l. side, spreads out over face; frequent nosebleed; red face.

‖For fourteen days neuralgia, comes on between 11.15 and 11.30 P.M., about fifteen or twenty minutes after lying down in bed; beginning in l. malar bone, extending down face sometimes to neck and only on l. side; pain shooting downward, with burning and throbbing, parts feel swollen; continues till about 3.15 or 3.30 A.M., when she gets to sleep; < lying, > directly she stands up; > by hard pressure, and either cold or warm applications; during day l. side of face feels as if it had been scorched, no actual pain, only a throbbing; pain > after eating.

‖A heavy cold in head developed into severe neuralgia of l. side of head and face, involving eye; pains seemed to start from l. occipital region and extend forward, sharp and tearing, especially in and around eye; much lachrymation, constant nausea and occasional vomiting of bile; least noise, even talking, < pain; light is intolerable.

‖Feeling as if all muscles of l. side of face from forehead to neck and l. axilla were pierced with red-hot needles; muscles of cheek and around eye spasmodically affected, muscles of eye contracted, making eye look smaller; dreadful banging, throbbing, burning, tearing pains; > when lying quietly on her face; < from coffee; after the pains affected side of face almost paralyzed; very weak, inclined to weeping; pain preceded by violent beating of heart; attacks renewed by eating.

‖Stinging, darting pains on l. half of face, commencing under l. eye, going downward to cheek bone, where they were severest, and toward l. side of nose and farther, radiating not so painful down to teeth of upper jaw; > from heat.

‖Facial neuralgia, l. side; zygomatic region and eyelids slightly reddened and swollen; conjunctiva injected, slight dacryorrhœa; pain commences near infraorbital foramen and extends into eye, temple, ear, nose and teeth, jerking and tearing; increased flow of saliva and increased temperature of parts, which are very sensitive to touch; usually commences in afternoon, rages until midnight, drives out of bed, and remits toward morning, when patient falls asleep from sheer exhaustion; during spell acceleration of pulse; præcordial anxiety; palpitation and great nervous agitation, with trembling of limbs; at first pain > by application of water, later this could not be borne; < in open, damp cold air; from lying upon affected side, and chewing; > from rest and wrapping up head.

|| Facial neuralgia of r. side; pain distributed about and within r. orbit, darted through from frontal to occipital region (> by *Cimicif.*, cured by *Spigel.*).

|| Facial neuralgia, l. side, suddenly coming and suddenly going, with palpitation of heart and sleeplessness.

|| Facial neuralgia, r. side; pain began in lower jaw, extending upward to ear and temple; hot feeling around eye; teeth feel too long; pain occurs whenever she lies down. θProsopalgia.

|| Severe tearing, burning pain shooting from l. side of forehead to temple, especially in l. supraorbital ridge with ptosis of l. upper lid.

▮ Prosopalgia from drinking tea.

▮ When moving muscles of face sensation as if skull would burst.

Stitches from upper maxilla to vertex.

Burning or tearing pressive pains in l. zygomatic region, leaving a dull sensation of swelling.

▮ Facial pains: < from stooping, slightest motion, concussion, noise and during stool.

Sweat on face.

9 **Lower Face.** Lips dry, pale, cracked.

Burning tension in upper lip during rest.

Burning in r. side of upper lip even on touch.

Tearing in lower jaw extending to ear and about it, as far as into nape of neck, so that he could not move head without pain.

Pain as if r. side of lower jaw would be torn out of its joint.

▮ Neuralgia radiating to nose, face, temples and neck.

10 **Teeth and Gums.** Painful jerks in nerve of a hollow tooth; tobacco smoke seemed to relieve.

▮ Toothache: throbbing, tearing in decayed teeth; pressing outward, teeth feel cold; > while eating and lying down; < after eating, from cold air and water, from stooping, at night, driving out of bed; from tobacco smoking.

|| Burning, twitching pains in carious teeth; they feel loose and too long; cold sensation when touched; pain < from pressure and stooping, extending into neck and toward r. ear and temple, so that she could not locate the pain; had hot, pale face, feet cold.

‖Sudden twitching pain in several teeth, r side, > from warmth of bed, < from slightest draft of air; > sitting quiet with eyes closed.

‖Toothache, r. side; free from pain all day, but when laying head upon pillow at night pain comes on, must sit up or walk about, pain then leaves but returns when she places head upon pillow.

|Throbbing toothache attended by a rending, burning pain in malar bone, paleness and swelling of face, with yellow rings under eyes; pain in eyes, frequent urging to urinate, with copious discharges, palpitation of heart, a sensation in chest resembling purring of a cat, chilliness and great uneasiness.

Digging pain in carious teeth.

|Toothache returns when thinking about it.

11 **Taste and Tongue.** Taste foul like putrid water.

Stammering, with abdominal ailments.

‖Repeats first syllable of a word three or four times. θHelminthiasis.

‖Tongue: coated yellow or white; burning, with blisters; cracked.

Fine stitches in r. side of tongue.

‖Stitches in r. side of tongue, < from least motion of tongue; formication in tongue extending into head; pain prevents her turning head to r. side; swelling below chin as large as a hazelnut, < mornings. θNeuralgia of tongue.

12 **Inner Mouth.** Breath fetid, putrid.

Mouth dry on awaking mornings, with stinging.

Mouth feels dry and pricks as from pins, yet filled with tenacious and nauseous saliva.

White or yellow mucus in mouth and throat.

‖Much spitting of frothy saliva, or slimy mucus. θRheumatic dyspepsia.

13 **Throat.** Sensation as of a worm rising in throat, > after eating. θHelminthiasis.

Tingling in œsophagus.

Sensation as if a half-fluid body were ascending in throat.

‖Neuralgic affection of pharynx. θSclerotitis.

‖Phlegm from choanæ drops down into throat.

14 **Appetite, Thirst. Desires, Aversions.** Ravenous hunger, with nausea and thirst.

Loss of appetite, with violent thirst.

Desire for alcoholic drinks.

15 **Eating and Drinking.** Better during, and generally after eating, excepting toothache.

Hiccough, Belching, Nausea and Vomiting. |Nausea: before breakfast, with sensation of a worm rising in throat; > after eating; sickly, pale face.

Vomits food, with sour rising like vinegar.

17 **Scrobiculum and Stomach.** ▮Pit of stomach sensitive to touch.

Dull stitches in pit of stomach and oppression of chest < on inspiration.

▮Pressure on stomach as from a hard lump.

▮Neuralgic pains in stomach.

▮▮Acrid, sour regurgitation after eating, followed by vomiting of food taken; constant severe pressing, corrosive pain in stomach; pressure in head and vertigo; stomach not sensitive to pressure; four years ago discharged a segment of tapeworm.

18 **Hypochondria.** Stitches in region of diaphragm, l. side, arresting breathing.

Heavy pressure in præcordial region, causing constriction and anxiety; with cutting and griping in bowels as from wind.

19 **Abdomen.** ▮Cutting colic at navel.

Pressure in umbilical region, as from a hard lump.

Stitches in abdomen.

Painful pressure in lower abdomen, as if it would burst, especially in evening before a soft stool, after which it was somewhat relieved.

Griping in abdomen as if all the intestines would be constricted, caused great anxiety and made respiration difficult.

Sharp stitches, like spleen stitches, in abdomen in region of os innominatum, only when walking, and disappearing after thirty or forty steps.

Lancinating pain in abdomen, with falling back of head and loss of senses.

▮▮Pinching and cutting pain in abdomen.

▮Intestinal irritation. θStrabismus. θHelminthiasis.

Noisy, sometimes painful borborygmus.

▮Swelling of abdomen.

Tension in groin.

▮Hernia inguinalis.

20 **Stool and Rectum.** Emission of fetid flatus.

▮Stools: of mucus, with tenesmus; large lumps of mucus, without feces; of feces, with masses of worms; hard, like sheep's dung, and enveloped in mucus; thin, mushy.

Frequent inefficient urging to stool.

▮Itching and tickling in anus and rectum; ascarides and lumbricoides.

Itching in anus and on coccyx.

▮▮Helminthiasis: dilated pupils; strabismus; putrid smell from mouth, itching of nose, griping pain in belly; throat inflamed, swallows often, pale redness in throat and swelling of mucous membrane; palpitation.

Boring stitch in perineum.

21 **Urinary Organs.** ▮Diabetes insipidus.

▮Urine: copious; with frequent urging, mostly at night; drips involuntarily, with burning in orifice of urethra; whitish sediment; watery, frequent, nervous.

22 **Male Sexual Organs.** Erections with voluptuous fancies, but without sexual desire.

Itching stitch in r. testicle and penis, from behind forward.

‖Prostatic fluid presses out of urethra.

Swelling of one-half of corona glandis.

Tingling around corona glandis.

24 **Pregnancy. Parturition. Lactation.** Stitches under either nipple.

‖Puerperal peritonitis.

25 **Voice and Larynx. Trachea and Bronchia.** Chronic hoarseness.

Catarrh with hoarseness; continuous coryza; dry heat without thirst; protruded eyes; violent headache; lachrymation.

Tickling in windpipe.

▮Influenza accompanied by facial neuralgia.

26 **Respiration.** ▮Short breath, < when talking, with red cheeks and lips.

▮▮Dyspnœa and suffocating attacks when moving in bed or raising arms; must lie on r. side or with head high. θHeart disease. θHydrothorax.

‖Hardly speaks or takes a deep breath for fear of aggravating the pain. θCardiac rheumatism or neuralgia.

▮Oppression of chest with palpitation when walking fast or from other bodily exertion. θInsufficiency of valves.

▮Suffocating spell from least motion. θCarditis.

27 **Cough.** ▮Cough: at night, with catarrh; dry, hard; with worm affections; with dyspnœa, < when bending forward; suffocating, as if from a quantity of water flowing into windpipe; dry, violent, hollow, from an irritation in trachea.

▮Catarrh of air passages with fever, hot skin, but no thirst or sweat.

28 **Inner Chest and Lungs.** ▮Constriction in chest, with anxiety and difficult breathing.

Violent pressure upon chest beneath l. clavicle, and on middle of chest.

Cutting constriction in chest, with anxiety.

Dull stitches in r. side of chest, only during inspiration.

▮▮Stitches in chest, < from least movement or when breathing.

Violent stitch in l. side, just beneath heart.

Dull sticking at point where beat of heart is felt.

Recurrent dull stitches, rhythmical with pulse, at point where impulse of heart is felt or rather more externally.

▮Sensation of tearing in chest.

Tearing boring pain, extending from within outward, beneath r. nipple, pain always extends to sternum and becomes a sharp pressive tearing pain.

Dull sticking pinching pain beneath r. nipple, in thorax, from within outward, violent only on inspiration.

ǀǀStitching needlelike pains in chest.

ǀǀCutting piercing pain through l. chest, near sternum to back; heart not beating, but an uninterrupted rush of blood through it; pulse not beating, but appeared to finger like a thread quickly pulled through artery; hands icy cold with cold sweat; great anguish expressed in face. θCardiac rheumatism.

▮Trembling feeling in chest on moving arms, or from any movement.

▮Can lie only on r. side, with head high. θHydrothorax.

▮▮Rheumatic troubles, especially in l. side of chest.

29 **Heart, Pulse and Circulation.** ▮▮Stitches about heart: synchronous with pulse; with anxiety and oppression; with commencing valvular disease, endocarditis, etc.; can only lie on r. side, or with head very high, least motion aggravates.

▮Stitches in heart, and violent throbbing motion of heart may be seen through clothing.

ǀǀDrawing sensation in region of heart. θAneurism.

▮Violent stitch in l. side, just under heart, returns periodically.

▮Stitches between heart and epigastrium.

▮Feeling as if heart were compressed or squeezed with a hand.

▮Purring feeling over heart; wavelike motion, not synchronous with pulse.

▮▮Palpitation: violent, < bending forward; high fever; when he sits down, after rising in morning; from deep inspiration or holding breath; from worms; from least motion; with anxious oppression of chest.

ǀǀViolent palpitation of heart and frequent attacks of fainting; blowing murmur with first sound of heart. θChlorosis.

▮Waving palpitation, not synchronous with pulse; purring feeling over heart; trembling of carotids.

ǀǀIn morning, as soon as he sat down, after rising from bed, heart began to beat violently, with great oppression and cutting pains in lower abdomen as from incarcerated flatulence.

▌Unusually violent palpitation, could hear pulsation, and beats could be seen through clothes.

ǀTremulous action of heart in nervous and hysterical disorders.

ǀǀSudden severe pain in l. side of chest, about region of heart, so violent it "almost knocks her down;" it then passes rapidly around body, from l. to r., seemingly on inside to scrobiculum cordis, where it remains about twelve hours; pain spasmodic, often induces vomiting; attacks every four weeks, but with no distinct regularity, for fifteen years. θAngina pectoris.

ǀǀSevere pains in all the limbs; hands stiff, cannot move them, particularly fingers; pressing cutting pain in abdomen, beneath floating ribs; terrible palpitation; audible beating of heart, causing pains in back; periodical cutting pains extending to shoulders, head and arms; constriction of chest; great dyspnœa, cannot get enough air, with great oppression of chest and anxious face; extreme emaciation; must be careful while eating lest pain be < to an intolerable degree. θArthritic rheumatism.

ǀǀAttacks of cramplike, grinding pain across chest; body convulsed; face pale; dyspnœa, nausea, anxiety and faintness accompanied attack, which lasted uninterruptedly for half an hour; rapid and strong beating of heart; bellows' sound during diastole, and friction sound during systole; < by slightest motion; pulse very feeble; extremely sensitive to cold. θRheumatic carditis.

ǀǀSevere stitching pains in cardiac region; violent palpitation, perceptible to eye; dyspnœa on moving in bed; oppression of chest; anxiety; slight cyanosis of upper lip; heartbeat weak; increased area of dulness on percussion; friction sounds; pulse weak, 120; had swelling of joints of r. thumb, knee, foot and elbow; dark brown sediment in urine; loss of appetite; sleeplessness. θPericarditis.

▌▌Acute pericarditis with anxiety and weight in præcordia.

▌Neurotic form of suffocative breast pang with cardiac hyperthophy.

ǀǀEndocarditis with insufficiency of mitral valve, after acute articular rheumatism, in a girl æt. 14; purring over region of heart, noise with first tick; throbbing of carotids and subclavian; violent nosebleed.

ǀǀStrong systolic blowing sound at apex of l. ventricle. θInsufficiency of mitral valves.

ǀǀConstant pressing, burning and ulcerative pain in

thorax; dyspnœa, with fear of suffocation on motion, so that she is afraid to get out of bed; tremulous sensation in chest and in temples, < from least motion of arms, particularly when raising them toward head, when there is a sensation as of something tearing in chest, with great dyspnœa and anxiety; flushing with sweat on face on touching epigastrium, she cannot bear pressure of clothing; at times cramping sensation, beginning in abdomen and extending into chest, causing dyspnœa; at times violent palpitation with sensation as if heart were being crushed, or with stitches and trembling sensation; at other times as if everything in chest were too short, loose and wabbling about; is very careful when moving and is filled with anxiety on seeing any one move quickly; frequent wabbling sensation in abdomen; head rests upon chest when lying and sitting, if she raises it she becomes anxious, feels as if something were tearing in chest and is seized with nervous spasmodic respiration, with violent and convulsive efforts at distension of chest, face becomes bluish-red and heart beats tumultuously, also violent pulsation in all the arteries; pulse 80 when lying, 93 sitting, and not synchronous with beat of heart; heartbeat weak, indistinct, one running into the other; change from systole to diastole indicated rather by a wavelike motion than by any distinct sound or impulse.

▮▮Systolic blowing at apex.

▮▮Rheumatic affections of heart.

▮Pulse: irregular; strong, but slow; trembling; weak and irregular, at one time rapid, at another slow; quicker than beating of heart; like a thread quickly pulled through artery; intermitting, every other beat drops out.

||Aneurism; a girl æt. 15, light complexion; a few itching pustules on forehead and chin; for two years, visible and felt by hand, a throbbing lump in second intercostal space; feels lump when stretching either arm backward; from stooping or lifting throbbing in chest, with vertigo; drawing in region of heart; stethescope over tumor reveals continuous rushing sound, more marked during heart's systole; first sound somewhat confused; second sound usually prolonged, and of increased intensity; a murmur upward from each side of sternum; frightened when examined; headache like band around head when stooping; nausea (*Spigel.* cured, assisted by *Carb. veg.* and later *Bryon.*).

30 **Outer Chest.** ▮Violent shootings in walls of chest, mostly on l., under clavicle or on a line with heart.

▮Painful contraction of muscles of chest.

31 **Neck and Back.** ▮Rheumatism of nape of neck with painful numbness; < lying on back.

Stitches in back; also when breathing.

Bruised feeling in spine, even during rest.

▮Throbbing of carotids and subclavian. θEndocarditis.

32 **Upper Limbs.** ▮Trembling of arms.

▮Stitches in bends of elbows and joints of hands and fingers.

Twitching in muscles of l. forearm just above wrist, only during rest.

Pressive pain above r. wrist, during rest.

Painful drawing on first joint of thumb where it unites with the metacarpal bone.

Tearing pain in phalanges of r. thumb.

Burning itching in palms.

‖Hands icy cold with cold sweat. θRheumatism.

▮Cold viscous sweat in hands.

Subcutaneous tubercles in palms of hands.

Hard, burning itching nodosities in hands.

Contraction of flexor of fingers.

33 **Lower Limbs.** Drawing tearing in r. thigh, while sitting.

Persistent tensive stitch in l. thigh, while walking, ceases on standing, returns on sitting.

Persistent itching stitch in l. thigh.

Tearing pain, like a sprain, in l. knee, only when walking, at times he limped because he could not bend knee as usual.

Stitching in calves, with jerking and pulsating, in both patellæ, if knees are held stiffly stretched out.

Stitches in joints of legs and feet, and in thigh.

Pulling in legs from below upward, with heat, or from above downward with coldness of feet.

Contusive pain in knee.

Sprain of foot (after *Arnica*).

Burning pain in instep, without redness.

Deep-seated and lancinating pain in sole of foot when resting body upon it.

Wartlike excrescences on toes.

34 **Limbs in General.** Constant restlessness during night.

Pressive, pulling or cutting pain in limbs, running lengthwise.

Stinging pain in limbs, principally in joints.

Trembling of limbs, lassitude and heaviness.

▮Stinging pain in limbs.

▮Stinging or stitching in joints.

Tearing pains in limbs, with great weakness of body; tearing in joints; rheumatism.

Acute inflammatory rheumatism; very sensitive to cold air and to touch; slightest jar or knock causes intense pain.

▮Twitching of limbs. θFracture of bones.

Hard nodosities on hands and toes.

35 **Rest. Position. Motion.** Rest: headache >; facial neuralgia >; burning tension of upper lip; bruised feeling in spine; twitching in muscles of forearm; pressive pain above r. wrist.

Lying: vertigo >; pressing pain in head >; headache very severe; causes suffocating fits; neuralgia in face <; on face, pains >; upon affected side facial neuralgia <; toothache >; head rests upon chest; pulse 80.

Lying on back: rheumatism of nape of neck <.

Laying head upon pillow at night: toothache comes on.

Lying with head high: pressing headache >.

Bolstered up in bed: suppressed intermittent >.

Must lie on r. side or with head high: heart disease; hydrothorax.

Sitting: vertigo; pain in forehead; headache >; toothache >; palpitation; head rests upon chest; pulse 93; tearing in thigh; stitch in thigh returns.

Standing: vertigo; pain in forehead; facial neuralgia <; stitch in thigh ceases.

Must sit up or walk about: toothache.

Knees stiffly stretched out: stitches in calves.

Rising: vertigo <; headache <; from a seat, body feels sore and heavy.

Bending forward: cough <; palpitation <.

Stooping: pressing pain in head <; headache as of a band; neuralgia <; pterygium <; toothache <; throbbing in chest.

Raising arms toward head: sensation of something tearing in chest.

Stretching arms backward: feels lump in intercostal space.

Motion: of eyes < vertigo; pressing headache <; violent pain in parietal bone; headache very acute; neuralgia <; rooting pain in head <; quick, as if brain were shaking in skull; quick, converts dull pain into acute; shaking in brain <; of eyes < pains; of eyes, dizzy; eyeball stiff; prosopalgia <; of muscles of face sensation as if skull would burst; of tongue pain <; in bed suffocating attacks; least, suffocating spells; stitches in chest <; of arms, trembling feeling in chest; palpitation; pain in chest <; in bed, dyspnœa; fear of suffocation; of arms, trembling sensation in chest and temples <; least, chill.

Very careful when moving.

Opening mouth: headache <.
Exertion: oppression and palpitation.
Walking: vertigo; pressing pain in head <; swashing in brain; pain in parietal bone; in open air, headache <; about room a long time, headache >; sharp stitches in abdomen disappeared after thirty or forty steps; fast, oppression of chest and palpitation; stitches in thigh; pain in knee; sensation of lightness in body; after, weakness.
Making misstep: violent pain in parietal bone.
Every step attended by violent jerks in head.
Resting body upon foot: pain in sole.
Lifting: throbbing in chest.

36 **Nerves.** Exaltation of special senses.
Great agitation of nerves.
Restlessness; cannot keep limbs still at night.
Body painfully sensitive to touch, it sends a shudder through whole frame; part touched feels chilly; tingling through body; if he knocks against any part there is a sudden painful crawling through whole body to head.
Body feels heavy and sore when rising from a seat.
Sensation of lightness in body when walking.
Weakness: in morning on waking; after walking.
Sense of weariness all over, with sensation of or real coldness of body.

37 **Sleep.** Sleepy by day, even mornings; goes to sleep late.
Sleep restless, unrefreshing.
Confused dreams, in which he seemed so busy that he felt weary in morning; could either indistinctly, or not at all, remember his dream.

38 **Time.** Morning: vertigo <; headache beginning; pterygium <; face bloated <; neuralgia of tongue <; mouth dry on waking; palpitation; weakness; sleepy; feels weary after dreaming.
Day: side of face as if it had been scorched; free from toothache; sleepy.
Noon: headache at height; headache suddenly disappears; prosopalgia <.
Afternoon: neuralgia commences, raging until midnight.
Toward evening: violent pain in parietal bone.
Evening: painful pressure in abdomen.
Night: pains through eyeballs <; choking; toothache commences; frequent urging; cough; constant restlessness; heat in flushes; sweat.

39 **Temperature and Weather.** Heat: pains in face >.
Warmth: headache <; toothache >.
Warm applications: > neuralgia.

Wrapping head up: facial neuralgia.
Open air: walking, headache <; eyes pain.
Slightest draft of air: toothache <.
Damp, rainy weather: neuralgia; migraine affecting supraorbital region; facial neuralgia <.
Water: applied in facial neuralgia > at first, afterward could not be borne.
Washing: stitches in head <; during, stitches >.
Cold water: pain in jaws <; head >.
Cold: neuralgia; air, < pain in jaws; applications > neuralgia; air, facial neuralgia <; rheumatic carditis, extremely sensitive.

40 **Fever.** Chill: often recurs at same hour each morning; alternating with heat or sweat, on some parts, others being hot; from least movement; spreads from chest.

▮ Heat: especially in back; flushes, at night, with thirst for beer; on face and hands, with chill in back; with desire to uncover.

▮ Sweat: chiefly on upper part of body; night sweats; offensive smelling, with heat at same time; clammy, on hands; cold.

41 **Attacks, Periodicity.** Alternate: chill and heat or sweat.
Periodical: pain in head; supraorbital neuralgia; deafness; prosopalgia; cutting pains to shoulders, head and arms.
3 A.M. for two or three hours: violent pain in eyes, continuing until 3 P.M.
From 10 A.M. to 3 P.M. pain increases.
Every morning: at sunrise, headache; attacks of excruciating pain in head at 4 o'clock; each succeeding morning attack <; chill at same hour.
From morning until sunset: prosopalgia.
Sunset: headache declines.
For half an hour: attacks of pain in chest.
For twelve hours: pain in scrobiculum.
For twenty-four hours: migraine.
For fourteen days: neuralgia comes on between 11.15 and 11.30 P.M., about fifteen minutes after lying down in bed.
Several times a week: headache.
For three weeks: rheumatic iritis.
For four weeks: inflammation of eye.
For four weeks: attacks of angina pectoris for fifteen years.
For two years: a throbbing lump in second intercostal space.
Ten years ago: struck over eye with a brick, extreme pain at irregular intervals.

42 **Locality and Direction.** Right: pressing pain in temple; tearing in frontal eminence; jerking tearing in zygoma;

pressive drawing in side of vertex and occiput; cutting pain in forehead and temple, extending over eye; eye inflamed; contractive burning pain in eyeball; sticking pain in eyeball; itching stitch in eyeball; shooting pain through eye; as if needles were thrust into eyeball; itching in concha; facial neuralgia; burning in side of upper lip; pain as if side of lower jaw would be torn out of its joint; pain from teeth into temple and ear; pain in teeth; stitches in side of tongue; cannot turn head to side on account of pain; itching stitch in testicle; dull stitches in side of chest; tearing boring pain beneath nipple; pinching pain beneath nipple; swelling of joints of thumb, knee, foot and elbow; pressive pain above wrist; tearing pain in phalanges of thumb; tearing in thigh.

Left: stitches in head and out of eye; headache spreading to side of head, temple and eye; violent pain in parietal bone; burning pain in side of frontal bone; violent stitches in temple; burrowing pain in vertex and forehead; violent pulsating pain in temple and over eye; neuralgia; violent throbbing shooting over eye; excruciating pain from deep in head affecting eye; cataract of eye; tensive pain in eyeball; rheumatic iritis; prosopalgia <; neuralgia, beginning in malar bone; side of face as if it had been scorched; as if muscles of side of face from forehead to neck and axilla were pierced with red-hot needles; stinging darting in half of face; facial neuralgia coming and going suddenly; tearing, shooting from side of forehead to temple < in supraorbital ridge, with ptosis of upper lid; tearing pain in zygomatic region; stitches in region of diaphragm; pressure upon chest beneath clavicle; violent stitch just beneath heart; piercing pain through chest; rheumatic troubles < on side of chest; severe pain in side of chest; systolic blowing sound at apex of ventricle.

Shooting in walls of chest, under clavicle or on a line with heart; twitching in muscles of forearm; stitch in thigh; itching stitch in thigh; tearing pain in knee.

From l. to r.: pain passes around body.

From within outward: boring in head; dull stitches on top of head; tearing, boring pain beneath nipple; pinching pain beneath nipple.

From without inward: pressure in temples.

From behind forward: pain through eyeball; stitch in testicle and penis.

From below upward: pulling in legs.

43 **Sensations.** As if he would fall; as if he would be obliged to go to stool; as if intoxicated; as if head would burst;

as of a band around head; as if head were tightly bound; as of electric sparks in temples; brain seemed to be loose; as if brain were shaking in skull; as if nerves were being cut by a fine instrument in forehead and temple; as if eye would be pushed out of head; head as if too large; as if hairs or feathers were on lashes; upper lids hang as if paralyzed; eyeballs as if too large; as if sand were in eyes; as if needles were thrust into eyeball; as if eye would be pressed out of socket; as if eye would fly into pieces; as if eye were being pulled forward and backward; pain in eye as if it would drive him crazy; as if ear were loosely stopped or a thick mist were in front of it; ears as if stuffed; as if back of nose were lightly touched by hairs, or as if a gentle wind were blowing across it; face feels as if it had been scorched; as if all muscles of l. side of face from head to neck and l. axilla were pierced with red-hot needles; teeth as if too long; as if l. side of lower jaw would be torn out off its joint; sensation resembling purring of cat; as of a worm rising in throat; as if a half fluid body were ascending in throat; as of a hard lump in stomach; as if abdomen would burst; as if all the intestines would be constricted; suffocating as if from a quantity of water flowing into windpipe; pulse as if a thread pulled through arteries; as if heart were compressed or squeezed with a hand; as if heart were being crushed; as if everything in chest were too short, loose and wabbling about; as if something were tearing in chest.

Pain: at cerebellum; in upper and lower jaw.

Excruciating pains: in eye.

Extreme pain: over eye.

Violent pain: in l. parietal bone.

Sudden severe pain: in l. side of chest, about region of heart.

Severe pains: in all the limbs.

Excruciating, burning, stitching pains: from deep in head to eye.

Dreadful banging, throbbing, burning, tearing pains: in face and neck.

Sharp, stabbing, sticking pains: through eyeball back into head.

Stabbing pain: through eye.

Lancinating pain: in abdomen; in sole of foot.

Violent throbbing, shooting pains: over l. eye.

Cutting, piercing pain: through l. chest, near sternum to back.

Cutting: in bowels; at navel; in abdomen; extending to shoulders, head and arms.

Pressing cutting pain : in abdomen.
Shooting pain : through forehead.
Shooting pain : through eye, back into head ; in walls of chest.
Darting pain : through eyeball.
Stinging, darting pains : in l. half of face.
Burning, twitching pains : in carious teeth.
Twitching pain : in several teeth.
Painful jerks : in nerves of a hollow tooth.
Violent stitch : in l. side, just below heart.
Severe stitching pains : in cardiac region.
Stitching, needlelike pain : in chest.
Stitching pain : in eye and temple ; in calves.
Sudden stitch : extending to eye, zygoma, jaw, teeth, throat.
Violent burrowing stitch : in middle of eye and in inner canthus.
Boring stitch : in perineum.
Pulsating stitches : in frontal protuberances.
Stitches : in l. side of head and out of l. eye ; dull, on top of head ; in l. temple ; from upper maxilla to vertex ; in region of diaphragm ; in abdomen ; under either nipple ; in chest ; about heart ; in heart ; between heart and epigastrium ; in back ; in bends of elbows and joints of fingers and hands ; in joints of legs and feet and in thigh.
Fine stitches : in l. temple ; in l. side of tongue.
Persistent itching stitch : in l. thigh.
Persistent tensive stitch : in l. thigh.
Itching stitch : in r. eyeball ; in r. testicle and penis.
Dull stitches : in pit of stomach ; in r. side of chest ; where heartbeat is felt.
A violent jerk : in head.
Very violent tearing : in occiput, forehead and temple.
Tearing pains : in occiput, in vertex and in forehead ; in lower jaw to ear and nape of neck ; in chest ; in phalanges of r. thumb ; in l. knee ; in limbs ; in joints.
Tearing, boring pain : beneath r. nipple.
Tearing : rooting up pain.
Tearing, lightning-like twitches : in head.
Jerking tearing : in r. zygoma.
Thrustlike tearing pain : in forehead.
Throbbing, tearing : in decayed teeth.
Burning or tearing pressive pain : in l. zygomatic region.
Tearing, burning pain : shooting from l. side of forehead to temple.
Burning, tearing pain : in brain.
Tensive, tearing pain : in forehead.

Drawing, tearing: in r. thigh.
Rending, burning pain: in malar bone.
Digging pain: in carious teeth.
Burrowing pain: in occiput.
Pinching pain: in abdomen.
Griping: in bowels.
Cramplike grinding pain: across chest.
Boring: in forehead, vertex, cerebellum.
Pinching, drawing, itching pain: in external ear.
Pulsating pain: in l. temple, and over l. eye.
Neuralgic pain: in and about eye; in face; radiating to nose, face, temple and neck.
Cutting constriction: in chest.
Constant pressing burning and ulcerative pain: in thorax.
Contractive, burning pain: in r. eyeball.
Burning pain: in r. side of forehead to eyes; in l. side of frontal bone; in face; in instep.
Pressive, corrosve pain: in stomach.
Contusive pain: in knee.
Sharp sticking: just behind and above frontal eminence.
Constant sticking pain: in r. eyeball.
Dull sticking: at point where beat of heart is felt; beneath r. nipple; in thorax.
Rheumatic pain: at nape of neck.
Tensive pain: in l. eyeball; in face.
Intolerable pressive pain: in eyeball.
Pressing pain: in top of head; in r. temple; in r. side of head and eye; in eyeballs; in ears; above r. wrist.
Numb pain: through head.
Stinging: in mouth; in limbs.
Smarting: in nose.
Burning: in r. side of upper lip; in orifice of urethra.
Burning tension: in upper lip.
Burning itching: in palms.
Soreness: of body.
Painfulness: of cerebellum.
Bruised feeling: in spine.
Soreness: of scalp.
Painful numbness: of nape of neck.
Cramping sensation: from abdomen into chest.
Violent pressure: in forehead; in both temples.
Painful drawing: on first joint of thumb.
Pressive drawing: in r. side of vertex and occiput.
Drawing sensation: in region of heart.
Jerking: in both patellæ.
Pulling: in legs.
Throbbing: in face; in teeth; in lump in second intercostal space; in chest; of carotids and subclavian.

Pulsating: in both patellæ.
Heat: in back; on face, and hands.
Dry heat and burning: in eyes.
Tingling: in œsophagus; through body.
Tension: of scalp; of groin.
Pressure: in stomach; in head; in præcordial region; in umbilical region; in lower abdomen; violent upon chest.
Constriction: in chest.
Heavy feeling: of body.
Weight: in præcordia.
Oppression: of chest.
Tickling: in nose; on back of nose; in anus and rectum; in windpipe.
Pricking: in lids.
Painful crawling: through whole body to head.
Dryness: of mouth.
Anxiety: in præcordia.
Discomfort: in abdomen and thorax.
Lightness: of body.
Wabbling sensation: in abdomen.
Swashing: in brain.
Purring feeling: over heart.
Trembling: of arms.
Trembling feeling: in chest.
Tremulous sensation: in chest and temples.
Formication: in tongue, extending up into head.
Itching: in r. concha; in nose; in anus and rectum; on coccyx; in pustules.
Coldness: of feet; of body.

41 **Tissues.** Neuralgic affections; sensitiveness to concussion or shock.
Dropsy of internal parts.
Painful glandular swellings.
Rheumatism attacking heart.

45 **Touch. Passive Motion. Injuries.** Touch: dull stitches in head <; headache <; scalp sore; eyeball sensitive; face during neuralgia sensitive; burning in upper lip; cold sensation in teeth; pit of stomach sensitive; on epigastrium, flushing with sweat on face; acute inflammatory rheumatism; sends a shudder through whole frame.
Lying on hand: headache >.
Wiping eyes: as if hairs were on lashes <.
Pressure: > pressing headache; headache >; neuralgia > by hard; toothache <; stomach not sensitive; of clothes unbearable.
Rubbing: itching stitch in eyeball returns.
Jar, every: headache <; or knock causes sudden painful crawling through whole body to head.

[46] **Skin.** Pale, wrinkled, yellow, earthy skin.

[47] **Stages of Life, Constitution.** Light hair, debilitated, pale, thin, bloated persons, complaining of weakness.

▮▮ Worse from every shaking, commotion, or concussion.

Adapted to anæmic, debilitated subjects, of rheumatic diathesis; scrofulous children afflicted with ascarides and lumbrici.

Boy, æt. 5; stuttering speech.

Boy, æt. 10, three years ago had an attack of rheumatism, a year thereafter another attack, followed by dropsy, six weeks ago a third attack; cardiac disorder.

Girl, æt. 14, after acute articular rheumatism; endocarditis.

Girl, æt. 15, suffering seven years; headache.

Boy, æt. 17, well developed, naturally vigorous and active, dark hair, blue eyes, fair complexion; rheumatic carditis.

Girl, æt. 19, suffering from chlorosis; headache.

Young man, æt. 19; iritis.

Miss R., æt. 23, complexion fair, hair dark, lymphatic temperament, after suppression of ague; supraorbital neuralgia.

Alice T., æt. 23, suffering a month; prosopalgia.

Miss W., æt. 23, suffering two years; mitral insufficiency.

Man, æt. 25, choleric-sanguine temperament, strong constitution; neuralgic headache.

Woman, æt. 26, ill since birth of last child, which was her fourth; cardiac disorder.

Woman, æt. 27, nervous, ill seven years; gastric disorder.

Woman, æt. 28, single, suffering four years; neuralgia of tongue.

Woman, æt. 35, suffering one month; conjunctivitis.

Woman, æt. 36, cook; toothache.

Laborer, æt. 36, after rheumatism pericarditis.

Man, æt. 38, German, ten years ago was struck over l. eye with a brick, since then suffering; supraorbital neuralgia.

A lady, æt. 38, a brunette, of robust habit, mother of several children, had always a tendency to nervous affections, especially when under external influences; neuralgia of face.

Miss H., æt. 44, suffering fourteen days; facial neuralgia.

Man, æt. 51, suffering from rheumatic iritis; ciliary neuralgia.

Shoemaker, æt. 52; toothache.

Lady, æt. 54; ciliary neuralgia.

Man, æt. 56; facial neuralgia.

Watchmaker, nervo-bilious temperament, always suffered when compelled to use persistently the eye-glass; facial neuralgia.

48 **Relations.** Antidoted by: *Aurum*, restlessness in limbs; *Coccul.*, *Pulsat.*
It antidotes: *Mercur.*
Compatible: *Acon.*, endocarditis; *Arsen.*, *Digit.*, *Kali carb.*, heart symptoms; *Iris*, prosopalgia; *Arnic.*, carbuncle; *Zincum*, heart disease.

SPONGIA TOSTA.

Common Sponge roasted. *Spongia.*

Introduced and proved by Hahnemann, assisted by F. Hahnemann, Gutmann, Hartmann, Haynel, Hornburg, Langhammer, Wagner, Wislicenus, Stapf and Lehmann, Hah. Materia Medica, vol. 2; Fincke, Am. Hom. Rev., vol. 1, p. 317; Bell, Am. Jour. of Hom. Mat. Med., vol. 2, 1869, p. 211; Berridge, N. E. Med. Gaz., vol. 9, p. 403.

Clinical Authorities.—*Basedow's disease*, Hirsch, H. Kl., 1870, p. 113; Allen, Norton's Oph. Ther., p. 171; *Diphtheria*, Baynum, Hah. Mo., vol. 14, p. 605; *Pain in abdomen*, Veit Meyer, A. J. H. M. M., vol. 3, p. 8, from A. H. Z., vol. 71, p. 197; *Constipation*, Goullon, A. H. Z., vol. 78, p. 199; Raue's Rec., 1870, p. 251; *Epididymitis, orchitis*, Hornby, A. H. Z., vol. 82, p. 88; *Orchitis*, Hartmann, Schmid, Rück. Kl. Erf., vol. 2, p. 210; Schmid, B. J. H., vol. 5, p. 277; Williamson, T. H. M. S. Pa., 1873; *Affection of testicle*, Dudgeon, B. J. H., vol. 13, p. 137; *Irritability of larynx*, Nankivell, Hom. Rev., vol. 15, p. 137; *Laryngitis*, Lobethal, Rück. Kl. Erf., vol. 3, p. 100; Hendricks, A. H. Z., vol. 105, p. 166; *Perichondritis laryngea*, Unsin, Rück. Kl. Erf., vol. 5, p. 740; *Laryngeal affections*, Lobethal, Rück. Kl. Erf., vol. 3, p. 172; *Catarrh of air-passages*, Käseman, Rück. Kl. Erf., vol. 3, p. 27; *Croup*, Elb, Müller, Schneider, Billig, Bolle, Rück. Kl. Erf., vol. 5, p. 765; Stapf, Tietze, Hartmann, Hartlaub, Weigel, B. J. H., vol. 5, p. 294; Käseman, Bosch, Schwarze, Hartmann, Frank, H. in F., Hartung, Rück. Kl. Erf., vol. 3, p. 137; Morgan, A. J. H. M. M., vol. 2, p. 240; McNeil, Org., vol. 1, p. 481; *Asthma*, Gaspary, A. J. H. M. M., vol. 2, p. 281; Gaspary, Rück. Kl. Erf., vol. 3, p. 198; Gee, Hom. Phys., vol. 7, p. 18; *Cough*, Schleicher, Rück. Kl. Erf., vol. 5, p. 696; Bell, A. J. H. M. M., vol. 1, p. 211; Berridge, A. J. H. M. M., vol. 4, p. 37; Chauvet, Bib. Hom., vol. 9, p. 47; Nash, Org., vol. 3, p. 94; Med. Couns., vol. 1, p. 181; *Chronic cough*, Williams, A. J. H. M. M., vol. 4, p. 267; *Pertussis*, A. R., Rück. Kl. Erf., vol. 5, p. 729; *Circumscribed gangrene of lung*, Koch, A. J. H. M. M., vol. 4, p. 123; *Use in phthisis*, Hathaway, Mass. Trans., vol. 4, p. 231; *Aneurism of aorta*, Fanning, A. J. H. M. M, vol. 3, p. 10; *Endocarditis*, Bell, A. J. H. M. M., vol. 4, p. 211; *Affection of heart*, Wells, Hering's Anal. Ther., vol. 1, p. 223; Hering, Wells, A. J. H. M. M., vol. 1, p. 134; *Goitre*, B. in D., Rück. Kl. Erf., vol. 4, p. 380; Bernard, T. H. M. S. Pa., 1883, p. 204; *Bronchocele*, (3 cases), Barlow, N. A. J. H., vol. 17, p. 111; also B. J. H., vol. 26, p. 670; *Enlargement of thyroid gland*, Stumm, A. J. H. M. M., vol. 3, p. 108; *Ringworm*, Müller, B. J. H., vol. 23, p. 373.

[1] **Mind.** Conscious, but unable to act upon her limbs.

▮Insensibility (loss of feeling) with the chills.

Mental dulness; difficult comprehension.

▮Irresistible desire to sing, excessive mirth, followed by sadness.

▮Paroxysms of anxiety or anguish. θCardiac troubles.

▮Fear of the future; tired of life. θChronic orchitis.

Aggravation from excitement.

॥Fancies appear on shutting eyes. θTyphus.

Taciturn and discontented mood, not disposed to talk.

▮Delirium: with the heat; when falling asleep, with the chills.

Crazy feeling, head feels blown up.

Feels awkward about her work, which she cannot accomplish satisfactorily.

Alternating merry, peevish, vexed and scolding mood.

Dulness with gloominess over root of nose.

Inconsolability, would rather die on the spot; with the heat.

▮Weeping and inconsolable mood.

▮Inclination to weep: with the dreams; with whooping cough; with heat; with sweat.

▮▮Anxiety: in features; looks around anxiously; with the dreams; and heat, suddenly; nausea, pallor, after exercise out-doors; restlessness; with attacks in throat; in croup; with dyspnœa; in typhus.

॥She is very fretful and anxious about her condition, fears she will die of suffocation.

▮Anxious sweat and faintness; with angina pectoris.

She is very timid, and is especially pursued and incessantly tormented by a frightful scene of some mournful event of the past.

She is very timorous, and starts at every trifle, which affects her feet, so as to make them feel heavy.

▮Timidity of mind with the sweat.

▮Terror and fear: of approaching death; that she will die of suffocation; with heart disease; with whooping cough; with the heat; with the sweat.

He is anxious, as if some misfortune would occur of which he has a presentiment.

▮Apprehension of a fatal termination of his disease.

▮Great alarm, agitation, anxiety, difficult respiration.

▮Fright awakens.

▮Nervous; desponding about loss of sexual power.

▮Satiety of life, with the heat.

Ill-humored; dislikes to talk and answer.

Out of temper and lazy; would rather rest, and is not disposed to talk.

Peevish, vexed and scolding mood.
Sulky, obstinate and improper behavior.
▮Obstinacy, with whooping cough.
▮▮Every excitement increases the cough.
Thinking of it increases one-sided heat of face.

[2] **Sensorium.** ▮Vertigo: with danger of falling; at night, when awaking, with nausea; when sitting, as if head would fall to one side, with a feeling of heat in head; as if one would fall backward; as if tipsy; after sleep, with the heat; with rush of blood to head.

▮Congestion of blood to head, with throbbing and pressure in forehead.

▮Heaviness and fulness in head, as if all blood were mounting to head, with vertigo.

[3] **Inner Head.** Stitches in temples.

Sharp stitches externally in l. temple, extending to forehead.

While lying feels a strong pulsation, < about ear on which she is lying.

Dull headache in r. side of brain, on coming into **warm** room from open air.

Headache as if skull would burst, in vertex and forehead.

Pressing sensation: in r. temple, from within outward; downward drawing pain in r. side of head and neck; outward on r. parietal bone, while lying.

Pressing headache in vertex.

▮Pressing headache in r. frontal eminence, from within outward, < while sitting, on entering warm room after walking in open air, and from looking at anything sharply; > when lying in horizontal position, especially when lying on back.

▮Forehead: blood accumulated, pressing out; burning heat; violent heat; pain; stitches from temples; pressure.

▮Occiput: headache; stitches; pain; heaviness before fever; stitch on turning head; burning.

▮Headache: when gazing steadily; on rising, > after washing and taking breakfast; from dry, cold weather; after intoxication; with the chill; with heat of face.

▮Congestion of blood to head, with pressing, knocking and pulsating in forehead; redness of face, with anxious mien; > when lying in a horizontal position.

While lying, she feels a dull, tremulous roaring (wuwwern), like a strong pulsation, each time with a double stroke, in head, in region of ear upon which she lies in bed; when turning on other ear she feels it in that side.

Bursting pain in head, with whooping cough.

▮Meningitis, scrofulous or tuberculous; congestion of blood

to head, with pressing, knocking and pulsating in forehead; redness of face with anxious mien; > when lying in horizontal position; heat in head; bending head backward, with tension in neck; eyes staring, lids wide open; double sight; face pale and cold, with heat, or alternately red and pale; twitching of muscles with fever; frequent waking with a start; tossing about; stupid slumber.

4 **Outer Head.** ▮▮Sharp stitches in l. temple, externally, extending into forehead.

Sharp stitches in scalp, with heat of scalp.

▮Sensation as if hair were standing on end on vertex; during chill.

Sharp pressure externally, at both temples.

Gnawing pain, externally on crown of head.

Forehead painful to touch.

Disagreeable sensitiveness of cranial integuments, particularly on moving scalp.

▮Violent itching on scalp.

▮Yellow, scabby eruption.

Turning head: a stitch in occiput; to right, neck pains; neck stiff; tensive pain in neck.

▮Bending head back: tension in neck; in croup and suffocative attacks.

Jerks head downward.

▮Bending backward and sinking of head, with painful stiffness of neck; piping, anxious inspiration, with dry, barking cough. θCroup.

Holding head in an upright position, > dull pressure in occiput.

5 **Sight and Eyes.** Sees visions on closing eyes.

Double vision; > lying down.

Pressing and stinging in eyes.

Coldness of eyes.

Lachrymation and headache, when looking fixedly at one spot.

Things appear in flames, at night.

Objects appear to move up and down.

Could not distinguish objects.

She can recognize distant objects only with great exertion

Looking sharply at anything increases headache and causes lachrymation.

Pressing in outer half of l. eye.

Tension about l. eye, near temple.

Tearing and stinging in l. eye, after fever.

Stinging about eye.

Stinging, finally pressing pain in both eyes, in evening.

Stinging itching under l. eye, > by rubbing.

Coldness or heat in eyes.
Redness of conjunctiva; eyes fill with puslike matter.
Burning in l. eye about eyeball.
▮Heaviness and nightly agglutination of lids.
Tears exude from between closed lids.
Sudden stinging drawing at outer canthus of l. orbit, which spreads around, above and below to inner canthus.
Tensive stinging pain in l. outer canthus, most severe on moving eyes; disappearing when touched.
Eyes close involuntarily, almost spasmodically.
Pressing under eyelids.
Burning pain on external surface of l. lower lid.
Itching of eyelids.
▮Redness of eyes, with lachrymation and burning.
▮Eyes protruding, staring, or deeply sunken.
||Inflammation with dryness of lids.
Eyes have a dull, swollen look, as after intoxication.
Pressing pain over r. eye, externally.
▮Maculæ of cornea.
||Eyeballs staring and perceptibly protruding; stitches in balls and burning around eyes, with lachrymation, > from any sudden light; often eye feels as if twisted around; there is constant flashing of colors, mostly deep red, with figures of light, etc., even when eye is closed, especially at night; thyroid gland is considerably hypertrophied; palpitation very marked, makes her uneasy, restless and easily frightened, especially at night. θBasedow's disease.

6 **Hearing and Ears.** Hardness of hearing.
Congestion of blood to ears; burning.
Dull ringing in ears; ringing in r. ear; hears a pulsating roar in ear upon which she lies; as if a battery of guns were discharged, at night.
Cramplike pain in l. ear, while walking in open air.
Pressure in ears, and crowding sensation in same.
Drawing pain in internal r. ear.
Earache of a contracting kind.
Fine stitches in r. ear, outwardly, as if passing through tympanum.
Digging stitches in depth of l. ear.
▮Heat in ears.
Burning: in ears from throat; behind ear.
▮Suppuration of external ear.
Pain in cartilages of ears.
Burning in orifice of r. ear.
An inflamed nodule finally covered with a scab, painful to touch and remaining several days, in l. concha,

close to entrance of meatus auditorius; tensive pain, creeping as if it would gather and break, at times stitches.

Red swelling of r. helix, with a pimple on same, exuding moisture like an ulcer, for nine days; painful on external pressure.

Boils on l. ear, painful to touch.

7 **Smell and Nose.** Bleeding of nose: when blowing it; during dinner; with whooping cough.

Dulness and sensation of gloominess over root of nose like that preceding a common cold.

Tensive constricting sensation above root of nose.

Tearing in nose.

Creeping stitches in l. nasal bone.

▮Nose stuffed up. θCoryza. θWhooping cough.

▮Coryza: fluent; hoarseness; croupy cough; after dry, cold winds; with chills; in measles.

▮▮Breathing through nose obstructed by a swelling in fauces.

▮Dryness of nose.

▮Retention and thickening of nasal mucus.

▮Nasal mucus viscous, grows thick. θMembranous croup.

▮Chronic dry nasal catarrh; nose entirely occluded.

▮▮Coryza; nose running, or stopped up, with fever; hoarseness; at same time catarrhal affection of larynx, with hollow or crouplike cough; respiration difficult, with a noise sounding as in laryngo-stenosis.

▮▮Nostrils wide open; fanlike motion.

▮Nose pinched; cold.

Eruption on point of nose, and on lips.

8 **Upper Face.** ▮Face: distressed, in croup; anxious; livid; pale and bloated; blue; pale, with sunken eyes; red, with anxious expression; alternately red and pale; ▮▮cold sweat.

Heat on one side of face, < when thinking of it.

Swelling of cheeks.

Itching and stinging in cheeks.

Cramplike pain from l. articulation of jaw to cheek; evenings, while eating or when walking in open air.

A vexed expression, with cough at night.

Coldness, pallor and sweat of face, with heat of body.

▮Cold sweat in face, in evening.

Flying heat in face and in blood, with excitement of nerves.

▮Herpes on face, especially in scrofulous persons, after a cold, with dry, croupy cough.

9 **Lower Face.** Tearing and stinging in l. cheek after fever.

Into cheeks throbbing, down from head; down from articulation of jaw; tearing from cheek to neck.

Pressing, tearing sensation in r. zygomatic arch.

||Pricking pains passing transversely across upper jaw.

Jerking fine stitch from posterior portion of r. upper jaw into r. internal ear, at night in bed.

||Cramplike pain extending from l. articulation of jaw, down cheek; evenings while eating.

Tension in articulation of l. jaw when walking in open air.

Pain in articulation of jaw as if dislocated.

Lower jaw drawn by cramp; painful to touch.

Swelling of cheeks.

Stinging, itching in l. cheek.

Fine stitches beneath lower lip.

||Mouth firmly closed, only slightly opened with a groaning breath.

Lips livid.

|Eruptions on lips; after fever.

|Swelling of maxillary glands, with tension.

After opening mouth wide, and then biting teeth firmly together, cramp in neck.

Protracted violent burning under r. angle of mouth, near chin, as if eruption were to appear; < on stretching skin.

Left side of chin to angle of mouth painful to touch, as if ulcerated.

|Numbness in chin.

Heat in chin.

Pimples beneath chin, on neck, painful to pressure.

10 **Teeth and Gums.** Teeth feel dull and loose when masticating.

Itching and stinging in teeth.

Pain as if something had got jammed between teeth in chewing.

Pain in posterior molars of r. lower jaw, as if gums and teeth were swollen and latter being lifted.

Burning pain in l. upper molars.

||Heat in teeth.

Itching in upper and lower teeth.

Gums painful while chewing, with swelling; thin white coating.

11 **Taste and Tongue.** |Taste: bitter, only in throat; bitter, with dry tongue; bitter, with chill; sweetish, in mouth; like glycerine; of fresh nuts; coffee is bitter and disgusting; tobacco has a scratchy, bitter taste in mouth and fauces.

|Tongue: brown, dry; dry and red; vesicles at edge of tongue, with soreness.

|Difficulty of speech.

12 **Inner Mouth.** Mouth raw.

Mouth and tongue full of vesicles, with burning and stinging pains, cannot eat solid food.

ǀǀMouth burning, dry. θCroup.

Saliva diminished; or with whooping cough, increased.

13 **Throat.** ▮Burning and stinging in throat; rawness and scratching.

▮Penetrating tickling in throat, toward ear.

▮▮Sore throat, < after eating sweet things.

▮Thyroid gland swollen, even with chin; at night suffocating spells, barking, with stinging in throat and soreness in abdomen.

▮Throat externally swollen; suffocating attacks.

▮Relief of throat symptoms, when lying on back.

Stitches in goitre, even when not swallowing.

Constantly recurring needlelike stitches above pit of throat, externally, in lower portion of goitre.

ǀǀPulse 100; respiration 50, wheezing, whistling, occasionally sawing; head thrown back, muscles of chest working, abdomen contracted under ribs with every effort to inflate lungs; cold, clammy sweat all over; lies quietly on side, anxious for breath; does not want to be fanned; eyes fixed, pupils dilated; does not notice attendants; loose involuntary discharge from bowels in morning. θDiphtheria.

π Tension and pressure in throat (relieved by *Calc*).

ǀǀPain in throat when coughing and speaking.

Stinging in throat, particularly after eating, and a sensation outside of throat as if something were being pressed out; < morning and evening.

▮Stitches in throat.

▮Dryness in throat; < by hawking.

Roughness of throat on coughing; in whooping cough.

Scraping in throat.

Quick and strong hawking ends a suffocating attack.

▮Tickling in throat causes cough.

Continual very bitter taste deep in throat, not in mouth.

Burning in throat, in front, and then in ears.

Attack of sudden burning and compression; drawing toward throat; and anxiety, passing off on sitting up in bed.

▮Frequent burning and dryness in throat.

▮Tonsils, soft palate and uvula somewhat swollen and highly reddened.

Painful pressure above thyroid cartilage, < by palpitation.

Very disagreeable sensation of relaxation in œsophagus and stomach, as if he had drunk a great deal of lukewarm water.

Heat in œsophagus.

||Swelling in fauces, with a broad basis, projecting from r. to l., allowing in l. but a small passage of food and obstructing breathing through nose; voice somewhat nasal; snoring and rattling breathing at night; wakes up several times during night with want of breath, increasing to suffocation; a slight cough and a numbness in chin and in front of throat.

||Deglutition prevented.

|Difficult swallowing. θCroup.

|On swallowing: stitches in neck pass off; violent straining pain; pain in goitre; a moving sensation in goitre.

14 **Appetite, Thirst. Desires, Aversions.** |Insatiable appetite and thirst; or diminished appetite, out of humor.

Desire for dainties.

|Thirstlessness; rarely thirst with the chill.

||Thirst, but is only able to swallow small quantity and with difficulty.

Violent thirst after smoking.

15 **Eating and Drinking.** ||Eating and drinking relieve cough.

|Drinking milk, ale or spirits, or cold or hot tea, or cold water brings on cough.

During dinner, nosebleed.

While eating, cramp in articulation of jaw.

On chewing: gums pain; pain in molars.

After eating: stinging in throat; sweet things < sore throat; fulness and distress; cutting in upper part of abdomen; colic.

16 **Hiccough, Belching, Nausea and Vomiting.** ||Hiccough.

Eructations: repeated; empty; sour; bitter.

Nausea: continuous; and vertigo, when waking; when smoking; and waterbrash.

Retching of mucus.

Sense of sickness and faintness at stomach as if one had drunk a quantity of warm water.

17 **Scrobiculum and Stomach.** She cannot endure tight clothing about body, particularly around epigastric region.

Pressure in epigastrium, in afternoon.

Internal sensation of coldness in epigastrium, with fulness in that region.

Pressing pain in gastric region, lasting all forenoon.

Beneath short ribs pain on coughing.

||Chill in pit of stomach.

|Pit of stomach drawn in during croup.

Ulcerative feeling in pit of stomach; must lie on back.

Drawing, as if growing together, in pit of stomach as far

as throat, when it seems to press windpipe so that she can hardly breathe.

▮Craves dainties; after eating has dyspeptic distress and fulness of stomach; > from warm drinks, particularly colicky pains in abdomen.

Cannot tolerate tight clothing about stomach.

Stitches in region of stomach.

||Stomach feels flaccid and as if standing open. θWhooping cough.

||Craving at stomach before menses.

▮Dyspeptic distress and fulness in stomach, after eating.

18 **Hypochondria.** ||Pressure in hypochondria. θWhooping cough.

||Chronic pancreatitis.

19 **Abdomen.** Rumbling in abdomen < evenings and mornings.

▮Violent action of abdominal muscles during inspiration.

▮Viscera drawn up against diaphragm.

▮Cannot bear tight clothing on abdomen. θWhooping cough. θDyspepsia.

||Pain in l. side of abdomen; digging and choking; > after discharge of wind; at times as if something alive were moving there.

▮Pain in abdomen, instead of catamenia.

Tensive pain from middle of hypogastrium to anus; cutting in hypogastrium, extending toward l. breast, in evening.

Boring stinging in l. hypogastrium on expiration, < on stooping.

Tense abdomen.

Tensive pain in upper abdomen while sitting or walking, < on stooping.

While sitting, painful constriction in l. side, beneath stomach, particularly when lying on r. side.

▮▮Cramps in abdomen; pinching colic.

Lower part of abdomen feels empty; viscera drawn up against diaphragm.

||Gurgling in abdomen, urging and rumbling before stool.

Sensation like a fine digging, as if something alive were beneath skin of abdomen, above l. hip in the side upon which he lies, in morning.

A twisting sensation in l. side of abdomen, < when pressed with hand.

Stitches in r. side of abdomen, in region of liver.

Fine stitch, externally, on navel.

▮Colic: before menses, before chill; with the sweat.

||Violent commotion of abdominal muscles during inspiration. θWhooping cough.

Squalmishness in abdomen, with frequent fluid stools, like diarrhœa.

When smoking tobacco, heat in abdomen rises into chest, rest of body chilly.

▮Heat in abdomen.

▮▮Peritonitis.

Cramplike pain in l. groin, while sitting.

Stitches below groin.

Pain in abdominal ring as in inguinal hernia.

Only while sitting, pressing, tearing pain in region of abdominal ring, on both sides.

Itching near groin.

Glandular swelling in r. groin, with tensive pain while walking.

Small boil in l. groin, very painful.

Swelling of inguinal glands.

20 **Stool and Rectum.** ▮Diarrhœic stools: with tenesmus; frequent, fluid; white.

▮After cholera, croup.

▮▮Occasional diarrhœa with a large number of ascarides, after which she always feels great relief.

▮▮Stools small and hard, with tenesmus.

▮Before stool: noise in abdomen; urging and rumbling; itching in anus.

During stool: pressure, caused by flatus in lumbar region; straining in anus as if diarrhœa would ensue; sore pain in anus lasting for some days.

After stool: blood passes from anus.

▮Costive; hard stool, insufficient, with tenesmus; soreness of anus.

▮▮Formication in rectum.

Pain from hypogastrium to anus.

▮Smarting in anus.

Stitches in anus, and snarling noise in abdomen, before each stool.

Itching, biting and soreness at anus, discharge of ascarides.

▮▮Ascarides with whooping cough.

21 **Urinary Organs.** Very thin stream of urine.

▮Frequent urging to urinate, with small discharges; at times without discharge; at others with discharges of acrid smelling urine, which deposited a dirty-white sediment.

Increased flow of urine.

▮Involuntary discharge of urine. θWhooping cough.

▮Urine frothy; sediment thick, greyish white or yellow.

22 **Male Sexual Organs.** Drawing, painful stitches, extending from body through glans penis.

Voluptuous itching at point of glans penis, for several hours, urging him to rub the part.

Itching, burning in scrotum and body of penis.
Total want of sexual desire.
❙❙Chronic enlargement of prostate gland.
❚Swollen, painful spermatic cords.
❙❙Stitches into spermatic cord; drawing.
Large, somewhat blunt stitch, shooting from testicle into spermatic cord.
Pressive swelling of testicles.
Simple pain in testicles, also when touched.
A pinching, bruised, squeezing pain in testicles.
❙❙Shooting up entire cord; any motion of bed or clothing brought on throbbing, in addition to constant, heavy, dragging pains.
❙❙Since two years swelling of l. testicle as large as a hen's egg, smooth and hard; obstruction of vasa efferentia; shooting pain from testicle into inguinal region.
❙❙After checked gonorrhœa orchitis, first r. then left.
❚Maltreated orchitis; also after checked gonorrhœa.
❙❙Right epididymis enlarged and hardened, with little pain; cord also thickened and hard; fistulous opening (in connection with lower part of epididymis), discharges a little thick, whitish matter; scrotum has an irregular and discolored appearance from a sinus and cicatrization of former abscesses and sinuses; urine always thick; total want of sexual desire; both testicles soft and small; nervous and despondent about loss of sexual power; apprehensive of a fatal termination.
❙❙Scirrhous testicle.
❚Heat in male genitals; in penis, scrotum, testicle and spermatic cords.

23 **Female Sexual Organs.** Enlargement and induration of ovaries.
❚Menses too soon, too profuse.
❚Before menses: colic, backache, soreness in sacrum and craving in stomach, palpitation.
❚During menses: drawing in all the limbs; awakes with suffocating spells.
Catamenia suppressed; at the time violent pains in small of back and abdomen.
❚Violent drawing in upper and lower limbs, during menses.

24 **Pregnancy. Parturition. Lactation.** ❙❙A particular condition of placenta seems only cause for protracted, painful and unsuccessful labor.
❙❙Twice, after a few doses of *Spongia* 200, miscarried at about six or eight weeks; a few doses brought on flowing like menses, continuing several days.

25 **Voice and Larynx. Trachea and Bronchia.** ❚❚Hoarseness, cough, coryza.

▮Hoarse, voice cracked or faint, choking sensation; whistling inspiration.

▮Hoarseness with soreness and burning.

▮Feeling of a plug in larynx; larynx sensitive to touch and when turning neck; talking hurts.

Pressure in larynx when singing.

Cracked voice in evening; increasing hoarseness, can only speak with difficulty.

▮Voice: nasal; hollow; low; lisping; weak; cracked; not clear; failing, when talking or singing; giving out, with chronic hoarseness.

▮Chronic catarrhal hoarseness.

▮Hoarseness: with coryza; with cough; whooping cough; typhus; sweat; measles; after laryngotomy.

▮Rough, crowing cry with the cough.

‖Aphonia in a boy, æt. 3, who had undergone laryngotomy for removal of a bean.

▮Chronic sore throat, < when reading aloud, talking or singing; < after eating sweet things.

▮▮Laryngeal phthisis.

▮Great dryness of larynx.

▮Laryngismus stridulus.

▮▮Talking, singing or swallowing hurts larynx.

▮Inflammation of larynx, trachea and bronchia.

▮Attacks of mucous rattling in windpipe; at times strangling.

▮Feeling of stoppage in windpipe.

▮Starts from sleep suddenly with contraction of larynx.

▮Region of thyroid gland indurated.

▮Contraction in larynx, constriction, suffocation; also during sleep.

▮As if a stopper or valve were in larynx. θCroup. θWhooping cough.

▮After plastic lymph has been deposited a foreign body is audible in larynx or trachea moving to and fro; child coughs up cutaneous masses or tough, thick phlegm.

Severe pressing inward in larynx, as if with a nail, when moving, in evening.

Drawing toward larynx and contraction therein, in evening.

Jerking, fine stitches externally in region of larynx.

▮Irritation in upper part of larynx.

▮Tickling in larynx, with whooping cough.

▮Burning, tickling in larynx and trachea.

▮Scraping, roughness, in larynx and trachea.

▮Dryness of larynx; < by hawking; with the sweat; with short barking cough, embarrassed breathing as if larynx and trachea were narrower; with difficult speech, hoarseness; expectoration of more or less yellow mucus, consisting of little lumps; beginning phthisis laryngea.

▮Laryngeal catarrh: with coryza; with dry cough, tormenting during night; with ulcers in larynx.

▮▮Larynx sensitive to touch. θCroup. θWhooping cough.

||Perichondritis laryngea; hollow, barking, dry cough, day and night, constriction in larynx; pain in larynx on touching it, and on turning neck; whistling breathing.

||Larynx elevated and depressed, during respiration. θCroup.

||Swollen larynx, almost protruding above chin.

▮Glandular swellings about larynx and trachea.

▮In trachea: pain; shock upward, like a suffocative paroxysm, starting out of sleep; contraction; burning; rattling; pain on coughing; dryness.

▮Catarrhal affections of air passages with dry cough and hoarseness, no fever, in grown persons.

||Fever and irritation in throat, with hoarse, croupy cough, < in evening; breathing wheezy; spells of choking in middle of night. θLaryngitis.

▮Dry bronchitis, with terrible, hard, dry, racking cough; much dyspnœa and slight expectoration; < in hot room, > by eating or drinking.

▮Spasmodic paroxysms of cough and dyspnœa; < from a sudden change of atmosphere, a wind arising or an unpleasant moral impression; wheezing, sibilant ronchi.

▮▮Cough dry and sibilant, sounding like a saw driven through a pine board. θCroup.

||Awoke with a violent, harsh, hollow-sounding cough; voice hoarse; respiration quick, little impeded, but with much rattling; high fever; skin hot and dry. θCroup.

||After cessation of coryza, hollow, barking, dry cough, with croupy sound; short attacks of rattling in windpipe while breathing; skin hot; frequent stretching and yawning; while coughing, makes faces and complains of pain under larynx; cough < in afternoon; lachrymose humor; pulse hard, rapid. θCroup.

||Sat up in bed; face bloated and bluish; anxious expression; breathing difficult, rattling, with much effort of chest and distortion of face; eyes project; head bent backward; cough whistling and resonant; seizes hold of nearest object, grasps at larynx, which is painful; anxious sweat; pulse 110; great heat, constant thirst; involuntary discharge of feces and urine while coughing. θCroup.

‖ Burning fever; face red; skin dry; violent thirst; constipation; hoarse, rough, deep, barking cough, which he tries to suppress; rattling, whistling respiration; starting up in sleep and anxious breathing; when lying bores head backward into pillow. θCroup.

‖ After a chill, at night burning heat of skin, redness of face, headache, delirium; violent, hoarse, hollow, barking cough, with great pain in larynx; rough, hoarse voice; rattling, whistling respiration. θCroup.

‖ High fever, frequent attacks of suffocation and cough; hoarse, rough voice; whistling respiration, audible at a distance; region of larynx painful; starting up in bed as if she would suffocate; boring backward of head; ill-humor, crying, indifference to everything. θCroup.

‖ Sudden attack of croup about 9 P.M.; threw back her head; face first red, then blue, cold and moist; eyes red and suffused; cough dry and painful; limbs cold and moist; during paroxysms struggled and writhed into erect position.

‖ Hoarseness, cough, and dryness of Schneiderian membrane for two days; sudden development of croup; child sits on mother's lap with head thrown back; fanlike motion of nostrils; laborious breathing, with a sawing sound; now and then sharp whistling cough; protrusion of eyes; eyelids wide open; great anxiety depicted on countenance.

‖ Sits up in bed; cannot lie on account of want of breath; eyes protruding, staring; nose pinched and cold; face pale and bloated; mouth firmly closed or only slightly opened, with a groaning breath; loss of voice; deglutition prevented; head drawn backward; swollen larynx almost protruding above chin; lower part of abdomen feels empty; viscera drawn up against diaphragm; groaning respiration without any motion of chest; pulse imperceptible; hands and feet cold; whole body covered with a cold, clammy sweat.

| A little girl, 2½ years old; aroused by cough, sits up suddenly in bed, looks around anxiously; gasps for breath as if it could not get any; in a short time a second attack, more violent than first, followed by repeated attacks, each more violent; infrequent dry cough; hoarseness; breathing somewhat accelerated and difficult; every quarter of an hour restlessness and anxiety increased; wanted to be carried about, threw its head back, or imploringly stretched out its hands for relief; face turned dark red when in height of attack; eyes protruded and neck commenced to swell rapidly; between attacks child showed signs of thirst,

but is unable to swallow but a small quantity, and with difficulty; frequent urging to urinate, at times without discharge, at others with discharge of normally colored, acrid-smelling urine, which deposited a dirty white sediment.

▮▮A young lady, æt. 24; three days after convalescence from cholera, face bluish-red, somewhat bloated, anxious and distorted; increased bodily temperature, with diminished warmth of extremities; tonsils, soft palate and uvula somewhat swollen and highly reddened; breathing very rapid and short; on deeper inhalation a whistling noise in larynx, with sinking in of intercostal spaces; weak, vesicular breathing; at times sudden, dull concussions of cough, ending in a long-drawn whistling inspiration; dyspnœa; anxiety; blueness of face; lisping voice; weak pulse, 100; violent straining pain on swallowing; pain in throat when coughing and speaking; larynx sensitive to touch; constant anxiety; great heat and feeling of exhaustion; thin, white coating on gums.

▮▮Croup < before midnight (< before morning, *Hepar*).

▮Cough rough, dull, hollow and barking; either perfectly dry, or difficult loosening of phlegm; breathing slow and drawing, noisy, whistling, sawing (when phlegm commences to rattle, *Hepar*).

▮Fair complexion; < before midnight; dry sound of breathing and cough.

▮▮Cough is dry and sibilant, or sounds like a saw driven through a pine board, each cough corresponding to a thrust of the saw; no mucous rattle; cough dry and hoarse, causes pain in throat. θCroup.

▮Wakes with suffocation about larynx on falling asleep, early at night.

26 **Respiration.** ▮Breathing: wheezing, anxious, < during inhalation, with violent laboring of abdominal muscles; piping, anxious; whistling, sawing between coughs, with whooping cough or croup; rattling; loud; snoring; noisy; weak, slow and drawn; accelerated and difficult; very rapid and short; very quick, gasping; laborious; gasping; panting; groaning, without motion of chest; slow, deep, as after exhaustion; as if through a sponge.

▮Dyspnœa: with palpitation; severe, on lying down; exhaustion in chest, < after every exertion; sudden weakness, tottering while walking, blood seems to rush into chest as if it would burst; with frothy, white sputa and much retching; an hour after slight coughing brings up grey lumpy mucus; > by bending body forward.

‖Asthma: from taking cold, cannot lie down; sibilant ronchi; after menses; breathing always tight, cannot inspire nor expire freely; in consequence of goitre; breathing, rattling and panting; after every slight motion loses her breath and becomes faint; blood rushes to her chest and head; hot in face, anxious; fears she will die of suffocation; spasmodic, with organic disease of heart; must throw head back; < at full moon.

|Awakes with suffocative sensation; wakes up choking when falling asleep.

‖Came slowly into office, walked stooped, sat down carefully, leaned forward and kept very quiet and seemed to be much exhausted; labored inspiration involving abdominal muscles, quite marked; had not slept for two nights, obliged to sit upright in his chair; leaning backward, lying down, or exertion takes his breath away.

|Dyspnœa and great weakness in chest, could hardly talk after exercise.

Suffocation on moment of falling asleep.

‖Wakes with suffocation about larynx; on falling asleep early at night; fair skin.

Suffocative paroxysm, with pain in chest.

‖On deep inhalation, whistling in larynx and sucking in of intercostal spaces.

On slow, deep inspiration, stitch in chest.

|On breathing, sensation of air passing into glands of neck. θGoitre.

On expiration, pain in hypogastrium.

27 **Cough.** ‖Cough: dry, barking, hollow, croupy; wheezing, asthmatic; caused by burning or tickling in larynx, sensation like a plug or valve, or by feeling of accumulation of mucus and weight in chest; dry, with burning in chest; loose, suddenly changing to dryness and hoarseness (typhus); without expectoration, with chill; incessant, from a place low down in chest, where it pains, as if sore and bloody; slight, from swelling in fauces, short, infrequent; short, dry, irritating, with feeling of roughness in larynx, and pains in chest; dry, rough, barking, with dyspnœa; sudden concussion; spasmodic; violent; dry, hollow, wheezing, < in evening; dry or sibilant, or sounds like a saw driven through a pine board, each cough corresponding to a thrust of the saw; hollow, with some expectoration, day and night; hollow in croup or remaining after croup; in measles; with a high crowing sound; sharp, whistling; exceedingly painful, in croup; hurting larynx.

‖Cough caused by tickling in throat; expectoration easy,

sometimes salty; < on rising from bed and when indoors; brought on by smoking, lying on back or r. side, drinking milk, ale, spirits, cold tea, or cold water; > by eating or by warm tea or warm coffee; disturbs sleep; < in wet weather; > in frosty weather.

▮Frequent night cough in paroxysms of two minutes, with a vexed expression.

‖Aneurism of descending aorta, a paroxysmal, dry, suffocative cough, coming at irregular intervals, but especially on lying down, or when drinking hot tea; dyspeptic distress and fulness in stomach after eating (relieved).

‖When coughing, sweat.

▮On coughing, pain in chest and trachea, with roughness of throat.

On coughing, painful pressure beneath short ribs.

▮Whooping cough, deep, hollow, barking. caused by sensation of a plug in larynx, with expectoration only in morning of small quantities of tough, yellow, hardened mucus, compelling one to swallow it again.

‖Cough caused by feeling of a plug in throat; brought on by movement and lying down, especially on r. side or back; > by sitting up or eating; dyspnœa < by talking or moving, or lying down, especially on r. side or back, and by bending back or stooping, or by lying with head low; > by bending forward slightly, by eating or by drinking warm cocoa; excited by a feeling of large accumulation of mucus and weight at chest; voice lost at times, subject to such attacks, in cold weather, for six years.

▮Chronic cough, violent attacks, brought up small, hard tubercle.

▮Expectoration: scanty, of saltish tasting mucus; scanty, tenacious, yellow, indurated, slightly sour-tasting; loosened mornings, but must be swallowed again; profuse, mucous, cannot lie down (pneumonia in stage of resolution); smelling like milk (whooping cough); of yellow mucus in little lumps; of cutaneous masses.

28 **Inner Chest and Lungs.** Pain in chest and bronchi, with rawness in throat when coughing.

After exertion suddenly exhausted, chest particularly affected, could hardly speak; heat in face and nausea; heaviness in head.

▮Oppression of chest.

Weight dragging down on r. chest; tightness of chest from a cold.

▮Constricting or contracting pain in chest; spasmodic constriction. θWhooping cough. θHeart disease.

Pressure in l. chest, sometimes stitches.

Pressing, cutting pain on deep inspiration, in l. side of chest.

Sudden pain, in chest and dorsal muscles of l. side, as if a broad body armed with points were pressing upward, a broad pressure with many fine stitches.

Drawing stitches beneath second rib of l. side of chest, only on walking.

Drawing stitches in l. side of chest, while sitting with back slightly bent, but particularly on slow, deep inspiration.

Severe intermittent stitches in l. side of chest.

Transient, painful stitches on r. side of chest; when the part is rubbed it seems as if a weight were dragging down in that place, under skin

Severe pricking pain in r. breast, from within outward.

Stinging, pinching, crawling pain in l. side of chest in region of sixth and seventh ribs, < from pressure.

A pinching jerk in l. side of chest, from without inward.

Boring stitch in r. costal muscles, continuous on inspiration and expiration.

▮Constrictive spasmodic pain through chest and larynx.

▮Stitches, resembling pleuritic stitches, in both sides.

▮Pain in chest on coughing.

A spot deep in chest causes coughing.

▮Heat in chest; sensation as if she had something hot inside of chest.

Heat from abdomen.

Burning in chest, with cough.

She grows weak after every trifling motion of body; blood rushes up into chest, face grows hot, body begins to glow, bloodvessels are hard and distended and she loses her breath; she recovers only after a long rest.

▮Burning, soreness, rawness, heaviness in chest.

▮Congestion to chest from least movement or exertion; dyspnœa, nausea, faintish weakness.

Orgasm of blood in chest after least exertion, with dyspnœa, anguish, nausea and faintish weakness.

After moderate motion out of doors, she suddenly grows weak and totters to a chair; amid great anxiety, nausea, pallor, short gasping breath, blood seems to rush from heart up into chest as if to burst out above; eyes close involuntarily, almost spasmodically, tears exude from between closed lids; she is conscious, but is unable to act upon her limbs by means of volition.

▮Bronchial catarrh: with dry cough and hoarseness, without fever; with measles.

▮Acute bronchitis, with profuse secretion of mucus; much oppression of breathing; all symptoms < by lying with head low; cough < by room getting too warm; > by eating, even eating a little.

▌Inflammation of air-passages, with dry, irritating cough and burning tickling in larynx.

▌Bronchitis: with continuous, dry, fatiguing cough; mucous râles subcrepitant, whistling and sonorous; following croup.

▌▌Chronic bronchitis, with a dry spasmodic cough.

A spot deep in chest as if raw and bloody from coughing.

▌Broncho and croupous pneumonia.

Pneumonia: in stage of resolution, with profuse secretion and expectoration of mucus; inability to lie down; cough > by eating and drinking.

▌Tuberculous consumption: beginning in apex of (l.) lung; severe dyspnœa on lying down; exhaustion after every exertion, especially of chest; hoarseness, with sudden aphonia while speaking; chilliness in back, not removed by artificial heat, yet if the room becomes too warm the cough is increased; cough < from evening until midnight, from cold air, from talking, singing or moving; > from eating or drinking.

29 **Heart, Pulse and Circulation.** ▌Constricting pain in cardiac region with anxiety; anxious sweat. θAngina pectoris.

Heart beating a double stroke; pulsating sound in ear.

πSuffering with an organic affection of heart, she ate and swallowed a piece of sponge, just roasted; sudden and terrible beating of heart and suffocation; lips livid; respiration violently gasping, great pain in heart; terror and fear of approaching death.

▌▌Attacks of oppression and cardiac pain; < lying with head low.

▌Rheumatic endocarditis, loud blowing with each heart-beat.

▌Stinging pressing pains in præcordial region.

▌▌Violent palpitation, awakens after 12 P.M.; sensation of suffocation; bellows' murmur; loud cough, which is hard, tight, dry; great alarm, agitation, anxiety, dyspnœa.

▌▌Palpitation: violent, with pain, gasping respiration; suddenly awakened after midnight, with suffocation, great alarm, anxiety; valvular insufficiency; before catamenia; with congestion to chest.

▌▌Rheumatism left lumbar muscles and seized heart (second similar metastasis); awakened between 1 and 2 A.M. by a sense of suffocation, accompanied by loud, violent cough, great alarm, agitation, anxiety and difficult respiration; action of heart violent and rapid, and each beat accompanied by a loud blowing as of a bellows.

‖Irregular action of heart, suffocating palpitation on making even slight exertion, or on going up stairs or ascending ground; if she raises arms above head she becomes faint; lay in bed with her head high; awoke often in a fright and felt as if she were suffocating; physical signs of valvular deposit unmistakable.

▮In fibrinous deposit upon valves of heart, it causes a gradual disappearance of valvular murmur.

▮Rheumatic endocarditis, valvular insufficiency (usually mitral), systolic murmur.

▮Valvular insufficiency; awaking at night with fear and terror.

▮▮Angina pectoris; contracting pain in chest, heat, suffocation, faintness, and anxious sweat.

‖Aneurism of descending aorta; paroxysmal, dry, suffocative cough, coming at irregular intervals, but especially on lying down or drinking hot tea; dyspeptic distress and fulness in stomach after eating (relieved).

Pulse: frequent, hard, full or feeble; rapid, full; very rapid, full and hard; hard, small, full; imperceptible.

▮Symptoms of circulation are <: from mental lassitude; from coughing; when lying on r. side; before menstruation; after lying down; sitting bent forward; from smoking; from going up stairs.

▮Congestion to head, ears, nose (nose bleeding), face, chest, abdomen, lower limbs.

▮Ebullition of blood, distension of veins.

30 **Outer Chest.** Fine stitches externally on chest and arms.

Stinging itching on l. breast near shoulder.

Induration of l. breast, a space of two inches in length by half inch thickness, painful to touch, coming on in evening and disappearing in morning.

Itching on breast.

▮Intercostal spaces sinking in with inhalation.

31 **Neck and Back.** ▮Pricking sensation above throat pit.

▮Numbness in front of throat.

Carotids pulsating perceptibly.

‖Throat pressed forward; croup.

▮External swelling of throat.

Glandular swellings under r. lower jaw hinder motion of neck and are painful to touch.

Pain as if cervical glands were swelling by side of trachea and larynx.

‖Swelling of glands of neck, with tensive pain on moving neck, or when pressing on them.

▮Scrofulous swelling and induration of cervical glands.

Painful sensation of stiffness in l. side of neck on turning head to r. side.

Stiffness of neck on stooping and turning head.

ǀPainful stiffness of muscles of neck and throat.

After opening mouth wide, and then biting teeth firmly together, a painful cramp in cervical muscles; violent drawing in lower jaw, with pain in articulation of jaw as if it would be dislocated.

Crampy pain in cervical muscles.

Frequently returning, pressing, cracking pain on l. posterior side of neck, near shoulder blade, not changed by any motion.

The back of neck snaps on stooping.

Intermittent, slow pressure on r. side of neck, as if skin were compressed between fingers; downward in region of carotid artery, also painful externally to touch.

Tension of cervical muscles, particularly of r. side, on bending head backward.

Painful tension in l. side of neck, near thyroid cartilage, on turning head to r. side.

Transient creeping sensation on neck.

Great, slow stitches in r. cervical muscles, just after waking from sleep, passing off while swallowing, but returning again soon afterward.

A transient stitch in l. side of neck.

Drawing pricking through l. side of neck.

Twitching of r. cervical muscles while lying.

ǀNeck cold in evening; distended veins.

Sensation in thyroid and cervical glands on breathing as if air were passing up and down those glands.

ǀThyroid gland very much swollen, painful on touching neck and on pressure.

Region of thyroid gland seems as if hardened.

Pressing sensation in goitre, several times daily.

πJerking pain in side where small goitre exists; throbbing in head, descends into cheeks, and extends thence into neck in shape of tearing pain.

πStinging pain in goitre on swallowing; slight pain when parts are at rest.

πStitches in goitre, when not swallowing.

πSensation in goitre as if everything were shaking and moving about in same, as if it were alive, particularly on swallowing.

ǀǀSensation in goitre like motion, a working about, distension and bracing.

ǀGoitre occurring with the inhabitants of valleys.

ǀǀGoitre; three years' growth, very large, unsightly, lumpy, irregular, hard, slightly tender, always on having a cold.

||Goitre; six years' growth, constantly increasing, becoming somewhat fuller, with some slight pain and tenderness on handling every time she has a cold.

||Goitre; of many years' standing, extremely unsightly and repulsive; larger than both her breasts; hard, knotty, somewhat tender.

||Goitre: from earliest youth (æt. 19) has attained a considerable size.

||Thyroid gland of both sides swollen, even with chin; at night suffocating spells and stinging in throat, with soreness in abdomen.

||For four years, large goitre, rather soft, located especially in r. lobe of thyroid body; menses profuse; nervous palpitation.

|Pressing pain in small of back.

Feeling of coldness in back, in region of last ribs.

Chill on back, in small of back.

Itching on back.

Pressing sensation passing up and down through spine, while sitting erect.

Pressure in lumbar region.

Dull stitch in r. lumbar muscles.

Dull pain in region of symphysis of r. ilium and sacrum, while standing.

A pressing pain in sacral region only while walking, and particularly on setting down l. foot.

Pressing pains in small of back with whooping cough.

A fine tearing pain in sacrum, while sitting only, passing from r. to l. side and upward.

Severe stitch in small of back.

|Pain in small of back instead of catamenia.

|Sacrum sore before menses.

Small of back and nates are very numb.

32 **Upper Limbs.** Very painful flying stitch on r. shoulder-blade.

||Muscular twitching about l. shoulder joint.

Burning on l. shoulder.

Pain in scapulæ as if a pointed instrument were thrust in, a continuous stabbing pain, combined with soreness.

Fine stitches in armpit, while sitting.

Continuous prickling itching in l. armpit, while sitting.

In l. armpit drawing pressure, by jerks, alternating with similar sensation in l. popliteal space.

Arms most tired.

Stretching of arms.

||Pains in upper limbs with chills.

Stinging drawing through upper arm.

Bruised pain in arms, almost like soreness.

Burning in arms and hands.
‖ Heat in upper limbs, shoulders and hands.
Beneath upper arms, itching.
Stitches in elbow joint on motion.
Stitches in point of elbow and then tearing in joint as long as he holds his arm bent.
Pressing pain in joint of l. elbow.
‖ Boring pain at elbow.
A cramplike pain, with slow throbbing, beneath elbow joint, at upper end of forearm, particularly on supporting arm.
Heaviness in forearms.
Trembling of forearms and hands.
Pain in l. forearm as if bones were being pressed together.
Pain from thumb into forearm.
Drawing pain in forearms.
Severe stitches, boring from within outward, in internal muscles of r. forearm.
| Drawing stitches in forearms and hands.
A feeling in and between wrists as if parts were weakened by decay.
Heaviness and trembling of forearms and hands.
Large vesicles on forearms.
Swelling of hands and stiffness of fingers.
Several stitches in r. wrist, during rest.
Severe drawing in l. wrist.
Drawing, pressing pain above r. wrist.
‖ Stretches hands out for relief.
Hands trembling.
‖ Stitches in hands.
| Hands: cold; cold and bluish, with chill; burning; hot, with chill; swollen, could not bend fingers.
‖ Cramplike pain in balls of thumbs.
| Redness and swelling of finger joints, with tension on bending them.
Painful drawing in posterior joint of l. thumb, extending into forearm.
A protracted stitch, combined with sore pain in anterior joint of thumb.
Itching in ball of l. thumb not dispelled by rubbing.
The tips of index fingers lose their feeling, without growing pale.
Pressing pain in metacarpal joint of middle finger of r. hand.
Middle joint of l. middle finger became thick and red and seemed tense on motion.
| Numbness of tips of fingers, with whooping cough.

33 **Lower Limbs.** Nates numb.

Rapid twitching of a portion of r. gluteal muscles.
Stitch near hip.
Thigh spasmodically drawn forward or backward.
Thighs numb, cold, with fever.
Thighs numb and chilly, while the rest of body is hot.
▮Numbness or coldness of thighs, with fever.
Tension as if a muscle were too short, in upper end of thigh, on stepping, accompanied each time by a stitch.
Protracted, drawing stitches at upper part of l. thigh, below groin, particularly when walking.
Itching, tickling on l. thigh, near groin, with desire to rub the part.
Severe stitches, boring outward in r. thigh, in front, near hip.
Fine, very sensitive stitch in skin of inner r. thigh.
In morning, while in bed, pulsating, sharp stitches through r. thigh, above knee.
Pain in inner side of thigh, above r. knee, pressing toward posterior part.
Pressing, stinging pain above r. knee, while sitting.
Pain from foot to thigh.
Heaviness in knee joints, felt on walking.
▮Feeling of lameness from r. knee to r. hip.
While walking, tiredness in knee as if they would give way, although he sets his foot down firmly.
Severe drawing in l. knee, followed by profuse sweat, for several nights.
Dull stinging in l. knee, in evening, while lying down.
Tearing in tibia all afternoon.
During rapid walking, a feeling at lower end of l. tibia as if a weight were hanging on it.
Pain in ankles extending up tibia.
Tearing from ankle to knee.
Drawing pressure, coming by jerks, in l. popliteal space, arising only on bending knee and alternating with a similar sensation in l. armpit.
Pressing pain in external tendon of flexor muscle, in popliteal space (r. leg), more violent on walking than while sitting.
Sharp stitches in r. calf, while walking.
Continuous prickling itching in popliteal spaces while walking, with desire to scratch parts.
Numbness, first of r. then of l. lower leg, after brief afternoon naps; when he tried to walk, l. lower leg was spasmodically drawn up to thigh; even when sitting he could not keep it stretched out, it was then drawn spasmodically backward.
▮Stiffness of legs.

Drawing, tearing from r. ankle joint to knee.
Tearing in ankles; feet heavy as lead, heaviness extending up tibia.
Pressing pain in r. heel, < while walking.
While standing, a severe stitch out at r. heel.
Stitches passing upward in r. heel while sitting.
Severe intermitting stitches in l. heel, from within outward, while standing, passing off on motion.
After a long walk, pricking as if from pins in heels.
Feet heavy as lead.
Her feet are affected; she starts at every trifle.
Feet feel heavy.
▮Heat in feet: veins distended; with the chill; particularly in heels.
Creeping in lower portion of l. foot.
Itching on feet.
Tiredness in lower limbs.
Great commotion and restlessness in both lower legs; is obliged to change his posture frequently.
▮Drawing pain from lower portion of r. foot to thigh; drawing during menses; pains in lower extremities with chill and fever.
Cold feeling in legs; legs are cold.
▮Chill on lower limbs, especially on thighs.

34 **Limbs in General.** ▮Stiffness in limbs.
▮Trembling in all the limbs.
Sense of weariness in upper portion of body as if bruised and of numbness in lower portion.
Stretching of limbs.
▮▮Hands and feet cold.
Protracted, exhausted and tired lameness of all limbs.

35 **Rest. Position. Motion.** Slight pain in goitre; stitches in wrist.
Lying: strong pulsation about ear on which she is lying; dull, tremulous roaring in head; double vision >; bores head backward; dyspnœa <; suffocative cough <; after, symptoms of circulation <; twitching of cervical muscles; stinging in knee.
Lying in a horizontal position: headache >; congestion of blood to head >.
Lying on back: pressing headache >; throat symptoms >; brings on cough; dyspnœa <.
Must lie on back: ulcerative feeling in pit of stomach.
Lying on r. side: painful constriction of l. side; brings on cough; symptoms of circulation <.
In side on which he lies: digging in hip.
Cannot lie: on account of want of breath; asthma; pneumonia.

Lying with head low: dyspnœa <; all symptoms of bronchitis <; attacks of oppression and cardiac pain <.

Sitting: as if head would fall to one side; pain in frontal eminence <; up in bed, sudden burning and compression passes off; tensive pain in abdomen; painful constriction in l. side; cramplike pain in l. groin; pressing tearing pain in region of abdominal ring; cough >; stitches in l. chest; fine tearing pain in sacrum.

Stitches in armpit; prickling in armpit; stinging above r. knee; could not keep leg stretched out; stitches in heels.

Sits up in bed: croup; suffocative paroxysm passes off.

Must sit up: on account of shortness of breath.

Stooping: stinging in l. hypogastrium <; tensive pain in abdomen <; dyspnœa <; stiffness of neck; back of neck snaps.

Bending body forward: dyspnœa >; symptoms of circulation <.

Bending back: dyspnœa <.

Holding head upright: dull pressure in occiput >.

Bending head backward; congestion of blood to head; tension in neck; in croup; tension of cervical muscles.

Bending fingers: tension.

Could not bend fingers: swollen.

When holding arm bent: tearing in joint.

Raising arms above head: becomes faint.

Erect position: writhed and struggled into with croup; pressing sensation up and down spine.

Standing: pain in ilium and sacrum; stitch out at heel.

Rising: headache; cough <.

Must change posture frequently: restlessness in legs.

Motion: of scalp, sensitiveness of cranial integuments; of eyes, < stinging pain; every slight, loses her breath and becomes faint; brings on cough; every trifling, grows weak; congestion to chest; after moderate, grows suddenly weak; cough <; of neck, pain in swollen glands; stitches in elbow joint; finger seemed tense; stitches in heel pass off.

After every exertion: dyspnœa <.

Exertion: suddenly exhausted; congestion to chest; exhaustion of chest; slight, suffocating palpitation.

Opening mouth wide, then biting teeth firmly together: cramp in neck.

Masticating: teeth feel dull and loose; gums painful; pain in molars.

Swallowing: stitches in neck pass off; violent straining pain; pain in goitre; a moving sensation in goitre; stinging pain in goitre; as if goitre were alive.

Turning head: stitch in occiput; neck pains; neck stiff; tensive pain in head; larynx sensitive; to r. side, stiffness of left.

Stepping: tension in thigh.

Walking: tensive pain in abdomen and r. groin; tottering; stitches beneath second rib; pain in sacral region, particularly setting down l. foot; stitches in thigh <; heaviness in knee joint; tiredness in knees; as if weight were hanging to tibia; stitches in calf; itching in popliteal space; l. lower leg spasmodically drawn up; pain in heel <; long time, pricking in heels.

Going up stairs: suffocating palpitation; symptoms of circulation <.

Ascending ground: suffocating palpitation.

After exercise: heat.

36 **Nerves.** Excitement of nerves.

▮Stiff, without ability to move.

Strange feeling all over.

Tendency to start.

||Twitching of muscles, with fever.

Unable to act upon her limbs by means of volition.

||Clumsiness of body.

▮Weak: after every trifling motion; suddenly, after motion out-doors; exhausted after exercise.

Tiredness of whole body, especially arms.

Great tiredness and inclination to sleep.

Lassitude of body and mind; prefers to be inactive and rest.

||As if she were going to faint, with heat in face, and anxiety.

▮Faint when losing her breath.

Feeling of numbness of lower half of body.

37 **Sleep.** ||Sleepiness with yawning.

Stupid slumber, with fever.

||When falling asleep, awakes choking.

▮Falling asleep early at night; suffocation awakens.

▮Lies asleep with head low.

Restless slumber after chills, with heat.

Sleeplessness until midnight.

Sleepless, with violent ebullitions.

Dreams: about murder and assassination; fatiguing; vexatious, with anxiety and disposition to weep; mournful.

As soon as he fell asleep, his mind wandered and he was delirious.

Spoke aloud in her sleep, but not anxiously.

Very short sleep, with many dreams, four consecutive nights; wakes at midnight, but cannot sleep again on account of restlessness; whenever he closes his lids, the most vivid pictures would immediately arise before his vision, while waking; it seemed to him as if a battery of guns were discharged, or as if everything were in flames; again scientific subjects forced themselves upon his mind, in short, a mass of subjects crossed each other in his imagination, disappearing at once when opening his eyelids, but reappearing as soon as the lids were closed.

▮▮Awakens in a fright and feels as if suffocating.

▮Awakening with fear and terror.

▮Frequent waking with a start.

▮Starting out of sleep toward morning from a shock in trachea upward like a suffocative paroxysm, passing off after sitting up in bed.

▮▮Awakened between 1 and 2 A.M. by sense of suffocation.

Tossing about at night.

After siesta legs numb.

▮▮Worse after sleep.

38 **Time.** Toward morning: starting out of sleep.

Between 1 and 2 A.M.: awakened by suffocation.

Morning: involuntary discharge from bowels; stinging in throat <; rumbling in abdomen <; digging in hip; expectoration only of small quantities of tough, yellow, hardened mucus; pulsating, sharp stitches through thigh; early, sweat.

Forenoon: pressing pain in gastric region.

Day and night: dry cough; hollow cough, with some expectoration.

Afternoon: pressure in epigastrium; cough <; tearing in tibia; after brief naps numbness of legs; chill <.

Evening: stinging and pressing pain in eyes; cramplike pain from jaw to cheek; cold sweat in face; stinging in throat <; rumbling in abdomen <; cutting in hypogastrium; cracked voice; pressing inward in larynx; contraction in larynx; croupy cough <; till midnight cough <; induration of breast comes on; neck cold; stinging in knee; chill <.

9 P.M.: sudden attack of croup.

Night: vertigo when awaking, with nausea; things appear in flames; figures of light; restless and easily frightened; as if a battery of guns were discharged in ears; a vexed expression, with cough; stitch from jaw to ear; suffocating spells; rattling breathing, terminating cough; in middle, spells of choking; after a chill burning heat of skin; suffocation about larynx; awakes in fear and terror; tossing about; chill <; heat; sweat.

Before midnight: croup <; dry sound of breathing and cough; sleepless until.

At midnight: wakes and cannot get to sleep again.
After 12 P.M.: awakes, violent palpitation; awakes with suffocation.

39 **Temperature and Weather.** Heat does not > chilliness of back.
Hot room: dry bronchitis <.
Hot tea: cough <.
Near warm stove: chill with shaking.
Warm room: coming into from open air, headache; cough <.
Warm drinks: distress in stomach >; cough >; dyspnœa.
In bed: chill <.
Indoors: cough <.
Open air: pain in l. ear; pain from jaw to cheek; tension in articulation of jaw; grows suddenly weak; after walking, chill.
Sudden change of atmosphere: spasmodic paroxysms of cough and dyspnœa <.
After taking cold: asthma.
Dry, cold weather: headache >.
Dry, cold winds: coryza.
Washing: headache >.
Wet weather: cough <.
Cold: tea or water brings on cough; weather, subject to attacks of dyspnœa; air, cough <.
Frosty weather: cough >.

40 **Fever.** Coldness: all over; of eyes; of neck; in epigastrium; of hands of thigh; pallor and sweat of face with heat of whole body.
Cold feeling: in head; in stomach; on back; on lower limbs; on small of back; on thighs.
When feeling cold an itching arises.
Shuddering across back.
▮Chill: with shaking, even near a warm stove; mostly across back; after walking in open air; < in bed; in afternoon; in evening; at night; with coryza; with internal heat; with heat at same time; alternating with heat.
▮Chill, then heat, then sweat.
▮▮Strong heat soon after chill, with dry, burning heat over whole body, with exception of thighs, which remain cold, numb and chilly.
▮Heat: with external chill; rises from abdomen, rest of body chilly; with thirst, at night; anxious, dry, with red face and weeping, and inconsolable mood, or with whooping cough; after exercise; in bed; with sweats.
He suddenly grows anxious and warm over whole body, with heat and redness in face, with sweat.

Daily several attacks of heat with anxiety, pain in region of heart, weeping and inconsolability; she would rather die on the spot.

| Dry, hot skin and congestion to head.

| Attacks of spreading, flying heat.

| Synochal fever, in croup.

Flushes of heat returning when thinking of them.

Heat, sweat and itching of skin.

| Sweat: anxious; cold, clammy; copious, during night; over whole body early in morning; with whooping cough; cool on face, evenings; of itching parts; profuse, follows drawing pain in knee; breaking out too easily.

| Stupid sleep with the sweat.

| Worse with the sweat; > after it.

‖ Want of perspiration.

| Typhus; loose cough suddenly changing to dryness and hoarseness, increasing to dyspnœa, with anxiousness.

41 **Attacks, Periodicity.** Alternately: face red and pale; pressure in armpit and popliteal space; chill and heat.

Attacks: repeated, of want of breath.

Frequent paroxysms of two minutes: cough.

For several hours: itching at glans penis.

Daily: several times, pressing sensation in goitre; several attacks of heat, with anxiety.

Nightly: agglutination of lids; wakes up several times with want of breath.

For two days: dryness of Schneiderian membrane.

For several nights: drawing in knee and sweat.

Four consecutive nights: very short sleep with many dreams.

For nine days: red swelling of r. helix.

For several days: sore pains in anus; flowing like menses.

Full moon: asthma <.

Since two years: swelling of l. testicle.

Three years' growth: goitre.

Four years' growth: goitre.

For six years: subject to attacks of dyspnœa.

Six years' growth: goitre.

Many years' standing: goitre.

42 **Locality and Direction.** Right: dull pain on side of brain; pressing sensation in temple; downward drawing pain in side of head and neck; pressing outward on parietal bone; pressing in frontal eminence; pressing pain over eye; ringing in ear; drawing pain in ear; fine stitches in ear; burning in orifice of ear; red swelling of helix; tearing in zygomatic arch; jerking fine stitch from upper jaw into internal ear; violent burning under angle of mouth; pain in molars of lower jaw;

stitches in side of abdomen; glandular swelling in groin; epididymis enlarged and hardened; weight dragging down in chest; painful stitches in chest; severe pricking in breast; crawling pain in side of chest; boring stitch in costal muscles; glandular swelling under lower jaw; slow pressure on side of neck; tension of cervical muscles; slow stitches in cervical muscles; twitching of cervical muscles; goitre in lobe of thyroid body; dull stitch in lumbar muscle; dull pain in region of symphysis of ilium and sacrum; flying stitch in shoulder blade; stitches in muscles of forearm; stitches in wrist; drawing pressing pain above; pressing pain in middle finger; rapid twitching of portion of gluteal muscles; stitches in thigh; stitch in inner thigh; pain in thigh above knee; pressing stinging above knee; lameness from knee to hip; stitches in calf; tearing from ankle joint to knee; pressing pain in heel; stitch at heel.

Left: stitches in temple to forehead; pressing in outer half of eye; tension about eye; stinging in eye; stinging itching under eye; burning in eye; sudden stinging drawing at external canthus of orbit; tensive stinging pain in external canthus; burning pain on external surface of lower lid; cramplike pain in ear; digging stitches in depth of ear; boils on ear; creeping stitches in nasal bone; cramplike pain from articulation of jaw to cheek; tearing stinging in cheek; tension in articulation of jaw; stinging itching in cheek; side of chin to angle of mouth painful to touch; burning pain in upper molars; pain in side of abdomen; cutting toward breast; boring stinging in hypogastrium; painful constriction in side; fine digging above hip; twisting sensation in side of abdomen; cramplike pain in groin; small boil in groin; swelling of testicle; pressure in chest; cutting in side of chest; broad pressure, with many fine points in side of chest; drawing stitches beneath second rib; pinching jerk in side of chest; consumption beginning at apex of lung; rheumatism in lumbar muscles; stinging itching on breast; induration of breast; stiffness in side of neck; cracking pain on posterior side of neck; tension in side of neck; transient stitch in side of neck; pricking through side of neck; setting down foot pain in sacral region; muscular twitching about shoulder joint; burning on shoulder; prickling itching in armpit; drawing pressure in armpit; drawing pressure in popliteal space; pressing pain in joint of elbow; pain in forearm; drawing in wrist; painful drawing in posterior joint of thumb; itching in ball of thumb; middle joint of middle finger; stitches in thigh; itching tickling in thigh; severe drawing in knee; dull stinging in knee, as if weight were hanging to tibia; leg drawn up when walking; stitches in heel; creeping in lower portion of foot.

From r. to l.: swelling in fauces; orchitis; pain in sacrum; numbness of legs.

From within outward: pressing in temple; pressing in frontal eminence; pricking in breast; stitches in r. forearm; stitches in thigh; stitches in heel.

From without inward: jerk in chest.

43 **Sensations.** As if head would fall to one side; as if one would fall backward; as if tipsy; as if all her blood were mounting to head; as if skull would burst; as if hair were standing on end; eye as if twisted around; as if a battery of guns were discharged in ears; stitches as if passing through tympanum; nodule in concha as if it would gather and break; jaw as if dislocated; as if eruption were to appear near chin; l. side of chin as if ulcerated; as if something had got jammed between teeth in chewing; as if gums and teeth were swollen, and latter being lifted; outside of throat as if something were being pressed out; as if he had drunk a great deal of lukewarm water, relaxation of stomach and œsophagus; pit of stomach as if growing together; stomaeh as if standing open; as if something alive were moving in abdomen; as if something alive were beneath skin of abdomen; as if diarrhœa would ensue; as of a plug in larynx; as of a stopper or valve were in larynx; as of a nail pressing in larynx; as if larynx and trachea were narrower; as if she would suffocate; as if child could not get breath; as if breathing through a sponge; as if chest would burst; chest as if sore and bloody; as of a plug in throat; as of a large accumulation of mucus and weight at chest; as if a broad body armed with points were pressing upward; as if a weight were dragging down in chest; as if she had something hot inside of chest; as if blood would burst out of chest; as if cervical glands were swelling; as if jaw would be dislocated; as if skin of neck were compressed between fingers; as if air were passing up and down thyroid and cervical glands; thyroid gland as if hardened; as if everything were shaking and moving about in goitre; as if goitre were alive; as if a pointed instrument were thrust into scapulæ; as if bones of forearm were being pressed together; as if parts in and between wrists were weakened by decay; as if a muscle were too short in upper end of thigh; as if knees would give way; as if a weight were hanging on lower end of tibia; as of pins in heels; as if she were

going to faint; as if everything were in flames; as if sweat would break out.

Pain: in vertex and forehead; in occiput; in neck; in cartilages of ears; in articulation of jaw; in posterior molars; in gums while chewing; in throat; in goitre; beneath short ribs; in l. side of abdomen; in abdominal ring; from hypogastrium to anus; in testicles; in larynx; in trachea; in chest; in bronchi; in small of back; in scapulæ; in upper limbs; from thumb into forearm; in inner side of thigh; from foot to thigh; in ankles up tibiæ; in lower extremities; in region of heart.

Violent pains: in small of back and abdomen.

Great pains: in larynx; in heart.

Sudden pain: in chest and dorsal muscles; of l. side.

Stabbing pain: in scapulæ.

Cutting: in upper part of abdomen; from hypogastrium to breast; in l. side of chest.

Tearing: in l. eye; in nose; in cheeks; from cheek to neck; in r. zygomatic arch; in elbow joint; in tibia; from ankle to knee; in ankles.

Fine tearing pain: in sacrum.

Pressing tearing pain: in region of abdominal ring.

Drawing tearing: from r. ankle joint to knee.

Bursting pain: in head; in trachea.

Pinching pain: in l. side of chest.

Pinching, bruised, squeezing pain: in testicles.

Boring pain: at elbow.

Boring stitch: in r. costal muscles.

Stitches: in temples; externally in l. temple; in forehead; in occiput; in scalp; in eyeballs; in nodule in concha; in goitre; above pit of throat; in throat; in region of stomach; in r. side of abdomen; below groin; in anus; into spermatic cord; in chest; in both sides; in goitre; in elbow joint; in point of elbow; in hands; near hip; in heel.

Severe stitch: in small of back; in internal muscles of r. forearm; in r. wrist; in r. thigh; out at heel.

Sharp stitches: in r. calf.

Flying stitch: on r. shoulder blade.

Transient, painful stitches: on r. side of chest; in l. side of neck.

Severe intermittent stitches: in l. side of chest; in heel.

Pulsating sharp stitches: through thigh.

Great slow stitches: in cervical muscles.

Protracted stitch: in joint of thumb.

Drawing painful stitches: from body through glans penis; beneath second rib of l. side of chest; in forearms and hands; at upper part of thigh.

Digging stitches: in depth of l. ear.

Jerking fine stitch: from posterior portion of r. upper jaw into r. internal ear; external, in region of larynx.

Fine stitches: in r. ear; beneath lower lip; externally on navel; externally on chest and arms; in armpits; in skin of inner thigh.

Large, somewhat blunt stitch: from testicle into spermatic cord.

Dull stitch: in r. lumbar muscles.

Creeping stitches: in nasal bone.

Itching stitch: as if caused by a very fine needle.

Shooting: up entire cord; from testicle into inguinal region.

Jerking pain; in side where goitre exists.

Pinching jerk: in l. side of chest.

Violent straining pain: on swallowing.

Pressing pain: in vertex; in r. frontal eminence; over r. eye; in gastric region; in l. side of chest; in præcordial region; in small of back; in joint of elbow; in metacarpal joint of middle finger; in tendon of flexor muscles; in heel.

Pressing cracking pain: on l. posterior side of neck.

Contracting pain: in ear; in chest.

Gnawing pain: on crown of head.

Heavy, dragging pains: in spermatic cord.

Drawing pain: in internal ear; in forearms; in joint of l. thumb; from lower portion of r. foot to thigh.

Colicky pains: in abdomen.

Painful cramp: in cervical muscles.

Cramp: lower jaw drawn; in neck; in abdomen.

Cramplike pain: in l. ear; from l. articulation of jaw to cheek; in l. groin; in cervical muscles; below elbow joint; in balls of thumbs.

Boring stinging: in l. hypogastrium.

Tensive stinging pain: in external canthus.

Stinging drawing: at external canthus of l. orbit; through upper arms.

Pressing stinging pain: above knee.

Stinging itching: under l. eye; on l. breast near shoulder.

Stinging: in eyes; about eye; in cheeks; in teeth; in mouth; in throat; in l. side of chest; in præcordial region; in goitre.

Biting: in anus.

Burning pain: on external surface of lower lid; in l. upper molars.

Violent burning: under r. angle of mouth.

Burning heat: in forehead; over whole body.

Burning: in occiput; in l. eye; in ears; in ears from

throat; behind ears; in orifice of r. ear; in mouth; in throat; in larynx and trachea; in chest; on l. shoulder; in arms and hands.

Itching burning: in scrotum and body of penis.

Heat: in head; in forehead; in scalp; in eyes; in ears; on chin; in teeth; in œsophagus; in male genitals; in chest; from abdomen in upper limbs, shoulders and hands; in feet.

Flying heat: in face; in blood.

Sore pain: in anus; in joint of thumb.

Bruised pain: in arms.

Itching biting: on breast, epigastrium, back and beneath arms; on feet.

Smarting: in anus.

Soreness: of tongue; of throat; in abdomen; of anus; in sacrum; in chest; of sacrum; of scapulæ.

Pricking pains: across upper jaw; in r. breast; above throat pit; in heels.

Crawling pain: in l. side of chest.

Tensive pain: in neck; from hypogastrium to anus; in upper abdomen; in r. groin; in l. side of neck.

Dull pain: in r. side of brain; in region of symphysis of r. ilium and sacrum.

Painful constriction: in l. side beneath skin; in chest; spasmodic, through chest and larynx; in cardiac region.

Severe drawing: in knee.

Drawing: in pit of stomach; in all the limbs; toward larynx; in l. wrist.

Drawing pressure: in armpit and popliteal space; above r. wrist.

Severe pressing: in larynx.

Pressure: in forehead; sharp, at both temples; in ears; in throat; above thyroid cartilage; in epigastrium; in hypochondria; in larynx; in l. chest; on r. side of neck; in lumbar region.

Pressing: in eyes; in outer half of l. eye; under eyelids.

Pressing sensation: in r. temple; in r. side of head and neck; on r. parietal bone; in r. zygomatic arch; in goitre; up and down spine.

Violent drawing: in upper and lower limbs; in lower jaw.

Tension: in neck; about l. eye, near temple; in articulation of l. jaw; of maxillary glands; in throat; of cervical muscles; in finger joints.

Tensive constrictive sensation: above root of nose.

Constriction: in larynx.

Heaviness: in head; in occiput; of lids; in chest; in forearms; in knee joints; of feet.

Crowding sensation: in ears.
Weight: dragging down on r. chest.
Oppression: of chest.
Fulness: in head; in epigastrium; in stomach.
Tightness: of chest.
Pulsation: about ear; in forehead.
Knocking: in forehead.
Twitching: of r. cervical muscles.
Throbbing: in forehead; into cheeks; in spermatic cord; in head, thence into cheeks and neck.
Twisting sensation: in l. side of abdomen.
Itching tickling: on l. thigh.
Prickling itching: in l. armpit; in popliteal space.
Drawing pricking: through l. side of neck.
Penetrating tickling: in throat, toward ear.
Tickling: in throat; in layrnx; in trachea.
Ulcerative feeling: in pit of stomach.
Irritation: in upper part of larynx.
Sensitiveness: of cranial integuments.
Rawness: of throat; in chest.
Roughness: of throat; in larynx and trachea.
Scratching: in throat.
Scraping: in throat; in larynx and trachea.
Dryness: of lids; of nose; of tongue; of throat; of larynx; in trachea; of Schneiderian membrane.
Moving sensation: in goitre.
Restlessness: in both lower legs.
Lameness: from knee to hip.
Stiffness: in neck; of muscles of neck and throat; of fingers; of legs; in limbs.
Strange feeling: all over.
Dyspeptic distress: in stomach.
Craving: in stomach.
Empty feeling: in lower abdomen.
Weariness: of upper portion of body.
Tiredness: in lower limbs; of whole body, especially arms.
Faintness: at stomach.
Weakness: in chest.
Relaxation: in œsophagus and stomach.
Numbness: on chin; in front of throat; of small of back and nates; of tips of fingers; of thighs; of lower legs; of lower portion of body.
Dulness: over root of nose.
Gloominess: over root of nose.
Creeping: in nodule in concha; on neck; in lower portion of foot; in skin.
Formication: in rectum.
Voluptuous itching: at point of glans penis.

Itching: violent, on scalp; of eyelids; in cheeks; in teeth; near groin; in anus; on breast; on back; beneath upper arms; in ball of thumb; on feet; of skin.

Cold feeling: in head; in stomach; on back; on lower limbs; on small of back; on thighs.

Coldness: of eyes; of nose; in epigastrium; of neck; in back; of hands; of thighs; in epigastrium.

44 **Tissues.** ▮Ebullitions; distended veins.

▮▮Swelling and induration of glands; goitre.

▮Dropsy in cavities of body.

▮Scrofulosis; skin and muscles lax; light hair.

▮Rheumatic affections of valves of heart; fibrous deposits upon valves.

▮Inflammation of larynx, trachea or bronchia.

▮Croup; bronchitis; tuberculous phthisis.

▮▮Tubercular diathesis.

45 **Touch. Passive Motion. Injuries.** Touch: forehead painful; nodule in l. concha painful; boils on ear painful; lower jaw painful; chin at angle of mouth painful; pain in testicle; larynx sensitive; pain in larynx; induration painful; swelling under lower jaw painful; r. side of neck painful; thyroid gland painful; goitre tender; skin sensitive.

Pressure: pimples beneath chin on neck painful; of hand < twisting sensation in abdomen; crawling pain in chest <; on glands causes pain; thyroid gland painful.

Cannot endure tight clothing about body, particularly epigastric region; and abdomen.

Rubbing: > itching under eye; seems as if weight were dragging down in r. side of chest; does not > itching in thumb; makes red spots; does not > itching stitch.

Scratching: does not diminish biting itching.

46 **Skin.** Sensitive to touch.

Red, itching blotches on skin.

Herpes.

Particularly when she feels cold, there arises an itching biting on breast, epigastrium, back and beneath upper arms, at other times it is only on feet; rubbing makes spot red, which seems to bite more severely for a short time, vesicles arise on these spots, which, however, soon vanish again.

▮Ringworm.

Here and there, about whole body, a protracted itching stitch, as if caused by a very fine needle, making it necessary to rub the part without being relieved thereby.

Burning itching, with desire to scratch.

▮Itching on skin: pricking with fever; as if sweat would break out; with heat and sweat.

First a creeping sensation in skin; then spot becomes red and hot, followed by biting itching, like a flea moving along (without stinging), upon which rashlike pimples appear; scratching does not dimish biting-itching, it appears to make it last longer.

▮Measles; barking cough, with hoarseness, coryza and bronchial catarrh.

▮Pruritus universalis; biting itching, in chronic cases.

❙❙Fistulous opening in scrotum; discharges little thick whitish matter.

❙❙Ulcers with scanty discharge; erysipelas; erythema.

47 **Stages of Life, Constitution.** Often indicated with children and women.

▮▮Light hair, lax fibre; fair complexion.

▮Scrofulous affections.

Child, æt. 6 months; croup.
Girl, æt. 6 months; croup.
Girl, æt. 11 months; irritability of larynx.
Boy, æt. 18 months, strong and lively; croup.
Girl, æt. 18 months, neck had been leeched and calomel given; croup.
Girl, æt. 2; croup.
Girl, æt. 2; croup.
Boy, æt. $3\frac{1}{4}$ years; croup.
Boy, æt. 4, scrofulous, cachectic-looking; croup.
Boy, æt. 5, robust, after a chill; croup.
Girl, æt. 6, frail, slender, dark hair and eyes; diphtheria.
Girl, æt. 19, lymphatic temperament, affected four years; goitre.
Young lady, æt. 19, well built, well nourished, scrofulous until her fourteenth year, has bronchocele; asthma.
Lady, æt. 23, suffering two years; enlargement of thyroid gland.
Miss M., æt. 25, healthy, plump, ruddy, weight 150, dark hair and eyes, affected three years; bronchocele.
Man, æt. 30, suffering eighteen months; pain in abdomen.
Lady, æt. 30, lymphatic constitution; Basedow's disease.
Lady, æt. 32, single, tall, slender, thick skin and thick lips, strumous, affected many years; bronchocele.
Man, æt. 35; affection of testicle.
Man, æt. 40, dark hair and complexion, after pneumonia; circumscribed gangrene of lung.
Woman, æt. 40; Basedow's disease.
Mrs. S., æt. 45, mother of six children, spare habit, scrofulous, affected six years; bronchocele.
Man, æt. 53, suffering fourteen years; cough.

48 **Relations.** Compatible: after *Acon.*, *Hepar;* before *Bromium*, *Carbo veg.*, *Hepar.*

SQUILLA.

Squills, Sea Onion. *Liliaceæ.*

A bulbous plant, bearing a long spike of whitish flowers, found on the sandy shores of the Mediterranean.

Introduced by Hahnemann, proved by himself, Becher, Hartmann, Hornburg, Mossdorf, Stapf, Teuthorn, Walther and Wislicenus, Mat. Med. Pura, vol. 3, p. 265.

CLINICAL AUTHORITIES.—*Affection of eye*, Sawyer, Med. Adv., June, 1889, p. 398; *Phlyctenule of conjunctiva*, Deady, Norton s Ophth. Therap., p. 171; *Enuresis nocturna*, Blaisdell, Stitson, A. H. O., vol. 12, p. 390; *Asthma*, Frank, N. A. J. H., vol. 9, p. 257; *Bronchitis*, Knorre, Rück. Kl. Erf., vol. 3, p. 27; Neidhard, Hah. Mo., vol. 20, p. 27; *Pertussis*, A. R., Rück. Kl. Erf., vol. 5, p. 729; *Whooping cough* Wesselhœft, A. J. H. M. M., vol. 4, p. 3; *Pneumonia*, Deschere, T. A. I. H., 1886, p. 323; *Dropsical affections*, Hahnemann, Hartmann, Rück. Kl. Erf., vol. 4, p. 355.

1 **Mind.** Great anxiety of mind, with fear of death.
Angry about trifles.
Aversion to mental or bodily labor.

2 **Sensorium.** Vertigo in morning, with nausea.
Head beclouded and dizzy.

3 **Inner Head.** Drawing lancinating headache.
Pulsation in head when raising it.
Headache in morning on waking, with pressing pains.
Contractive pain in both temples.
Quickly passing pain in occiput, from l. to right.
Stitching pain in r. side of forehead.
Affections of brain: child rubs its face and eyes a great deal, especially its eyes, as if to relieve itching; profuse or scanty urination.

4 **Outer Head.** Painful sensitiveness of vertex, mornings.

5 **Sight and Eyes.** I Staring look, eyes wide open.
II Left eye looks smaller than right; upper eyelid swollen.
Contraction of pupils.
The eyes feel as if swimming in cold water.
II For two weeks a large phlyctenule of conjunctiva on outer side of cornea; sensation as of cold water in eye, when in a cold wind.

6 **Hearing and Ears.** Tearing pain back of l. ear.

7 **Smell and Nose.** I Sneezes during cough; eyes water; rubs eyes and nose. θMeasles.
I Acrid, corrosive, fluent coryza, in morning; a regular general snizzle; coryza; mucous cough, with spurting of urine, and even of watery stools.

‖ Nostrils painful as if sore, with violent coryza.
Humid eruptions under nose, with stinging itching.

[8] **Upper Face.** Changeable expression and color of face.
During heat, redness of face, followed by paleness, without coldness.
Distorted countenance, with red cheeks, no thirst.

[9] **Lower Face.** Lips: twitch and are covered with yellow crusts; black and cracked.
Humid spreading eruption on upper lip.

[11] **Taste and Tongue.** Food tastes bitter, especially bread; or sweetish, especially soup and meat.

[12] **Inner Mouth.** Open, dry mouth.
Much viscid mucus in mouth.
Burning in mouth and throat.

[13] **Throat.** Burning in palate and throat; dryness in throat.
‖ Irritation in throat, with heat and tickling, causing constant cough.
Irritation to cough in pit of throat, in upper part of trachea.

[14] **Appetite, Thirst. Desires, Aversions.** Insatiable appetite.
Desire for acids.
Thirst for cold water, but dyspnœa allows her to take but a sip at a time.

[16] **Hiccough, Belching, Nausea and Vomiting.** Empty eructations.
Nausea: during morning cough; continuous in pit of stomach, alternating with a pain in abdomen, as with diarrhœa.
‖ Excessive nausea.
‖ Nausea in back of throat, almost constant accumulation of saliva in mouth.
Nausea in pit of stomach, alternating with pain in abdomen, or sensation as if diarrhœa would set in.

[17] **Scrobiculum and Stomach.** Pressure in stomach as from a stone.

[19] **Abdomen.** Cutting pain in abdomen as from flatulence.
Painful sensitiveness of abdomen and region of bladder.

[20] **Stool and Rectum.** Frequent discharge of very fetid flatus.
Diarrhœa, stools very offensive, watery, during measles, or looking black.
‖ Stools: dark-brown or black, slimy, fluid, in frothy bubbles; very offensive; painless; involuntary (when coughing, sneezing or passing urine).
Painless constipation.

[21] **Urinary Organs.** Continuous, painful pressure on bladder.
Tenesmus of bladder after micturition.
Frequent calls to urinate, especially at night, with scanty or profuse discharge of pale urine.

Sanguinolent urine with a deposit of red sediment.

Violent urging to urinate, with frequent emission of pale, limpid urine, looking like water. θDiabetes insipidus.

▮▮Involuntary micturition, especially when coughing.

||Continuous painful pressure on bladder and inability to retain urine. θEnuresis nocturna.

Unable to retain urine, because the amount is too large.

▮Urine: increased, pale, with frequent urging; involuntary, scanty, dark-red. θHydrothorax.

When urinating feces escape.

23 **Female Sexual Organs.** Atony of cervix uteri.

26 **Respiration.** Moaning, with open mouth; wheezing; rattling, with pleurisy, must sit up; short, with least exertion.

Dyspnœa, cannot drink; child seizes cup eagerly, but can drink only in sips.

Difficult or embarrassed respiration.

Frequently obliged to take a deep breath, which provokes cough.

▮Dyspnœa and stitches in chest, most distressing on inspiration.

Oppression across chest, as if it were too tight.

Shortness of breath from every exertion, especially when ascending.

Difficulty of breathing, with stitches in chest when breathing and coughing.

||Dry asthma for three years, and persistent panting respiration, no actual loss of breath at first; finally was obliged to get out of bed and sit at open window; could not lie on r. side without bringing on oppression; drawing pain through both hypochondriæ; urine scanty, reddish-yellow and neutral.

27 **Cough.** ▮▮Cough: dry, night and morning; short, rattling, disturbing sleep; spasmodic, from mucus in trachea, or tickling creeping sensation in chest; with headache, dyspnœa, spurting of urine, stitches in chest or pain in abdomen; caused by cold drinks; during measles; after eating; from every exertion; by changing from warm to cold air.

▮Frequent irritation to a short dry cough in four or five shocks caused by tickling beneath thyroid cartilage.

▮A violent sudden cough in morning, with stitch in side with every cough, with expectoration.

▮Cough, in morning, with profuse slimy expectoration.

▮▮Constant expectoration of mucus.

Cough in morning, with copious expectoration of thin, frequently reddish-colored mucus.

▮▮The loose cough in morning is more fatiguing than the dry in evening.

||Cough seems to proceed from lowest ramifications of bronchial tubes, with wheezing in lower part of lungs. θBronchitis.

|Every fit of coughing winds up with sneezing and involuntary urination.

|Sputa: white or reddish mucus; sweetish, or empyreumatic or offensive in odor; in small round balls, very difficult to expectorate.

||Dry spasmodic cough, brought on by taking a deep inspiration, causing pain in abdomen as from a shock and sensation as if intestines would burst out through abdomen, with retching, stitches in sides, pressure upon bladder and involuntary escape of urine; white, slimy, often sweetish-tasting expectoration in morning; none in evening; rattling of mucus before onset of paroxysm. θPertussis.

||Cough less troublesome in daytime, yet somewhat spasmodic and with whooping, but every night at 11 o'clock, or between 11 and 3 o'clock, she has a sudden attack of suffocation; it is very severe and compels her to spring to her feet and stand on tiptoe on her bed, stretching her body and arms upward in her agony; she cannot gain her breath for many seconds; anxiety and fear is extreme; at length the breath returns, with a whooping sound on inspiration; this is soon followed by a milder attack; the rest of the night is comparatively quiet; but drinking of cold water always brings on severe cough.

28 **Inner Chest and Lungs.** ||Stitches in chest, especially when inhaling and coughing; in sides of chest; pleurisy.

Compressive pain in r. side of chest, ending in a stitch.

Broad pressive stitches beneath last ribs of both sides.

|On inspiration, jerking stitches in r. and l. sides of chest, not far from sternum.

|Stitches in l. and r. true ribs, at same time.

Drawing stitch from last true rib to shoulder.

|Broad blunt stitches in last ribs of l. side, in morning in bed, that awakened him.

A contracting stitch in l. side, just beneath last ribs.

Drawing pain in chest.

Sharp stitches in scapular end of clavicle during inspiration and expiration.

Severe stitches near sternum, extending downward so that he could with great difficulty get his breath.

|Pains in chest < in morning.

|Heaviness on chest; congestion of blood to chest.

|Chronic catarrh, profuse secretion of tenacious white

mucus, which is only expectorated after severe cough; especially in children.

|| Circle of size of palm of hand, dull on percussion, in chest of a young lady.

|| Pneumonia r. side; cough very painful; high fever; breathing short and anxious, with general anxiety; dulness over r. lung on percussion, fine whistling breathing on auscultation; in some places no respiratory murmur; excessive dyspnœa, suffering during cough making child almost frantic; could take no nourishment on account of cough not allowing him to swallow; during fits of coughing, in his agony would rub his face all over briskly with his fist.

▮ Especially suitable in pneumonia and pleurisy, after bloodletting.

29 **Heart, Pulse and Circulation.** Pulse small and slow, slightly hard.

31 **Neck and Back.** Stiffness of neck.

Painful jerking above l. scapula.

Painless drawing in l. scapula.

32 **Upper Limbs.** Sweat in armpits.

Convulsive twitching in arms; cold hands.

33 **Lower Limbs.** Convulsive twitching of legs.

Cold foot sweat.

Sweat only on toes.

Soles red and sore when walking.

34 **Limbs in General.** Tearing and restlessness in upper and lower extremities.

Convulsive twitching and motions of limbs, < morning and evening and during motion.

Soreness in bends of joints.

Dull rheumatic pain; < when exercising, > while at rest.

35 **Rest. Position. Motion.** Rest: rheumatic pains >.

Could not lie on r. side without bringing on oppression.

Raising head: pulsation in it.

Must sit up: pleurisy.

Sitting: chilliness ceases.

Motion: twitching of limbs <.

Least exertion: short respiration; cough.

Ascending: shortness of breath.

Walking: soles red and sore; chilliness.

Exercising: rheumatic pains <.

37 **Sleep.** Frequent yawning, without sleepiness.

Restless sleep with much tossing about.

38 **Time.** Morning: vertigo and nausea; headache; painful sensitiveness of vertex; fluent coryza; nausea during cough; dry cough; violent sudden cough in morning; cough, with profuse expectoration; loose cough, very

fatiguing; stitches in ribs; pains in chest <; twitching of limbs <.

Daytime; cough less troublesome.

Afternoon: great heat in body.

Toward evening: chilliness.

Evening: dry cough; sweetish expectoration; twitching of limbs <; great heat in body.

Night: frequent calls to urinate; dry cough; internal chill.

39 **Temperature and Weather.** From warm to cold air: cough.

Aversion: to being uncovered, with heat.

Must get out of bed and sit at open window.

Cold wind: sensation as of cold water in eye.

Cold drinks: caused cough.

40 **Fever.** Chill internally at night, with external heat.

Chilliness toward evening when walking, not when sitting.

Icy-cold hands and feet, with warmth of rest of body.

Icy-cold feet.

Heat dry, burning, mostly internally.

Heat of whole body, with cold hands and feet, with aversion to being uncovered; face pale after heat.

Sensation of great heat in body, in afternoon and evening, generally with cold feet.

Whenever he uncovers himself during heat, he suffers from chilliness and pain.

Sweat wanting.

41 **Attacks, Periodicity.** Alternating: nausea in pit of stomach, with pain in abdomen.

Every night at 11 o'clock or between 11 and 3: sudden attacks of suffocation.

For three years: dry asthma.

42 **Locality and Direction.** Right: pain in forehead; compressive pain, side of chest; blunt stitch in last ribs; pneumonia, dulness over lung.

Left: eye smaller than right; pain back of ear; stitch in side; jerking above scapula; drawing on scapula.

From l. to r.: pain in occiput.

Right and left: stitches in side of chest; stitches in true ribs at same time.

43 **Sensations.** Eyes as if swimming in water; nostrils as if sore; as if diarrhœa would set in; as if chest were too tight; as if intestines would burst through abdomen.

Pain: in abdomen; in chest.

Tearing pain: back of l. ear; in upper and lower limbs.

Cutting pain: in abdomen.

Drawing lancinating pain: in head.

Severe stitches: near sternum.

Sharp stitches: in scapular end of clavicle.
Jerking stitches: in r. and l. side of chest.
Stitches: in chest; in side; in l. and r. true ribs.
Contracting stitch: in l. side.
Drawing stitch: from last true rib to shoulder.
Broad pressive stitches: beneath last ribs.
Broad blunt stitches: in last rib of r. side.
Stitching pain: in forehead.
Contractive pain; in both temples; in occiput.
Compressive pain: in r. side of chest.
Drawing pain: through both hypochondriæ; in chest.
Pressing pain: in head.
Dull rheumatic pains: in limbs.
Painful jerking: above scapula.
Painful pressure: on bladder.
Painful sensitiveness: of abdomen and region of bladder.
Soreness: of soles; in bends of joints.
Burning: in mouth and throat; in palate.
Great heat: in body.
Dryness: of mouth; of throat.
Pulsation: in head.
Painless drawing: on scapula.
Stiffness: of neck.
Pressure: in stomach, as from a stone.
Heaviness: on chest.
Tickling creeping sensation: in chest.
Stinging itching: under nose.
Icy-coldness: of hands; of feet.

46 **Skin.** Eruptions like itch, with burning, itching.
Excoriation in bends of limbs.

47 **Stages of Life, Constitution.** Boy, æt. 9, negro; pneumonia.
Miss H., æt. 15, fleshy, light complexion, blue eyes, large for her age, recovering from varicella; affection of eye.
Man, æt. 25, suffering two weeks; phlyctenule of conjunctiva.
Widow, æt. 63, suffering three years; asthma.

48 **Relations.** Compatible: after *Bryon.*

STANNUM.

Tin. *The Element.*

Trituration of the pure metal.

Introduced by Hahnemann, proved by himself, Franz, Gross, Guttmann, Hartmann, Haynel, Herrmann, Langhammer, Wislicenus, Chronische Krankh., vol. 5.

CLINICAL AUTHORITIES.—*Headache*, Dudgeon, B. J. H., vol. 29, p. 610; Schrön, B. J. H., vol. 11, p. 301; Rück. Kl. Erf., vol. 5, p. 193; *Ciliary neuralgia*, Nash, Org., vol. 3, p. 94; Nash, Med. Couns., vol. 1, p. 181; *Facial neuralgia*, Guernsey, Hom. Phys., vol. 6, p. 172; *Toothache*, Villers, A. J. H. M. M., vol. 1, p. 148; W. V. R., Hah. Mo., vol. 24, p. 391; *Gastralgia*, Hartmann, Lobethal, Rück. Kl. Erf., vol. 1, p. 663; Miller, Hah. Mo., vol. 10, p. 161; *Solar neuralgia* (5 cases), Jones, T. H. M. S. Pa., 1880, p. 197; *Colic*, Lilienthal, N. A. J. H., vol. 9, p. 447; Köck, A. H. Z., vol. 103, p. 161; *Hernia*, Guernsey, Hah. Mo., vol. 5, p. 63; *Use in tapeworm*, Hahnemann, Rückert, Hartmann, Rück. Kl. Erf., vol. 1, p. 809; *Leucorrhœa*, Miller, Hah. Mo., vol. 8, p. 44; *Complaints during pregnancy*, Kunkel, A. H. Z., vol. 83, p. 176; *Affection of larynx*, Wurda, Rück. Kl. Erf., vol. 3, p. 173; *Asthma*, Cheney, Med. Inv., vol. 9, p. 56; B. J. H., vol. 30, p. 415; *Affection of larynx simulating phthisis*, Müller, Rück. Kl. Erf., vol. 5, p. 790; *Asthma*, Cheney, Med. Inv., vol. 9, p. 56, also Br. J. H., vol. 30, p. 415; *Asthma, and Albuminuria*, Villers, Med. Adv., vol. 20, p. 108; *Cough*, Spooner, Hah. Mo., vol. 11, p. 107; Grant, Hom. Phys., vol. 8, p. 539; *Pertussis*, A. R., Rück. Kl. Erf., vol. 5, p. 729; *Affections of chest*, Kunkel, A. H. Z., vol. 107, p. 20; *Chronic catarrhal affection of chest*, Diez, Rück. Kl. Erf., vol. 3, p. 28; Müller, Rück. Kl. Erf., vol. 5, p. 790; *Phthisis*, B. in A., Gross, Rückert, Schreter, Diehl, Schulz, Schubert, Rück. Kl. Erf., vol. 3, p. 399; Müller, Rück. Kl. Erf., vol. 5, p. 843; Brigham, C. M., vol. 6, p. 96; *Intercostal neuralgia*, Villers, A. J. H. M. M., vol. 1, p. 149; *Scrivener's cramp*, Battmann, Rück. Kl. Erf., vol. 4, p. 615; *Neuralgia*, Villers, N. A. J. H., vol. 8, p. 79; B. J. H., vol. 17, p. 165; Rückert, A. H. Z., vol. 8, p. 77; *Spasms, Epilepsy*, Altmüller, Caspari, Hartmann, Attom., Rück. Kl. Erf., vol. 4, p. 592; *Hemiplegia*, Hartmann, Rück. Kl. Erf., vol. 4, p. 484.

1 **Mind.** Sadness, with aversion to men and disinclination to talk.

Continued restlessness and anxiety.

ııUneasy, does not know what to do with himself, pains > by walking, yet so weak he soon must rest. θAnæmia.

Sullen, answers unwillingly and shortly.

Her distress of mind ceases as soon as menses begin to flow.

ııA woman, æt. 39, pregnant in fourth month; continued anxiety and restlessness; must keep in bed not only on account of bodily weakness, but also on account of her inability to do anything, as she cannot muster sufficient courage, and is forgetful and absent-minded; feels like crying all the time, but crying makes her feel worse; great palpitation of heart and anxiety, especially if she has to give directions in her domestic affairs; thinking makes her feel wretched, and she cannot get rid of what once gets fixed in her mind; oversensitive smell; vertigo on moving head; visions in morning and through day of all kinds of fancied things; drawing pains in different places; difficult evacuation even of soft stool; urging to stool; urine profuse and pale and then scanty and brown, sometimes white like milk; flatus; dry, tiresome cough; lies always upon her back with one leg stretched and the other drawn up. θPregnancy.

2 **Sensorium.** Vertigo: when reading, with loss of thought; < walking in open air or raising head; it seems as if all objects were too far off; dizzy pressure through head; head feels heavy, with sadness.

3 **Inner Head.** Sharp jerking pains in anterior lobe of brain above orbit.

Headache in frontal region.

Pain as if forehead were shattered.

Dull pressure from within outward, in forehead.

Pressive tearing: in forehead; in r. half of forehead, at intervals; < by stooping.

▮Pressure in l. temple beginning slight, then increasing and so again diminishing as if forehead would be pressed inward.

Crushing pain, like a pressing inward in temples, all day.

▮Painful jerks through l. temple, forehead and cerebellum, leaving a dull pressure, < during rest, > from motion.

▮Throbbing headache in temples.

Stupefying, aching pain in brain.

Constriction and sudden pressure in whole upper part of head, slowly increasing and decreasing.

▮Heaviness in head, during rest and motion, evenings.

▮Headache every morning, over one or other eye, mostly l., gradually extending over whole forehead, increasing and decreasing gradually; often with vomiting.

‖Soon after rising, dull, stupefying pain over eyes, sometimes more over l., increasing gradually in intensity and involving whole forehead, attaining its climax in about two hours, after which it as gradually subsided and in **about two** hours was quite gone; pain of a pressing in, **cramping,** crushing character.

‖**Regularly** at 5 A.M. awakened by headache, occupying forehead and both eyes; severe pressive or grinding pains, < from motion; great sensitiveness to noise and light; pain not particularly severe at first, but it gradually inc**reased, maintained its intensity when at** its height for some time (generally from 8 to 9), then **gradu**ally diminished, finally disappeared.

||Violent, glowing, beating pain, extending from upper part of forehead to vertex; felt as if head would burst from inward blows; skin of forehead seems swollen, eyelids were forced together and could be but slightly opened; least noise increased pain to an intolerable degree, so that he crept to farthest corner of house; daily paroxysm lasting from 10 A.M. to 4 P.M., attaining its greatest intensity about noon.

||For a week past has had a slight cold, sneezing, some heated excoriating water running from nose and eyes; after third day of this cold he had an aching pain over l. eye, in l. temple, coming on about 4 A.M., very gradually increasing until 11 A.M., and from 3 P.M. as slowly decreasing, until by 6 P.M. it was entirely gone, not to return until 4 A.M.; at first, pain only aching, but after a few days it became sharp, cutting and boring, with a terrible sense of fulness; by end of a week so excruciating at its acme that patient, whose ability to bear pain was more than ordinary, would roll or toss over bed, exhibiting usual expressions of greatest agony; lachrymation of eye on affected side, with slight excoriation of lower lid; pain > for a time by pressure. θSolar neuralgia.

||Neuralgia of head; begins lightly and increases gradually to its highest point and then gradually declines.

4 **Outer Head.** Burning in forehead, with nausea, > in open air.

5 **Sight and Eyes.** Sees a rainbow about the candlelight.

Weak, sunken, lustreless eyes.

Pupils contracted.

||Neuralgia in l. eye, gradually increasing from 10 A.M. to noon, then gradually decreasing, with lachrymation during pain.

Biting in eyes, as from rubbing with a woolen cloth.

Agglutination of lids at night.

Pressure in l. inner canthus as from a stye, with lachrymation.

Pustular swelling at inner canthus of l. eye; like a lachrymal fistula.

Pressive pain in r. inner canthus.

Burning stitches in eyelids. θStyes.

||Blennorrhœa of lachrymal sac; profuse yellow-white discharge.

||Ptosis from sympathetic paralysis; returning every Tuesday.

6 **Hearing and Ears.** Ringing in l. ear.
Shrieking noise in ear when blowing nose.
Ulceration of ear-ring hole.

7 **Smell and Nose.** Oversensitive smell.
Stuffed feeling and heaviness, high up in nostrils.
Dry coryza on one side, with soreness, redness and swelling of nostril.

8 **Upper Face.** | Flushes of heat in face from any movement, > in open air; one cheek hot and red.
| Face pale, eyes sunk, mind dull.
| Face pale and sunken, sickly, features elongated.
| Face pale, sickly-looking, flushing easily on exertion.
Drawing pain in face, in malar bone and orbits.
Malar bone painful to touch before menses, during the flow it is painful even to move muscles of face.
Contusive pain in region of malar bone during menses.
‖ Prosopalgia: pains increase and decrease gradually; after suppressed chills by quinine.
| Intermittent supraorbital neuralgia from 10 A.M. to 3 or 4 P.M., gradually increasing until attaining its acme, and then again decreasing as gradually; after abuse of quinine.
‖ Violent neuralgia of face and head, pains stealing on in a "slow-and-sure" fashion, requiring hours to reach its maximum, then beginning its decrease, which is quite as slow.

10 **Teeth and Tongue.** Teeth feel loose, elongated, with painful jerking shortly after eating.
‖ Neuralgia from temples down over upper and lower maxilla and lips, a drawing, gnawing pain, begins at a certain hour for several days, rises up to its greatest severity and then decreases again gradually (from morning until evening).
‖ Pain in upper incisors for four days; pains severe, coming at first lightly, gradually increasing in intensity, and then gradually subsiding.
‖ Epileptiform convulsions from teething; child is more comfortable by lying with abdomen across some hard substance; clenching of thumbs.

11 **Taste and Tongue.** | Taste: sour; sweet; offensive; everything bitter but water.
‖ Difficult, weak speech, occasioned by weakness, particularly in chest.
Tongue: red; yellow; coated with yellowish mucus.

12 **Inner Mouth.** | Fetid smell from mouth.

13 **Throat.** Permanent rawness and dryness in throat; during deglutition a painful feeling of being denuded.
Extreme rawness and dryness of throat, without thirst,

these sensations are much more painful during deglutition; thick greyish or greenish mucus adheres to throat; strong efforts are required to raise it, and these excite inclination to vomit.

▮Rawness in throat, in morning. θChronic catarrh.

▮Stinging dryness in throat.

Cutting in throat as from knives, when swallowing.

▮Hawks mucus, with soreness in throat; voice then becomes clearer for singing.

Inclination to hawk up much mucus from throat, in evening, followed by a sore pain in throat.

▮Mucus sticks in throat, efforts to raise it excite vomiturition.

Thick, grey-green mucus, mixed with blood, is detached from throat.

15 **Appetite, Thirst. Desires, Aversions.** ▮Canine hunger during day, with loss of appetite in evening.

Appetite irregular, with hypochondriasis.

Aversion to beer; it tastes flat or bitter.

16 **Hiccough, Belching, Nausea and Vomiting.** Eructations: bitter, after eating; sour.

Nausea after eating, followed by vomiting of bile, or undigested food.

Vomiting: of blood; of bile and mucus on awaking in morning; of water on smelling cooking.

17 **Scrobiculum and Stomach.** ▮Sinking, gone feeling in epigastrium.

▮▮Pressure and obstruction in pit of stomach.

▮Heavy pressure in stomach, with soreness of it to touch.

▮Oppression of stomach in hysterical women, with nausea, pale face, great weakness, phlegmatic temperament.

▮Uneasy, knows not what to do with himself; pains > by walking, yet so weak he must soon rest.

▮Cardialgia, pains gradually come and go, extend to navel and are > from hard pressure; sickly expression; uneasy, does not know what to do with himself; > by walking, yet so weak he must soon rest.

▮Gastralgia; clawing, kneading pain, extending to umbilicus; epigastrium sensitive to pressure; tension, pressure, shortness of breath, with anxiety and nausea; chronic diarrhœa; frequent bitter belching; distension of stomach; hunger.

▮Hæmatemesis, < when lying, > from pressure on stomach; slight touch causes a feeling of subcutaneous ulceration.

18 **Hypochondria.** Occasionally through day great epigastric weakness and hunger, but cannot eat.

▮▮Burning in hepatic region; cutting pains about navel; pain as if from an ulcer; empty feeling after eating.

Burning in hepatic region; stinging.
Boring stitches in l. hypochondrium.
Hysteric spasms in region of diaphragm.

19 **Abdomen.** Empty feeling, even after eating.
Sensation of soreness in whole abdomen, < by touch.
|| Digging in abdomen before every stool.
| Cutting about navel; with bitter eructations, hunger and diarrhœa; > from hard pressure.
| Sensitiveness of abdomen to touch; sore as from subcutaneous ulceration.
| Stitches from both sides through hips; < from slightest motion, or touch, and when lying on r. side; > by bending double against a chair or table; vomiting of water when smelling any kind of cooking. θColic.
|| Colic and twisting pains in region of spleen, lasting about six hours; usually coming on at night, and when going off leaving a soreness, which wears off during course of week; for last few days pains were constant; pain commences lightly, gets worse and worse until it reaches its acme and then decreases, leaving a feeling as if there were a hole in his side.
Spasmodic colic above and below navel.
| Colic > by hard pressure or by laying abdomen of child across knees, or against shoulder.
|| Babe 4 months old, double inguinal hernia; diarrhœa of green, curdy stools and much colic, > by laying its abdomen across nurse's knee, or against point of shoulder.

20 **Stool and Rectum.** | Stools: green, curdy, with colic; mucous; with bitter eructations; hard, dry, knotty or insufficient, with renewed desire afterward.
| Diarrhœa: in nursing infants; it is exhausting to talk much or read aloud; it is more difficult to descend than to ascend, to sit down than to rise up; although stool has been fully accomplished does not feel relieved.
Before stool: motion, pinching and distension in abdomen.
During stool: cutting in anus; drawing from back through thighs; rigors.
| Rectum inactive; much urging even with soft stool.
| Constipation; stool hard, dry, knotty, or insufficient and green.
|| Constipation appearing every Monday or on days after a fete, but only in winter, while for the rest of the week the stools were regular; fulness in lower part of abdomen, with swelling, malaise, great heat in head, > in open air, returning when in house, with ill-humor and sadness; felt hungry at noon but no appetite in evening.

▮Passes worms; lumbrici; colic; sickly face; spells of abdominal pain, during which wishes to lean over on something hard for relief.

▮Tænia.

21 **Urinary Organs.** Urine: profuse and pale, then scanty, brown, and sometimes white like milk; scanty and loaded with phosphates.

After urination continued urging.

Urging to urinate is wanting as if there were no sensation in bladder; only a sensation of fulness indicates necessity to urinate; atony of bladder.

22 **Male Sexual Organs.** ▮Voluptuous sensation in genitals, ending in an emission.

▮Irritation, with great weakness and nocturnal emissions; marked neurasthenia.

▮Spermatorrhœa with excessive prostration.

ǀǀEmissions without lascivious dreams.

23 **Female Sexual Organs.** ▮Excited sexual desire; easy orgasm.

▮Scratching arm produces an intolerable sensation of pleasure in genital organs which extends to uterus and produces sexual orgasm. θNeurasthenia.

▮▮Bearing down in uterine region; prolapsus uteri and vaginæ; $<$ during stool; feels so weak must drop down suddenly, but can get up readily. θNeurasthenia.

▮Prolapse strangulated, tends to gangrene.

▮Menses: too early and too profuse; preceded by melancholy; pain in malar bones, continues during menses.

▮▮Leucorrhœa: with great debility; weakness, seems to proceed from chest; of yellow, white or transparent mucus; thin, watery, in debilitated subjects; profuse white or yellow, causing great general debility.

24 **Pregnancy. Parturition. Lactation.** ǀǀMelancholia. See Chapter 1.

▮Spasmodic labor pains; they exhaust her, she is out of breath.

Child refuses mother's milk.

25 **Voice and Larynx. Trachea and Bronchia.** ▮Voice husky, deep, hoarse, hollow; clearer or higher after hawking up mucus.

▮Roughness and hoarseness, momentarily $>$ by coughing.

▮▮Talking weakens, particularly the chest.

ǀǀCannot read to her children, it causes aching in throat, chest and deltoids.

ǀǀComplete aphonia; pain in larynx; severe cough, with profuse purulent expectoration; hectic fever; debilitating night sweats; diarrhœa.

▮Hoarseness, weakness and emptiness in chest on beginning to sing, so that she was constantly obliged to stop and take a deep breath; at times a few expulsive coughs removed hoarseness for a moment.

▮Rawness in larynx.

▮Irritation to cough in trachea, as from mucus, on breathing, with a cough neither loose nor dry, felt more while sitting bent over than when walking.

▮Mucus in trachea, in forenoon, easily expelled by a forcible cough, with great weakness of chest as if eviscerated; weakness of body and limbs, in which sensation of weakness extended upward and downward, several mornings in succession.

▮Bronchial dilatations, with purulent expectoration.

❘❘Cough, tickling in throat, loss of appetite, fever, debilitating night sweats; deglutition gradually became more difficult, caused severe cough and attacks of suffocation, expectoration more and more profuse, at first mucous, finally purulent, more than a pint in twenty-four hours; hoarseness; emaciation; epiglottis ulcerated, edges eaten away.

▮▮Laryngeal phthisis, with constant short hacking cough and aphonia; empty feeling in chest.

▮▮Accumulation of great quantities of mucus in trachea, easily thrown off by coughing. θBronchitis.

26 **Respiration.** Disposition to take a deep breath, causing a feeling of lightness.

Crowing, snoring respiration.

▮Oppressed breathing: from every movement; when lying down; in evening; from coughing.

Short, difficult respiration, caused by weakness of respiratory organs, with great emptiness in chest, though without dyspnœa.

▮Dyspnœa and want of breath on ascending steps and on slightest motion.

▮Evening dyspnœa; must loosen clothing.

❘❘Mrs. ——, æt. 37, spare, brunette, subject to asthma for many years; attacks, preceded by symptoms of ordinary cold, usually set in about 4–5 A.M., lasting from thirty-six to forty-eight hours; attacks increase and decrease gradually.

❘❘A man, æt. 40, had for a year and a quarter asthmatic attacks which, day or night, did not permit him to lie down; paroxysms increased and decreased gradually; retinitis albuminurica; albumen in urine and œdema of feet.

27 **Cough.** ▮▮Cough: in fatiguing paroxysms; epigastric region painful, as if beaten; violent, shattering, deep; short, from time to time, as from weakness in chest, with a

hoarse, weak sound; tickling as from soreness low down in trachea, a scraping extending upward into throat; constant inclination to hack, as if caused by much mucus in chest, with an internal sensation of scraping and rattling; frightful, with expectoration and spitting of blood; dry, in evening in bed; concussive in paroxysms of three coughs; caused by mucus in chest and by stitches in trachea, and dryness; with copious, green, salty sputum, most profuse in morning.

Scraping cough, with greenish expectoration of an offensive sweetish taste, < in evening before lying down with a hoarse voice; a sore sensation in chest and trachea after every cough (the irritation which provokes it is low down in trachea).

I Accumulation of much mucus in trachea, easily thrown off by coughing; afterward, soreness or stitches in chest.

I Cough caused by talking, singing, laughing, lying on side and from drinking anything warm.

II Phthisis pituitosa.

II Cough, particularly during day, with shortness of breath; profuse, white, thick, tasteless expectoration, without effort.

II Cough, returned every February and lasted until Summer or warm weather; had measles three years before, and taken cold; severe racking cough; inclination to vomit during cough; < in morning; expectoration of yellowish mucus of a sweetish taste.

I Whooping cough, with hoarseness, loss of breath, soreness and heaviness in chest, inclination to breathe deeply, sore or empty sensation in epigastrium, profuse offensive or salty tasting, yellowish or greenish expectoration, < at night lying down, face pale and emaciated, eyes sunken.

Expectoration of a globular, greyish lump of thick mucus, containing a clot of black blood, and appearing to come from throat.

II Sputum: like white of an egg; yellow green pus; sweetish; putrid, sour or saltish; during day.

28 **Inner Chest.** Oppression of chest as if it were internally constricted.

Distressing oppression in upper part of chest, was frequently obliged to take a deep breath, with a sensation of great emptiness in pit of stomach.

I Tension across upper part of chest with emptiness in lower.

I Constriction of chest with anxiety in evening.

II Chest so weak he cannot talk; empty feeling in chest.

Great dyspnœa, with anxiety, in evening, compelling one to loosen clothing.

Drawing a long breath causes a pleasant sensation of lightness, for a short time.

| Great sore feeling in chest; bruised pain.

Stitches in chest and sides hinder respiration.

Sudden, sharp, knifelike stitches in l. side of chest.

| Stitches in l. side of chest, when breathing or lying on that side.

Sudden drawing beneath l. breast on rising up in bed, followed by sharp knifelike stitches, extending thence into clavicle, toward shoulder, where pain persisted, and into l. side, extending downward into lower abdomen, < by bending inward, pressing upon it, and especially by inspiration and hacking which also caused a painful shock.

Itching tickling in chest.

Tension in chest. θHydrothorax.

|| After great fright, and in consequence of a severe cold, dull paralyzing pain in l. arm which on continuing to walk extended to l. side of chest, obstructing respiration and forcing him to stand still, pain then soon diminished, but was soon obliged to make another halt; during night suddenly aroused by violent pain at a point in l. breast which could not be definitely pointed out; pain increased gradually and was accompanied by an indescribable terror which drove him out of bed; could find relief in no position; profuse, cold sweat on head and upper part of trunk; when pain was at its height was unable to make a motion or utter a sound; for an hour was obliged to remain sitting, with head and trunk bent forward, with gasping, noisy respiration, spasmodically clutching arms of a chair; pain then diminished as gradually as it had increased and disappeared by morning. θNeuralgia of l. phrenic nerve.

|| Several days after a fright, while walking, an unusual feeling of weakness which appeared to proceed from chest and obliged her to loosen her dress and lie down; after remaining quiet for an hour the attack disappeared, but returned in a few days and gradually changed into a gnawing pain, seated at middle of sternum, commencing gently, gradually increasing for two hours and then disappearing just as gradually; at beginning of paroxysm, which returned more and more frequently, irresistible inclination to lie down, and at the height of attack was unable, for half an hour, to make any motion or sound; she became more chlorotic and menses more scanty and pale. θNeuralgia.

|| Hæmoptysis; tendency to copious expectoration.

|| Weakness in chest: with copious expectoration; as if

eviscerated, with weakness of whole body and limbs; and emptiness on beginning to sing, she was constantly obliged to stop and take a deep breath.

▮Chronic catarrhal affections of chest, with copious expectoration of yellowish, greenish, offensive-tasting mucus; great prostration; emaciation; œdema of limbs.

▮▮Shortness of breath; profuse but difficult expectoration of thick, offensive, salty-tasting mucus; expectoration entirely absent for nine or ten weeks, then recurs and lasts for five or six weeks; oozing of a watery clear fluid from umbilicus during the periods when she expectorates; sleep disturbed; sleeps upon back with head flexed upon chest; cannot lie upon side; stooping posture; great prostration; large mucous and whistling râles in chest; after a pneumonia several years previously.

▮▮Profuse expectoration; wheezing, oppressed breathing, < from motion; cough day and night, with nausea; expectoration white, thin, slimy; frequent stitches in sides of chest, < from breathing and coughing; prostration; cannot sleep on account of shortness of breath: can do no work; menses and stool normal.

▮▮Cough with copious, greenish, or yellowish offensive-tasting expectoration; cough generally dry in evening and at night, or else expectoration is difficult, while during day and in morning it is profuse and easy. θPhthisis.

▮▮Pulse 150 to 160; hectic fever; racking, exhausting cough day and night; expectorating every twenty-four hours about a quart of tough glairy mucus, mixed with purulent matter; large cavity in upper third of r. lobe; *Calc.* 30 reduced pulse to 120 and diminished sputa about one-fourth; in four or five weeks pulse quickened and improvement ceased, *Stannum* then cured. θPhthisis.

▮▮Cough which seemed to come from low down in chest, < at night, with profuse expectoration; tension across chest; dyspnœa < from motion; cannot lie down at night; rattling of mucus in chest; anorexia; night sweats; prostration; weakening of limbs; emaciation. θPhthisis.

▮▮Teeth loose, feel too long; accumulation of much mucus in throat; scratching in throat in evening; hoarseness; tickling cough; cough with greenish expectoration, of offensive whitish taste, < evenings; constriction of chest and anxiety in evening; shortness of breath, < from least motion; must unloosen clothing; stool scanty, greenish; intense burning of hands and feet;

general prostration; very tired and sleepy; profuse sweats every morning at 4 o'clock; emaciation; despondent, will not talk, is dissatisfied. θPhthisis.

|| Cough day and night, copious expectoration; great emaciation; pulse weak, rapid; burning heat of palms of hands, < in afternoon; profuse sweats early in morning; tongue red; severe diarrhœa; great prostration, compelling her to stay in bed. θPhthisis.

|| Prostration; pain in all limbs; constant irritation to cough; frequent shivering during day, and profuse sweats early in morning in bed; is no longer able to get up; constant cough; copious expectoration of masses of tasteless white mucus; unquenchable thirst; craving for sour things. θPhthisis.

|| Pale and emaciated; respiration rapid, short; cough often dry, often with profuse greenish-yellow sweetish-tasting mucus; < morning and evening; stitching pains in head, < in forehead, < after paroxysms of cough; abnormal appetite; pressure in stomach after eating; scanty stool; heaviness, coldness and swelling of hands and feet; in evening transient flushes of heat and thirst. θPhthisis.

▮ Mucous expectoration in first stage of consumption, or when a neglected catarrh or grippe threatens to pass into phthisis; can talk only a few words at a time for want of breath; more or less hoarseness; roughness of throat and sore pain in chest; feeling of weakness in chest as if deprived of its contents after expectorating or talking; constriction of chest and constant chilliness, alternating with flushes of heat; profuse night sweats; pressure and bloatedness of stomach always after eating; great lassitude, hands and feet heavy and cold or else burning hot. θPhthisis.

▮▮ Phthisis mucosa, with the characteristic cough, weakness and sputa; profuse sweats.

29 **Heart, Pulse and Circulation.** Pulse frequent and small.

30 **Outer Chest.** || A lady, æt. 50, formerly healthy, suffers since her climaxis from disease of liver; looks yellow, has no appetite, nauseous taste, tongue coated yellow, obstinate constipation; tongue villous, yellow, heavily coated, somewhat dry; weak voice, sounds of heart slow, weak, hardly 60 to minute, but regular; urine strongly saturated with sour secretion and vermilion precipitate firmly adhering to walls of vessels; some withered varices on anus; whole appearance anæmic; every Saturday morning wakes up with nausea and choking; feels a shock in region of liver, leaving behind, along second and third false ribs, a spas-

modic pain, which increases gradually in severity up to 3 or 4 P.M., when she vomits up food taken day before, and then pain decreases gradually so that by 10 o'clock in evening she is entirely relieved; next two days so weak that she is obliged to keep in bed; next four days tolerably well, until Saturday brings on return of her sufferings; during paroxysm passes a large quantity of watery urine. θIntercostal neuralgia.

31 **Neck and Back.** Weakness of nape of neck.

Stitches in back, in small of back and into limbs.

32 **Upper Limbs.** Jerking in muscles of arm when resting it; fingers jerk when holding pen.

Weakness and heaviness of arms, especially r.; < from motion.

Paralytic weakness of arms, if he holds a light weight for only a short time.

❚The arms easily become fatigued from moderate exercise, so that everything he holds is allowed to fall.

Aching in deltoids from reading.

Swelling of hands evenings.

❚Weakness and trembling of hands.

❚Cramping of fingers of writers and shoemakers; on attempting to pick up a small object, as a needle or a pen, or when they have been used a long time, fingers become suddenly rigid, distorted, spread out or contracted, in which position they remain for some time; the spasm can often be ended by opening fingers with unaffected hand; usually r. hand is affected; the toes in one case were also affected.

Burning in hands.

Chilblains on hands.

Painful hangnails.

33 **Lower Limbs.** Weakness and heaviness, especially of thigh and knee joint, must sit down.

❚❚Paralytic heaviness and weakness, especially in thighs and knee joints.

Stiffness and tension in bends of knees.

Swelling of ankles, evenings.

Burning of feet.

34 **Limbs in General.** ❚Paralytic heaviness of limbs; < using arms or walking, particularly descending.

❚Insupportable restlessness of all the limbs.

Swelling of hands and feet in evening.

❚Pains in limbs increase gradually and decrease in same manner.

35 **Rest. Position. Motion.** Rest: pains in head <; heaviness in head; of arm, jerking in muscles.

Lying: hæmatemesis <; asthma does not permit; whooping cough <.

Lying on back: one leg stretched, other drawn up during pregnancy; head flexed on chest; shortness of breath.
Lies on stomach: when asleep.
Lying on r. side: pain through hips <; causes cough.
Constantly wishes to lie or sit down: excessive prostration.
Must lie down: weakness of chest.
Cannot lie down: phthisis.
Obliged to remain sitting with head and trunk forward: pain in l. breast.
Sitting bent over: irritation to cough >.
Bending double against chair or table: > pains through hips.
Bending inward: stitches in abdomen <.
Must sit down: weakness and heaviness of thighs and knee joint.
Stooping: tearing in forehead <; with shortness of breath.
Raising head: vertigo <.
Rising up in bed: drawing beneath l. breast.
Rising from bed: sudden weakness.
Motion: pains in head >; heaviness in head; headache <; flushes of heat in face; stitches through hips <; oppressed breathing; want of breath; impossible from pain in breast; impossible, neuralgia of chest; wheezing <; dyspnœa <; shortness of breath <; weakness of arms <.
Walking: pains >, but must soon rest: vertigo <; pain goes from arm to chest; heaviness of limbs <; great lassitude.
Ascending steps: want of breath; weariness of body <.
Descending more difficult than ascending, sitting than rising; heaviness of limbs <.
Going down stairs: faintness.
Exertion: face flushes easily.
Exercise: arm easily fatigued; slow trembling <.

36 **Nerves.** Feels as if she would faint.
Faintness from going down stairs.
▮Great lassitude when walking.
▮Weariness of whole body, especially after ascending steps.
Was suddenly attacked by weakness; she could scarcely breathe, while dressing, after rising from bed.
▮Great weariness during day; was obliged to lie down.
Excessive prostration; constantly wishes to sit or lie down, and when about to sit down falls upon chair because she has not the power to sit down slowly.
▮Extreme exhaustion of mind and body.
▮Loss of power as if limbs were beaten.
▮▮Very much exhausted from talking or reading aloud.

▮▮Great sense of weakness in larynx and chest, thence all over body.

▮Trembling, < from slow exercise.

▮▮Neuralgia; the pain increases gradually to a very high degree, and decreases again as slowly.

▮Hysterical spasms, with pain in abdomen and in diaphragm.

Hysteria with frightful pains in head; full of notions.

▮Renewal of convulsions with cutting of every tooth; also in consequence of worms; child is weak; looks miserable.

▮Epilepsy: with tossing of limbs, clenching thumbs; opisthotonos; unconsciousness; with sexual complications; during dentition, with symptoms of worms; in evening; paleness of face, twitching of hands and eyes.

▮Hemiplegia, paralyzed parts constantly moist from perspiration; especially on l. side, with a feeling of a heavy load in affected arm and corresponding side of chest, and frequent night sweats.

▮Paralysis, from worms, onanism, spasms, emotions.

37 **Sleep.** ▮▮Sleeplessness.

▮Sleepy during day; goes to sleep late at night.

Restless, child moans during sleep, or supplicates in a timid manner.

So weak on waking it puts her out of breath to dress.

38 **Time.** Morning: visions of all kinds of fancied things; rawness in throat; vomiting of bile and mucus; mucus in trachea; inclination to cough <; expectoration easy; debilitating sweats; sweat < after 4 A.M.

10 A.M.: finger tips numb.

During day: canine hunger; great epigastric weakness and hunger; copious green salty sputa; cough <, with shortness of breath; expectoration easy; cough exhausting; frequent shivering; great weariness; sleepy.

Afternoon: burning heat of palms of hands <.

Evenings: heaviness in head; inclination to hawk up much mucus from throat; loss of appetite; dyspnœa; dry cough; cough < before lying down; constriction of chest; dyspnœa; scratching in throat; cough, with expectoration <; swelling of hands; swelling of ankles; swelling of feet; epilepsy.

Night: agglutination of lids; colic comes on; whooping cough <; cough exhausting; cough <; goes to sleep late; debilitating sweats.

39 **Temperature and Weather.** Warm drinks: cause cough. Open air: while walking vertigo <; burning in forehead >; flushes of heat in face >.

40 **Fever.** Chill: 10 A.M., finger tips numb; in evening, over

back; only on head, with thirst; slight, but with chattering teeth, as from convulsions, of masseter muscles; over whole body, lasting half an hour.

▮Heat: from 4 to 5 P.M., with sweat; burning, in limbs, mostly in hands, every evening; anxious, as if sweat would break out.

▮Sweat: smells mouldy, musty; debilitating, night and morning, most profuse on neck; debilitating, from least movement; profuse, after 4 A.M., every morning; in morning, mostly on neck, nape of neck and forehead.

Sweat principally on forehead and nape of neck, in morning after 4 A.M.

▮Hectic fever.

▮▮Worm fever, in a very excitable and restless boy; pain in stomach, lay upon stomach when asleep.

41 **Attacks, Periodicity.** Increasing and decreasing gradually: headache over eyes; cramping, crushing pain in head; grinding or pressive pains; neuralgia of head; neuralgia in l. eye; colic and pain in region of spleen; paroxysms of asthma; pain in l. breast; weakness in chest; spasmodic pain in region of liver; pains in limbs.

Alternating: chilliness and flushes of heat.

Every morning: headache; profuse sweat at 4 o'clock.

Several mornings in succession: weakness of body and limbs.

At 5 A.M.: regularly awakened by headache.

Daily: paroxysms from 10 A.M. to 4 P.M.

Every evening: heat in limbs.

Half an hour: chill lasts.

From 4 to 5 P.M.: heat.

For six hours: colic or twisting pains in region of spleen.

Every twenty-four hours: expectorates about a quart.

For four days: pain in upper incisors, increasing and decreasing gradually.

Several days after a fright: weakness in chest.

Every Monday: constipation.

Every Tuesday: ptosis from sympathetic paralysis.

Every Saturday morning: wakes up with nausea and choking.

For nine or ten weeks: expectoration absent, then recurs and lasts for five or six weeks.

Every February: cough returned.

For a year and a quarter: asthmatic attacks.

42 **Locality and Direction.** Right: tearing in half of forehead; pressive pain in inner canthus; heaviness and weakness of arm; spasm of hand.

Left: pressure in temple; jerks through temple; headache < over eye; aching over eye and in temple; neuralgia in l. eye: pressure in inner canthus; pustular swelling at inner canthus; ringing in ear; boring stitches in hypochondrium; stitches in side of chest when lying on side; drawing beneath breast; paralyzing pain in arm, thence to side of chest; violent pain at a point in breast.

From within outward: pressure in forehead.

43 **Sensations.** As if all objects were too far off; as if forehead were shattered; as if forehead would be pressed inward; pain as if from an ulcer in hypogastrium; as if there were a hole in his side; as if there were no sensation in bladder; chest as if eviscerated; epigastric region as if beaten; tickling as from soreness in trachea; inclination to hawk as if mucus were in chest; as if it were internally constricted; as if chest were deprived of its contents; as if she would faint; as if limbs were beaten; as of a heavy load in affected arm and side of chest; as if sweat would break out.

Pain: in frontal region; in upper incisors; larynx; in all limbs; in abdomen and in diaphragm; in stomach.

Violent pain: at a point in l. breast.

Frightful pains: in head.

Sharp jerking pains: above orbit.

Beating pain: from forehead to vertex.

Throbbing pain: in temples.

Cutting pain: in forehead and eyes; in throat; about navel; in anus.

Pressive tearing: in forehead; in r. half of forehead.

Boring pain: in forehead and eyes.

Crushing pain: in temples.

Stitches: from both sides through hips; in trachea; in chest; in l. side of chest; in back; in small of back and into limbs.

Burning stitches: in eyelids.

Boring stitches: in l. hypochondrium.

Sharp, knifelike stitches: in l. side of chest; from chest into clavicle.

Stitching pains: in head.

Bruised pain: in chest.

Gnawing pain: seated at middle of sternum.

Twisting pains: in region of spleen.

Pinching pain: in abdomen.

Grinding pain: in forehead and eyes.

Clawing, kneading pain: about umbilicus.

Digging: in abdomen.

Severe pressive pain: forehead and both eyes.

Pressive pain: in r. inner canthus.

Stupefying pain: in brain; over eyes.
Dull paralyzing pain: in l. arm.
Neuralgic pain: in l. eye; of face and head; from temples to lower maxilla and lips.
Glowing pain: from forehead to vertex.
Aching pain: in brain; over l. eye; in l. temple; in throat; in deltoids.
Drawing pain: in different places; in face, in malar bone and orbits; beneath l. breast.
Painful jerks: through l. temple and cerebellum.
Sore pain: in chest.
Contusive pain: in region of malar bone.
Biting: in eyes.
Stinging: in throat; in hepatic region.
Soreness: in nostrils; in throat; of stomach; in abdomen; in chest.
Burning: in forehead; in hepatic region; of hands and feet; of palms of hands; of feet.
Heat: in head.
Scraping: in throat.
Rawness: in throat; in larynx.
Pressure: dizzy, through head; in forehead; in l. temple; in l. inner canthus; in pit of stomach; in stomach.
Sudden pressure: in whole upper part of head.
Constriction: in upper part of head; of chest.
Tension: across upper part of chest; in bend of knees.
Heaviness: in head; in nostrils; in chest; of hands and feet; of arms; in thighs and knee joints; of limbs.
Distressing oppression: in upper part of chest.
Weakness: in chest; of body and limbs; in nape of neck; of arms; in larynx and chest.
Stuffed feeling: in nostrils.
Empty feeling: in epigastrium.
Gone feeling: in chest; in epigastrium; in pit of stomach.
Dryness: in throat; in trachea.
Pleasant lightness: by drawing a long breath.
Insupportable restlessness: of all the limbs.
Fulness: in abdomen.
Itching tickling: in chest.
Coldness: of hands and feet.

45 **Touch. Passive Motion. Injuries.** Touch: malar bone painful; stomach sore; slight, causes feeling of subcutaneous ulceration; soreness of abdomen <; pain through hips <.

Pressure: headache > for a time; cardialgia; pains go to navel, are > by hard pressure; epigastrium >; on stomach >; hæmatemesis >; hard >, colic; stitches in abdomen <.

Must loosen dress: weakness in chest.

Lying across something hard: abdomen more comfortable.

47 **Stages of Life, Constitution.** Child, æt. 4 months; hernia.

Girl, æt. 15; phthisis.

Girl, æt. 18, weak, poorly nourished, suffering ten weeks; cough.

Girl, æt. 18, of remarkable beauty, somewhat scrofulous in early childhood, temperament lively and cheerful, after a violent shock; neuralgia.

Miss W. P., æt. 18, plump, healthy, active; solar neuralgia.

Mr. M. E., æt. 22, hardy, active, muscular, accustomed to outdoor exercise; solar neuralgia.

Man, æt. 25, kicked by a horse in region of spleen thirteen years ago, since then suffering; colic.

Man, æt. 25, just recovered from typhoid fever, after a cold; affection of larynx.

Man, æt. 27; cough.

Lady, æt. 30, good constitution, somewhat reduced by the exhausting mode of life peculiar to St. Petersburg, and by domestic troubles; headache.

Man, æt. 30, bottlemaker; headache.

Man, æt. 30, for several years had cough; phthisis.

Man, æt. 32, ill two years; phthisis.

Woman, æt. 36, single, five months ago had severe catarrh of chest; phthisis.

Woman, æt. 36, for several years had cough in Spring and Autumn; phthisis.

Man, æt. 36; phthisis.

Mrs. ——, æt. 37, spare, brunette, suffering many years; asthma.

Man, æt. 37, ill two years; phthisis.

Mr. E. J., æt. 38, fleshy, hearty, plethoric; solar neuralgia.

Mrs. ——, æt. 39, four months pregnant; disorders of pregnancy.

Man, æt. 40, suffering fifteen months; asthma.

Woman, æt. 40, nurse, suffering several weeks; headache.

Mrs. W. S., æt. 42, somewhat broken down by other diseases, suffering many days; solar neuralgia.

Man, æt. 45, large frame, six feet high; solar neuralgia.

Man, æt. 50, tall, thin; phthisis.

Man, æt, 50, powerful, after a violent fright; neuralgia

Lady, æt. 50, formerly always healthy, suffering since climaxis with supposed disease of liver; intercostal neuralgia.

Woman, æt. 53, single, weak, irritable, after la grippe; phthisis.

Man, æt. 54, had itch, in consequence of much scratching foot became ulcerated, for five years was subjected to heroic treatment, and constitution was finally completely ruined, had many digestive disturbances, jaundice, dyspnœa, etc.; affection of larynx simulating phthisis.

Woman, æt. 59, several years ago had pneumonia, since then suffering; affection of chest.

Woman, rather stout, sanguine bilious temperament, lost her husband a few months previously, after having a scrofulous tumor discussed from neck by iodine; phthisis.

48 **Relations.** Antidoted by: *Pulsat.*

Compatible: after *Caustic.*, *Cina.*

Complementary: *Pulsat.*